The Domestic Dog

Its Evolution, Behavior and Interactions with People

Second Edition

Why do dogs behave the way they do? Why did our ancestors tame wolves? How have we ended up with so many breeds of dog, and how can we understand their role in contemporary human society? Explore the answers to these questions and many more in this study of the domestic dog.

Building on the strengths of the first edition, this much-anticipated update incorporates two decades of new evidence and discoveries on dog evolution, behavior, training, and human interaction. It includes seven entirely new chapters covering topics such as behavioral modification and training, dog population management, the molecular evidence for dog domestication, canine behavioral genetics, cognition, and the impact of free-roaming dogs on wildlife conservation. It is an ideal volume for anyone interested in dogs and their evolution, behavior, and ever-changing roles in society.

James Serpell is Professor of Animal Ethics and Welfare at the School of Veterinary Medicine, University of Pennsylvania. His research focuses on the behavior and welfare of companion animals, the development of human attitudes to animals, and the history and impact of human–animal relationships.

The Domestic Dog

Its Evolution, Behavior and Interactions with People

Second Edition

Edited by
JAMES SERPELL

Pencil illustrations by
PRISCILLA BARRETT

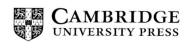
CAMBRIDGE
UNIVERSITY PRESS

CAMBRIDGE
UNIVERSITY PRESS

University Printing House, Cambridge CB2 8BS, United Kingdom

One Liberty Plaza, 20th Floor, New York, NY 10006, USA

477 Williamstown Road, Port Melbourne, VIC 3207, Australia

314-321, 3rd Floor, Plot 3, Splendor Forum, Jasola District Centre, New Delhi - 110025, India

79 Anson Road, #06-04/06, Singapore 079906

Cambridge University Press is part of the University of Cambridge.

It furthers the University's mission by disseminating knowledge in the pursuit of education, learning and research at the highest international levels of excellence.

www.cambridge.org
Information on this title: www.cambridge.org/9781107024144

First published 1995
Second edition 2017

A catalogue record for this publication is available from the British Library

Library of Congress Cataloging in Publication data
Serpell, James, 1952– editor.
The domestic dog / edited by James Serpell ; pencil illustrations
  by Priscilla Barrett.
[Second edition]. | New York : Cambridge University Press, 2016.
LCCN 2016024594 | ISBN 9781107024144
LCSH: Dogs – Behavior. | Dogs. | Human-animal relationships.
LCC SF433 .D66 2016 | DDC 636.7–dc23
LC record available at https://lccn.loc.gov/2016024594

ISBN 978-1-107-02414-4 Hardback
ISBN 978-1-107-69934-2 Paperback

In memory of Juliet Clutton-Brock
(1933–2015)

CONTENTS

Color plates are to be found between pp. 230 and 231

CONTRIBUTORS

Giorgio Andreoli, D. Biol, *Agriconsulting SpA, Rome, Italy*

Luigi Boitani, D. Biol, *Dept. of Biology and Biotechnology, University of Rome "La Sapienza," Rome, Italy*

John Bradshaw, PhD, *Anthrozoology Institute, Animal Welfare and Behaviour Group, School of Veterinary Science, University of Bristol, UK*

Geoffrey M. Carr, PhD, The Economist, *London, UK*

Paolo Ciucci, PhD, *Dept. of Biology and Biotechnology, University of Rome "La Sapienza," Rome, Italy*

Juliet Clutton-Brock

Raymond Coppinger, PhD, *School of Cognitive Science, Hampshire College, MA, USA*

Carlos A. Driscoll, DPhil, *Section of Comparative Behavioral Genomics, Laboratory of Neurogenetics; National Institute on Alcohol Abuse and Alcoholism; National Institutes of Health, MD, USA*

Deborah L. Duffy, PhD, *Department of Clinical Studies, School of Veterinary Medicine, University of Pennsylvania, Philadelphia PA, USA*

Francesco Francisci, D Biol, *ECOSOLUZIONI S.n.c., Cortona (AR), Italy*

Benjamin L. Hart, DVM, PhD, *School of Veterinary Medicine, University of California, Davis, CA, USA*

Lynette A. Hart, PhD, *Department of Population Health & Reproduction, School of Veterinary Medicine, University of California, Davis, CA, USA*

Elly F. Hiby, PhD, *Cambridge, UK*

Lex R. Hiby, *Cambridge, UK*

Robert Hubrecht, PhD, *Universities Federation for Animal Welfare (UFAW), Herts, UK*

Joelene Hughes, PhD, *Department of Zoology, University of Oxford, Recanati-Kaplan Centre, Oxford, UK*

J. Andrew Jagoe, MVB, PhD, *Abington Park Veterinary Group, Northampton, UK*

James Kirkwood, BVSc, PhD, *Universities Federation for Animal Welfare (UFAW), Herts, UK*

Randall Lockwood, PhD, *ASPCA, New York, NY, USA*

Kathryn Lord, PhD, *School of Cognitive Science, Hampshire College, Amherst, MA, USA*

David W. Macdonald, DSc, *WildCRU, Department of Zoology, University of Oxford, Recanati-Kaplan Centre, Oxford, UK*

Friederike Range, PhD, *Messerli Research Institute, Veterinärmedizinische Universität Wien (Vetmeduni Vienna), Wien, Austria*

Pamela Reid, PhD, *ASPCA, New York, NY, USA*

Ilana Reisner, DVM, PhD, *Reisner Veterinary Behavior & Consulting Services, PA, USA*

Nicola Rooney, PhD, *Anthrozoology Institute, Animal Welfare and Behaviour Group, School of Veterinary Science, University of Bristol, UK*

Richard A. Schneider, PhD, *Department of Orthopaedic Surgery, University of California at San Francisco, CA, USA*

James Serpell, PhD, *Department of Clinical Studies, School of Veterinary Medicine, University of Pennsylvania, Philadelphia, PA, USA*

Linda van den Berg, PhD, *Rotterdam, the Netherlands*

Zsófia Virányi, PhD, *Messerli Research Institute, Veterinärmedizinische Universität Wien (Vetmeduni Vienna), Wien, Austria*

Bridgett M. vonHoldt, PhD, *Department of Ecology and Evolutionary Biology, Princeton University, NJ, USA*

Stephen Wickens, PhD, *Universities Federation for Animal Welfare (UFAW), Herts, UK*

Mariko Yamamoto, PhD, *Ibaraki, Japan*

Stephen Zawistowski, PhD, *Gouldsboro, PA, USA*

1 Introduction

JAMES SERPELL

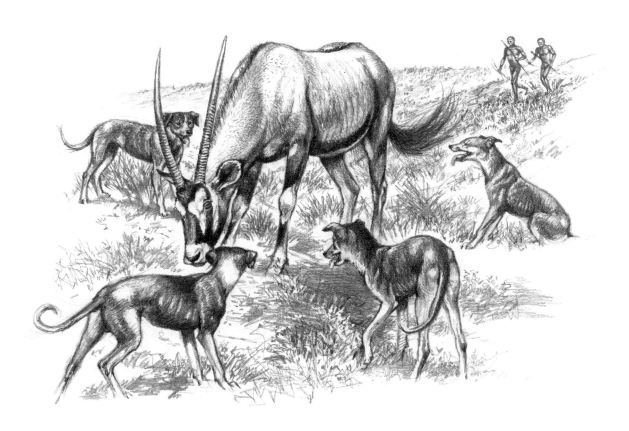

In the Introduction to the first edition of this book – published some 20 years ago – I bemoaned the general lack of objective and reliable scientific information about the domestic dog, and attributed this dearth of knowledge to scientific chauvinism. "Most modern biologists and behavioral scientists," I wrote:

> seem to regard domestic animals as "unnatural" and therefore unworthy or unsuitable as subjects for serious scientific investigation. According to this stereotype, the domestic dog is essentially a debased and corrupted wolf, an abnormal and therefore uninteresting artifact of human design, rather than a unique biological species (or superspecies) in its own right, with its own complex and fascinating evolutionary history. (Serpell, 1995, p. 2)

I am happy to report that this statement no longer rings true. Indeed, the domestic dog has become something of a scientific celebrity in recent years, and I would like to believe that the material presented in the first edition contributed to this change of heart. Numerous, highly respected, "high impact" scientific journals now regularly publish scholarly articles on the evolutionary origins of the dog, its molecular genetics, its social behavior and cognitive capacities, and its complex interactions with human society. Major international conferences are devoted exclusively to "canine science," while innumerable TV documentaries, books and blogs have done a remarkable job of conveying all of this new dog science to a seemingly insatiable popular audience. At the same time, the dog's success as a social companion and working partner has continued to grow, not only among developed nations but also in many developing countries. In 1995, for example, when the first edition came out, an estimated 55 million dogs lived in the USA. Now the figure is closer to 80 million. And, as people's attachments for dogs as family members and valued assistants have grown, so too has concern for the health and welfare of these animals.

Celebrity, however, comes at a price. More people may know more about dogs than ever before, but it is often a shallow sort of knowledge that is easily exploited by self-styled dog experts for personal gain. The carefully edited antics of these charismatic but frequently ill-informed dog gurus and "whisperers" may be entertaining to watch on TV but, ultimately, it is the dogs who suffer when their owners imbibe too much of this quasi-scientific "snake oil." A major goal of this book is to serve as an antidote to these popular depictions by providing a state-of-the-art scientific assessment of what we truly know – and what we don't know – about the evolution, natural history, and behavior of *Canis familiaris*. The field of canine science has come a long way since 1995 but, as readers of this book will discover, many aspects of the biology and behavior of dogs and their relations with people still remain mysterious.

The remarkable scientific progress in our understanding of dogs in the last 20 years means inevitably that some of the material presented in the original edition of *The Domestic Dog* is no longer current or correct. Scientific advances have also identified some important gaps in the previous volume, notably in areas where research has developed most rapidly in the last two decades. In the process of bringing their chapters up to date, and incorporating so much new information, many of the original contributors to the book have accomplished extraordinary feats of revision and synthesis in their revised chapters. The addition of seven entirely new chapters, addressing research topics that barely existed 20 years ago, has also successfully filled the more obvious holes in the original structure of the book.

For convenience, this new edition is divided into four parts. Part I (*Origins and evolution*) addresses two fundamental questions: Where did the domestic dog come from? And how, in evolutionary terms, did it get to where it is today? Chapter 2 explores the latest archaeological evidence for dog origins and domestication, and Chapter 3 examines the growing body of molecular evidence of where the dog came from and when. Chapter 4 reassesses the evolutionary mechanisms underlying the transformation of the earliest dogs into some of the working breeds we see today, each with its own distinctive behavior and morphology.

Part II (*Behavior, cognition and training*) is devoted to the topic of domestic dog cognition and behavior, as well as addressing so-called "behavior problems" and their treatment. Chapter 5 looks at the complex world of canine behavioral genetics and what is known about the inheritance of behavioral traits in different breeds, and Chapter 6 reviews the extensive literature on behavioral development in dogs, particularly with regard to the long-term effects of early experience. Chapter 7 explores methods of identifying and quantifying breed and gender differences in behavior, while Chapter 8 addresses the topic of canine social and communicatory behavior as well as exploring differences in social behavior between wolves and dogs. Chapter 9 presents a timely review of the literature on canine aggression, including the contentious issue of breed-specific legislation, and Chapter 10 discusses the extensive new literature on the domestic dog's cognitive and emotional capacities. Chapters 11 and 12 both address the topic of dog training and behavior modification; first from the viewpoint of veterinary behavior, and second, from an applied ethology perspective.

Part III (*Dog–human relationships*) focuses on the dog's roles, welfare, and status in human society. Chapter 13 considers the remarkable physical and psychosocial benefits that humans appear to derive from canine companionship. In contrast, Chapter 14 summarizes the many welfare problems confronting dogs in their various relationships with humans. Chapter 15 addresses cultural diversity in human attitudes towards the domestic dog, and the surprising degree of ambivalence that dogs excite despite their extraordinary contribution to human lives and livelihoods.

Part IV (*Life on the margins*) examines the lives of dogs living on the fringes of human society, the various problems they face and cause, and the possible solutions to those problems. The ecology and social life of free-roaming and feral dogs is described in Chapters 16 and 17, while Chapter 18 is devoted to the various impacts of free-roaming dogs on wildlife populations. Chapter 19 discusses the contentious issue of how to accomplish dog population management in ways that are both culturally sensitive and humane. Finally, Chapter 20 provides a brief overview of some of the key issues and remaining gaps in our knowledge of the domestic dog and its relations with people.

Each of the new chapters contributed to this edition of *The Domestic Dog* has been subjected to critical peer review prior to publication. I am extremely grateful to Cristian Bonacic, Crista Coppola, Katinka DeBalogh, Göran Ericsson, Elena Garde, Suzanne Hetts, Alexandra Horowitz, Greger Larson, Evan MacLean, Ann McBride, Guillermo Perez, Peter Savolainen and Stephen Zawistowski for volunteering their valuable time and expertise to this effort. I am also hugely indebted to Priscilla Barrett for once again enhancing the text with her elegant chapter illustrations. I wish to thank all of the eminent contributors to this book, and the staff at Cambridge University Press, for their patience and forbearance during this volume's somewhat lengthy production. Lastly, I am profoundly grateful to Jacqui, Oscar and Ella for all of their love, support and forbearance.

References

Serpell, J. A. (1995). *The Domestic Dog: Its Evolution, Behaviour and Interactions with People*. Cambridge: Cambridge University Press.

Part I

Origins and evolution

2 Origins of the dog: The archaeological evidence

JULIET CLUTTON-BROCK

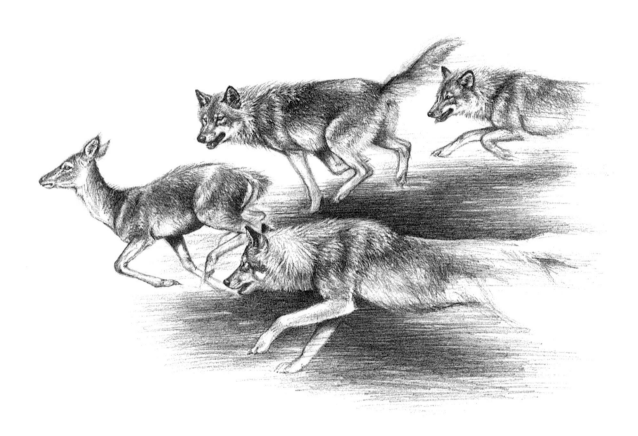

2.1   Introduction

After more than a century of argument and discussion, it is now generally agreed that the single progenitor of all domestic dogs, ancient and modern, was the grey wolf, *Canis lupus*, but when and where domestication first took place is still much argued about. Was the wolf domesticated in one part of the world or in many regions over its huge range covering the Northern Hemisphere, and what exactly constitutes a domestic dog? The word "domestic" means simply "of the home," so any tamed animal may be said to be domestic, but if the term is to be used as a scientific descriptive it must have a biological definition, and there must be a clear separation between a wild species and its domestic derivative. A domestic dog is not a tamed wolf but is it a separate species?

To paraphrase the most frequently used definition (see e.g. Lawrence, 1995, p. 551): a species is a population of animals that breeds freely and produces fertile offspring. If the hybrid offspring are infertile then the parents are separate species, for example the horse and the donkey. However, many animals that are normally considered to be separate species will interbreed with fertile offspring, as will all the wild species of the genus *Canis*, these being the wolf, coyote, and the several species of jackal. A more useful definition is the biological species concept which states that, "species are groups of interbreeding natural populations that are reproductively isolated from other such groups" (Mayr, 1966, p. 19). Using this definition, all fully domesticated animals can be classified as separate species from their wild progenitors, from which they are reproductively isolated. The dog is no longer a tamed wolf but, as a result of selective breeding under human control, it has evolved into a new species, named by Linnaeus, *Canis familiaris*, which by further reproductive isolation and under the influence of both natural and artificial selection produces new breeds (Clutton-Brock, 2012).

2.2   Precursors of the dog

With the increasing care and advanced technology used in the excavation of archaeological sites during the second half of the twentieth century, the bones of wolves have been found in association with those of early hominins[1] from as early as the Middle Pleistocene period. Examples include the cave of Lazeret near Nice in the south of France, dated at 150 000 years bp[2] (de Lumley, 1969), Zhoukoudian in North China, dated at 300 000 years bp (Olsen, 1985), and the 400 000-year-old site of Boxgrove in Kent, England (Robert & Parfitt, 1999). As these associations demonstrate, the sites of occupation and hunting activities of humans and wolves must often have overlapped, but these finds are dated to before the appearance of anatomically modern humans (*Homo s. sapiens*), and there is no physical evidence of social interaction between the two species of hunters. During the 1990s, however, molecular studies were beginning to be applied to archaeozoology and, in 1997, Carles Vilà and his colleagues published their dramatic thesis suggesting that the wolf and the dog became separate breeding populations at least 135 000 years ago (Vilà *et al.*, 1997). This conclusion was

---

[1] Hominin is the taxonomic term encompassing modern humans, extinct human species and all immediate ancestors, e.g. *Australopithecus*. The term hominid is now given a wider use and includes all modern and extinct great apes as well as modern humans and chimpanzees etc.

[2] bp denotes the radiocarbon date expressed as radiocarbon years before present (taken as AD 1950). When written in capitals, BP denotes that the radiocarbon date has been calibrated to provide the true or calendar age of the sample.

arrived at by comparing the number of genetic changes or substitutions in the control region of mitochondrial DNA derived from samples of wolves, dogs and coyotes. It was found that dog and wolf mtDNA differed by a maximum of 12 substitutions and an average of 5.3, whereas the DNA of wolves and coyotes (*Canis latrans*) differed by at least 20 substitutions. Wolves and coyotes are believed, on fossil evidence, to have diverged about one million years ago, so the scientists used this figure to calculate the rate of gene substitution assuming that such mutations occur at a steady rate over time. This led them to conclude that dogs and wolves could have diverged more than 100 000 years ago.

The assumptions from this molecular evidence are no longer considered to be valid and this extraordinarily early date for the emergence of the first "dogs" must be discounted (see vonHoldt & Driscoll, Chapter 3). But dating from about 100 000 years after this period, but before the peak of the Last Glacial Maximum (hereafter LGM), around 26 000 to 20 000 years ago, a tranche of canid remains has been identified from cave sites in Europe, the Ukraine and Siberia in which the skulls and teeth appear to show what are assumed to be the characteristics of incipient domestication. These characters include a reduction in overall size, a shortening of the jaws and widening of the snout, often without reduction in size of the teeth so that the cheek teeth are compacted. When a wild canid is found with these abnormalities it is sometimes an animal that has been kept in captivity under stress and fed on an improper diet. Based on the presence of these known characters, Mietje Germonpré and her colleagues have identified more than six skulls which they claim as Palaeolithic dogs from faunal assemblages that include large numbers of wolf remains together with the bones of their prey, particularly mammoth. The sites are the caves of Goyet in Belgium, Předmostí in the Czech Republic, and two sites in the Ukraine dating from before the LGM (Germonpré et al., 2009, 2012),

From the Ice Age cave of Razboinichya in the Altai Mountains, Nikolai Ovodov and colleagues (2011) have identified another "incipient dog," which they suggest represents, "an early Holocene lineage of wolf domestication." All these canid remains that have been identified as "dog" have been dated to before the LGM; that is, to around 30 000 years ago. Interestingly, however, although more than 190 skulls of cave bears have been recorded from the 30 000 year-old cave of Chauvet in the Ardèche, and the walls are covered with a great many depictions of lions, there is not a single authentic record of a wolf, either as a skull or in the rock art. At this time, there is no published verification for the statement of Garcia (2005) and Germonpré et al. (2009, p. 481) that, "in the deepest part of the cave, a track of footprints from a large canid is associated with those of a child," or that torch wipes made by this child were dated at c. 26 000 bp, nor that, "based on the short length of medial fingers in the footprints the canid track was interpreted as being made by a large dog."

The early hypothesis that domestication originated from the practice of capturing and taming young wild individual animals was generally replaced in the second half of the twentieth century by the theory that wild animals became associated with human groups and were thereby habituated and tamed from their own volition (see e.g. Budiansky, 1992). Wolves would have scavenged around human settlements and would slowly have become enfolded into human societies; a process that could have occurred in any area where both wolves and humans lived, and in any period from the Middle Pleistocene up to the present (for a map see Larson et al., 2012). It is further predicted that young wolves, which no longer hunted megafauna but scavenged for food around human camps, would fail to develop the skulls and jaws of hunters and would exhibit the less powerful musculature and skull structure of domestic dogs, as was shown with measurements of the skulls of captive wolves as long ago as 1894 (Wolfgramm, 1894). This is the basis for the assumption by Germonpré and her colleagues that the canid skulls they identified from

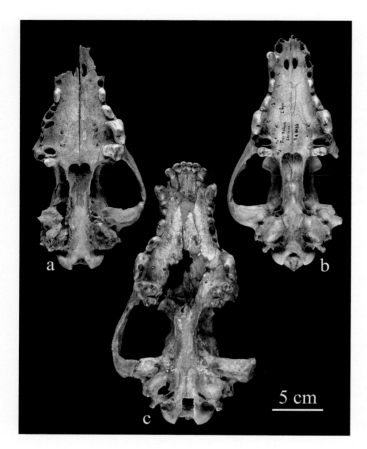

Figure 2.1 Ventral view of skulls identified as (a) "dog," and (b) and (c) wolves. (Reprinted from *Journal of Archaeological Science*, **36**, Germonpré M., Sablin, M.V., Rhiannon, E. *et al.*, Fossil dogs and wolves from Palaeolithic sites in Belgium, the Ukraine and Russia: osteometry, ancient DNA and stable isotopes, pp. 473–90 (2009), Elsevier and the Royal Belgian Institute of Natural Sciences, reprinted with permission.)

5 cm

Pleistocene caves were incipient dogs (see Figure 2.1). However, these "dog-like" characters do occur in wild canids as a result of ecological stress and inbreeding, as shown in the skulls of Arctic wolves (Clutton-Brock *et al.*, 1994; Federoff, 1996) and sporadically in other wild canids as figured by Miles & Grigson (2003). It is quite unknown how often abnormalities of this type occur in the skulls of modern wolves, let alone their relative numbers in wolves of Pleistocene date. There is also the crucial point, noted by Crockford & Kuzmin (2012), that the caves in which Germonpré and colleagues' six putative dog skulls were found range over thousands of kilometres and at least 19 000 years in age.

It could well be that, from time to time, Palaeolithic hunters reared tame wolf cubs in their communities and it is possible that the skulls of these canids can be and have been identified as incipient "dogs." However, there is no evidence at present that these tamed wolves would have bred in reproductive isolation from the rest of their species and thereby produced future generations of domestic dogs (Crockford & Kuzmin, 2012; Larson *et al.*, 2012). The latest potentially tamed wolf to be identified from the Pleistocene period, at present, is from the site of Avdeevo, an open air site on the Russian Plain near the city of Kursk, and dated between 20 000 and 21 000 years ago (Germonpré *et al.*, 2012, p. 185). After this time the extreme climate of the Last Glacial Maximum may well have driven away all hunters and their prey from northern Europe and Asia for around 5000 years.

2.3   Morphology and domestication

After a few generations, the puppies of wolves living by scavenging as commensals in a human community would exhibit a general reduction in the size of the body and head, and this trend is marked in the remains of the earliest domestic dogs. Reduction in size is a characteristic feature of the early stages of domestication not only in canids but in many different species of mammal (Tchernov & Horwitz, 1991; Clutton-Brock, 1999). The small overall size of early domestic mammals would have been partly a result of progressive stunting caused by malnutrition from the time of conception. Stunted growth has been demonstrated in young animals kept on an inadequate diet, as in the experiments on pigs by McMeekan in the 1930s (see Hammond, 1940). There would also have been strong natural selection for diminution, since small animals would have survived better on little food. Tchernov & Horwitz (1991, p. 69) argued that diminution of size in the early dogs was also a response to the changed ecological regime of the domestic state and they suggested that:

The relief of selective pressures associated with domestication set in motion a cyclical reaction of accelerated maturation, increased reproductive capacity with a tendency for litter sizes to be larger, and shortened generation time. This resulted in smaller sized, younger parents with smaller sized offspring.

During the process of domestication in the dog, the facial region (muzzle and snout) became shorter and wider with consequent crowding and displacement of the cheek teeth.[3] Tooth crowding occurred in the early stages because evolutionary reduction in the size of the teeth took place at a slower rate than the shortening of the maxillary and mandibular bones. However, the teeth did become smaller in time, and modern dogs have teeth that are very much smaller than those of wolves, even in giant breeds such as the Great Dane. The teeth may also be misplaced, or even increased in number over the normal for the canid dental formula (see Miles & Grigson, 2003, pp. 84–8). The shape of the mandible became more curved, and an angle developed between the facial region and the cranium, called the "stop" in modern breeds. The eyes became rounded and more forward-looking and the frontal sinuses became swollen, while the bones of the skull became thinner. The tympanic bullae were reduced in size and flattened.

It is probable that the colour of the coat would have changed from the tawny grey of the wolf to the yellow of the dingo quite early on in the first dogs, and maybe, before long, this will be established by molecular research, as it has been by Ludwig *et al.* (2009) for the first domestic horses. All these morphological changes are unlikely to have had much to do with intentional selection but occurred slowly as the result of physiological and hormonal changes associated with the transition to domestic existence (Crockford, 2006; Morey, 1992; Lord *et al.*, Chapter 4).

In the well-known experiments on the domestication of silver foxes in Russia that were begun by D. K. Belyaev in the 1950s and continue to the present day, all the above changes occurred in a short time without a change of diet, but simply as a result of fox cubs being strictly selected for the physical and behavioral features of domestication. However, these remarkable results were achieved by intense artificial selection on animals that were the progeny of foxes that had been reared in small cages for the fur trade for about 50 years (Statham *et al.*, 2011). Whereas, as recognized by Trut *et al.* (2004, p. 644), the domestication of wolves would have been determined by natural selection for

---

[3] Almost no whole skulls of the earliest domestic dogs have survived, so it is not possible to investigate relative changes in the different parts of the skull. The work of Wayne (1986) suggests that, while the muzzle may have widened, the length of the facial region, although shortened, would have remained in proportion to the reduced cranial length.

coexistence with human hunters who, "were only one factor that shifted the direction of selection to behavior and the ability to exist in the new, anthropogenic environment."

2.4   The first dogs

Apart from the possible precursors to the dog, dating from before the LGM, archaeological evidence indicates that the dog was the first species of animal to be domesticated with certainty. This occurred towards the end of the last Ice Age when all human subsistence still depended on hunting, gathering and foraging. The record for the earliest directly dated canid remains that can be identified as definite domestic dog, goes to a right maxillary fragment with cheek teeth from Kesslerloch Cave in Switzerland (Figure 2.2). This cave is one of the major Magdalenian sites in Central Europe and was first excavated in 1898/9. Recently, a reappraisal of the faunal remains from the cave was carried out by archaeozoologists, and a fragment of canid upper jaw was identified as dog and not wolf. This was confirmed from its small size and from the morphology of the upper carnassial and first molar. A sample of the dog maxilla was directly dated to 12 225 ± 45 bp (KIA-33350) or c.14 100–14 600 BP (Napierala & Uerpmann, 2012).

Until the identification of the maxilla from Kesserloch the earliest find of a dog was of a mandible from the late Palaeolithic grave of an old man and a young woman at Bonn-Oberkassel in Germany (Nobis, 1981). This dog is dated through closely associated material to around the same date as the Kesserloch maxilla, that is c.12 100 bp. After this period, the identification of the bones and teeth of dogs on prehistoric sites and their separation from those of wolves has become relatively straightforward, as it was, for example, with the skulls of a dog and a wolf from the Early Mesolithic site of Star Carr in Yorkshire, England.

The well-known site of Star Carr is the most important Mesolithic site in Britain. The site was occupied around a waterlogged lakeside for around 350 years from c.10 700–10 350 BP during the preboreal and boreal climatic periods. The Ice Age had ended and temperatures were close to those of recent times, although the sea levels had not yet risen enough to separate Britain from the

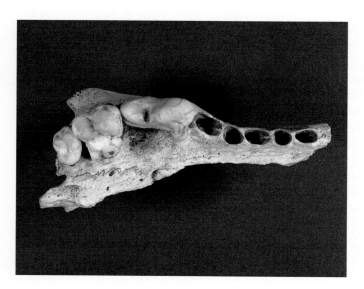

Figure 2.2 The right maxilla identified as domestic dog from the Magdalenian cave of Kesserloch, Switzerland. (From Napierala, H. & Uerpmann, H-P (2012), © 2010 John Wiley & Sons, Ltd, reprinted with permission.)

Continent. A huge number of organic artifacts were preserved in the peat, including nearly 200 harpoon points made of red deer antler. The site was first excavated by J. G. D. Clark in 1949–51, the faunal remains were studied by Fraser & King (1954), and the dog was described in detail by Magnus Degerbøl (1961), but work has continued on the site and on the artifacts and faunal remains ever since.

In 1985, during excavations at the nearby Mesolithic site of Seamer Carr, the neck vertebrae of a dog were retrieved that match in age and size the skull of the Star Carr dog (Clutton-Brock & Noe-Nygaard, 1990). A fragment of one of these vertebrae has provided a radiocarbon accelerator date of 9940 ± 110 bp [Oxa-1030]. It is conceivable that the skull and neck came from one individual dog, but they could also be from two dogs from the same litter or from unrelated dogs of the same size and age. These are the only remains of dogs that have so far been identified from Mesolithic Britain (of which there are a large number of sites), so it is probable that the number of dogs during this very early period was quite small. They were probably inbred and displayed little variation in size amongst individuals.

Another remarkable feature of the dog vertebrae from Seamer Carr is that two samples of bone yielded stable carbon isotope ratios of −14.67% and −16.97%. These ratios reveal that the dog obtained a significant part of its food from marine fish. Clutton-Brock & Noe-Nygaard (1990) have therefore postulated that the sites of Star Carr and Seamer Carr were hunting camps that were visited by people who lived for much of the year nearer to the coast and obtained most of their food by fishing.

The skull of a fully adult dog very similar in size and proportions to the Star Carr skull has been excavated from another Mesolithic wetland site at Bedburg-Köningshoven in Germany (Street, 1989). Similar remains of dogs have also been found from the numerous waterlogged Mesolithic sites in Denmark where the period is known as the Maglemosian. The similarity in size and osteological characteristics of the remains of these first domestic dogs found on prehistoric sites in northern Europe may indicate that all these early dogs were the result of dispersal from a single founder population. The skull of the dog from Bedburg-Köningshoven, for example, is closer in size and morphology to the remains of the earliest dogs from western Asia than it is to the very large European wolves, as exemplified by the Mesolithic wolf skull from Star Carr. However, wolves must have lived close to human settlements in many parts of the world, and a single litter of puppies from any one of these could have provided the founders for an independent domestication event that subsequently became very widespread.

The dogs that have been identified from these Mesolithic sites in northern Europe come from a similar time period to the sites in western Asia from where a cluster of canid remains has been identified as belonging to *Canis familiaris*. These sites belong to the cultural period known as the Epipaleolithic or Natufian and they are associated with a dramatic change in human hunting strategies. During the Paleolithic period, animals were killed by direct impact from heavy stone axes and spears. During the Natufian, and the corresponding Mesolithic period of Europe, arrows armed with tiny stone blades called microliths came into widespread use (Mithen, 2003). The success of these long-distance projectiles would have been enhanced by the new partnership with dogs that could help to track down and bring to bay wounded animals. This cooperative hunting technique would thus have resulted in greater hunting efficiency, as it does among some contemporary hunting societies (Koster, 2008; Lee, 1979).

During the 1930s, a small number of canid skulls from Natufian sites in Palestine were identified as those of dogs by Dorothea Bate; the most notable of these being a nearly complete skull from the cave of Wady el-Mughara at Mount Carmel (Bate, 1937). Thirty years later, in the 1960s, I re-examined the skulls from Mount Carmel, Shukbah, Zuttiyeh, and Kebarah that are held in the

Natural History Museum, London, and questioned their domestic status. Measurements showed that they were very similar to the skulls of living Arabian wolves, except that they were slightly smaller and rather wider in the palate (Clutton-Brock, 1962). In western Asia the wild wolf, *Canis lupus arabs*, is, at the present day, the smallest of the subspecies that range over the northern hemisphere. This makes the identification of fragments of canid bone from later archaeological sites difficult because there is very little reduction in size from the wolf to the dog (Harrison, 1973). However, as described by Dayan (1994) and Tchernov & Valla (1997), the fossil remains of wolf from Natufian and earlier sites are from very large individuals, while the canids that have been identified from sites of this period as dogs are as small as the Mesolithic dogs from Europe. The realization that the early Holocene wolves of western Asia were as large as those in Europe has made a crucial difference to the acceptance of the small canids from sites of equivalent date as dogs, and it is now generally agreed that Bate's identification of the canids from her early sites as dogs was correct. But were they descended from the large wolves that inhabited the region at that time or had these dogs been imported from somewhere else?

In the 1970s the discovery of a Natufian site with the burial of a human skeleton with its hand on the remains of a puppy became the best-known early evidence for the domestication of the dog in the Near East (Davis & Valla, 1978). The site is near the Huleh Lake in the upper Jordan valley in Israel, and is dated at 12 000 years ago. Its inhabitants were hunter-gatherers who were on the verge of becoming agriculturalists. They lived in round stone dwellings, used basalt pestles and mortars for grinding cereals, and buried their dead in stone-covered tombs. In one of these, at the entrance to a dwelling, the skeleton of an elderly human was found together with that of a puppy of between four and five months of age. The human skeleton lay on its right side, in a flexed position, with its hand on the thorax of the puppy (Figure 2.3). Since the finding of this human and canid burial at Ein Mallaha, another Natufian burial with canid skeletons was excavated at the cave of Hayonim Terrace, Israel. This burial is late Natufian in date and held the remains of three humans and two dogs (Tchernov & Valla, 1997).

The canid remains in these graves have been widely accepted as those of the earliest dogs on cultural grounds, that is, their close association with the human skeletons must imply that in life they were highly valued animal companions and that therefore they must be domestic dogs. However, the remarkable discovery of a fox skeleton buried with a human in a pre-Natufian grave throws the identification of these "dogs" based on the cultural evidence alone in doubt and reopens the question of whether these canid skeletons are really those of domestic dogs. The skulls are not morphologically similar to those of jackals (*Canis aureus*) but what else could they be?

'Uyun al-Hammam is a pre-Natufian site in northern Jordan, with elaborate human burials associated with animal remains. Eleven human skeletons had been buried in at least eight graves, as described in the excavation report by Lisa Maher and her colleagues (2011). It is clear from the careful interpretation of the burials that one of these humans had been buried with the body of a fox (*Vulpes vulpes*), and later when this grave was opened again and the partly decomposed human skeleton was moved to a bed of red ochre in another area nearby, the head of the fox was moved with it. Maher *et al.* describe the association thus:

It is possible that the link between fox and human was such that when the human died the fox was killed and buried alongside. Later, when the graves were re-opened, these links were remembered and bones moved so that the dead person would continue to have the fox with him or her in the afterlife.

The burial of the fox in close association with a human, as well as the burials of "dogs" in Natufian graves in Israel, supports the view that, throughout their evolution, humans have possessed a unique instinct for nurturing members other species of animals, irrespective of their potential "uses." Thus,

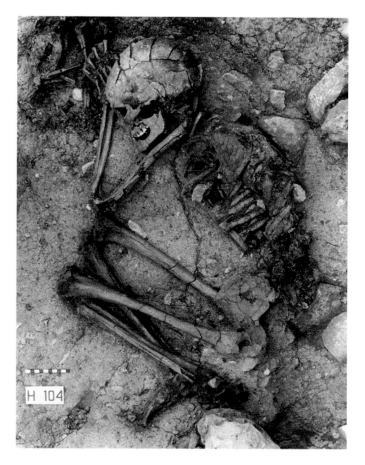

Figure 2.3 Burial of a human with a puppy from the Natufian site of Ein Mallaha, Israel. (© Simon Davis, reprinted with permission.)

the biological and semantic divisions between the wild and the domestic, as we view them today, may have taken thousands of years to become established.

Contemporary and later sites in other countries of western Asia have also yielded canid remains that have been identified as dogs (see, for example, Clutton-Brock, 1969 and Stanley Olsen's *Origins of the Domestic Dog*, 1985, pp. 71–9). Notable amongst these is a small mandible with compacted teeth from the site of Palegawra in Iraq, dated at around 12 000 years ago (Turnbull & Reed, 1974). From the following Neolithic period, between 9000 and 7000 years ago, remains of dogs become ubiquitous in archaeological sites from many parts of the world, and in these, the dog-like features of the skull and teeth are fully developed. One hundred and thirteen fragments of skulls, teeth and skeletal bones have been identified as those of large domestic dogs from the early Neolithic site of Jarmo in Iraq (9250–7750 bp) by Lawrence & Reed (1983). In China there are Neolithic dogs from 7000 years ago (Olsen, 1985).

Remains of dogs have been found with those of the extinct Japanese wolf, *Canis lupus hodophilax*, from the rock shelter site of Tocibara in Japan, dating at around 8000 bp (Miyao *et al.*, 1984). Olsen (1977, 1985) considered that the small Chinese wolf, *Canis lupus chanco*, was the ancestor, not only of early Chinese dogs, but also of those that moved with the early human immigrants across the Bering Straits into North America. However, molecular analysis has now provided two conflicting theses for the origin of all dogs, worldwide: first, that of Leonard *et al.* (2002) and vonHoldt *et al.* (2010) who claim that all past and present domestic dogs in the world, including all those from the Americas, ultimately descended from the grey wolf of the Middle East, although out-breeding with local wolves (including the North American wolf) also occurred in the early history of specific lineages. This claim supports the evidence from archaeozoology of the past 50 years. The second claim of Jun-Feng Pang and colleagues (2009) argues for a single origin of all dogs worldwide from wolves that lived in China, south of the Yangtze River (see vonHoldt & Driscoll, Chapter 3, for discussion).

2.5   Origin of dogs in the Americas

The first authentic description of the great variety of American aboriginal dogs was published by Glover Allen (1920), who divided the kinds of North and South American native dogs into 17 groups: Eskimo, Plains Indian, Sioux, long-haired Pueblo, larger or common Indian, Klamath Indian, short-legged Indian, Klallam Indian, Inca, long-haired Inca, Patagonian, Mexican hairless, small Indian or Techichi, Hare Indian, Fuegian, short-nosed Indian, and Peruvian pug-nosed. The earliest reliably dated remains of dog in North America come from the burial of the complete skeletons of four dogs in the Koster site in Illinois dated to around 8500 years ago. In South America, the earliest presumed dog remains are from Fell's Cave in the southernmost tip of Chile. However, the very early date of 10 700–6500 years ago has led to their identification being questioned, for there are several extinct and living, wild species of indigenous canid that are possible candidates for these remains. However, since flake tools and quantities of other animal remains have been excavated from the earliest levels at Fell's Cave, there is no reason why these early American hunters would not also have had dogs (Clutton-Brock, 1988).

As well as being valuable haulage animals, it is clear from archaeozoological reports that dogs in North America were important providers of meat. This has been evaluated from the early levels of the Preclassic (1200 BC–AD 250) site of Cuello in Belize where the faunal remains showed that dogs had been bred for food and killed at the end of their first year of life. The dogs were small, falling within the size range of the "small Indian dog or Techichi" of Allen's groups. They did not belong to the hairless, xoloitzcuintli, since none of the mandibles showed the congenital lack of anterior teeth, which is genetically linked with hairlessness (Clutton-Brock & Hammond, 1994).

Apart from the xoloitzcuintli, which is known to have been kept purebred since ancient times, there are no known living breeds of indigenous native American dogs, for all have interbred, either accidentally or by design, with immigrant European dogs. This includes the Eskimo dog and the modern breed known as the Native American Indian Dog (Schwartz, 1997). However, the many different breeds that were owned by the First Nations are well known from historical images and written accounts, as well as from their buried remains and from artifacts and clothing made from dog skins and hair.

An unusual and distinct breed, known as the Salish wool dog, has been described from the south west coast of British Columbia by European accounts in the late 1700s. They were small, long-haired, white dogs that were bred exclusively for their thick soft fur. The wool dogs were kept reproductively isolated from all other dogs in houses for most of the year but taken to off-shore islands, with buried dried fish for food, during the summer salmon fishing season. They were owned by women, and the thick fleeces of the dogs were sheared several times a year. The wool was woven into Salish blankets. Following the arrival of sheep with European colonists, the wool dogs became extinct (Schulting, 1994).

2.6   Origin of dogs in Africa south of the Sahara

Because dogs overlap in size with the endemic African jackals (*C. aureus, C. adustus and C. mesomelas*) it is not easy to distinguish their skeletal remains on archaeological sites. However, the spread of dogs southward with livestock herders can be shown by the few authenticated finds of their remains from the north to south sequence of archaeological sites: Esh Shaheinab and Kerma in Sudan, c. 3300–2000 BC; Ntusi in Uganda, AD 895–1025; Iron Age Kalomo in Zambia, AD 950–1000; south of the Limpopo River in southern Africa after AD 600 (Clutton-Brock, 1993, p. 64).

In South Africa there were two main groups of inhabitants before the southward expansion of Bantu-speaking peoples. They were the indigenous Khoi people who belonged to a single linguistic group but were divided into the Khoisan (Bushmen) who were hunter-gatherers and who survive today in very small numbers, and the Khoikhoi (Hottentots) who were pastoralists who herded cattle and sheep, but who were almost all exterminated by European colonists in the nineteenth century.

It is not known whether dogs first travelled south with Bantu-speaking herders from Central Africa in the early Iron Age, or whether they arrived earlier in the South with the Khoikhoi pastoralists who are believed to have originated further north in East Africa. The Khoikhoi would have met the Khoisan who were hunter-gatherers, and who were the indigenous people living in South Africa, and who survive today in small communities in arid areas of southern Africa, notably in the Kalahari (Botswana). They keep dogs that may be direct descendants of the ancestral stock and are still a very important element in the social and economic life of these hunter-gatherers. In his now classic work on the !Kung San of the Kalahari Desert, Richard Lee (1979) recorded the use of dogs for hunting and found that between a third and three-quarters of the animals killed during his study period were obtained with the help of dogs that were often highly trained. Lee described the typical !Kung dog as, "a small animal (50 cm tall at the shoulder) of undistinguished appearance. It is a short-haired breed varying in colour from all black to all buff with many piebald forms" (Lee, 1979, p. 143). However, before the arrival of the colonists, dogs appear to have been more popular with the Khoi pastoralists than with the hunters. In the ancient rock art of southern Africa, there are rather few images of dogs and these are usually shown following people, rather than in a hunt.

Indigenous village dogs are everywhere in Africa today and when not interbred with imported greyhounds and other breeds of European dogs they are remarkably similar in conformation throughout their range. Towards the end of the twentieth century, a few dog-owners and biologists realized that these dogs represent an ancient genetic lineage that should be preserved (see Larson *et al.*, 2012). In 1998 a meeting was held to discuss the conservation of traditional African dogs. They were given the name Africanis, and the Africanis Society of Southern Africa was founded (Gallant, 2002).

2.7   Origin of the dingo and New Guinea singing dog

Archaeological evidence indicates that humans first reached Australia more than 40 000 years ago. The earliest dingoes arrived less than 12 000 years ago; a deduction based on the fact that there are no remains of dogs from Tasmania, which became geographically isolated from mainland Australia by the formation of the Bass Strait at about this time. Significantly, the Indigenous Australians never acquired domestic pigs, and this would suggest that the dog was taken to the continent before the earliest domestication of the pig. New archaeological and dating evidence indicates that pigs were not taken to New Guinea and Melanesia before 3000 BP (O'Connor *et al.*, 2011).

In skeletal anatomy, the dingo closely resembles the small wolf of India, *Canis lupus pallipes,* and the pariah dogs of Southeast Asia. Based on mitochondrial DNA sequences analyzed by Savolainen and colleagues (2004), the dingo is now considered a direct descendant of a small founder population of domesticated dogs that were introduced to Australia, possibly on a single occasion, around 5000 years ago. The earliest radiocarbon date obtained for dog remains from Australia is 3450 ± 95 bp (Milham & Thompson, 1976). Although the dog was never used for traction in Australia, as it was by the Native Americans, it was greatly valued by the Aborigines as a hunting partner, companion, bed-warmer and occasional item of food. After arriving in Australia, the dogs became feral, spread rapidly, and have lived as part of the wild mammal fauna ever since.

Early accounts by Europeans of the Indigenous Australians and the dingo describe a relationship that was probably not dissimilar to that of hunter-gatherers and wolves all over Eurasia some 12 000 years ago, in the pre-agricultural period. The great majority of dingoes in the nineteenth century lived and hunted as wild carnivores and may have been as widespread as wolves in the early Holocene of Eurasia and North America. Aboriginal families kept some dingoes as pets, used some as hunting partners, ate them when meat was scarce, and also showered them with affection. Meggitt (1965) has described the associations between the Aborigines and the dingo. These varied from hunting the adult dogs for their tails, which were worn as headdresses, to capturing young pups which, if strong, were reared as hunting partners, or, if weak, were eaten. Meggitt quoted a comment from Lumholtz (1889, p. 179), writing about the dingo in northern Queensland: "its master never strikes, but merely threatens it. He caresses it like a child, eats the fleas off it, and then kisses it on the snout." These tamed dingoes were, however, very poorly fed. Apart from being given bones, they were left to scavenge for themselves, so that in the past a tame dingo could always be distinguished from a wild one by its poor condition (Meggitt, 1965). More recent relationships between the Indigenous Australians, dingoes and introduced domestic dogs have been reviewed by Smith & Litchfield (2009).

For the last hundred years the dingo has been regarded as vermin and persecuted because it kills sheep. Those that remain in the wild are in great danger of losing their purebred status through interbreeding with free-roaming European dogs (Ginsberg & Macdonald, 1990, pp. 52–4). The extermination of the purebred dingo would be a great loss because it is part of the living heritage of hunter-gatherer culture, as well as being part of Australian history.

Dogs may have been taken to New Guinea at around the same time as to Australia to provide meat and hides and fur in a land that was dominated by wild birds. It may be assumed that the dogs became feral here also and spread rapidly into the forests and high altitude mountains. Here they bred under natural selection and evolved into a distinct ecomorph with the tawny-yellow coat of the dingo and the unique singing howl, which carries over great distances.

2.8   Conclusions

To every part of the world where people have travelled for perhaps 10 000 years, they have taken their dogs with them, as they still continue to do. Today, genetics and archaeology have come together to open an entirely new window on the history of the interactions between humans and animals. It is now possible not only to discover when and where domestication of each species occurred but also from which particular genetic race of progenitor species they were first descended, and how and when they were moved around the world. However, none of these amazingly detailed facts can be deduced without the expertise of the archaeologist who excavates the animal remains, and the archaeozoologist who identifies and interprets the species.

References

Allen, G. M. (1920). Dogs of American Aborigines, *Bulletin of the Museum of Comparative Zoology, Harvard University*, 63: 431–517.

Bate, D. M. A. (1937). Palaeontology: the fossil fauna of the Wady-el Mughara Caves. Vol. 1, Part II, In *The Stone Age of Mount Carmel*, eds. D. A. E. Garrod & D. M. A. Bate. Oxford: Clarendon Press, pp. 139–237.

Budiansky, S. (1992). *The Covenant of the Wild: Why Animals Chose Domestication*. New York: William Morrow.

Bulmer, S. (2001). Lapita dogs and singing dogs and the history of the dog in New Guinea. In *The Archaeology of Lapita Dispersal in Oceania: Papers from the Fourth Lapita Conference, Canberra*, eds. G. R. Clark, A. J. Anderson & T. Vunidilo. Canberra: Pandanus Books, pp. 183–201.

Clutton-Brock, J. (1962). Near Eastern canids and the affinities of the Natufian dogs. *Zeitschrift für Tierzüchtung und Züchtungsbiologie*, 76: 326–33.

Clutton-Brock, J. (1969). Carnivore remains from the excavations of the Jericho Tell. In *The Domestication and Exploitation of Plants and Animals*, eds. P. J. Ucko & G.W. Dimbleby. London: Duckworth, pp. 337–45.

Clutton-Brock, J. (1988). The carnivore remains excavated at Fell's Cave in 1970. In *Travels and Archaeology in South Chile by Junius B. Bird*, ed. J. Hyslop. Iowa City: University of Iowa Press, pp. 188–95.

Clutton-Brock, J. (1993). The spread of domestic animals in Africa. In *The Archaeology of Africa: Food, Metals and Towns*, eds. T. Shaw, P. Sinclair, B. Andah & A. Okpoko. London: Routledge, pp. 61–70.

Clutton-Brock, J. (1999). *A Natural History of Domesticated Mammals*, 2nd edition. Cambridge: Cambridge University Press/The Natural History Museum.

Clutton-Brock, J. (2012). *Animals as Domesticates: A World View Through History*. East Lansing, MI: Michigan State University Press.

Clutton-Brock, J. & Hammond, N. (1994). Hot dogs: comestible canids in Preclassic Maya culture at Cuello, Belize. *Journal of Archaeological Science,* 21: 819–826.

Clutton-Brock, J., Kitchener, A. C. & Lynch, J. M. (1994). Changes in the skull morphology of the Arctic wolf, *Canis lupus arctos*, during the twentieth century. *Journal of Zoology, London*, 233: 19–36.

Clutton-Brock, J. & Noe-Nygaard, N. (1990). New osteological and C-isotope evidence on Mesolithic dogs: companions to hunters and fishers at Star Carr, Seamer Carr and Kongemose. *Journal of Archaeological Science*, 17: 643–53.

Crockford, S. J. (2006). *Rhythms of Life: Thyroid Hormone and the Origin of Species*. Victoria, B.C.: Trafford.

Crockford, S. J. & Kuzmin, Y. V. (2012). Comments on Germonpré et al., Journal of Archaeological Science 36, 2009 "Fossil dogs and wolves from Palaeolithic sites in Belgium, the Ukraine and Russia: osteometry, ancient DNA and stable isotopes", and Germonpré, Lázkičková-Galetová, and Sablin, Journal of Archaeological Science 39, 2012 "Palaeolithic dog skulls at the Gravettian Předmostí site, the Czech Republic". *Journal of Archaeological Science*, 39: 2797–801.

Davis, S. J. M. & Valla, F. R. (1978). Evidence for domestication of the dog 12,000 years ago in the Natufian of Israel. *Nature*, 276 (5688): 608–10.

Dayan, T. (1994). Early domesticated dogs of the Near East. *Journal of Archaeological Science*, 21: 633–640.

Degerbøl, M. (1961). On a find of a Preboreal domestic dog (*Canis familiaris* L.) from Star Carr, Yorkshire, with remarks on other Mesolithic dogs. *Proceedings of the Prehistoric Society*, 27: 35–55.

de Lumley, H. (1969). Une Cabane de chasseuse acheuleenes dans la Grotte du Lazaret à Nice. *Archeologia*, 28: 26–33.

Federoff, N. E. (1996). Malocclusion in the jaws of captive bred Arctic Wolves. *Canis lupus arctos*. *Canadian Field-Naturalist*, 110: 683–687.

Fraser, F. C. & King, J. (1954). Faunal remains. In *Excavations at Star Carr an Early Mesolithic Site at Seamer near Scarborough, Yorkshire*, ed. J. G. D. Clark. Cambridge: Cambridge University Press, pp. 70–95.

Gallant, J. (2002). *The Story of the African Dog*. Pietermaritzburg: University of Natal Press.

Garcia, M. A. (2005). Ichnologie generale de la grotte Chauvet. *Bulletin de la Societé Prehistorique Française*, 102: 103–108.

Germonpré, M., Láznicková-Galetová, M., Mikhail, V. & Sablin, M. V. (2012). Palaeolithic dog skulls at the Gravettian Predmostí site, the Czech Republic. *Journal of Archaeological Science*, 39: 184–202.

Germonpré, M., Sablin, M. V., Stevens, R. E. *et al.* (2009). Fossil dogs and wolves from Palaeolithic sites in Belgium, the Ukraine and Russia: osteometry, ancient DNA and stable isotopes. *Journal of Archaeological Science*, 36: 473–490.

Ginsberg, J. R. & Macdonald, D. W. (1990). *Foxes, Wolves, Jackals, and Dogs: an Action Plan for the Conservation of Canids*. Gland, Switzerland: International Union for Conservation of Nature and Natural Resources.

Hammond, J. (1940). *Farm Animals*. London: Edward Arnold.

Harrison, D. L. (1973). Some comparative features of the skulls of wolves (*Canis lupus* Linn.) and pariah dogs (*Canis familiaris* Linn.) from the Arabian Peninsula and neighbouring lands. *Bonner Zoologische Beiträge*, 24: 185–91.

Hemmer, H. (1990). *Domestication: the Decline of Environmental Appreciation*. Cambridge: Cambridge University Press.

Koster, J. M. (2008). Hunting with dogs in Nicaragua: An optimal foraging approach. *Current Anthropology*, 49: 935–944.

Larson, G., Karlsson, E. K., Perria, A. *et al.* (2012). Rethinking dog domestication by integrating genetics, archeology, and biogeography. *Proceedings of the National Academy of Sciences*, http://doi/10.1073/pnas.1203005109

Lawrence, B. & Reed, C. A. (1983). The dogs of Jarmo. In *Prehistoric Archaeology along the Zagros Flank*, eds. L. S. Braidwood, R. J. Braidwood, B. Howe, C. A. Reed & P. J. Watson. Chicago, IL: The Oriental Institute of the University of Chicago, pp. 485–94.

Lawrence, E. Ed. (1995). *Henderson's Dictionary of Biological Terms*, 11th edition. London: Longman Group.

Lee, R. B. (1979). *The !Kung San: Men, Women, and Work in a Foraging Society*. Cambridge: Cambridge University Press.

Leonard, J. A., Wayne, R. K., Wheeler, J. *et al.* (2002). Ancient DNA evidence for Old World origin of New World dogs, *Science*, 298: 1613–16.

Ludwig, A., Pruvost, M., Reissmann, M. *et al.* (2009). Coat color variation at the beginning of horse domestication. *Science*, 324: 485.

Maher, L. A., Stock, J. T., Finney, S. *et al.* (2011). A unique human-fox burial from a pre-Natufian cemetery in the Levant (Jordan). *PLoS ONE*, 6: e15815.

Mayr, E. (1966). *Animal Species and Evolution*. Cambridge, MA: Belknap Press.

Meggitt, M. J. (1965). The association between Australian Aborigines and dingoes. In *Man, Culture, and Animals: the Role of Animals in Human Ecological Adjustments*, eds. A. Leeds & A. P. Vayda. Washington, DC: American Association for the Advancement of Science, No. 78, pp. 7–26.

Miles, A. E. W. & Grigson, C. eds. (2003). *Colyer's Variations and Diseases of the Teeth of Animals*, revised edition. Cambridge: Cambridge University Press.

Milham, P. & Thompson, P. (1976). Relative antiquity of human occupation and extinct fauna at Madura Cave, south-eastern Australia. *Mankind*, 10: 175–80.

Mithen, S. (2003). *After the Ice: A Global Human History 20,000–5000 BC*. London: Weidenfeld & Nicolsen.

Miyao, T., Nishizawa, T., Hanamura, H. & Koyasu, K. (1984). Mammalian remains of the earliest Jomon period at the rockshelter site of Tochibara, Nagano Pref., Japan. *Journal of Growth*, 23: 40–56.

Morey, D. F. (1992). Size, shape and development in the evolution of the domestic dog. *Journal of Archaeological Science*, 19: 181–204.

Musil, R. (1984). The first known domestication of wolves in central Europe. In *Animals and Archaeology: 4. Husbandry in Europe*. eds. C. Grigson & J. Clutton-Brock. Oxford: BAR International Series, 227, pp. 23–6.

Napierala, H & Uerpmann, H-P. (2012). A "new" Palaeolithic dog from Central Europe. *International Journal of Osteoarchaeology*, 22: 127–37.

Nobis, G. (1981). Das älteste Haustier des Menschen. *Unterkiefer eines hundes aus dem Magdaléniengrab von Bonn-Oberkassel*. Bonn: Das Reinische Landesmuseum.

O'Connor, S., Barham, A. & Aplin, K. *et al.* (2011). The power of paradigms: examining the evidential basis for early to mid-Holocene pigs and pottery in Melanesia. *Journal of Pacific Archaeology*, 2: 1–25.

Olsen, S. J. (1977). The Chinese wolf, ancestor of New World dogs. *Science*, 197: 553–5.

Olsen, S. J. (1985). *Origins of the Domestic Dog: the Fossil Record*. Tucson, AZ: University of Arizona Press.

Ovodov, N. D., Crockford, S. J., Kuzmin, Y. V. *et al.* (2011). A 33,000 year-old incipient dog from the Altai Mountains of Siberia: Evidence of the earliest domestication disrupted by the Last Glacial Maximum. *PLoS ONE*, 6: e22821. http://doi:10.1371/journal.pone.0022821

Pang, J-F., Kluetsch, C., Zou, X-J. *et al.* (2009). MtDNA data indicate a single origin for dogs south of Yangtze River, less than 16,300 years ago, from numerous wolves. *Molecular Biology and Evolution* 26: 2849–64.

Robert, M. B. & Parfitt S. A. A. eds. (1999). Boxgrove: A Middle Pleistocene hominid site at Eartham Quarry, Boxgrove, West Sussex. *English Heritage Archaeological Report*, 17. London: English Heritage.

Savolainen, P., Leitner, T. & Wilton, A. N. *et al.* (2004). A detailed picture of the origin of the Australian dingo, obtained from the study of mitochondrial DNA. *Proceedings of the National Academy of Sciences*, 101: 12387–90.

Schulting, R. (1994). The hair of the dog: the identification of a coast Salish dog-hair blanket from Yale, British Columbia. *Canadian Journal of Archaeology*, 18: 57–76.

Schwartz, M. 1997. *A History of Dogs in the Early Americas*. New Haven, CT & London: Yale University Press.

Smith, B. P. & Litchfield, C. A. (2009). A review of the relationship between indigenous Australians, dingoes (*Canis dingo*) and domestic dogs (*Canis familiaris*). *Anthrozoös*, 22: 111–28.

Statham, M., Trut, L. N., Sacks, B. N. *et al.* (2011). On the origin of a domesticated species: identifying the parent population of Russian silver foxes (*Vulpes vulpes*). *Biological Journal of the Linnean Society*, 103: 168–75.

Street, M. (1989). *Jäger und Schamen: Bedburg-Königshoven ein Wohnplatz am Niederrhein vor 10000 Jahren*. Mainz: Römisch-Germanischen Zentralmuseums.

Tchernov, E. & Horwitz, L. K. (1991). Body size diminution under domestication: unconscious selection in primeval domesticates. *Journal of Anthropological Archaeology*, 10: 54–75.

Tchernov, E. & Valla, F. F. (1997). Two new dogs, and other Natufian dogs, from the southern Levant. *Journal of Archaeological Science*, 24: 65–95.

Trut, L. N., Plyusnina, I. Z. & Oskina, I. N. (2004). An experiment on fox domestication and debatable issues of evolution of the dog. *Russian Journal of Genetics*, 40: 644–55.

Turnbull, P. F. & Reed, C. A. (1974). The fauna from the terminal Pleistocene of Palegawra Cave, a Zarzian occupation site in northeastern Iraq. *Fieldiana Anthropology*, 63: 81–146.

Vilà, C., Savolainen. P., Maldonado, J. E. *et al.* (1997). Multiple and ancient origins of the dog. *Science*, 276: 1687–9.

vonHoldt, B. J., Pollinger, P., Lohmueller, K. E. *et al.* (2010). Genome-wide SNP and haplotype analyses reveal a rich history underlying dog domestication, *Nature*, 464: 898–902.

Wayne, R. K. (1986). Cranial morphology of domestic and wild canids: The influence of development on morphological change. *Evolution*, 40: 243–61.

Wolfgramm, A. (1894). Die Einwirkung der Gefangenschaft auf die Gestaltung des Wolfsschädels. [The influence of captivity on the development of wolf skulls.] *Zoologische Jahrbucher*. Jena Abteilung fur Systematik Bd. 3: 773–822.

3 Origins of the dog: Genetic insights into dog domestication

BRIDGETT M. VONHOLDT AND CARLOS A. DRISCOLL

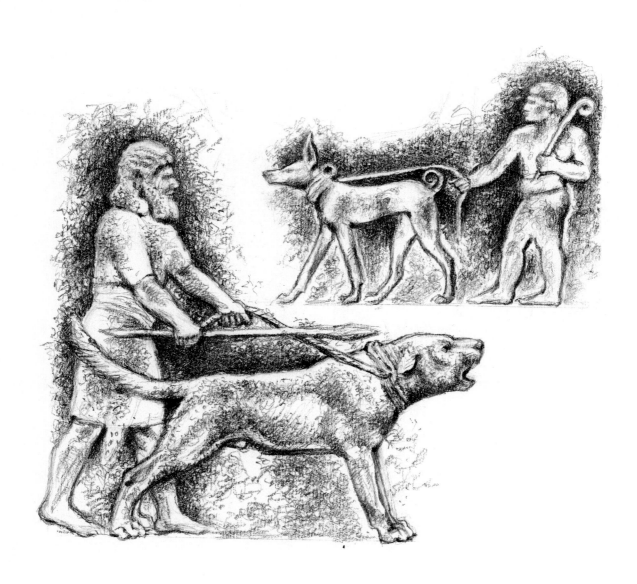

3.1   Introduction

Dogs are the oldest domesticated animal and today are second only to cats as the most popular pet in western societies (Boyko, 2011; Leonard *et al.*, 2006; Wayne and vonHoldt, 2012). The dog has taken on many significant roles in human society, ranging from companion, sentry, and hunting partner to its more recent function as a model for understanding human disease. By exploring the genetic and evolutionary history of our canine companions, we can better understand not only the natural history of dogs but also our own evolutionary history.

Inquiries into the dog's natural history are now enlightened by molecular and genetic data to an overwhelmingly greater degree then they were 20 years ago when the first edition of this book was published. This trend towards increasing molecular inference will certainly continue, though morphology and archaeology will remain vitally important in completing our understanding of the cultural context of the changes wrought by domestication.

3.2   The wolf, ancestor of the dog

The dog and its ancestor, the wolf (*Canis lupus*), belong to the family Canidae. The 34 living species of canids are grouped into four clades: a red fox-like clade, a South American clade, a wolf-like clade, and a clade comprising only the gray and island fox (*Urocyon cinereoargenteus* and *U. littoralis*, respectively) (Lindblad-Toh *et al.*, 2005; Perini *et al.*, 2009) (Figure 3.1). Canids are found in all terrestrial habitats and, with the human-assisted introduction of dogs and foxes to Australia and New Zealand, Antarctica is now the only continent without a resident population. Currently, seven species belong to the dog-like genus *Canis* (Figure 3.2), which arose nearly six million years ago (mya) in North America and, along with a number of other carnivore species, expanded into Eurasia (4 mya) via the Beringian land bridge, and subsequently into Africa (3 mya) (Wang & Tedford, 2008). The archaeological record indicates that the modern-day gray wolf (*Canis lupus lupus*) evolved in Eurasia around 3–4 mya, re-invading North America about 500 000 years ago (Wang & Tedford, 2008). Supremely adaptable, the wolf inhabits nearly every habitat and environmental condition (Mech & Boitani, 2003). Wolves vary greatly in size depending on their environmental distribution, from the gracile 13 kg wolves of the Middle Eastern deserts to the large robust individuals (over 78 kg) of the Arctic tundra.

Members of the genus *Canis* vary in appearance, behavior and degree of sociality (Mech & Boitani, 2003; Packard, 2003). Based on recent molecular genetic studies and corroborating morphological evidence, it is now agreed that the sole ancestor of the dog is the gray wolf, *Canis lupus*. Though this verdict settles hundreds of years of speculation on dog origins (e.g. Clutton-Brock, 1981; Darwin, 1868), resolving which particular group of wolves was directly ancestral to the dog still proves challenging (Ding *et al.*, 2012; Franz *et al.*, 2016; Freedman *et al.*, 2014; Pang *et al.*, 2009; Savolainen *et al.*, 2002; Shannon *et al.*, 2015; vonHoldt *et al.*, 2010; Wang *et al.*, 2016). Establishing an evolutionary timeframe for the initial domestication process is similarly problematic, though estimates based on archaeological records and mitochondrial DNA indicate 16 000 and 12 000 years ago, respectively (Clutton-Brock, Chapter 2; Larson *et al.*, 2012). The taxonomic status of the dog remains contentious in some quarters, with a minority calling for the dog to be listed as a separate species, *Canis familiaris*, while others consider it a subspecies of the gray wolf (i.e. *Canis lupus familiaris*).

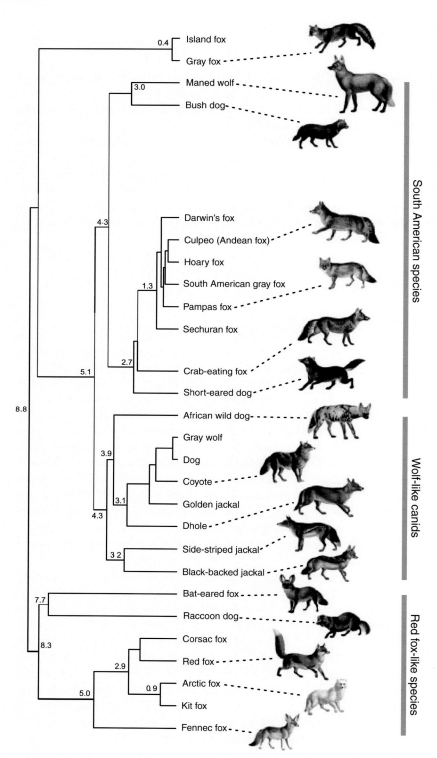

Figure 3.1 *Canidae* phylogeny with estimated dates of divergence in millions of years indicated on the branches. (Adapted by permission from John Wiley & Sons: *Journal of Evolutionary Biology* (Perini, F. A. *et al*., The evolution of South American endemic canids, etc.), copyright 2009.) (A black and white version of this figure will appear in some formats. For the color version, please refer to the plate section.)

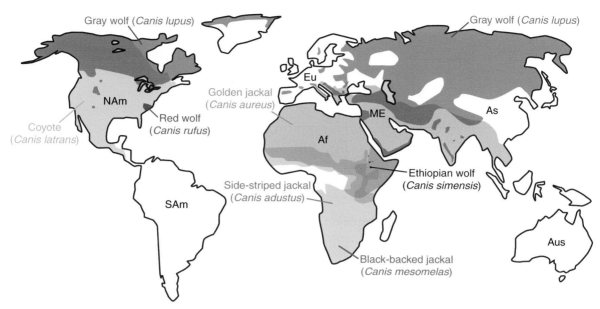

Figure 3.2 Species of *Canis* from the wolf-like clade and their current geographic distribution (IUCN, 2012). Distributions may overlap. Wolves were historically widespread across the Old and New Worlds, with current fragmentation a result of humans. Abbreviations: Af, Africa; As, Asia; Aus, Australia; Eu, Europe; ME, Middle East; NAm, North America; SAm, South America. (A black and white version of this figure will appear in some formats. For the color version, please refer to the plate section.)

3.3   The human handprint: Canine domestication

Just what is meant by domestication? *Domestic* is a colloquial term applied to many animals habitually used by humans or habituated to human places. Domestication, in contrast, is a biological process that leads to the development of unique human–animal relationships that vary greatly both in quality and intensity. To borrow a concept from ecology, we could describe the relationship that many people today believe they have with their dogs as a *mutualistic* one – i.e. one in which both parties benefit from the association. But we can also recognize dog–human relationships that might be better described as *commensal* – i.e. cases in which one member (the dog) benefits from the association while the other is more or less unaffected. Both represent examples of domestication but clearly to different degrees.

Domestication is fundamentally different from *taming*, which is the habituation of an individual animal to human presence. Domestication alters the genetic (and morphological) characteristics of a breeding population and, unlike taming, these changes are heritable (Coppinger *et al.*, 2009). The domestication of wolves was an evolutionary process that favored any heritable predisposition to tameness in a restricted population of ancestral wolves when in close proximity to human populations (see Box 3.1). Subsequently, the process of domestication mandates a degree of genetic isolation from the parent species in order to segregate alleles controlling the suite of behaviors and morphology encompassing the "domestication syndrome" (see below).

For our purposes here, domestic dogs are wolves that have undergone a process of selection, crucially relating to behavior and cognition, but also including morphology and metabolism, which has resulted in heritable genetic changes in allele frequencies. There continues to be much debate and speculation as to how this selection process occurred but, either way, it is likely to have happened in a series of stages (Diamond, 2005; Driscoll *et al.*, 2009; Lord *et al.*, Chapter 4; Vigne, 2011; Zeder, 2012):

1. Selective affiliation of wolves with humans predisposed to tolerance and lower levels of aggression and fear in proximity to humans; a process shaped by a combination of natural selection and human acceptance.
2. Fitness advantages accrue to those wolves that reproduce successfully in, or in close proximity to, the human environment, probably reinforced by a degree of human provisioning (transition from natural to unconscious artificial selection).
3. Early selection for "utility" leading to the initial emergence of primitive dogs by an unconscious process of artificial selection.
4. Prehistoric type formation based on landraces or specific utilities (e.g. coursing, baying, short legs, etc.) (a transition from unconscious to deliberate artificial selection).
5. Modern era of genetic isolation and rapid radiation of highly specialized breeds, often based on physical conformation, rather than strict utility (methodical artificial selection).

Not all domestic dogs have been subjected to all five of these stages. Some are best described as *semi-domestic* in the sense that they have not been subjected to conscious selective breeding but have, due to long association with humans and their environment, and long reproductive isolation from their wolf ancestors, plainly become domestic animals (that is, they are clearly part of a human landscape and are derived from it). Examples of such semi-domestic dogs include the dingo and New Guinea singing dog, neither of which has been subjected to the kind of conscious selective breeding associated with the modern radiation (stages 4–5) but which have experienced the early stages of domestication (stages 1–3).

Box 3.1 Natural versus artificial selection

Charles Darwin discussed artificial selection as an analogue of evolution by natural selection (Darwin, 1868), but both selection processes require that the desired traits are heritable with some more advantageous than others. Natural selection is the environmentally driven mechanistic process that works to preserve only the adaptive variants; artificial selection works in a similar way, but with the key difference that humans determine which traits are to be passed on to the next generation of pups (Diamond, 2005; Driscoll *et al.*, 2009). Human-imposed selective breeding of only a subset of dogs shapes the canine population, shifting the frequencies of morphological and behavioral traits. Therefore, the domestication of a species is an evolutionary process accomplished through artificial selection.

The dingo has been isolated in Australia for approximately 5000 years (Larson *et al.*, 2012; Savolainen *et al.*, 2004). During this time, dingoes have evolved primarily through natural selection post-domestication, since they have never been subjected to the highly managed breeding found among modern purebred dogs. As a result, the dingo is still readily socialized or habituated to human proximity and has, historically, participated in mutually beneficial hunting parties with Australian Aborigines, but it is also capable of living altogether independent of humans in self-sustaining

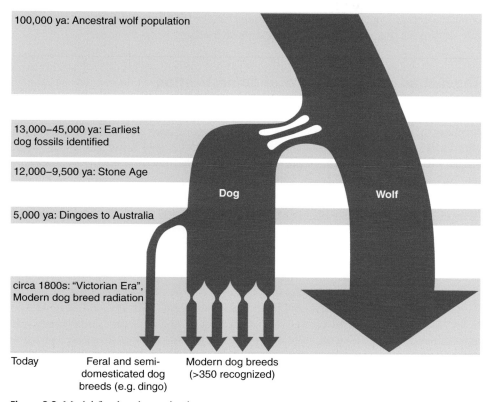

100,000 ya: Ancestral wolf population

13,000–45,000 ya: Earliest dog fossils identified

12,000–9,500 ya: Stone Age

Dog   Wolf

5,000 ya: Dingoes to Australia

circa 1800s: "Victorian Era", Modern dog breed radiation

Today   Feral and semi-domesticated dog breeds (e.g. dingo)   Modern dog breeds (>350 recognized)

Figure 3.3 Model for dog domestication.

populations. Dingoes have also experienced some admixture with modern domestic dogs following the arrival of European colonists, leaving a genetic fingerprint that has influenced the interpretation of their evolutionary history (Figure 3.3) (Larson *et al.*, 2012; Savolainen *et al.*, 2004).

Likewise, the African village dogs recently described by Boyko *et al.* (2010) are a cryptic population of dogs living in association with humans that have not experienced the artificial selection associated with modern breed formation. The term "cryptic" here refers to populations that are morphologically indistinguishable from the surrounding population but which are still genetically distinct, indicating that some degree of genetic isolation is being enforced either ecologically or geographically. As a result of the absence of conscious artificial selection on these semi-domestic populations, some hypothesize that such dogs harbor a closer representation of the early, domestic dog genome, though this remains controversial.

Regardless of where wolf domestication occurred, the inter-specific bond between early dogs and humans was probably loose enough to permit dogs to form transitory associations with local gray wolves (Anderson *et al.*, 2009; Randi, 2008; Vilà and Wayne, 1999; Vilà *et al.*, 2005). This fraternization allowed these dogs to hybridize with wolves, enriching the dog genome during early phases of domestication, and thereby providing new genetic and phenotypic variants. A genome-wide genetic study has confirmed these secondary contacts with local wolf populations, providing new sources of genetic diversity to the genomes of early dogs (vonHoldt *et al.*, 2010). Over succeeding generations, dogs acquired important status in human society, and often received benefits from being part of the human "pack," likely in the form of protection, access to resources, and companionship. Dogs were quickly integrated into human culture, while breeding practices gradually shaped the dog's function and form with each successive generation.

3.4   The human cultural context of domestication

Domesticated dogs come from one or more lineages of gray wolves that have been modified by chronic exposure to humans and human environments. A highly social species, the wolf relies upon cooperative living and it is therefore easy to imagine that the first proto-dogs were born to wolves that had a propensity to associate with or tolerate some degree of proximity to human groups. As these tolerant wolves reproduced, their pups inherited the genes for their parents' temperament and these proto-dogs established the first population of early dogs (see Box 3.2). The stories of these first dogs can be deciphered from the fossil record and from the cultural context of human burial sites. It seems that, rather than being domesticated in direct association with Near Eastern agriculture roughly 10 000 years ago, as were other species (e.g. cattle, goats, pigs, and sheep), the archeological record suggests that dogs may have appeared in an earlier hunter-gatherer past, and in a region including Europe and eastern Siberia (Driscoll *et al.*, 2009; Crockford & Kuzmin, 2012; Germonpré *et al.*, 2009; Ovodov *et al.*, 2011; Sablin & Khlopachev, 2002; Zeder, 2008) (Figure 3.3). However, in the Epipaleolithic (late Stone Age, ~ 15 kya), humans shifted towards a sedentary and eventually agrarian-based society (Dayan, 1999; Morey, 1994). In these early civilizations humans were accompanied by their dogs, presumably fulfilling various practical roles in local villages and fields, perhaps serving as companions, and probably traded or bartered along trade routes (Sundqvist *et al.*, 2006).

Dating these early dog populations can be challenging. Although dates may be derived from genetic data by invoking a "molecular clock," these analyses often result in large margins of error. For this reason, archaeologists tend to rely on carbon dating of fossil remains. The challenge then is in the differentiation of dog fossils from those of other closely related canine species (see Clutton-Brock, Chapter 2).

Box 3.2 The Russian farm-fox experiment

In one of the most interesting experiments of the last century, silver foxes (*Vulpes vulpes*) have undergone experimental domestication at a Russian breeding center in Siberia (Belyaev, 1969; Trut, 1999; Trut *et al.*, 2009). This "farm-fox experiment" provides some important clues as to how domestication might have proceeded, and serves as a remarkable resource for understanding how selective breeding can shape phenotypes.

The experiment was initiated in the 1950s by the scientist Dmitry Belyaev at the Russian Academy of Sciences's Institute of Cytology and Genetics (Belyaev, 1969; Spady and Ostrander, 2008; Statham *et al.*, 2011; Trut, 1999; Trut *et al.*, 2009). The goal was to selectively breed the foxes to become tamer. However, as the tame lineage of foxes were producing tamer kits, the researchers noticed physical changes in the foxes' appearance: size variation increased; their coats became more diverse in coloration and fur structure (e.g. appearance of wirehair and curly); ears flopped over; tails became shortened and curly, and females became polyestrous, allowing for multiple litters per year (Trut, 1999). Many if not all of these traits have been noted in other domesticated species (including cattle, goats, pigs and sheep) and are now referred to as the "domestication syndrome" (Driscoll *et al.*, 2009; Trut, 1999; Trut *et al.*, 2009) (Table 3.1). Surprisingly, within 10 generations of selectively breeding the foxes for tame behavior, they began to closely resemble domesticated dogs in both physical and behavioral phenotypes (Figure 3.4) (Hare *et al.*, 2005; Kukekova *et al.*, 2010; Spady and Ostrander, 2008; Statham *et al.*, 2011).

Table 3.1 The domestication syndrome – a suite of physical traits common to domesticated species (adapted from Driscoll *et al.*, 2009; Dobney and Larson, 2006; Hare *et al.*, 2005; Kukekova *et al.*, 2010; Spady and Ostrander, 2008; Trut, 1999; Trut *et al.*, 2009).

Domesticated species	Dwarf/giant size variety	Piebald spotting	White spotting	Wavy or curly hair	Curly or rolled tails	Shortened tails	Floppy ears	Change in reproduction
Cat	•	•				•	•	•
Cow	•	•	•				•	•
Dog	•	•	•	•	•	•	•	•
Donkey	•	•		•				•
Goat	•	•	•	•			•	•
Guinea pig	•	•		•				•
Horse	•	•	•	•			•	•
Mouse	•	•		•				•
Pig	•	•	•	•	•		•	•
Rabbit	•	•	•				•	•
Sheep	•	•	•	•		•	•	•

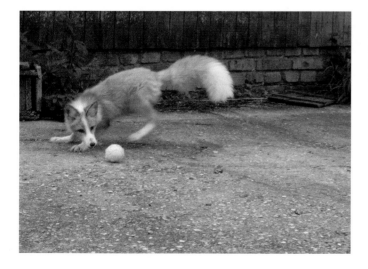

Figure 3.4 Tame-bred foxes have many physical and behavioral traits that are dog-like. This tame adult fox is playing with a ball. Photograph courtesy of Anna Kukekova (see Spady and Ostrander, 2007).

3.5   The canine genetic toolkit

In 2003, the entire nuclear DNA sequence from a Standard Poodle was made publicly available. In 2005 the genome of a different dog, a Boxer, was published (Kirkness *et al.*, 2003; Lindblad-Toh *et al.*, 2005). From these DNA sequences researchers identified specific sites where nucleotides varied within and between individuals. So far, over 2.5 million of these variants, referred to as single nucleotide polymorphisms or "SNPs," have been catalogued in the dog genome (Kirkness *et al.*, 2003; Lindblad-Toh *et al.*, 2005).

As researchers began exploring the genetics of domesticated animals, a few basic statistical methods were standardized in order to unravel the genetic history of species. Many researchers relied upon DNA sequence data and theories from evolutionary genetics to infer relationships or *phylogenies*. For example, if the goal is to infer which population is the wild ancestor of a domesticate, then the phylogenetic tree would provide a type of "family tree" in which the wild and domesticated groups are expected to be more closely related then either is to more distantly related species. This method has been applied towards understanding evolutionary relationships among wild and domesticated species, including the dog (Dobney & Larson, 2006; Driscoll *et al.*, 2007; Frantz *et al.*, 2016; Parker *et al.*, 2004; Savolainen *et al.*, 2002; Shannon *et al.*, 2015; Vilà *et al.*, 1997, 2005; vonHoldt *et al.*, 2010; Wang *et al.*, 2016; Zeder *et al.*, 2006).

3.6   Molecular evidence of the ancestral wolf populations

Moving a step beyond the analysis of archaeological remains from burial sites and dating of fossils through radioactive decay methods, advancing technologies allow for detailed genetic analyses of individuals from distinct geographic origins and evolutionary time periods. In addition to geography and timing, we can also begin to assess the number of wolves involved in the early stages of domestication (i.e. the number of founders), how many separate domestication events likely occurred, and the genetic changes that can be linked to the physical changes wolves experienced in the process of domestication.

A number of recent molecular studies have sought to determine which geographic population(s) of wolves is genetically closest to modern-day domestic dogs; doing so supplies strong inferential evidence for the geographic and cultural origin of dogs. Several theoretical approaches have been employed. One early study was based on analyzing matrilineal mitochondrial DNA from a handful of Eurasian wolves and hundreds of dogs representing various geographic regions (Africa, America, Europe, Asia, Siberia, and India) as well as ancestries (e.g. purebred, semi-domestic dogs, mixed breed, stray, mongrels) (Savolainen *et al.*, 2002). By inferring phylogenetic relationships and assessing genetic diversity, this and subsequent studies have concluded that all dogs share a common ancestry with wolves from East Asia, specifically in the region south of the Yangtze River (Pang *et al.*, 2009; Savolainen *et al.*, 2002; Wang *et al.*, 2016). The study relied upon measures of genetic diversity as an indication of the geographic center of domestication. Based on the assumption that as individuals disperse from a large population they take with them only a subset of the original genetic diversity, the source population is presumed to be more diverse than that found in the colonizing offshoots (Barrett & Schluter, 2008; Biswas & Akey, 2006; Innan & Kim, 2004).

An alternative approach has been to survey the genetic variation and genomic structure of primitive and semi-domestic dogs, such as the dingo, New Guinea singing dog, and the African village dog. The genomes of these dogs are often considered to represent surviving versions of "ancestral" dog genomes, some of which exist in isolation from wild canids (e.g. dingoes and New Guinea singing dogs) while others may survive as endogamous, cryptically differentiated populations that do not currently interbreed with recently derived dog breeds, though they may have experienced inter-breeding in the past (Boyko *et al.*, 2009). Additionally, village dogs thrive as free-roaming commensals within local human communities and have not been subjected to strong selective breeding. Therefore, a genetic survey of these unique dogs may provide insight into a putatively "ancestral" dog genome. However, care needs to be taken to properly distinguish true village dogs (which may have existed for millennia) from introduced free-roaming dogs of recent European derivation, since results will likely be misinterpreted if these dogs are mistakenly included.

The collection and analysis of genome-wide single nucleotide polymorphism (SNP) data across village and semi-domestic dogs has revealed a surprising result. When the genetic diversity was assessed in African village and domesticated dogs from around the globe, researchers found comparable levels of diversity to that of East Asian dogs from previous studies, calling into question the view that dogs originated in East Asia (Boyko *et al.*, 2009; Shannon *et al.*, 2015). A subsequent study that genetically surveyed 85 dog breeds determined that wolves from the Middle East contributed the most variation to the genome of the domestic dog, with other dog-specific genetic variants only found in this wolf population (Gray *et al.*, 2010; Parker *et al.*, 2009; vonHoldt *et al.*, 2010). The apparent association with this geographic region is not surprising since it tends to corroborate earlier theories that most domesticated animals have at least one point of origin in the Fertile Crescent (Dayan, 1999; Driscoll *et al.*, 2009; Zeder, 2008; Zeder *et al.*, 2006) (see Box 3.3).

Recently, Freedman *et al.* (2014) utilized whole genome sequencing to survey representative individuals from the three putative centers of wolf domestication – China, the Near East, and Europe – in addition to genome sequences from the supposedly ancient, semi-domestic dog breeds, the Basenji and dingo. They inferred that numerous bottlenecks through dog domestication history have occurred, as well as instances of post-divergence gene flow, with the initial process of domestication estimated to have started around 11 000–16 000 years ago, predating the agricultural revolution. Moreover, the study found that modern wolves form a monophyletic sister clade to domestic dogs, implying that the direct ancestor of dogs is extinct, impossibly confounding any attempt at resolving the geographic origin of dogs when examining only extant lineages. This result was recently corroborated by an independent study of a fossil dog specimen from a cave in the Altai Mountains of Siberia (Druzhkova *et al.*, 2013). This study analyzed the mtDNA from a 33 000-year-old Pleistocene fossil dog and identified that it showed an affinity with modern dogs and prehistoric wolves from North America. Due to the lack of phylogenetic proximity with any contemporary wolf population, it is proposed that the population of wolves directly ancestral to modern day dogs is indeed extinct. Further support for a European origin of domestic dogs comes from Thalmann *et al.*'s (2013) recent sequencing of mitochondrial genomes from ancient and modern canids. Bayesian phylogenetic and dating analyses identified that all modern dogs are more closely related to ancient European canids, with the onset of dog domestication occurring between 18 800 and 32 100 years ago. This domestication event, they propose, coincides with the evolutionary time when humans preyed upon megafauna as hunter-gatherers. In fact, their findings suggest that the conditions for domestication are not unique. Many early lineages of proto-dogs were likely initiated but with many failing to survive to modern day, thereby populating the fossil record with aborted episodes of domestication.

Most recently, genomic analyses have confirmed deep evolutionary divergence between two geographically disparate wolf populations (Fan *et al.*, 2016; Frantz *et al.*, 2016). Frantz and colleagues (2016) suggest this may represent two independent dog domestication events. They suggest that eastern dogs dispersed westward alongside their human counterparts between 6400 and 14 000 years ago. The arrival of these eastern dogs replaced the indigenous Paleolithic dog population in western Europe. This potential genetic replacement through admixture presents challenges for inferring the history of dog domestication.

Box 3.3 New World origins?

In the Americas, fossils reliably identified as dog are significantly younger (ca. 9000–10 000 ya) than those in the Old World (15 000–33 000 ya) although dogs were common in the New World at the time of European colonization (Clutton-Brock, Chapter 2; Larson *et al.*, 2012; Leonard *et al.*, 2002). An obvious question is whether these New World dogs represented a separate lineage of domesticated dogs (i.e. domesticated in the Americas from American wolves) or if they accompanied early humans in crossing the Bering land bridge, presumably between 20 000 and 11 000 ya. To answer this question, DNA sequence of pre-Columbian dog fossils from both the Old and New Worlds were analyzed and compared to modern day dogs and gray wolves. Phylogenetic analyses revealed that fossil New World dogs were more closely related to the European-derived modern dog breeds and thus did not represent a unique and separate domestication (Goebel *et al.*, 2008; Leonard *et al.*, 2002; Waters *et al.*, 2007).

3.7 Breeds

The origin and relationships among domesticated dog breeds, whose histories are often anecdotal or only partially documented, has been a persistent interest of genetic research long before the release of the dog genome sequence. Early natural historians considered each dog breed to be derived from a local canid population, be it wolf, coyote, jackal, or fox (Darwin, 1868). In Europe, dog breeds have existed since at least the 1300s (certainly even earlier accounts of distinct varieties have been described in classical Greek literature), mostly for hunting; a different dog breed was employed for each different quarry: badger hounds, wolfhounds, otter hounds, and deer hounds, for example. Note, however, that this is not the first formation of dog varieties; sighthound-type coursing dogs and mastiff-type hunting dogs represent two breed types of antiquity (Clutton-Brock, 1981 and Chapter 2). There was, at that time, no evidence of strong line breeding: dogs being bred to task in the fashion of a true working dog such that any dog with desirable qualities, regardless of parentage, was introduced into the line. By the mid 1800s, however, dog breeding was driven primarily by a focus on form rather than function.

The Victorian view of what a breed should be changed to emphasize conformation and pedigree, and the weight given to actual functionality was often greatly lessened. This is where modern dog breeding has its roots. Breed organizations, such as the American Kennel Club (AKC), established strict regulations to control breeding practices in order to achieve and preserve specific desired aesthetics or function (Figure 3.3), and virtually mandated the practice of line-breeding (Ritvo, 1989). As universal breeding standards were applied, the number of dogs allowed to reproduce quickly decreased and only show champions of a breed that possessed an outstanding award-winning record became popular sires. With the same champion being used many times in a pedigree, inbreeding was frequently commonplace. A major consequence of this strong line-breeding practice is an increased occurrence of medical conditions and breed-specific diseases (see Hubrecht *et al.*, Chapter 14). Because breeders could select mutations with obvious phenotypes (e.g. dwarfism, see below) to include in their lineage, and because fanciers tend to select for the extremes of a phenotype, such breeding practices did allow for the rapid development of new sizes, shapes, colors, and behavioral features. As a result, there are currently about 175 distinct breeds recognized by the AKC, while over 350 breeds have worldwide recognition (Lindblad-Toh *et al.*, 2005; Parker *et al.*, 2004; Spady & Ostrander, 2008; Young & Bannasch, 2006).

In an early genetic study designed to identify individual breed histories, researchers surveyed the dog genome and identified repetitive DNA elements called *microsatellites*. Based on a survey of 96 microsatellites in over 400 dogs representing 85 breeds, genetic relatedness-based measurements were used to cluster individual breeds into larger breed "groups" related in heritage, such as mastiff-related breeds, breeds convergent on the herding behavioral trait, and Nordic breeds, for example (Parker *et al.*, 2004). These breed groups often represented major "functional categories" and have been confirmed by a more recent study (Parker, 2012; vonHoldt *et al.*, 2010) (Figure 3.5). However, inferences based on relatedness present a statistical challenge as the domesticated and wild groups can interbreed and produce viable offspring. Such hybridization events between distinct lineages increase the levels of gene-sharing and genetic diversity, which will ultimately bias evolutionary interpretations.

Any analysis of dog breeds is complicated by the fact that breed histories are characterized by periods of admixture between lines, followed by strict line breeding. Any occurrence of mixing across breeds will inflate genetic diversity and skew the resulting inferences of ancestral relationships (AKC, 2006; Parker *et al.*, 2004, 2010; Parker & Ostrander, 2005; Sutter & Ostrander, 2004). Therefore, scientists must rely upon additional analytical methods if they are to avoid making incorrect inferences based solely on the measurement of genetic similarity and diversity.

Studies of morphological changes as documented from archaeological and burial sites have described variations in skeletal sizes, proportions, and dentition, but assessing the genetic changes in similar specimens will provide information about the molecular changes associated with artificial selection under domestication (see Box 3.2).

3.8   Genetic studies: the evolution of dog morphology

Domesticated dogs display a breadth of phenotypic variability not observed in gray wolves, or indeed in any other domesticated animal (Stockard, 1941). Conversely, significant traits exist in wolves that are lacking in their domestic derivatives. Female wolves, for example, experience one estrous cycle per year, with the pups reared in a pack consisting of relatives (e.g. siblings, cousins) in addition to unrelated adults that forego reproduction and provide regurgitated food for the pups (vonHoldt *et al.*, 2008). Upon maturation, pups disperse out of their natal pack in an attempt to find a mate and potentially establish their own pack. Dogs, on the other hand, have had many of their natural history traits altered through the domestication process in a way that distinguishes them from their wild relatives (Spady & Ostrander, 2008; Statham *et al.*, 2011; Trut, 1999; Trut *et al.*, 2009) (see Box 3.2). Dogs reach sexual maturity more quickly than wolves (<1 versus 2 years, respectively), and will continue to bark throughout their lives, a behavioral trait that is rare in adult wolves (Clutton-Brock, 1981; Morey, 1994). Also, critical to dogs' survival among humans is the reduction

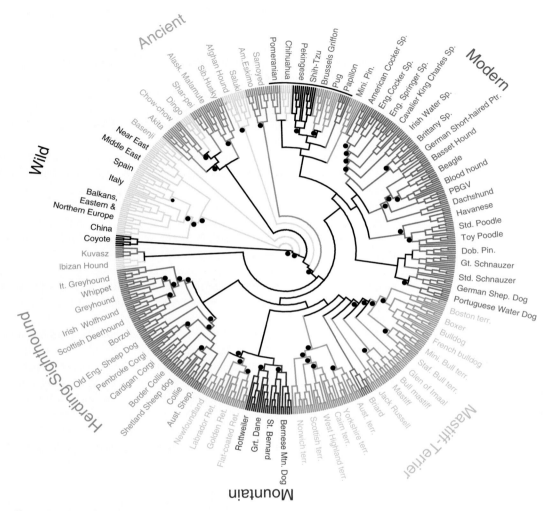

Figure 3.5 Breed phylogeny, where the colors of branches indicate a "functional" breed group: yellow, ancient breeds; brown, spitz breeds; black, toy breeds; blue, mastiff-like breeds; red; modern breeds; gray, wild canids; green, herding-sighthounds; purple, mountain breeds. Black bar indicates Toy breeds. Ancient breeds were as defined in vonHoldt *et al.* (2010) and Parker (2012). Dots on internal branches indicate >95% confidence. (Adapted from vonHoldt *et al.*, 2010; Parker, 2012.) (A black and white version of this figure will appear in some formats. For the color version, please refer to the plate section.)

of hunting impulses (at least in most breeds) that make it possible for dogs and domestic livestock to live together peacefully.

With the development of genome resources in the past decade, many researchers have conducted genome-wide analyses concomitantly and uncovered a large number of shared genomic regions across various dog breeds that are associated with typical "dog-specific" phenotypes; that is, the collection of traits that make a dog (Akey *et al.*, 2010; Boyko *et al.*, 2010; Chase *et al.*, 2009; Freedman *et al.*, 2016; Jones *et al.*, 2008). Surprisingly, it turns out that seemingly complex traits in dogs (e.g. body dimensions, dentition, skeletal proportions) are due to a small handful of genes that explain each trait, unlike the hundreds of genes required for the expression of similar traits in humans and non-domesticated animals (Flint & Mackay, 2009; Visscher, 2008; Voight *et al.*, 2006; Wellcome Trust Case Consortium, 2007). Additional studies have focused on very specific traits that are shared among a handful of dog breeds. Here, we focus on three examples of trait-specific mapping efforts and their evolutionary implications (see Box 3.4).

Box 3.4 Gene mapping

Gene mapping is a method in which scientists search for particular gene variants that are statistically associated with a phenotype. In the case of diseases, such variants may serve as therapeutic targets for treatment. Mapping a gene variant in humans is a complex statistical challenge, often requiring genetic samples from thousands of individuals. The method relies upon a set of genetic markers located across the genome, and then testing these markers statistically for a non-random association with a phenotype of interest, such as a disease or physical trait, across individuals with the trait (case) and those lacking it (controls) (see also van den Berg, Chapter 5). Despite the high degree of line breeding (and lack of genetic diversity) in the dog genome, genetic variants will exist as a result of random mutations, a subset of which are associated with specific phenotypes (e.g. disease, curly tail, pigmentation patterns). For example, consider a dog breed that segregates two phenotypes (e.g. a bull terrier of both the piebald and solid pigmented variety; see Barsh, 2007) (Figure 3.6). After locating and sampling a number of solid and piebald bull terriers, we would scan each of the 38 canine chromosomes in search for a region that is shared among all piebald bull terriers but lacking in the solid pigmented dogs. We could further improve our chances of locating this genomic region if we expand our search to other breeds that segregate the piebald phenotype (Figure 3.6).

3.8.1   Domestic trait 1: How to make a toy

The initial stages of dog domestication resulted in a dog that was proportionally reduced in size, a distinct phenotype along the spectrum of *dwarfism*, or proportional reduction in size. Dwarfed dog breeds are easily recognizable, and are collectively referred to as "Toy" breeds by the AKC based on the sharing of one distinguishing feature: miniature body size. The genetics behind body size variation was originally investigated in the Portuguese water dog, as this breed was recently established with detailed pedigree records and is sexually dimorphic (the female is smaller in size than the male) (Chase *et al.*, 2002, 2005, 2009). An initial genetic survey identified a large region (15 million bases or nucleotides long) on chromosome 15 containing the insulin-like growth factor 1 gene (*IGF1*) that was significantly associated with canine body size (Chase *et al.*, 2005). The function of this gene is well described in humans as a growth factor that regulates postnatal skeletal growth (Baker *et al.*, 1993; Laron, 2001; Yakar *et al.*, 2002).

To further understand how this gene region is associated with small body size, a follow-up fine-mapping analysis focused on the region in detail in search of a genetic change that produces the trait of interest (body size) (Sutter *et al.*, 2007). The mapping study categorized dogs as giant (>30 kg) and toy (<9 kg) breeds based on breed standards and searched for a fragment of DNA

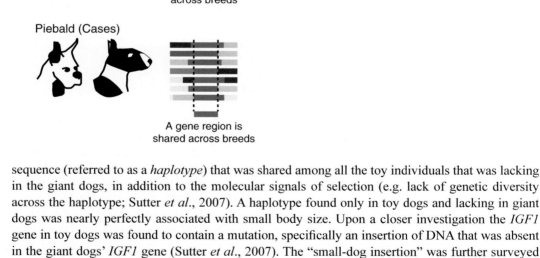

Piebald Boxer

Chromosome 20

Boxer 1
Boxer 2
⋮
Boxer 7

Shared gene region

Non-piebald Boxer

No gene region shared

Piebald Bullterrier

Shared gene region

Non-piebald Bullterrier

No gene region shared

Solid (Controls)

No gene region is shared
across breeds

Piebald (Cases)

A gene region is
shared across breeds

Figure 3.6 Conceptual framework of gene mapping through association. Here, the trait being mapped is piebald coloration across two breeds, the boxer and the bull terrier. Each colored segment is considered a different allele or variant on the chromosome. (Adapted by permission from Macmillan Publishers Ltd: *Nature Genetics* (Barsh, G.S., How the dog got its spots), copyright 2007.) (A black and white version of this figure will appear in some formats. For the color version, please refer to the plate section.)

sequence (referred to as a *haplotype*) that was shared among all the toy individuals that was lacking in the giant dogs, in addition to the molecular signals of selection (e.g. lack of genetic diversity across the haplotype; Sutter *et al.*, 2007). A haplotype found only in toy dogs and lacking in giant dogs was nearly perfectly associated with small body size. Upon a closer investigation the *IGF1* gene in toy dogs was found to contain a mutation, specifically an insertion of DNA that was absent in the giant dogs' *IGF1* gene (Sutter *et al.*, 2007). The "small-dog insertion" was further surveyed across global wolf populations, in order to better understand its evolutionary history. The insertion was found only among toy dogs, and was absent from the wolf genome, confirming that this mutation occured post-domestication and is a toy dog-specific genetic variant (Gray *et al.*, 2010). Interestingly, when looking at the larger genomic region containing the *IGF1* gene, all domesticated dogs have closer kinship with Middle Eastern wolves than other wolf populations, corroborating the earlier findings of genomic contribution (Gray *et al.*, 2010; vonHoldt *et al.*, 2010).

Only a handful of genes, when altered, result in the miniaturized version of a dog. A breeder can take advantage of this genetic variant with large phenotypic effect by crossing the miniature dog with other non-miniature dogs in order to shop around this subset of size-altering genes. This strict nature of controlled dog breeding allows for goal-directed changes in phenotypes, as is the case for the miniature breeds found today (Sutter *et al.*, 2007).

3.8.2   Domestic trait 2: How to make shortened limbs

Just as in the case of miniature-sized dogs, many short-legged breeds were created for various functional purposes, such as burrow hunting, traversing through thick brush, and finding scents low to the ground. Many genes (specifically *growth factors*) have been described that help regulate overall body size and skeletal proportions in humans (Giustina *et al.*, 2008; Lefebvre & Bhattaram, 2010; Su *et al.*, 2008). However, only recently was the genetic basis of canine leg length uncovered from a genetic screen of short-legged and regularly sized dogs. All dogs with the short-legged phenotype carried a single extra copy of the fibroblast growth factor 4 (*FGF4*) gene, whose effects halted the elongation of the long bones in limbs during embryonic development (Parker *et al.*, 2009). This second full-length identical copy of *FGF4* has a unique origin as a retrogene copy established through a gene duplication event called *retrotransposition*.

Specific types of DNA elements (a subset called *retrotransposons*) can undergo self-replication, with the new copy inserting into a new location in the genome (Cordaux & Batzer, 2009; Kazazian, 2004; McClintock, 1956). The replication process of retrotransposons can be at times error-prone, sometimes incorporating with their new copy bits of other DNA sequences. In the case of short-legged dogs, the retrotransposon copy contained the entire protein-coding sequence of the *FGF4* gene and, upon inserting this copy over 30 million nucleotides away, was a new identical copy of the gene but under new regulatory controls. Short-legged breeds then not only carry the original parental gene of the parental *FGF4* gene, but also an additional copy. Researchers also found that this new gene copy functioned independently, with the over-expression of this new copy linked to the termination of long-bone growth prematurely in development, producing short legs (Parker *et al.*, 2009).

The part of the chromosome that contains the *FGF4* retrogene copy was additionally surveyed in wolves from across the globe in order to help infer when this retrogene was likely to have first inserted and the first short-legged dog appeared. Using the haplotype around the retrogene, the major finding is that all short-legged breeds, no matter where they originated geographically, share this same retrogene. Therefore, all short-legged dogs share a common ancestor with one origination event of this retrogene duplication and insertion, which has been passed around to various dog lineages by deliberate cross-breeding.

3.8.3   Domestic trait 3: How to change hair type and structure

From smooth, long fur to coarse furnished (eyebrow and mustache growth) wirehair, dogs exhibit a breadth of fur structure and type not found in their wild counterparts (Cadieu *et al.*, 2009). When a genetic screen was conducted across 108 AKC-recognized breeds, seven hair phenotypes were found to segregate with variants of three genes: fibroblast growth factor 5 (*FGF5*; nucleotide mutation), R-spondin-2 (*RSPO2*; 167 nucleotide insertion), and a keratin (*KRT71*; nucleotide mutation) (Cadieu *et al.*, 2009). Each permutation of the genetic variants accounted for the vast majority of canine coat texture/patterning. Regarding the evolutionary timing of these fur phenotypes, only one is considered ancestral (short hair lacking curl, wirehair and furnishings), whereas the other six phenotypes are *derived*, and have a more recent evolutionary history. The derived variants were surveyed in the wolf genome and found to be lacking, further reinforcing the view that the canine ancestral fur phenotype is short, straight, smooth and without furnishings (Cadieu *et al.*, 2009).

As with each of the domestic traits discussed, these phenotypes are exclusive to dogs compared to their wild relatives and they likely arose only once (due to the genetic relationships among breeds and the concordance of phenotype with genotype), with humans dispersing those mutations within and across breed lineages through their selective breeding practices. These efforts were the primary driving forces by which the appearance of dog diversity was created despite a paucity of genetic diversity found in their genomes.

3.9   Conclusions

The origin of the domestic dog is a complex story, including many unresolved details on location and timing. The aspects most clearly resolved are the genetic changes linked to the evolving canine phenotype: the traits that are unique to domestic dogs. Many features of the dog phenotype can now be viewed as an array of genetic variants, each influencing the size, shape and function of the animal. As our genetic sequencing technologies decrease in costs, we are better able to search multiple dimensions of the genome for links to what makes a dog a dog. This is an exciting time for canine geneticists who embark on the journey to understand the differences between the dog and wolf genomes, and identify variants linked to behavior and disease, many of which have human analogs.

References

AKC (American Kennel Club) (2006). *The Complete Dog Book*, 20th edition. New York, NY: Ballantine Books.

Anderson, T. M., vonHoldt, B. M., Candille, S. I. *et al.* (2009). Molecular and evolutionary history of melanism in North American gray wolves. *Science*, 323: 1339–43.

Akey, J. M., Ruhe, A. L., Akey, D. T. *et al.* (2010). Tracking footprints of artificial selection in the dog genome. *Proceedings of the National Academy of Sciences USA*, 107: 1160–5.

Baker, J., Liu, J. P., Robertson, E. J. & Efstratiadis, A. (1993). Role of insulin-like growth factors in embryonic and postnatal growth. *Cell*, 75: 73–82.

Barrett, R. D. H. & Schluter, D. (2008). Adaptation from standing genetic variation. *Trends in Ecology & Evolution*, 23: 38–44.

Barsh, G. S. (2007). How the dog got its spots. *Nature Genetics*, 39: 1304–6.

Belyaev, D. K. (1969). Domestication of animals. *Science*, 5: 47–52.

Biswas, S. & Akey, J. M. (2006). Genomic insights into positive selection. *Trends in Genetics*, 22: 437–46.

Boyko, A. R. (2011). The domestic dog: man's best friend in the genomic era. *Genome Biology*, 12: 216.

Boyko, A. R., Boyko, R. H., Boyko, C. M. *et al.* (2009). Complex population structure in African village dogs and its implications for inferring dog domestication history. *Proceedings of the National Academy of Sciences USA*, 106: 13903–8.

Boyko, A. R., Quignon, P., Li, L. *et al.* (2010). A simple genetic architecture underlies morphological variation in dogs. *PLoS Biology*, 8: e1000451.

Cadieu, E., Neff, M., Quignon, P. *et al.* (2009). Coat variation in the domestic dog is governed by variants in three genes. *Science*, 326: 150–3.

Chase, K., Carrier, D. R., Adler, F. R. *et al.* (2002). Genetic basis for systems of skeletal quantitative traits: principal component analysis of the canid skeleton. *Proceedings of the National Academy of Sciences USA*, 99: 9930–5.

Chase, K., Carrier, D. R., Adler, F. R., Ostrander, E. A. & Lark, K. G. (2005). Interaction between the X chromosome and an autosome regulates size sexual dimorphism in Portuguese Water Dogs. *Genome Research*, 15: 1820–4.

Chase, K., Jones, P., Martin, A., Ostrander, E. A. & Lark, K. G. (2009). Genetic mapping of fixed phenotypes: disease frequency as a breed characteristic. *Journal of Heredity*, 100: S37–41.

Clutton-Brock, J. (1981). *Domesticated Animals from Early Times*. Cambridge: Cambridge University Press.

Coppinger, R., Spector, L. & Miller, L. (2009). What, if anything, is a wolf? In *The World of Wolves: New Perspectives on Ecology, Behaviour and Management*, eds. M. Musiani, L. Boitani and P. Paquet. Calgary, Alberta: The University of Calgary Press, pp. 51–65.

Cordaux, R. & Batzer, M. A. (2009). The impact of retrotransposons on human genome evolution. *Nature Reviews Genetics*, 10: 691–703.

Crockford, S. J. & Kuzmin, Y. V. (2012) Comments on Germonpré et al., Journal of Archaeological Science 26, 2009 "Fossil dogs and wolves from Palaeolithic sites in Belgium, the Ukraine and Russia: osteometry, ancient DNA and stable isotopes", and Germonpré, Lázkicková-Galetová, and Sablin, Journal of Archaeological Science 26, 2012 "Paleolithic dog skulls at the Gravettian Predmostí site, the Czech Republic". *Journal of Archaeological Science*, 39: 2797–801.

Darwin, C. (1868). *The Variation of Animals and Plants under Domestication*. London: John Murray.

Dayan, T. (1999). Early domesticated dogs of the Near East. *Journal of Archaeological Science*, 21: 633–40.

Diamond, J. (2005). *Guns, Germs, and Steel*. New York: Norton and Company, Inc.

Ding, Z., Oskarsson, M., Ardalan, A. et al. (2012). Origins of domestic dog in Southern East Asia is supported by analysis of Y-chromosome DNA. *Heredity*, 108: 507–14.

Dobney, K. & Larson, G. (2006). Genetics and animal domestication: new windows on an elusive process. *Journal of Zoology*, 269: 261–71.

Driscoll, C. A., Macdonald, D. W. & O'Brien, S. J. (2009). From wild animals to domestic pets, an evolutionary view of domestication. *Proceedings of the National Academy of Sciences*, 106: S9971–8.

Driscoll, C. A., Menotti-Reymond, M., Roca, A. L. et al. (2007). The Near Eastern origin of cat domestication. *Science*, 317: 519–23.

Druzhkova, A. S., Thalmann, O., Trifonov, V. A., Leonard, J. A., Vorobieva, N.V., Ovodov, N. D., Graphodatsky, A. S. & Wayne, R. K. (2013). Ancient DNA analysis affirms the canid from Altai as a primitive dog. *PLoS One*, 8: e57754.

Fan, Z., Silva, P., Gronau, I., Wang, S., Serres Armero, A., Schweizer, R. M., Ramirez, O. et al. (2016). Worldwide patterns of genomic variation and admixture in gray wolves. *Genome Research*, 26: 163–73.

Flint, J. & Mackay, T. F. C. (2009). Genetic architecture of quantitative traits in mice, flies and humans. *Genome Research*, 19: 723–33.

Frantz, L. A., Mullin, V. E., Pionnier-Capitan, M., Lebrasseur, O., Olliver, M., Perri, A. et al. (2016). Genomic and archaeological evidence suggest a dual origin of domestic dogs. *Science*, 352: 1228–31.

Freedman, A. H., Gronau, I, Schweizer, R. M. et al. (2014). Genome sequencing highlights the dynamic early history of dogs. *PLoS Genetics*, 10: e1004016

Freedman, A. H., Schweizer, R. M., Ortega-Del Vecchyo, D., Han, E., Davis, B. W., Gronau, I. et al. (2016). Demographically-based evaluation of genomic regions under selection in domestic dogs. *PLoS Genetics*, 12: e1005851

Germonpré, M., Sablin, M., Stevens, R. et al. (2009). Fossil dogs and wolves from Palaeolithic sites in Belgium, the Ukraine and Russia: osteometry, ancient DNA and stable isotopes. *Journal of Archaeological Science*, 36: 473–60.

Giustina, A., Mazziotti, G. & Canalis, E. (2008). Growth hormone, insulin-like growth factors, and the skeleton. *Endocrine Reviews*, 29: 535–59.

Goebel, T., Waters, M. R. & O'Rourke, D. H. (2008). The late Pleistocene dispersal of modern humans in the Americas. *Science*, 319: 1497–502.

Gray, M. M., Sutter, N. B., Ostrander, E. A. & Wayne, R. K. (2010). The IGF1 small dog haplotype is derived from Middle Eastern gray wolves. *BMC Biology*, 8: 16.

Hare, B., Plyusnina, I., Ignacio, N. et al. (2005). Social cognitive evolution in captive foxes is a correlated by-product of experimental domestication. *Current Biology*, 15: 226–30.

Innan, H. & Kim, Y. (2004). Pattern of polymorphism after strong artificial selection in a domestication event. *Proceedings of the National Academy of Sciences USA*, 101: 10667–72.

IUCN (2012). The IUCN Red List of threatened species. Version 2012.1 [Online]. Available: www.iucnredlist.org

Jones, P., Chase, K., Martin, A., Ostrander, E. A. & Lark, K. G. (2008). Single-nucleotide polymorphism-based association mapping of dog stereotypes. *Genetics*, 179: 1033–44.

Kazazian, H. (2004). Mobile elements: drivers of genome evolution. *Science*, 303: 1626–32.

Kirkness, E. F., Bafna, V., Halpern, A. L. et al. (2003). The dog genome: survey sequencing and comparative analysis. *Science*, 301: 1898–903.

Kukekova, A. V., Trut, L. N., Chase, K. et al. (2010). Mapping loci for fox domestication: Deconstruction/reconstruction of a behavioral phenotype. *Behaviorial Genetics*, 41: 593–606.

Laron, Z. (2001). Insulin-like growth factor 1 (IGF-1): a growth hormone. *Molecular Pathology*, 54: 311–16.

Larson, G., Karlsson, E. K., Perri, A. et al. (2012). Rethinking dog domestication by integrating genetics, archeology, and biogeography. *Proceedings of the National Academy of Sciences USA*, 109: 8878–83.

Lefebvre, V. & Bhattaram, P. (2010). Vertebrate skeletogenesis. *Current Topics in Developmental Biology*, 90: 291–317.

Leonard, J. A., Vilà, C. & Wayne, R. K. (2006). From wild wolf to domestic dog. In *The Dog and Its Genome*, eds. E. A. Ostrander, U. Giger & K. Lindblad-Toh. Cold Spring Harbor, NY: Cold Spring Harbor Laboratory Press, pp. 95–118.

Leonard, J. A., Wayne, R. K., Wheeler, J. et al. (2002). Ancient DNA evidence for Old World origin of New World dogs. *Science*, 298: 1613–16.

Lindblad-Toh, K., Wade, C. M., Mikkelsen, T. S. et al. (2005). Genome sequence, comparative analysis and haplotype structure of the domestic dog. *Nature*, 438: 803–19.

Mech, L. D. & Boitani, L. (2003). Wolf social ecology. In *Wolves: Behavior, Ecology, and Conservation*, eds. L. D. Mech & L. Boitani. Chicago, IL: The University of Chicago Press, pp. 1–34.

McClintock, B. (1956). Controlling element and the gene. *Cold Spring Harbor Symposia on Quantitative Biology*, 31: 197–216.

Morey, D. F. (1994). The early evolution of the domestic dog. *American Scientist*, 82: 336–47.

Ovodov, M. D., Crockford, S. J., Kuzmin, Y. V. *et al*. (2011). A 33 000 year-old incipient dog from the Altai Mountains of Siberia: Evidence of the earliest domestication disruption by the last glacial maximum. *PLoS One*, 6: e22821.

Packard, J. M. (2003). Wolf behavior: Reproductive, social, and intelligent. In *Wolves: Behavior, Ecology, and Conservation*, eds. L. D. Mech & L. Boitani. Chicago, IL: The University of Chicago Press, pp. 35–65.

Pang, J. F., Kluetsch, C., Zou, X. J. *et al*. (2009). MtDNA data indicate a single origin for dogs south of Yangtze River, less than 16,300 years ago, from numerous wolves. *Molecular Biology & Evolution*, 26: 2849–64.

Parker, H. G. (2012). Genomic analyses of modern dog breeds. *Mammalian Genome*, 23: 19–27.

Parker, H. G., Kim, L. V., Sutter, N. B. *et al*. (2004). Genetic structure of the purebred domestic dog. *Science*, 304: 1160–4.

Parker, H. G. & Ostrander, E. A. (2005). Canine genomics and genetics: running with the pack. *PLoS Genetics*, 1: e58.

Parker, H. G., vonHoldt, B. M., Quignon, P. *et al*. (2009). An expressed fgf4 retrogene is associated with breed-defining chondrodysplasia in domestic dogs. *Science*, 325: 995–8.

Parker, H. P., Shearin, A. L. & Ostrander, E. A. (2010). Man's best friend becomes biology's best in show: genome analyses in the domestic dog. *Annual Review of Genetics*, 44: 309–36.

Perini, F. A., Russo, C. A. & Schrago, C. G. (2009). The evolution of South American endemic canids: a history of rapid diversification and morphological parallelism. *Journal of Evolutionary Biology*, 23: 311–22.

Randi, E. (2008). Detecting hybridization between wild species and their domesticated relatives. *Molecular Ecology*, 17: 285–93.

Ritvo, H. (1989). *The Animal Estate: The English and Other Creatures in the Victorian Age*. Cambridge, MA: Harvard University Press.

Sablin, M. & Khlopachev, G. (2002). The earliest Ice Age dogs: evidence from Eliseevichi I. *Current Anthropology*, 45: 795–819.

Savolainen, P., Zhang, Y. P., Luo, J., Lundeberg, J. & Leitner, T. (2002). Genetic evidence for an East Asian origin of domestic dogs. *Science*, 298: 1610–13.

Savolainen, P., Leitner, T., Wilton, A. N., Matisoo-Smith, E. & Lundeberg, J. (2004). A detailed picture of the origin of the Australian dingo, obtained from the study of mitochondrial DNA. *Proceedings of the National Academy of Sciences USA*, 101: 12387–90.

Shannon, L. M., Boyko, R. H., Castelhano, M., Corey, E., Hayward, J. J., McLean, C. *et al*. (2015). Genetic structure in village dogs reveals a Central Asian domestication origin. *PNAS*, 112: 13639–44.

Spady, T. C. & Ostrander, E. A. (2008). Canine behavioral genetics: pointing out the phenotypes and herding up the genes. *American Journal of Human Genetics*, 82: 10–18.

Statham, M. J., Trut, L. N., Sacks, B. N. *et al*. (2011). On the origin of a domesticated species: indentifying the parent population of Russian silver foxes (*Vulpes vulpes*). *Biological Journal of the Linnean Society*, 103: 168–75.

Stockard, C. R. (1941). *The Genetic and Endocrinic Basis for Differences in Form and Behavior: As Elucidated by Studies of Contrasted Pure-line Dog Breeds and their Hybrids*. Philadelphia, PA: The Wistar Institute of Anatomy and Biology.

Su, N., Du, X. & Chen, L. (2008). FGF signaling: its role in bone development and human skeleton diseases. *Frontiers in Bioscience*, 13: 2842–65.

Sundqvist, A. K., Bjornfeldt, S., Leonard, J. A. *et al*. (2006). Unequal contribution of sexes in the origin of dog breeds. *Genetics*, 172: 1121–8.

Sutter, N. B., Bustamante, C. D., Chase, K. *et al*. (2007). A single IGF1 allele is a major determinant of small size in dogs. *Science*, 316: 112–15.

Sutter, N. B. & Ostrander, E. A. (2004). Dog star rising: the canine genetic system. *Nature Reviews Genetics*, 5: 900–10.

Thalmann, O., Shapiro, B., Cui, P. *et al*. (2013) Complete mitochondrial genomes of ancient canids suggest a European origin of domestic dogs. *Nature*, 342: 871–4.

Trut, L. (1999). Early canid domestication: the farm-fox experiment. *American Scientist*, 87: 160–9.

Trut, L., Oskina, I. & Kharlamova, A. (2009). Animal evolution during domestication: the domesticated fox as a model. *Bioessays*, 31: 349–60.

Vigne, J. D. (2011). The origins of animal domestication and husbandry: a major change in the history of humanity and the biosphere. *Comptes Rendus Biologie*, 334: 171–81.

Vilà, C., Savolainen, P., Maldonado, J. E. *et al*. (1997). Multiple and ancient origins of the domestic dog. *Science*, 276: 1687–9.

Vilà, C., Seddon, J. & Ellegren, H. (2005). Genes of domestic mammals augmented by backcrossing with wild ancestors. *Trends in Genetics*, 21: 214–18.

Vilà, C. & Wayne, R. K. (1999). Hybridization between wolves and dogs. *Conservation Biology*, 13: 195–8.

Visscher, P. M. (2008). Sizing up human height variation. *Nature Genetics*, 40: 489–90.

Voight, B. F., Kudaravalli, S., Wen, X. & Pritchard, J. K. (2006). A map of recent positive selection in the human genome. *PLoS Biology*, 4: e72.

vonHoldt, B. M., Pollinger, J. P., Lohmueller, K. E. *et al*. (2010). Genome-wide SNP and haplotype analyses reveal a rich history underlying dog domestication. *Nature*, 464: 898–902.

vonHoldt, B. M., Stahler, D. R., Smith, D. W. *et al*. (2008). The genealogy and genetic viability of reintroduced

Yellowstone gray wolves. *Molecular Ecology*, 17: 252–74.

Wang, G.-D., Zhai, W., Yang, H.-C., Wang, L., Zhong, L., Liu, Y.-H., *et al.* (2016) Out of southern East Asia: the natural history of domestic dogs across the world. *Cell Research*, 26: 21–33.

Wang, X. & Tedford, R. H. (2008). *Dogs: Their Fossil Relatives and Evolutionary History*. New York, NY: Columbia University Press.

Waters, M. R. & Stafford, T. W. Jr. (2007). Redefining the age of Clovis: implications for the peopling of the Americas. *Science*, 315: 1122–6.

Wayne, R. K. & vonHoldt, B. M. (2012). Evolutionary genomics of dog domestication. *Mammalian Genome*, 23: 3–18.

Wellcome Trust Case Consortium (2007). Genome-wide association study of 14,000 cases of seven common diseases and 3,000 shared controls. *Nature*, 447: 661–78.

Yakar, S., Rosen, C. J., Beamer, W. G. *et al.* (2002). Circulating levels of IGF-1 directly regulate bone growth and density. *Journal of Clinical Investigation*, 110: 771–81.

Young, A. & Bannasch, D. (2006). Morphological variation in the dog. In *The Dog and Its Genome*, eds. E. A. Ostrander, U. Giger & K. Lindblad-Toh. Cold Spring Harbor, NY: Cold Spring Harbor Laboratory Press, pp. 47–65.

Zeder, M. A. (2008). Domestication and early agriculture in the Mediterranean Basin: origins, diffusion, and impact. *Proceedings of the National Academy of Sciences USA*, 105: 11597–604.

Zeder, M. A. (2012). The domestication of animals. *Journal of Anthropological Research*, 68(2): 161.

Zeder, M. A., Emshwiller, E., Smith, B. D. & Bradley, D. G. (2006). Documenting domestication: the intersection of genetics and archaeology. *Trends in Genetics*, 22: 139–55.

4 Evolution of working dogs

KATHRYN LORD, RICHARD A. SCHNEIDER AND RAYMOND COPPINGER

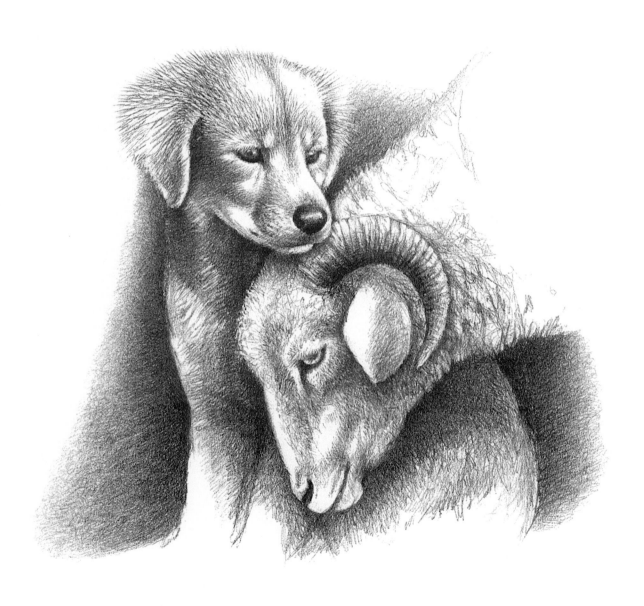

4.1   Introduction

When we think of dogs, we tend to think of animals that were selected for behavior performed in the service of people. Dogs pull sleds, guard property, herd sheep, guide the blind, track and retrieve game, and so on. We also think of dogs in terms of breeds, and often try to identify the breeds that make up some mongrel, as if all dogs had unadulterated, purebred ancestry. Many see their favorite breed woven into the Bayeux Tapestry or carved into the walls of an ancient tomb. Some think of breeds as if they were ancient species, separately derived from different strains of wolves, jackals or even coyotes. And people are often amazed at the many different sizes, colors, shapes, faces, and behaviors dogs come in.

Dogs' practical service to people is frequently overstated. Of the billion or so dogs in the world, only a tiny percentage of them work or hunt. Pure breeds of dogs for the most part are modern inventions (Larson *et al.*, 2012).

Frequently it is stated that the breeds were "selected" to perform some specific behavior, implying that changes have come about through a gradual accumulation of traits, by a process similar to natural selection. Darwin (1858) used domestic animals as an example of "artificial" selection analogous to natural selection. However, discoveries in the last hundred years have suggested other evolutionary mechanisms underlying the morphological and behavioral conformation of domesticated animals.

This chapter distils our observations and experiments on the subject of breed-specific behavior. It is divided into two sections. Section 4.2 focuses on the functional morphology and behavior of three "types" of working dogs. First are the livestock guarding dogs, which evolved in pastoral societies, where the only selection by humans is for behavior designed to repel or eliminate animals they don't like. Second are the sled dogs, which are bred to pull. Any animal can be taught to pull, but in sled dogs there is intense selection for a superior conformation that can efficiently perform the task. Third are the livestock herding dogs, bred to conduct livestock. There is little selection for physical conformation in herding dogs, but rather intense selection for a behavioral conformation including attention to the quality, frequency, and sequencing of specific motor patterns. Section 4.3 discusses and reviews the various evolutionary mechanisms that created dogs in general, and these working dogs in particular. We are interested in the stages of evolution that created and continue to create the background population of dogs. Dogs from this population were and still are adopted, bred, and modified to produce dogs that, in some sense, enter into a mutualistic relationship with humans. Looking at these phenotypes in detail provides insights into the derivation of breed-specific behavior. It also gives insight as to why breeds have breed-specific shapes, faces, colors, and sizes.

4.2   Morphology and behavior of working dogs

4.2.1   Livestock guarding dogs

Livestock guarding dogs may be the most populous working dog in the world. They are ubiquitous in pastoral cultures. Indeed, it is virtually impossible to find a pastoral culture where they are not present. They are better described as *landrace* dogs, meaning they are locally adapted to the environment and the task. They vary greatly in size, color, and shape. They tend to be smaller in equatorial and desert scrub, increasing in size with increasing latitude and altitude. The dogs of

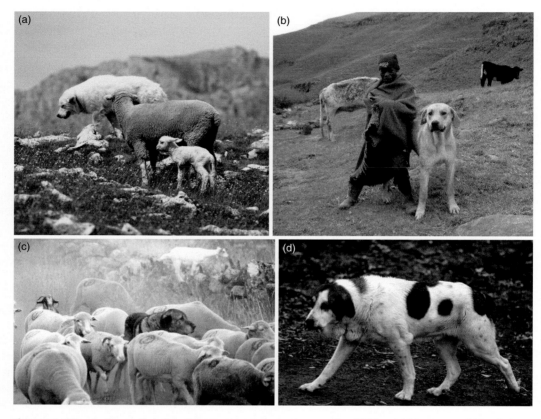

Figure 4.1 Livestock guarding dogs in some areas can reach upwards of 30 kg: (a) Maremma; (b) Maluti mountain dog; (c) Spanish mastiff; (d) Slovakian shepherd dog. (Photos a, b & d by Raymond Coppinger, photo c by Lorna Coppinger.)

the transhumance migrations reach sizes of 20–30 kg (Figure 4.1). From these regional landrace populations a few representative individuals have been removed, sexually isolated, and registered as breeds with international kennel clubs: examples include the French Great Pyrenees, Turkish Anatolian shepherds, and Italian maremmas. Landrace dogs are the product of natural selection and post-zygotic selection; that is, the culling or disposal of unwanted dogs with no direct control over the dog's reproduction. Breeds, in contrast, are the result of pre-zygotic selection – the deliberate mating together of preferred animals to perpetuate an observable breed-specific phenotype.

Livestock guarding dogs must be attentive, trustworthy, and protective of livestock. These behaviors are not trainable in terms of operant conditioning, but are rather the result of early socialization (Figure 4.2). The proper environment during the critical period of socialization (Fox & Bekoff, 1975; Scott & Fuller, 1965; Serpell *et al.*, Chapter 6) is the key to the development of the trustworthy, attentive, and protective behavior of a livestock guardian. During its first year, a pup passes through several neurological growth stages. During these stages developing neurons are particularly sensitive to the pup's external environment. By manipulating the environment one achieves the desired behavior (Coppinger & Coppinger, 2001, 2016).

The critical period of socialization begins at four weeks in dogs. During this period the pup forms its social bonds, sometimes referred to as species recognition patterns. Dogs easily form

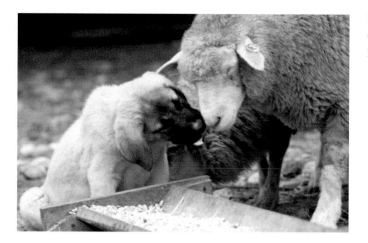

Figure 4.2 Socialization of livestock guarding dog. (Photo by Jay Lorenz, reprinted with permission.)

inter-specific social bonds with other species (Cairns & Werboff, 1967; Fox, 1969, 1971; Freedman *et al.*, 1960; Stanley & Elliot, 1962). Therefore, pups born in pastoral communities with frequent exposure to livestock are "naturally" attentive to the species they grow up with.

Guardian dogs are rendered untrustworthy when they display disruptive behaviors such as play routines or the onset of the predatory motor patterns: eye/stalk, chase, or bite. Disruptive behavior can be diminished by correction, by removal of the stimulus that elicited the display, or, in many cultures, by simply culling the dog. Livestock guarding has little to do with the legendary brave companion fiercely protecting its master's property. Rather, guarding dogs protect by disrupting predators through the performance of behaviors that are ambiguous or contextually inappropriate, such as barking and mobbing (Lord *et al.*, 2009), tail-wagging, social greeting, play, and occasionally aggression. Many species of predator will terminate a hunting sequence if disrupted, and "discovery" by a dog or dogs is often enough to avert depredation.

Livestock guarding dogs are an adjunct to the pastoral community. They "work" continuously without commands and there is no need even to name them; their genealogy is not important to shepherds. What the shepherd chooses is observable behavior. What they get are essentially village dogs with weakened adult stereotypical behavior sequences. They display non-predatory motor patterns toward the livestock with which they have been socialized. Since many sheep-raising communities have historically been transhumant or nomadic, gene flow occurs between livestock guarding dogs and the village dogs of the different regions through which they pass. Females in estrus are not usually penned, and so mate with other flock attending dogs and also with non-working dogs. Mongrelization tends to disrupt stereotypic behavior, and thus does not necessarily decrease working abilities, and may at the same time improve genetic health via hybrid vigor (Coppinger *et al.*, 1985). In the southwestern United States, Navajo shepherds have dogs that look very much like village dogs and appear very effective in protecting livestock (Black & Green, 1985).

Regional phenotypes do exist because of adaptation via natural selection to the regional environment, and due to capricious post-zygotic selection by humans for aspects of appearance. These animals are often erroneously identified as breeds. This type of artificial selection is usually based on a preferred coat color. For example, the Italian Maremmano–Abruzzese (maremma) is usually white. An Italian shepherd, asked why the Maremanno was white, claimed that only the white puppies were raised, the unwanted colored ones were culled. In spite of these regional variations in color, we have found no significant differences in guarding abilities of stock guardians in countries from Western Europe all the way to eastern Asia (Coppinger *et al.*, 1988).

Increased interest in pet and show dogs in the United States, as well as in Western Europe, led to the selling of regional landrace dogs, defining them as breeds, and sexually isolating them. In several countries "landrace dogs" have become a focus of national pride, which also increases their value, making it possible and profitable for shepherds to sell the type-form dogs. These dogs become the foundation for the "breed" and then further selection leads to companion or show animals.

4.2.2 Sled dogs

Sled dogs need not have a specific behavior profile. They are simply trained to perform the working task. Many species of mammals and even birds have been trained and used to pull some device. The size and shape of a draft animal depends specifically on the size, shape, and speed of the device that needs to be pulled. A team of dachshunds can be trained to pull a sled but not at sled-dog racing speeds.

Modern racing sled dogs are a good illustration of how working dogs evolve. Early sled dog races were recreational tests of the prowess of hardworking, trap line, freight-pulling dogs that transported people, cargo, and mail on the snowy frontiers of North America and Asia. Collections of dogs arriving at fur-buying centers were rapidly selected into competitive teams that raced for prize money. Teams and dogs were selected for speed over specific distances, and not for freight-hauling abilities. The goal became to complete the course in the shortest amount of time, compared to other teams, which would leave the starting line at regular intervals. Racing dogs were selected to be morphologically efficient, minimizing mass and motion while maximizing speed.

In the early part of the twentieth century, five-minute miles were enough to win a 25-mile race. By mid-century the speed had increased to four-minute miles. In the last years of the twentieth and the beginning of the twenty-first century, winning teams were competing sometimes at just under three-minute miles. In long races of 1000 miles, sled dogs must be able to trot for many hours a day, often covering more than 100 miles, day after day. The 1100-mile Iditarod race has a record time of eight days – which means the dogs are running almost six marathons a day for over a week. Easily, the racing sled dog is the fastest land mammal in the world over marathon distances.

The need for sled dogs became critical during the Alaskan Gold Rush that began in 1896. Few dogs were kept by native Alaskans before colonization by outsiders, and, although Native American dogs carried packs, moved cargo, and hunted, they may have been just as important as sources of food and fur (Lantis, 1980). Not until the expansion of the Thule culture during the eighth and ninth centuries does evidence appear of dogs hitched to the sled in a fan arrangement (MacRury, 1991). The concept of tandem harnessing and the use of a specialized lead dog came much later, perhaps introduced to the New World by Europeans.

The few dogs belonging to fur trappers or indigenous Alaskans at the turn of the twentieth century were supplemented, during the Gold Rush, by an influx of dogs from other parts of North America and Russia. As a result, teams were composed of a variety of sizes, shapes, and breeds, including bird dogs, retrievers, hounds, and forms resembling Newfoundlands. By 1908, in the first All-Alaska Sweepstakes race in Nome, breed differences were still apparent, although the best teams showed a uniformity of size and conformation (Coppinger, 1977). The 1911 race was won by Scotty Allan, whose dogs were remarkably uniform, while still displaying the phenotypic characteristics of a variety of breeds. The modern racing husky is a product of hybridization, post-zygotic culling, and eventually selection of individuals being bred for racing qualities. Breeding between good dogs was often a result of proximity rather than planning. Occasionally, a few individuals were chosen for

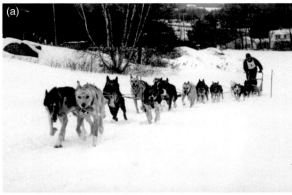

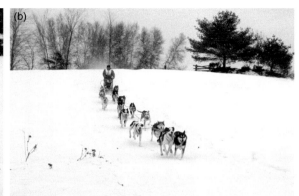

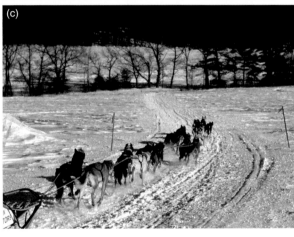

Figure 4.3 (a)–(c) World champion teams. Modern racing huskies look like a "breed" showing a uniformity of breed-like characteristics, but they are strongly dependent on the diversity of hybridization. (Photos by Lorna and Raymond Coppinger.)

some capricious reason and sexually isolated from the larger population and registered with a kennel club to create a breed, such as the Siberian husky.

Today's best racing dogs are the product of an acquisition and culling process based not on their looks or strength but on their ability to run fast on groomed trails, and to behave themselves on a team (Figure 4.3). Racing dogs are purchased from other racers or bred from high-performance dogs. Top working females are often not bred because pregnancy and lactation interrupts their racing careers. Females in heat also induce behavioral displays by males that are not appropriate on a team. Dogs from a given kennel often acquire distinctive phenotypes and are referred to as "Belford dogs" or "Lombard dogs," after the mid-century champions, Charles Belford and Roland Lombard. Pride in their abilities with dogs has led Native Americans to pool their resources. George Attla, one of the best Alaskan drivers of the 1970s, selected dogs annually from native villages. It was an honor to have one's dog picked for his team and to have that dog distinguished as an "Attla dog." Dogs purchased from champion drivers become valuable as breeding animals simply because they pass through the most successful kennels. Locally superior dogs, once they become known to a wider audience, may acquire the name of their region, e.g. Alaskan husky, Quebec hound. At some point they might be referred to as landrace dogs rather than breeds. But this breed-producing process resembles that of other working breeds that bear the names of the original breeder or region, such as the Jack Russell terrier, Doberman pinscher, German shepherd, Saint Bernard, Catahoula leopard cow hog dog, and so on.

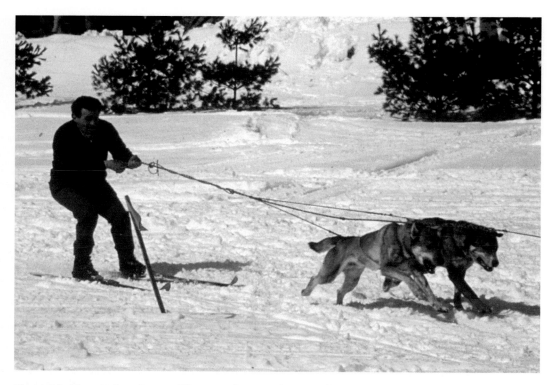

Figure 4.4 Almost mirror images. These two dogs are almost perfect, except the dog on the left has its left front foot on the ground while the dog on the right side has its left hind foot down. (Photo by Lorna Coppinger.)

Sled dogs are acquired and bred because of their gait. Top drivers know that gait in detail. Dogs developed for marathon distance races lope with at least one foot always in contact with the ground (Figure 4.4). In long races, dogs trot or pace with two feet in contact with the ground.

Speed is attained not only by rapidity of movement, but also by the length of the gait – known as reach. This length is determined by the dog's size and shape: all other things being equal, the larger the dog the longer the reach. The slope of the pelvis, the distance between the shoulder blades and the length of the back, all allow for maximum extension of both the front and rear legs. Good drivers say that a dog runs with its back, and as every human racer or dancer knows, the most fatiguing activity is pulling the (hind) legs forward, much of which is done with back muscles (the psoas).

As important as speed, dogs paired in harness need to have matched gaits, preferably mirror images of each other. The physics of pulling a sled can be explained fairly simply. The single dog on a one-dog team pulls 100% of the load, while each dog on a two-dog team pulls about 85%. Harness vectors, plus the resulting torque on the sled, create an inefficiency that prevents any better distribution of work (ideally, 50–50 for a two-dog team). Each dog on a six-dog team actually pulls about half the load. More than 12 dogs add no net gain. On open-class teams, 14–16 dogs are run to provide "spares" in case dogs have to be dropped during the race due to injuries or fatigue, since no new dogs can be added once the race has begun. By matching the dogs' gaits, drivers can reduce the energy lost to vector forces and increase the speed, because the distance the sled and lines have to move is shortened (Figure 4.4).

Many drivers know their dogs' characteristics without understanding the underlying biology. For example, although bigger dogs are potentially faster because of their longer stride, drivers know

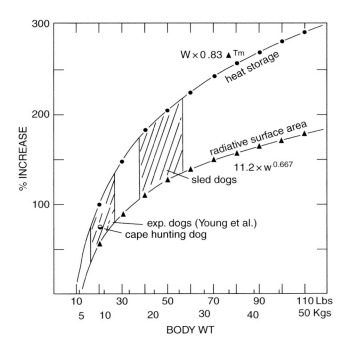

Figure 4.5 Relation between body weight and heat storage capacity in dogs. The chart shows that large dogs cannot radiate heat fast enough to run long distances, and that small dogs have problems conserving heat. (From Phillips *et al.*, 1981.)

that dogs over 25 kg have less endurance. Running sled dogs will attain rectal temperatures of 105°F (40°c) or more; larger dogs cannot dissipate heat quickly enough and become heat-exhausted (Figure 4.5). Another trait understood by drivers is that the feet of some dogs "snowball"; that is, ice and snow collect on foot hairs, and produce pain and injury as the dogs run (Figure 4.6). This condition seems to be caused by excessive sweating through the footpad. Such sweating is universal in dogs, although arctic wolves do not have functional merocrine or apocrine glands (Sands *et al.*, 1977). Most drivers, unaware of the underlying physiology and anatomy, just select those animals that can go the distance without being in pain when they run.

Dogs do not pull sleds because they are forced to. Running on a team is not a typical conditioned response, for there is no obvious reward for the performance. After a race or training session the dog is removed from harness and put into its travel box. Feeding is done at a given hour each day,

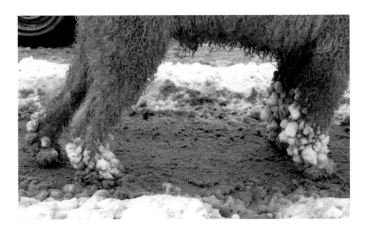

Figure 4.6 Snowballing. (Photo by Raymond Coppinger.)

usually in the early evening so as not to interfere with the day's activities. Dogs are not punished if they do not run well. Whipping or abusive treatment can damage a dog, decreasing its abilities and, worst of all, creating a "sulker." If severe, the dog is likely to quit. Cracking a whip or making novel noises may increase the speed for the moment, but to overdrive a team beyond its pace may deprive the dogs of enough energy to finish the race, and is also likely to lead to quitting, a sled dog driver's worst fear. Good drivers guard against ever having a dog quit, for if a dog learns to quit at stressful times, it cannot be relied upon and cannot be raced. Instead of punishment, good drivers keep dogs out of situations where they might misbehave.

Good drivers, for example, avoid circumstances where dogs are likely to fight. Dogs that routinely display aggressive behavior are not used. Fighting can be reduced by pairing males with females but this also means selecting against sexual dimorphisms in order to preserve uniformity of gait. Lead dogs are often run in pairs and are often female and chosen mainly to set the pace, since other dogs on a team know the commands. A team with "deep" talent will have dogs that can be switched during a race to relieve fatigued leaders. The driver's job is to supervise the process. The method is one of establishing a routine; there are few commands. There is, however, considerable social facilitation between individuals, and a dog's demeanor at harnessing time could best be described as "major excitement." Dogs left behind will bark continuously and show other signs of distress.

Where did sled dog behavior come from? The selection and training procedure just described is similar to Jack London's description in his novel, *Call of the Wild*. London was right in making "Buck" a cross between a Saint Bernard and a Scottish sheepdog, stolen in one of the lower 48 states. However, Buck and his fellow captives were dog derivatives, not wolf derivatives. Sled dogs behave like dogs, not wolves. Lead dogs are in that position because the driver sees their ability to run fast, to stay out in front, and to take commands. They are not chosen because they establish dominance over the rest of the team. The driver is not a substitute leader forcing the dogs to submit, but an observant manager trying to reduce wasted energy, and select dogs that perform well. The driver's chief job is to anticipate problems and prevent conditions that disrupt the performance.

When sled dogs run, they are playing. They are exhibiting non-functional, internally rewarded behavior, as in the classical definition of play. They are not chasing food or even another team. The classic analogy that they are operating with highly evolved social pack behavior inherited from wolves is not only not true of dogs but turns out probably not true for wolves either. Wolves are more likely using simple rules to perform complex pack behaviors (see Muro *et al.*, 2011). No serious sled dog driver would hybridize a sled dog with a wolf, because the offspring would have traits counter-productive to racing fast on a team: an increase in size, improper gait, unmanageable behavior, and little tendency to "play" at racing. MacRury (1991) presents good evidence that Inuit dogs are not hybrid wolves, and that these people show little desire to produce such hybrids.

4.2.3   Herding dogs

Herding dogs (like livestock guarding dogs, but unlike sled dogs) need not have any specific size or shape, but (unlike livestock and sled dogs) depend entirely on a behavioral conformation of specific motor patterns. Fentress and McLeod (1986) explain a motor pattern as follows, "it is through the production of integrated sequences of movement that animals express rules ... ." The rules are different for a border collie than they are for a pointer, which is why you can't train one to do the other's job (Coppinger & Feinstein, 2015).

Herding dogs conduct livestock from one place to another by causing fear-flocking and flight behavior. They are known in the trade as "chase and bite" dogs. The various breeds have been selected for specific behavior patterns, primarily those motor patterns that are directed toward livestock. Herding dogs are generally divided into headers, heelers, and catch dogs, depending on their tendency to either circle livestock and bring them toward the handler, drive livestock away from the handler in a trailing pattern, or actually stop the livestock by taking them off their feet. There are also breed differences in how far away from the handler they will work. Australian shepherd dogs and New Zealand huntaways work with their heads up, and vocalize while they chase sheep. Border collies and kelpies are silent and use a circling out-run followed by a head-down eye, stalk, and chase. Blue heelers bite at the hocks of cattle, a behavior that is generally not acceptable for dogs that herd the more vulnerable sheep. In early eighteenth and nineteenth century England, butchers had catch dogs to control range cattle in pens and congested areas. These dogs became the bull-baiting dogs of the sports arena (Jones, 1988). In the American southwest, they are called catch dogs and are used to herd wild range cattle. Catahoula leopard cow hog dogs are used in groups, forcing range cows into tight herds that are then driven with cracking whips by horsemen, while the dogs prevent individuals from leaving the herd.

It is generally thought that herding dogs are using motor patterns homologous to the predatory behavior patterns of the ancestral canids. These include the orientation posture (head above shoulders, ears up, eyes and nose focused towards potential prey item) (Figure 4.7a), followed by eye

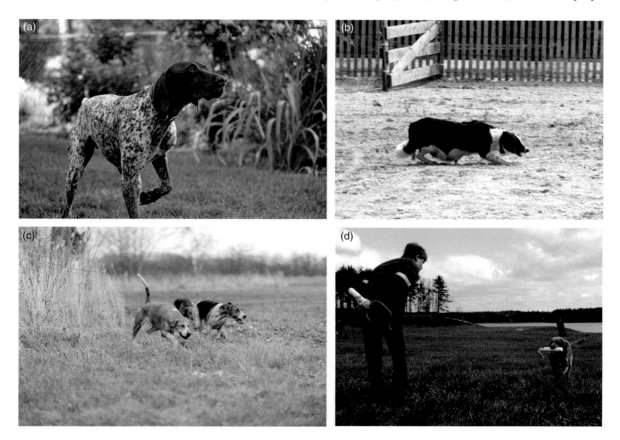

Figure 4.7 Hunting motor patterns: (a) pointer orienting (photo by Moon Wymore); (b) border collie "eye-stalking" (photo by Lorna Coppinger); (c) walking hounds chasing (photo by iStock/Getty Images Plus); (d) Chesapeake Bay retriever grab-bite (photo by Lorna Coppinger).

(head position at or below level of shoulders, ears flat or forward, eyes and nose focused on potential prey item) (Figure 4.7b), stalk (body posture, legs bent, while moving forward or standing still) (Figure 4.7b), chase (running after potential prey) (Figure 4.7c), grab-bite (initial bite to prey: in a large prey animal this is often to a flank, and may be substituted with a forefoot stab in smaller prey) (Figure 4.7d), kill-bite, often called crush-bite (a bleeding bite directed towards the jugular region, sometimes substituted with a head-shake), and finally, dissect (pulling apart the prey animal). In many wild carnivores, predatory motor patterns are so stereotyped that a field biologist can look at a kill and know immediately the species of the predator.

The different breeds of herding dog display different motor patterns at different frequencies. The intensity of the display varies to the extent that some breeds are easier to train to display (or not to display) a particular behavior. It is difficult, for example, to train corgis and heelers not to nip at flying hocks and, therefore, they can be miserable companions for joggers. Although the emergence of the motor patterns during development is variable, training of herding dogs does not, and really cannot, begin until after the onset and sequencing of eye, stalk, and chase. Training consists of directing the animal to the environment where the motor pattern is elicited.

Experiments at Hampshire College showed that the release of the eye/stalk behavior in adult border collies was stimulated in part by anticipation of movement of the "prey." When chickens were sedated just enough so that they stood motionless and inactive to the approaching dog, border collies were unable to hold the eye motor pattern, and would resort to displacement activities (conflict behaviors) such as play-bowing or barking (Lord *et al.*, 2009). They resumed the eye posture at any suggestion of motion (Coppinger *et al.*, 1987).

Showing of eye seems to provide its own reward. Once the onset of the motor pattern occurs ontogenetically, the only way to keep most collies from showing it is to remove them from the stimulus. The same is true of other behavior patterns necessary for a good herding dog, because the dog seeks the rewards, and modifying the behavior is difficult. The solution to the problem of too much or too little correct behavior is often to get a different dog.

Because the eye, stalk, and out-run behavior patterns seem to be so strictly heritable, once the proper quality and frequency of display are established for a particular task, then the breed cannot be improved by crossing with other breeds, as can be done in guarding and sled dogs. Appropriately, discussions of genealogy are common among people who rely on their dogs to herd. Like sled dog drivers, sheep herders tend to get their dogs from other, well-known herders. Border collie breeders know exactly what a dog is like if it is related to MacKnight's Gael or Greenwood's Moss. Conversations between owners tend to be entirely about behavior and breeding, and scarcely ever about what the dog looks like. Because their job requires precise movement, herding dogs tend to be of a more uniform conformation than livestock guarding dogs, but not as uniform as racing sled dogs.

The one caveat to the above discussion that should be mentioned is that the herding behavior illustrated is that of trial dogs. As with the sled dogs, the beginnings of competition trials changed the nature of the dog. It is doubtful that the trial performing dog would be of much use to the majority of pastoralists nor would the average shepherd have the time, skill, or inclination to train such a dog.

4.3   The origins of working dog morphology and behavior

The three kinds of working dogs described above would appear to have three different kinds of phyletic histories. Our task now is to describe the evolutionary processes that created these specialists.

Each kind of working dog is a specialist for a particular task, rendering each of them poorer at performing the task for which the other breeds are specialized. The average livestock guarding dog or herding dog can be trained to pull sleds but cannot be trained to do it well. Both herding dogs and sled dogs, even if socialized properly, make poor livestock guarding dogs because of their active dispositions and inappropriate displays of innate motor patterns. Herding livestock depends upon the display and sequencing of specific predatory motor patterns not found in guarding dogs or sled dogs.

Worldwide, livestock guarding dogs are technically landrace dogs adapted to local pastoral societies and specific pastoral landscapes. Their particular sizes, shapes, faces, and behaviors are products of natural selection. Humans have little or no control over their reproduction, but contribute to selection by eliminating unwanted individuals. When and where did livestock guarding dogs evolve? Most likely, it had to be after the appearance of livestock and pastoral societies. Ancient writings such as Homerian legends (2500 ya) and biblical writings (~2000 ya) have lush illustrations of pastoralists at work. Before that there is anthropological evidence of sheep, goats and dogs back to roughly 6000 ya (Hole & Wyllie, 2007; Le Quellec, 2006).

Racing sled dogs are more clearly products of artificial selection in the Darwinian sense. The process starts by sorting through some background populations of dogs, and collecting and testing individuals for their abilities to accomplish some task. Superior working individuals become valuable to the owner and are purposefully bred together or simply tend to breed with other superior working individuals because of proximity, creating offspring that are more likely to display the working phenotype and behavior.

When did people first start to use sled dogs? It should be remembered that activities such as sledding, once accomplished by some person or group, might not be continuous over time even within the group. Although Malamute Indians had a history of dog sledding, a new system appeared in the region, created by the early twentieth century gold rushers. Their dogs were imported from out of state. The methodology of freighting on pre-packed trails was new, and the invention of the lead dog, was not only new to the region but adopted by the Native Americans. An example of this is provided by Lantis (1980), who claims that serious sledding didn't take place in North America until the Thule culture displaced the Dorsets across the continent between 700 and 300 years ago.

Herding dogs are not very common in pastoral societies. There are few dogs that take commands such as the border collie, Australian kelpie, or New Zealand huntaway. The vast majority of herding "breeds" such as the heelers (corgis or blue heelers), or the catch dogs (bull dogs), are drovers' dogs, and referred to as "chase and bite" dogs.

When did herding dogs first appear? The legends and the behaviors indicate that they appear and reappear as cross-breeds between the landrace pastoral dogs and hunting breeds. There are many examples from the nineteenth and twentieth centuries. The New Zealand Huntaway is purportedly a cross between a sheep dog, a black Labrador, and hounds. Similarly, in the nineteenth century, the German shepherd dog was purposely created by a breeder who crossed sheep dogs with other breeds. Legend has it that the border collie was created by crossing landrace sheep dogs with pointers.

The question of whether the "original" dog was domesticated to perform some helpful function such as guarding sheep or houses, pulling sleds, or herding livestock, is essentially moot. There are no firm data at all that the first dogs were domesticated by humans. "Domestic dog" simply means "living with people" and does not imply any intentional process. In addition, no clear evidence exists as to when domestic dogs first lived with people. Archaeological material in the form of dogs drawn with leashes and collars on pottery fragments shows good evidence of people hunting with dogs 6000 years ago (Hole and Wyllie, 2007). Dogs must have existed before 6000 ya but there is surprisingly little hard evidence that they did. Archeologists find canids buried with people that could be dogs, or skulls and bones that could be dogs. But the emphasis must be on the "could be." The

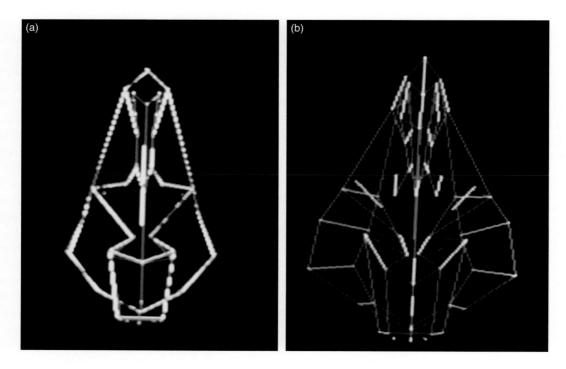

Figure 4.8 An overlay of (a) a wolf skull with a border collie skull and (b) a borzoi skull with a pug skull. (Photos by Richard A. Schneider.)

problem is that there are not good diagnostic differences between dogs and the other members of the genus (but see Clutton-Brock, Chapter 2). We would also argue that one cannot reliably distinguish mesaticephalic dog skulls (an average length to width skull ratio), from wolves, if age and size are taken into account. Small breeds such as border collies, have faces and head shapes which vary little from yearling wolves, suggesting that the "original" dogs were <15 kg animals (Figure 4.8). Similarly, geneticists do not have a methodology yet that can reliably date the divergence of dogs from their ancestors (Coppinger *et al.*, 2010; vonHoldt & Driscoll, Chapter 3). Additionally, evolution acts at the level of populations. Finding one individual that varies from the ancestral phenotype does not constitute domestication. Larson (2011, p. S491) expressed these problems well when he wrote, "Thus, molecular clock efforts so far simply lack the precision to date Holocene phenomena. And this is true even after putting aside the issue of what a domestication date actually means."

Whatever the speculations on dog origins, either in the Mesolithic or Neolithic, there is no evidence that dogs were purposefully domesticated, which precludes any discussion that the original dogs were employed in the performance of any task. The three types of working dogs we analyzed here certainly were not direct descendants of some wild canid. For the two kinds of livestock dogs one has to postulate the origin of livestock. Attempts to train wolves to pull sleds are hilariously funny (Zimen, 1987).

One could ask if there are some other working tasks for which dogs were purposefully domesticated, such as serving as hunting companions? We would argue that this is implausible. Hunting dogs, like our other working dogs, are adopted from the background population of dogs. It might be noted that a purposefully bred hunting dog takes almost two years to train and socialize before they perform appropriately. The written histories of existing hunting dogs, like those of the other working dogs, describes their development from some background population of dogs.

Price (1984) points out that domestication is a two-stage process involving, first, genetic adaptations to living in the domestic environment and, second, socialization of individuals in each generation. The evidence with our three types of working dogs would support that notion. Each type of working dog has a phenotype (including the behavioral phenotype) that is an adaptation to the environment (including the task to be performed). But each individual has to develop the proper behavior.

4.3.1   Direct trait-by-trait selection

A common assumption is that changes between dogs and their ancestors, or between breeds of dog, are the product of a gradual process of trait-by-trait selection akin to natural selection. However, it is difficult to accept that some breed-specific traits (e.g. the short limbs of the dachshund, or basset hound) were ever initially selected for in terms of an adaptionist scheme. Little evidence exists of breeders choosing among dogs for a gradual accumulation of a character, such as shorter and shorter legs, in order to produce a short-legged dog that could walk into a hole and extract a rabbit. Rather, these traits were more likely inadvertent outcomes of single gene mutations subsequently preserved and reinforced through artificial selection (see vonHoldt & Driscoll, Chapter 3). Nor are the selective advantages of floppy ears, curly tails, jowls or variegated coat colors immediately obvious. Bemis (1984, p. 304) pointed out that, "the observation of evolutionary change by itself is insufficient evidence that adaptation actually occurred." When considering the diversity of dog breeds, it is unreasonable to propose, "rational adaptive explanations to account for each of these changes … Rather, some, perhaps most of the changes are interpreted as the product of selection operating on a restricted set of characters" (Bemis, 1984, p. 303), affecting what Coppinger & Smith (1990, p. 360) called the, "whole package of behavior and morphology." Darwin observed that, "if man goes on selecting, and thus augmenting, any peculiarity, he will almost certainly modify unintentionally other parts of the structure, owing to the mysterious laws of correlation" (cited in Løvtrup, 1987, p. 105). If there is selection for just one trait, many others may be altered in the process (Geist, 1971).

Gradualism is not the only mechanism for the evolution of new species. Punctuated equilibrium, initially proposed to account for the lack of fossil evidence for gradual change, suggests that a species stays the same for millions of years until a relatively rapid change in taxonomic characteristics as a result of genetic mutation leads to a new species (Eldredge & Gould, 1972). Even with a theory like "punctuated equilibrium" there does not seem to be enough time in the 8000 years since dogs first appeared to collect all the mutations necessary to produce the hundreds of breeds existing today.

Geist (1987, p. 1067) concurred with others (Løvtrup, 1977, 1987; Waddington, 1957) in the rejection of gradualism, stating that, "the gradualist model, in its selectionist forms, fails to address the fact that phenotypes, not genotypes, are the raw material of natural selection." Here we extend this concept to include the behavioral phenotype. In the case of our three working types, it was the ability to perform particular behaviors that was selected for, with little notion of what the resulting dogs would or should look like. Thus, we suggest that working dogs were selected for by breeding together the most effective dogs rather than via the gradual selection for particular traits such as those that appear in the modern breeds.

4.3.2   Hybridization

Of the 200–400 recognized breeds – pick your favorite number – the majority have been created since the late nineteenth century by cross-breeding (Larson *et al.*, 2012). New forms or saltatory changes can be produced quickly by hybridization (Stebbins, 1959). Not only does hybridization cause a disruption of eco-specific behavior in wild forms but, more importantly, such systems as predation, courtship, territory, social hierarchy and pack formation, tend to fragment and sometimes disappear (Coppinger *et al.*, 1985; Lord *et al.*, 2013). Our understanding about the development of breeds is expressed well by Haldane (1930, p. 138) who stated that there is, "every reason to believe that new species may arise quite suddenly, sometimes by hybridization, sometimes perhaps by other means." We believe the same is true of breeds of dogs.

As an evolutionary mechanism, hybridization can lead to morphological diversification and "structural disharmonies" (Stockard, 1941, p. 17); a concept reminiscent of Belyaev's (1979) term "destabilization." Alberch (1982, p. 20) viewed diversification and adaptation as independent processes, with the former inherently preceding the latter. He stated:

the role of development in evolutionary processes of morphological change is twofold. On one hand, the structure of the developmental program defines the realm of possible novelties … while, on the other, the regulatory interactions occurring during ontogeny can accommodate genetic and environmental perturbations and result in the production of an integrated phenotype.

In other words, the shape of the animal and its behavior is not predetermined by the genes, but rather the genes interacting with the developmental environment allows for a range of phenotypic outcomes.

Thus, hybridization can form Stockard's "structural disharmonies" by altering the timing of "the developmental program," proposed by Albrech. However, the limits of these structural disharmonies depend on the organism's ability to accommodate the changes. Accommodation is the fitting together of the various organ and behavioral systems. A simple example was given by Twitty (1966), an embryologist who transferred the eye germ cells from a big salamander species into a tiny species, resulting in little salamanders with great big eyes. Remarkably, the little salamanders grew eye sockets to fit their new eyeballs and added extra brain cells to "accommodate" their large eyes. It is interesting to note that the eye itself maintained the size it would have had in its donor, suggesting that the eye is intrinsic rather than accommodative. In other words, the eye grew to a specific genetically determined size regardless of the new information coming from its surrounding host environment.

As with the salamander, the dog's skull has features that have not been selected for but are simply the accommodation of one organ system to another. Pugs, maremmas, and borzois, which have differences in the timing of the developmental program of the nasal bones, illustrate the accommodation of the teeth and bones to each other to make a workable skull.

4.3.3   Origin of size, shape, face, and color

It has become a cliché that the domestic dog is the most variable mammalian species. If asked to describe what distinguishes domestic dogs from their wild counterparts, and separates modern breeds from one another, most people would point to the striking differences found in body size, facial form, coat pattern, and behavior. Similar anatomical and colorful variations in facial features are found in various species of birds. Explanations for such variations in dogs have in the past ranged

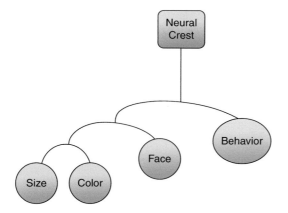

Figure 4.9 Size, color, face shape, and behavior are all interconnected through the neural crest. Thus, like a mobile, if you alter one it affects all of the others.

over a number of topics including selection for puppy-like qualities such as cuteness and tameness (Coppinger & Coppinger, 1982; Fox, 1965, 1978; Frank & Frank, 1982; Goodwin *et al.*, 1997). But these "structural disharmonies" of characteristics such as the face, color, size, and behavior are relatively easy to change developmentally. This is simply because they tend to change together, since they develop in the same embryological cascade of events. These size, color, behavior, and facial traits have co-evolved together simply because they arise from a common set of embryonic building blocks of cellular and molecular mechanisms that connect and counterbalance one another internally like elements in a kinetic mobile.

Imagine a mobile with four strings dangling from acentric arms balancing connections to size, color, face, and behavior. If you pull (select for) any one trait, the others will move (change) (Figure 4.9). This was obvious when Dmitry Belyaev performed his fox study. In an experiment to develop a more manageable animal, Belyaev (1979, p. 305) bred only those silver foxes that consistently displayed tame behavior and found that after 20 years of intense selection, "quite new morphological characters appeared that are not found in wild animals but are quite characteristic of some breeds of dog: a peculiar position of the tail … and finally, the drooping ears characteristic of young dogs." Unlike wild types, some of these foxes had black-and-white piebald coats (Figure 4.10) and even a diestrous breeding cycle. Careful to mitigate the effects of inbreeding, Belyaev selected from over 10 000 foxes and outbred to numerous farms. He also demonstrated that these traits were not due to simple Mendelian gene segregation. Therefore, when Belyaev selected for tame behavior he also got changes in skull shape, coloration, and behaviors unrelated to tameness (see also vonHoldt & Driscoll, Chapter 3).

Experimental studies on a variety of animals, especially birds, have revealed that the facial and integumentary (skin, hair/feathers, color, etc.) systems, as well as the biogenetic pathways that control behavior, are all highly integrated by an embryonic population of cells called the neural crest. Selection for changes in one system can have rapid and inadvertent consequences for the others. Understanding where and when the facial, integumentary, and behavioral systems become linked during development explains how the domestic dog has changed shape so dramatically, quickly and continuously during its short evolutionary history. The embryonic cells of the neural crest have turned out to play a critical role in this process (Crockford, 2002; Sánchez-Villagra *et al.*, 2015; Wilkins *et al.*, 2014).

Much of the information on the role of the neural crest cells comes from transplant experiments that use different organisms. During the development of the face and jaws, neural crest cells generate all of the skeletal and connective tissues, including bone, cartilage, and the dentine of teeth (Couly & Le Douarin, 1988; Couly *et al.*, 1992, 1993, 1995; Le Lièvre & Le Douarin, 1975; Noden, 1978,

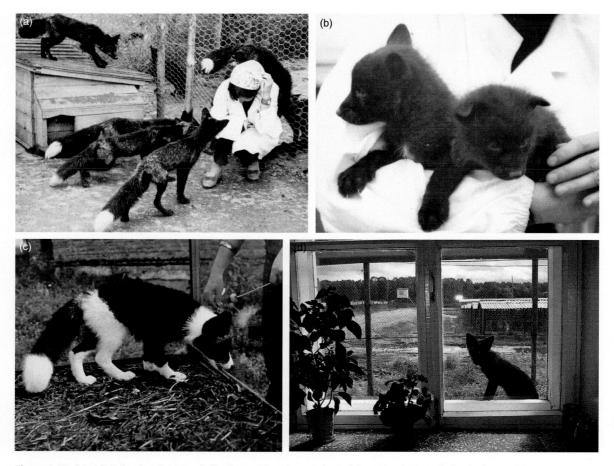

Figure 4.10 (a)–(d) Selection for tame behavior produced a number of dog-like characteristics in foxes. (Photos courtesy of D. Belyaev, reprinted with permission.)

1983; Webb & Noden, 1993). In experiments similar to Twitty's (1966) neural crest cells destined to become the beak (intrinsic) of a quail were transplanted into a duck. The little duck grew up with a quail bill. Here is the perfect hybrid – a duck with a quail face (Eames & Schneider, 2008; Schneider & Helms, 2003). What is most interesting is that all of the patterning information for beak size and shape comes from the quail donor neural crest and the duck host has to *accommodate* this new face and attach all its muscles and blood vessels to this hybrid bill – which it does, making a perfect but novel fit. The new face has not been selected for except in the sense that the embryological processes are designed to produce a workable face.

Interestingly, the cells that form the back and base of the skull come from a different embryonic source called the mesoderm. Thus, there is a boundary in the skull that separates those bones and cartilages in the face and jaws that are derived from the neural crest and those in the back and base of the skull that form from the mesoderm (Noden & Schneider, 2006; Schneider, 1999). Probably because of this, the posterior portion and base of the skull remains highly conserved even in the most extreme dog breeds (Drake, 2011). In contrast, the greatest shape changes that have occurred during the evolution of dogs are found in the face and jaws, and they correspond precisely to the neural crest-derived region of the skull (Coppinger & Schneider, 1995; Schneider, 2005, 2015).

The neural crest also makes all of the pigment-producing melanocytes and is the source of color and pattern in the skin and hair (Bronner-Fraser, 1994; Cramer, 1991; Eames and Schneider, 2005; Hirobe, 1995; Le Douarin & Dupin, 1993; Rawles, 1948). Likewise, the neural crest produces the cells in the adrenal gland that secrete adrenaline, noradrenaline, and dopamine, and give rise to the pigmented dopaminergic neurons in the substantia nigra, a region of the brain closely associated with learning and reward (Arons & Shoemaker, 1992; Richardson & Sieber-Blum, 1993).

Thus, changes in the neural crest are simultaneously the major source of evolutionary variation in the facial skeleton, the integument, and in behavior (Eames & Schneider, 2005; Schneider, 2005). In terms of dog evolution, the neural crest acts as a conduit through which breed-specific adaptations are implemented. In a manner analogous to the production of chimeras, new breeds of dogs can be created by hybridizing two or more breeds together. When Max von Stephanitz created the German shepherd dog at the end of the nineteenth century, he cross-bred at least six different breeds of dogs, each with a face of its own. The result is a new breed of dog with a novel face created by an accommodation of all those faces into one new one. The possibilities are endless. Simply breeding large breeds to small can create animals with phylogenetically bizarre faces (Fox, 1975). Hybridizing large dogs to small dogs or other extremes of size, face shape, color, or behaviors will produce new or phylogenetically bizarre forms. As the list of dog breeds grows, the possibility for creating new sizes, shapes, and colors also increases.

The arguments reviewed by Coppinger & Schneider (1995, p. 38) that the face and head shape of dogs was indicative of selective retardation (neoteny) for more juvenile behavior appear overly simplistic in retrospect. One can select for (perceived) puppy-like morphological and behavioral characteristics, but the resulting shape is only superficially paedomorphic. For example, the pug has a shorter snout, but its skull looks nothing like the skull of a wolf pup. Rather than leading to a puppy-like adult, retardation of development (or any change in developmental timing) is most likely to lead to a novel shape and behavior. Furthermore, while it may be the result of a change in the timing of development (heterochrony), this superficially puppy-like "breed" is not necessarily the result of neoteny, the slowing of developmental timing. In fact, Drake (2011) has shown that breed differences are not simply the result of selective retardation.

4.4   The origin of working dog behavior

We have described three types of working dogs – livestock guarding dogs, sled dogs, and herding dogs. For the sake of simplicity, we call them breeds, while remaining aware that technically they do not always exist in sexually isolated populations. Each is supposed to behave in a characteristic "breed-typical" way, much as different species are said to display "species-typical" behavior. These are not the general personality traits listed in breed standards, but rather frequency, sequencing and contexts of specific motor patterns (units of behavior). The big question here is: How do these breed-typical behavioral differences evolve?

Ethologists measure behavior with ethograms, which are inventories of motor patterns. As mentioned earlier we can think of motor patterns as having rules for when, where, and how they are expressed. Our first assumption is that each of the working breeds is behaving according to different sets of rules. Motor patterns are measured by their quality or shape (Figure 4.10), their frequency and duration, and the sequences and contexts in which the movements are performed. Like faces or coat colors, dog motor patterns can be signature qualities of the breed, i.e. clearly identifiable intrinsic characteristics. Wolves and dogs display the same or homologous motor patterns, but at different frequencies and in different sequences. Adult wolves display a complete, functional, foraging motor pattern sequence: orient > eye > stalk > chase > grab-bite > kill-bite > dissecting-bite. Adult border collies show only the beginning portion of this sequence: orient > eye > stalk > chase, while grab-bite and kill-bites are considered faults in this breed. In contrast, German shepherds bred for Shutzhund work display orient > chase > grab-bite.

As neonates, all breeds of dogs and all species of *Canis* display the same neonatal foraging behaviors: orient > root > attach > suckle > tread (Fuller & Dubuis, 1962; Levy, 1934; Rosenblatt, 1983; Scott, 1963). Adult foraging motor patterns first appear in the context of play during the critical period of socialization (Fox, 1969; Fox *et al.*, 1976; Scott & Marston, 1950; Serpell *et al.*, Chapter 6). Coppinger & Smith (1990) and Burghardt (2005) have suggested that play is the result of juveniles mixing together neonatal motor patterns (that are turning off) with adult motor patterns (that are turning on). As a general rule, the earlier these adult motor patterns appear during development the greater the likelihood that they will be displayed in the adult repertoire.

Lord (2010) tested this hypothesis by recording the first appearance, frequency, and sequencing of the hunting motor patterns in 11 wolves, 28 Shutzhund lineage German shepherds, and 13 herding lineage border collies. She found that foraging motor patterns that have an earlier onset are displayed at higher frequencies in intra-specific social and play behaviors. Environment appears to play some role in the onset of motor patterns. "Eye" appears significantly earlier in mother-reared German shepherds than in hand-raised German shepherds, suggesting that a particular environment initiated the first performance.

The evidence from our studies suggests that breed-typical behavior is the result of alterations in the onset of motor patterns. An early onset of a motor pattern increases the frequency in the adult behavior, whereas a late onset tends to reduce the frequency of display in adult behavior. Adult German shepherds that have a hypertrophied display of grab-bite show a very early onset of this motor pattern (29.5 days) (Lord, 2010), while livestock guarding dogs that rarely display grab-bite display this motor pattern for the first time at 6 months or later (Coppinger & Coppinger, 1993). Thus, just as with the face, a change in the timing of the development of motor patterns results in a novel adult behavior not a recreation of juvenile wolf behavior.

There is a misconception in the dog world that looking more like a wolf means that a dog will act more like a wolf and *vice versa*. Dog behavior only superficially resembles juvenile wolf behavior in that dogs do not show the adult wolf functional motor pattern sequence. While selection for a particular shape leads to a change in behavior there is no direct correlation between how much a dog looks like a wolf and how much it acts like a wolf. To say one novelty is more or less wolf-like is missing the point. All breeds evolved from the original dog and therefore no one dog breed is more closely related to the wolf. All breeds are new variations on the original dog theme.

The context in which these behaviors are displayed is largely determined by early experience. For example, livestock guarding dogs form species recognition patterns inter-specifically when raised with livestock animals during the critical period of social development. Similarly, border collies will not show the eye–stalk–chase behaviors toward species they have been socialized with during their critical period, although they will continue displaying these motor patterns at high frequencies toward species they were not raised with. Therefore, differences in the timing of this critical period could alter behavior.

The critical period of socialization has three developmental components: (1) onset of motor coordination; (2) onset of sensory systems; and (3) onset of fear. Altering the ontogenetic timing (heterochrony) of these components has a significant effect on the emerging adult behavior.

The critical period of socialization begins with the ability to walk and explore (Scott & Marston, 1950). Wolves begin to walk and explore at two weeks of age. Dogs begin to explore at four weeks of age (Fox, 1964; Rheingold, 1963; Scott & Fuller, 1965). Despite this two-week difference in the beginning of the critical period, the sensory development of both dogs and wolves is identical (Lord, 2013). Dogs and wolves are deaf until three weeks and functionally blind until they are four weeks old. Two-week-old wolves cannot see or hear and are exploring their environment with their noses (Figure 4.11a) (Lord, 2013). At the onset of a dog's critical period, it is exploring with scent, sound, and sight (Figure 4.11b).

The critical period of socialization is brought to a close by the avoidance of novelty (Scott & Fuller, 1965). This occurs at eight weeks in dog pups (Freedman *et al.*, 1960; Scott & Marston, 1950), and six weeks in wolf pups (Fentress, 1967; Woolpy & Ginsberg, 1967; Zimen, 1987). Previous literature has referred to the avoidance of novelty as the onset of fear, but this is a misnomer because

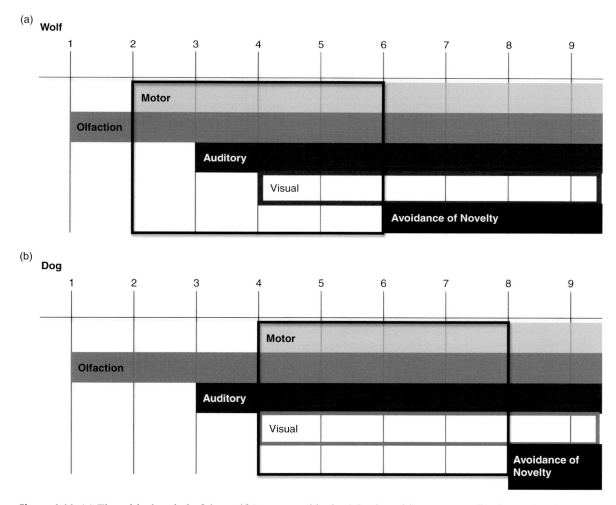

Figure 4.11 (a) The critical period of the wolf (represented by box) begins with motor coordination and ends with the avoidance of novelty, shown in relationship to the ability to smell, hear and see. (Modified from Lord, 2013.) (b) The critical period of the dog (represented by box) also begins with motor coordination and ends with avoidance of novelty, but has a very different relationship to the ability to smell, hear and see. (Modified from Lord, 2013.)

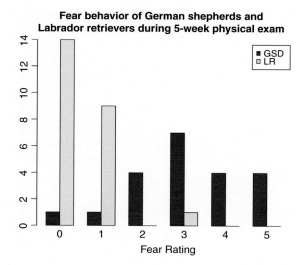

Fear behavior of German shepherds and Labrador retrievers during 5-week physical exam

Fear Rating

Figure 4.12 More German Shepherds showed higher levels of fear during their 5-week physical exam than Labrador retrievers, suggesting that German shepherds are closer to the end of their critical period than Labradors at this age.

fear starts weeks earlier and gradually increases until it reaches a threshold at which the animal avoids novelty. This confusing term, along with the inability to socialize wolves after the age of three weeks, has led some authors to suggest that the critical period in wolves closes at three weeks (see review in Miklósi, 2007). However, the so-called "fear" responses occurring at three weeks are based on the startle response triggered by the opening of the ears and not the avoidance of novelty (see Lord, 2013; Udell *et al.*, 2014).

This small two-week difference in the critical period results in a large change in early experience during a time when such experience can exert a dramatic influence on dogs' and wolves' adult behavior. Dogs have four weeks to explore their world using olfaction, audition and vision. Wolves, on the other hand, have four weeks to explore their world using olfaction, but only three weeks to explore it using audition, and two weeks to explore it using vision. Thus, species recognition by wolves is primarily olfactory, while dogs develop social recognition and attachments by smell, sound and sight (Hall *et al.*, 2015; Lord, 2013).

Smaller but similar differences in the critical period likely occur between breeds. In an unpublished study by Lord, 45 institutionally raised puppies, which included four litters of German shepherds (21 pups) and four litters of Labrador retrievers (24 pups) were observed at their first physical examination (a novel experience) at five weeks of age. Fear reactions were coded on a six-point scale, with zero being no fear reaction, and five being catatonic. German shepherd pups displayed fear more often and to a greater extent than Labrador retrievers. Moderate to extreme fear was exhibited by 90% of the German shepherds, while only 4% of the Labrador retrievers displayed even moderate fear (Figure 4.12).

These data suggest that these German shepherd pups were quickly reaching the avoidance of novelty (end of the critical period) ahead of schedule. Thus, German shepherds are more likely to reach the avoidance of novelty before they leave their institutional kennel environment. Labradors, on the other hand, are more likely to reach the end of the critical period after they arrive in a home, where they can experience varied novel stimuli such as children, car-rides, stairs, and traffic noise. Therefore, given the same rearing environment, the German shepherds would be more reactive and more fearful as adults than Labrador retrievers. This evidence has recently been supported by Morrow *et al.* (2015).

4.5 Conclusion

Several breeds of working dogs that perform tasks in concert with humans provide illustrations of how evolution can function effectively to give rise to new and specialized populations of animals. Darwin noted that some characteristics tended to change together, and concluded that the resulting condition was due to the "mysterious laws of correlation." Recent research has shown that the "mysterious laws" are governed by embryological developmental processes originating in neural crest cells, a concept that advances our understanding of how the unique behavior and shapes of working dogs could evolve so quickly.

Breeds of dogs are often referred to as if they were species – and why not? Dog breeds vary enormously in size, shape, color, and behavior – as if they were distinct species. Specialized working and hunting breeds give us an interesting view of how species-typical characteristics evolve. Point by point selection for new and unique behaviors will result in new and unique sizes, faces, and colors. Selection for some specific task or performance such as livestock guarding, pulling sleds, or herding has essentially rearranged the onset of motor patterns during the critical period or, indeed, the onset and offset of the critical period itself. Evolutionary changes in the ontogeny of motor patterns and in the onset and duration of the critical period have also, inadvertently, produced new and original colors and faces.

Acknowledgements

We want to thank Lynn Miller, Clive Wynne, and Ramon Escobedo Martinez for reviewing an earlier draft of the manuscript and making helpful comments. A special thanks to Lorna Coppinger for her help on reworking this chapter. In 1995 we singled out Valerius Geist for inspiring many of our thoughts on these difficult subjects. He continues to do so.

References

Alberch, P. (1982). The generative and regulatory roles of development in evolution. In *Environmental Adaptation and Evolution*, eds. D. Mossakowski & G. Roth, pp. 19–36. New York: Gustav Fischer.

Arons, C. D. & Shoemaker, W. J. (1992). The distributions of catecholamines and beta-endorphin in the brains of three behaviorally distinct breeds of dogs and their F$_1$ hybrids. *Brain Research*, 594: 31–9.

Belyaev, D. K. (1979). Destabilizing selection as a factor in domestication. *Journal of Heredity*, 70: 301–8.

Bemis, W. E. (1984). Paedomorphosis and the evolution of the Dipnoi. *Paleobiology*, 10: 293–307.

Black, H. L. & Green, J. S. (1985). Navajo use of mixed-breed dogs for management of predators. *Journal of Range Management*, 38: 11–15.

Bronner-Fraser, M. (1994). Neural crest cell formation and migration in the developing embryo. *The Journal of the Federation of American Societies for Experimental Biology*, 8: 699–706.

Burghardt, G. M. (2005). *The Genesis of Animal Play*. Cambridge, MA: The MIT Press.

Cairns, R. B. & Werboff, J. (1967). Behavior development in the dog: an interspecies analysis. *Science*, 158: 1070–2.

Coppinger, L. (1977). *The World of Sled Dogs*. New York: Howell Book House.

Coppinger, L. & Coppinger, R. P. (1982). Livestock-guarding dogs that wear sheep's clothing. *Smithsonian Magazine*, April, 64–73.

Coppinger, L. & Coppinger, R. P. (1993). Dogs for herding and guarding livestock. In *Livestock Handling and Transport*, ed. T. Grandin. Cambridge, MA: CAB International, pp. 179–96.

Coppinger, R. P., Coppinger, L., Langeloh, G., Gettler, L. & Lorenz, J. (1988). A decade of use of livestock guarding dogs. In *Proceedings of the Vertebrate Pest Conference*, Vol. 13, eds. A. C. Crabb & R. E. Marsh. Davis, CA: University of California, pp. 209–14.

Coppinger, R. P. & Coppinger, L. (2001). *Dogs: A Startling New Understanding of Canine Origin, Behavior & Evolution*. New York: Scribner.

Coppinger, R. P. & Coppinger, L. (2016). *What is a Dog?* Chicago, IL: University of Chicago Press.

Coppinger, R. P. & Feinstein, M. (2015). *How Dogs Work*. Chicago, IL: University of Chicago Press.

Coppinger, R. P., Glendinning, J., Torop, E., Matthay, C, Sutherland, M. & Smith, C. (1987). Degree of behavioral neoteny differentiates canid polymorphs. *Ethology*, 75: 89–108.

Coppinger, R. P. & Schneider, R. (1995). Evolution of working dogs. In *The Domestic Dog: Its Evolution, Behaviour and Interactions with People*, ed. J. Serpell. Cambridge: Cambridge University Press, pp. 21–47.

Coppinger, R. P. & Smith, C. K. (1990). A model for understanding the evolution of mammalian behavior. In *Current Mammalogy*, Vol. 2, ed. H. Genoways. New York: Plenum, pp. 335–74.

Coppinger, R. P., Smith, C. K. & Miller, L. (1985). Observations on why mongrels may make effective livestock protecting dogs. *Journal of Range Management*, 38: 560–1.

Coppinger, R. P., Spector, L. & Miller, L. (2010). What if anything is a wolf? In *The World of Wolves: New Perspectives on Ecology, Behaviour and Management*, eds. M. Musiani, L. Boitani & P. Paquet. Calgary, Canada: University of Calgary Press, pp. 41–67.

Couly, G. F., Coltey, P., Eichmann, A. & Le Douarin, N. M. (1995). The angiogenic potentials of the cephalic mesoderm and the origin of brain and head blood vessels. *Mechanisms of Development*, 53: 97–112.

Couly, G. F., Coltey, P. M. & Le Douarin, N. M. (1992). The developmental fate of the cephalic mesoderm in quail-chick chimera. *Development*, 114: 1–15.

Couly, G. F., Coltey, P. M. & Le Douarin, N. M. (1993). The triple origin of skull in higher vertebrates: a study in quail-chick chimeras. *Development*, 117: 409–29.

Couly, G. F., & Le Douarin, N. M. (1988). The fate map of the cephalic neural primordium at the presomitic to the 3-somite stage in the avian embryo. *Development*, 103: 101–13.

Cramer, S. F. (1991). The origin of epidermal melanocytes. Implications for the histogenesis of nevi and melanomas. *Archives of Pathology & Laboratory Medicine*, 115: 115–19.

Crockford, S. J. (2002). Animal domestication and heterochronic speciation. In *Human Evolution through Developmental Change*, eds. N. Minughpurvis & K. J. McNamara. Baltimore, MD: Johns Hopkins University Press, pp. 122–53.

Darwin, C. (1858). Abstract of a Letter from C. Darwin, Esq., to Prof. Asa Gray, Boston, U.S. dated Down, September 5th, 1857. *Proceedings of the Linnean Society of London, Zoology*, 3: 50–3.

Drake, A. G. (2011). Dispelling dog dogma: an investigation of heterochrony in dogs using 3D geometric morphometric analysis of skull shape. *Evolution & Development*, 13: 204–13.

Eames, B. F. & Schneider, R. A. (2005). Quail-duck chimeras reveal spatiotemporal plasticity in molecular and histogenic programs of cranial feather development. *Development*, 132: 1499–509.

Eames, B. F. & Schneider, R. A. (2008). The genesis of cartilage size and shape during development and evolution. *Development* 135: 3947–58.

Eldredge, N. & Gould, S. J. (1972). Punctuated equilibria: an alternative to phyletic gradualism. In *Models in Paleobiology*, ed. T. J. M. Schopf. San Francisco, CA: Freeman Cooper, pp. 82–115.

Fentress, J. C. (1967). Observations on the behavioral development of a hand-reared male timber wolf. *American Zoologist*, 7: 339–351.

Fentress, J. C. & McLoed, P. J. (1986). Motor patterns in development. In *Handbook of Behavioral Neurobiology. Vol. 8 Developmental Psychobiology and Developmental Neurobiology*, ed. E. M. Blass. New York: Plenum Press, pp. 35–97.

Fox, M. W. (1964). The ontogeny of behaviour and neurologic responses in the dog. *Animal Behaviour*, 12: 301–310.

Fox, M. W. (1965). *Canine Behavior*. Springfield, IL: Charles C. Thomas.

Fox, M. (1969). Behavioral effects of rearing dogs with cats during the "critical period of socialization." *Behaviour*, 35: 273–280.

Fox, M. W. (1971). *Integrative Development of Brain and Behavior in the Dog*. Chicago, IL: University of Chicago Press.

Fox, M. W. (1975). Behavior genetics of F1 and F2 coyote-dog hybrids. *Applied Animal Ethology*, 1: 185–95.

Fox, M. W. (1978). *The Dog: Its Domestication and Behavior*. New York: Garland STPM Press.

Fox, M. W. & Bekoff, M. (1975). The behaviour of dogs. In *The Behaviour of Domestic Animals*, 3rd edition, ed. E. S. E. Hafez. London: Baillière Tindall, pp. 370–409.

Fox, M. W., Halperin, S., Wise, A. & Kohn, E. (1976). Species and hybrid differences in frequencies of play and agonistic actions in Canids. *Zeitchrift fur Tierpsychologie*, 40: 194–209.

Frank, H. & Frank, M. G. (1982). On the effects of domestication on canine social development and behavior. *Applied Animal Ethology*, 8: 507–25.

Freedman, D. G., King, J. A. & Elliot, O. (1960). Critical period in the social development of dogs. *Science*, 133: 1016–17.

Fuller, J. L. & Dubois, E. M. (1962). The behavior of dogs. In *The Behavior of Domestic Animals*, ed. E. S. Hafez. Baltimore, MD: The Williams & Wilkins Company, pp. 415–52.

Geist, V. (1971). *Mountain Sheep: A Study in Behavior and Evolution*. Chicago, IL: University of Chicago Press.

Geist, V. (1987). On speciation in ice age mammals, with special reference to cervids and caprids. *Canadian Journal of Zoology*, 65: 1067–84.

Goodwin, D., Bradshaw, J. W. S. & Wickens, S. M. (1997). Paedomorphosis affects agonistic visual signals of domestic dogs. *Animal Behaviour*, 53: 297–304.

Haldane, J. B. S. (1930). *The Causes of Evolution*. London: Longmans Green.

Hall, N., Lord, K., Arnold, A., Udell, M. & Wynne, C. (2015). Assessment of attachment behaviour to human caregivers in wolf pups (Canis lupus lupus). *Behavioural Processes*, 110: 15–21.

Hirobe, T. (1995). Structure and function of melanocytes: microscopic morphology and cell biology of mouse melanocytes in the epidermis and hair follicle. *Histology and Histopathy*, 10, 223–37.

Hole, F. & Wyllie, C. (2007). The oldest depictions of canines and a possible early breed of dog in Iran. *Paléorient*, 33: 175–85.

Jones, M. (1988). *The Dogs of Capitalism; Book 1: Origins.* Austin, TX: Twenty First Century Logic.

Lantis, M. (1980). Changes in the Alaskan Eskimo relation of man to dog and their effect on two human diseases. *Arctic Anthropology*, 17: 2–24.

Larson, G. (2011). Genetics and domestication: important questions for new answers. *Current Anthropology*, 52: S485–95.

Larson, G., Karlsson, E. K, Perri, A. *et al.* (2012). Rethinking dog domestication by integrating genetics archeology, and biogeography. *Proceedings of the National Academy of Sciences of the United States of America*, 109: 8878–83.

Le Douarin, N. M. & Dupin, E. (1993). Cell lineage analysis in neural crest ontogeny. *Journal of Neurobiology*, 24: 146–61.

Le Lièvre, C. S. & Le Douarin N. M. (1975). Mesenchymal derivatives of the neural crest: analysis of chimaeric quail and chick embryos. *Journal of Embryology & Experimental Morphology*. 34: 125–54.

Le Quellec, J. L. (2006). Rock art and cultural responses to climatic changes in the Central Sahara during the Holocene. In *Exploring the Mind of Ancient Man*, ed. P. C. Reddy. New Delhi: Research India Press, pp. 173–88.

Levy, D. M. (1934). Experiments on the sucking reflex and social behavior of dogs. *American Journal of Orthopsychiatry*, 4: 203–24.

Lord, K. (2010). A heterochronic explanation for the behaviorally polymorphic genus Canis: a study of the development of behavioral differences in dogs (*Canis lupus familiaris*) and wolves (*Canis lupus lupus*) (Doctoral Dissertation). Retrieved from Electronic Doctoral Dissertations for Umass Amherst. Paper AAI3409623.

Lord, K. (2013). A comparison of the sensory development of wolves (*Canis lupus lupus*) and dogs (*Canis lupus familiaris*). *Ethology*. 119: 110–20.

Lord, K., Feinstein, M. & Coppinger, R. (2009). Barking and mobbing. *Behavioural Processes*, 81: 358–68.

Lord, K., Feinstein, M., Smith, B. & Coppinger, R. (2013). Variation in reproductive traits of members of the genus Canis with special attention to the domestic dog (*Canis familiaris*). *Behavioural Processes*, 92: 131–42.

Løvtrup, S. (1977). *The Phylogeny of Vertebrata.* London: John Wiley.

Løvtrup, S. (1987). *Darwinism: The Refutation of a Myth.* London: Croom Helm.

MacRury, I. K. (1991). The Inuit Dog: its provenance, environment and history. Unpublished M.Phil. Thesis, Scott Polar Research Institute, University of Cambridge.

Miklósi, A. (2007). *Dog Behaviour, Evolution, and Cognition.* Oxford: Oxford University Press.

Morrow, M., Ottobre, J., Ottobre, A. *et al.* (2015). Breed-dependent differences in the onset of fear-related avoidance behavior in puppies. *Journal of Veterinary Behavior*, 10: 286–94.

Muro, C., Escobedo, R., Spector, L. & Coppinger, R. P. (2011). Wolf-pack (*Canis lupus*) hunting strategies emerge from simple rules in computational simulations. *Behavioural Processes*, 88: 192–97.

Noden, D. M. (1978). The control of avian cephalic neural crest cytodifferentiation. I. skeletal and connective tissues. *Developmental Biology*. 67: 296–312.

Noden, D. M. (1983). The embryonic origins of avian cephalic and cervical muscles and associated connective tissues. *The American Journal of Anatomy*, 168: 257–76.

Noden, D. M. & Schneider, R. A. (2006). Neural crest cells and the community of plan for craniofacial development: historical debates and current perspectives. *Advances in Experimental Medicine and Biology*. 589: 1–23.

Phillips, C. J., Coppinger, R. P. & Schimel, D. S. (1981). Hyperthermia in running sled dogs. *Journal of Applied Physiology*, 51: 135–42.

Price E.O. (1984) Behavioral aspects of domestication. *Quarterly Review of Biology*. 59, 1–32

Rawles, M. E. (1948). Origin of melanophores and their role in the development of color pattern in vertebrates. *Physiological Reviews*, 28: 383–408.

Rheingold, H. L. (1963). Maternal behavior in the dog. In *Maternal Behavior in Mammals*, ed. H. L. Rheingold. New York: John Wiley & Sons, Inc., pp. 169–202.

Richardson, M. K. & Sieber-Blum, M. (1993). Pluripotent neural crest cells in the developing skin of the quail embryo. *Developmental Biology*, 157: 348–58.

Rosenblatt, J. S. (1983). Olfaction mediates developmental transitions in the newborn of selected species of mammals. *Journal of Neurobiology*, 14: 347–75.

Sánchez-Villagra, M. R., Geiger, M. & Schneider, R. A. (2015). The taming of the neural crest: a developmental perspective on the origins of morphological covariation in domesticated mammals. *Royal Society Open Science*, 3: 160107.

Sands, M. W., Coppinger, R. P. & Phillips, C. J. (1977). Comparisons of thermal sweating and histology of sweat glands of selected canids. *Journal of Mammalogy*, 58: 74–8.

Schneider, R. A. (1999). Neural crest can form cartilages normally derived from mesoderm during development of the avian head skeleton. *Developmental Biology*, 208: 441–55.

Schneider, R. A. (2005). Developmental mechanisms facilitating the evolution of bills and quills. *Journal of Anatomy*, 207: 563–573.

Schneider, R. A. (2015). Regulation of jaw length during development, disease, and evolution. *Current Topics in Developmental Biology*, 115: 271–98.

Schneider, R. A. & Helms, J. A. (2003). The cellular and molecular origins of beak morphology. *Science*, 299: 565–8.

Scott, J. P. (1963). The process of socialization in canine and human infants. *Monographs of the Society for Research in Child Development*, 28: 1–47.

Scott, J. P. & Fuller, J. L. (1965). *Genetics and the Social Behavior of the Dog.* Chicago, IL: University of Chicago Press.

Scott, J. P. & Marston, M. (1950). Critical periods affecting the development of normal and mal-adjustive social behavior of puppies. *The Journal of Genetic Psychology*, 77: 25–60.

Stanley, W. C. & Elliot, O. (1962). Differential human handling as reinforcing events and as treatments influencing later social behavior in basenji puppies. *Psychological Reports*, 10: 775–88.

Stebbins, G. L. (1959). The role of hybridization in evolution. *Proceedings of the American Philosophical Society*, 103: 231–51.

Stockard, C. R. (1941). The genetic and endocrinic basis for differences in form and behavior. *American Anatomical Memoirs*, 19: Philadelphia, PA: Wistar Institute of Anatomy and Biology.

Twitty, V. C. (1966). *Of Scientists and Salamanders.* San Francisco, CA: W. H. Freeman.

Udell, M., Lord, K., Feuerbacher, E. & Wynne, C. (2014). What is a human from a dog's perspective. In *Dog Behavior and Cognition*, ed. A. Horowitz, New York, NY: Springer, pp. 221–40.

Waddington, C. H. (1957). *The Strategy of the Genes.* London: George Allan and Unwin.

Webb, J. F. & Noden D. M. (1993). Ectodermal Placodes: Contributions to the development of the vertebrate head. *American Zoologist*, 33: 434–47.

Wilkins, A. S., Wrangham, R. W., & Fitch, W. T. (2014). The "domestication syndrome" in mammals: a unified explanation based on neural crest cell behavior and genetics. *Genetics*, 197: 795–808.

Woolpy, J. H. & Ginsburg, B. E. (1967). Wolf socialization: a study of temperament in a wild social species. *American Zoologist*, 7: 357–63.

Zimen, E. (1987). Ontogeny of approach and flight behavior toward humans in wolves, poodles and wolf-poodle hybrids. In *Man and Wolf*, ed. H. Frank. Dordrecht, Netherlands: Dr. W. Junk Publishers, pp. 275–92.

Part II

Behavior, cognition and training

5 Genetics of dog behavior

LINDA VAN DEN BERG

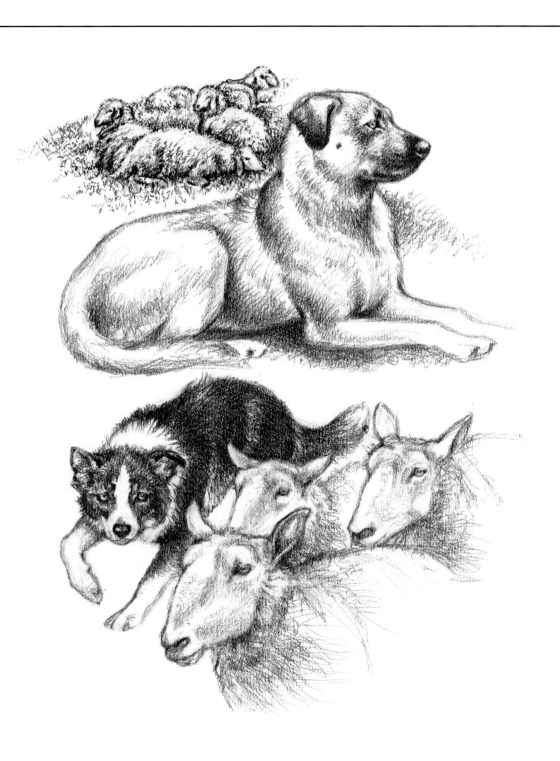

5.1   Introduction

Selection for behavior has played a key role in the history of dog domestication and breeding. Early dog domestication probably involved selection for tameness. A few generations of selection for tameness in the famous Russian silver fox experiments led to a domesticated strain of foxes that showed dog-like behavior and displayed curly tails, drop ears, and loss of pigment (Trut *et al.*, 2009). The early domestication of dogs was followed by the formation of dog breeds. Different aspects of ancestral wolf behavior have been selected for in different breeds: dogs have been bred to guard, herd, hunt, pull sleds, and to provide companionship. Selection for physical appearance became more important at a later stage when people began breeding dogs for show. Extreme population bottlenecks,[1] founder effects,[2] drift[3] and strong artificial selection for desired traits during breed formation have resulted in a dog population that is a collection of genetic isolates with highly diverging morphology, disease susceptibility, and behavioral characteristics (Sutter & Ostrander, 2004).

Scott and Fuller (1965) performed a pioneering study of breed differences and inheritance of canine behavior. Their experiment involved dogs of five breeds: basenji, beagle, American cocker spaniel, Shetland sheepdog and wire-haired fox terrier. Breeds and their crosses were compared for reactivity, trainability and problem-solving behaviors. Scott and Fuller observed behavioral differences between the breeds in the majority of their behavioral tests; for instance, in playful aggression and dominance. Wire-haired fox terriers were the most aggressive, consistently "ganging up" on group members. These attacks were so serious that victims had to be removed in order to prevent serious injury. More recently, Svartberg (2006) compared the behavior of 31 dog breeds using data from a standard behavioral test. Significant breed differences were observed for all investigated traits (Figure 5.1). Dog breeds also differ in the prevalence of problem behavior. For instance, certain breeds are predisposed to obsessive-compulsive behaviors: bull terriers frequently exhibit tail chasing, while Doberman pinschers are prone to acral licking.

The fact that breed differences in behavior exist, and that behavioral dispositions can be selected for, suggests that there is a genetic basis for behavior. Behavioral genetics is the study of the individual variation in behavior due to genetic differences between animals. Behavioral genetic studies in dogs have traditionally been studies of breed differences, selection studies, and population-based heritability studies. More recently, researchers have attempted to identify genetic variants that explain behavior at the molecular level. This chapter reviews both the earlier heritability studies and the more recent molecular genetic studies of behavioral traits in dogs.

---

[1]A population bottleneck is a marked reduction in population size followed by the survival and expansion of a small random sample of the original population. Many dog breeds experienced bottlenecks at times of war and economic depression.

[2]When a species invades a new area, the original, small population is called a founder population. The term is usually applied in a context of subsequent population growth. Recent founder populations exhibit reduced genetic variation due to the population bottleneck. Many dog breeds were established from a small number of founders. Genetic homogeneity is maintained in dogs by the "breed barrier rule," i.e. no dog may become a registered member of a breed unless both its parents are registered members of the same breed. In other words, dog breeds are genetic isolates.

[3]Drift refers to changes in allele frequency over generations due to random factors. It leads to lower genetic variation, especially in small populations. All dog breeds have been subject to drift.

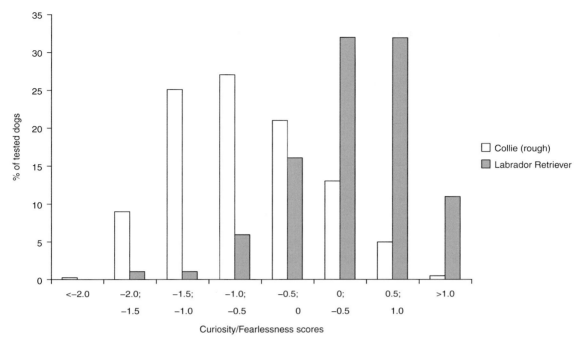

Figure 5.1 Results of the study of breed-typical behavior (Svartberg, 2006). The distribution of curiosity/fearlessness scores in the Dog Mentality Assessment (DMA) behavioral test is shown for two dog breeds: collies and Labrador retrievers. Labradors were the highest ranking breed for this trait and collies ranked the lowest. Despite substantial within-breed variation, the means of the distributions of the two breeds are shifted with respect to each other. (Figure reprinted from Svartberg (2006) with permission from Elsevier.)

5.2   Quantifying the genetic influence on behavior: Heritability

5.2.1   Principles of heritability studies

People that use dogs as working animals are obviously interested in knowing the degree to which behavioral variation is correlated with genetic variation. Heritability (h^2) is a measure of the relative contribution of additive genetic effects[4] to the total variance observed in a trait (Bourdon, 1997; Nicholas, 2003). It can also be described as the proportion of the parental deviation from the population average that is transmitted to the offspring. Total variance in a trait is comprised of a genetic part and a non-genetic part. The latter arises from environmental effects and is often called environmental variance or residual variance.[5] Heritability estimates are ratios and can thus

[4]The term "additive genetic effects" refers to the effect of independent genes. Non-additive genetic effects are gene combination effects, i.e. dominance or epistasis.

[5]Environment in behavioral genetics refers to all factors other than inherited factors. Examples in dogs include prenatal circumstances (such as stress in the pregnant bitch) and early experiences such as maternal care (Scott & Fuller, 1965), living conditions at the home of the breeder (Appleby *et al.*, 2002), illness as a puppy (Podberscek & Serpell, 1997), and socialization (Appleby *et al.*, 2002; Houpt and Willis, 2001; Scott & Fuller, 1965; see also Serpell *et al.*, Chapter 6).

be influenced by changes in environmental variation. For instance, h^2 estimates will increase if animals are assessed in a consistent manner because this will lead to reduced experimental variation. The estimates also often differ between male and female dogs. Strictly speaking, h^2 estimates only apply to the population from which they were derived in the time period when they were assessed. In spite of these limitations, h^2 estimates can provide a broad guide to the relative contributions of genetic and environmental influences on population variance of a trait. Heritabilities may predict the consequences of various selection procedures. Highly heritable traits are expected to respond well to direct selection and performance testing. Traits with a low h^2 may require progeny selection[6] or the use of crossbreeding to produce genetic advantages.

Heritability estimations are based on resemblances between relatives. Family, adoption, and twin designs have been used to estimate the h^2 of behavioral traits in humans (Boomsma *et al.*, 2002). Such studies have shown that there is a significant genetic influence on the majority of human behaviors examined. Heritability estimates for some mental disorders in humans are very high, e.g. 0.90 for autism (Burmeister *et al.*, 2008). Older heritability studies in dogs often used paternal half-sib correlations, i.e. correlations between the performances of different progeny sired by a particular father.[7] Only the performance of the progeny is required, not that of the sire. An alternative method is offspring-parent regressions, using either one parent (usually the sire) or the average of both parents (termed offspring-midparent regressions). The performance of both offspring and parents are used in these types of study. Modern heritability studies use data about all available individuals by applying Best Linear Unbiased Prediction (BLUP) techniques (Henderson, 1975). In BLUP, breeding values of individual dogs are calculated based on phenotypic information on the dog itself, its parents, siblings, half-siblings, its progeny, as well as more distantly related dogs. Several reviews discuss the heritability of behavioral traits in dogs, particularly in relation to working behavior, temperament, and behavior problems (Hall & Wynne, 2012; Houpt & Willis, 2001; Hradecká *et al.*, 2015; Mackenzie *et al.*, 1986; Ruefenacht *et al.*, 2002). Heritability estimates for canine behavioral traits are mostly in the low to moderate range. This is no surprise because traits that have undergone selection in the past are expected to show reduced additive genetic variance (Fisher, 1930).

5.2.2 Heritability of canine working behavior

Dogs were originally selected for working behavior, e.g. herding, guarding, hunting, and pulling sleds. As a result, retrievers retrieve and pointers point. The results of selection for working behavior can also be observed in the canine genome. For instance, Huson *et al.* (2010) observed that the genetic profile of Alaskan sled dogs bred for sprint racing differs from that of Alaskan sled dogs bred for running long-distance races. Many publications present heritability estimates of performance in canine working tests (see Ruefenacht *et al.*, 2002; Hall & Wynne, 2012 for reviews). In most of these studies, large numbers of dogs were exposed to a range of standard situations, and their behavior scored by trained test leaders. Heritability estimates for these kinds of scored traits are mostly in the low to moderate range, e.g. between 0.09 and 0.24 in the German shepherd field behavior test (Ruefenacht *et al.*, 2002), between 0.1 and 0.4 in the flat-coated retriever hunting behavior test (Lindberg *et al.*, 2004), between 0.14 to 0.50 for herding behavior in border collies (Arvelius *et al.*, 2009), between 0.07 and

---

[6]Progeny selection indicates choice of breeding animals based on phenotypes of their offspring. This differs from direct selection, where breeding animals are chosen based on their own phenotype.

[7]This is typically a study design with several sires that are each mated to several different dams. Progeny of a single dam are full siblings (sibs). Progeny produced by different dams, but from the same sire, are half-siblings.

0.18 for defense abilities in Belgian shepherd dogs (Courreau & Langlois, 2005), and between 0.15 and 0.32 for service dog performance (Wilsson & Sundgren, 1997a). For some traits, higher heritabilities were found. For example, "waiting passively in a group" in the hunting behavior test of the Swedish flat-coated retriever club had an estimated h^2 of 0.74 (Lindberg *et al.*, 2004).

5.2.3   Heritability of dog personality

Personality or temperament can be defined as "underlying behavioral tendencies that differ across individuals, that are consistent within individuals over time, and that affect the behavior that is expressed in different contexts" (Stamps & Groothuis, 2010, p. 302). The Swedish dog mentality assessment test (DMA) is designed to provide insight into canine personality traits. The DMA is a standardized behavioral test that consists of 10 subtests, during which dogs are exposed to several different situations. The reactions of the dogs are recorded for 33 behavioral variables. Svartberg & Forkman (2002) collected DMA data from 1175 dogs of 47 breeds. The investigators performed factor analysis[8] on these variables and extracted five primary factors: (1) playfulness; (2) curiosity/ fearlessness; (3) chase-proneness; (4) sociability; and (5) aggressiveness. Svartberg (2006) analyzed DMA scores from 13 097 dogs of 31 breeds and reported substantial breed differences in personality (Figure 5.1). Higher order factor analysis showed that all factors except aggressiveness were related to each other, creating a broad factor that influences behavior in a range of situations. This broad factor is comparable to the shyness-boldness axis in humans, which reflects a tendency to approach novel objects and a willingness to take risks (Wilson *et al.*, 1994). This broad dimension is supported by the results of earlier dog studies, and a similar dimension was also detected in silver foxes (Kukekova *et al.*, 2011a). It was found to be related to performance in working tests (tracking, searching, delivering messages, handler protection): high-performing dogs were bolder than low-performing dogs (Svartberg, 2002). Saetre *et al.* (2006) estimated the heritability of the DMA behavioral traits using 10 000 German shepherd and Rottweiler dogs that all completed the DMA. Their results suggest that there is shared genetics behind all behavioral traits except in those related to aggression. Heritabilities were generally low, ranging from 0.04 (remaining fear) to 0.19 (tug-of-war). The heritability of shyness–boldness was estimated to be 0.25 in these two different breed samples. Several smaller heritability studies have used measures other than the DMA for personality traits. Ruefenacht *et al.* (2002) reviewed these studies and reported that heritability estimates for traits related to canine personality range from 0 to 0.58 with an average of 0.20.

5.2.4   Heritability of problem behavior

Canine behavioral problems such as aggression, anxiety and obsessive compulsive behaviors pose serious threats to canine welfare. Behavioral problems accounted for 24% of dogs euthanized in Danish veterinary practices in a study of Mikkelsen and Lund (2000). Problem behavior is usually normal behavior manifested in extreme or inappropriate ways. An example is fearfulness. Fear is an instinctive natural response to a threat. For the majority of dogs, fear is of short duration and increases the chance of escaping danger. For dogs with an anxiety disorder, the state of fear lasts much longer and the dog may become extremely sensitive to any perceived threat. The most

---

[8]Factor analysis is a statistical method that aims to reduce a large number of variables to a smaller number of underlying variables (factors) based on the pattern of correlation between the variables.

common anxiety disorders in dogs are separation anxiety, noise phobia, thunderstorm phobia, and generalized anxiety (Bamberger and Houpt, 2006). Selection experiments and studies of breed differences suggest that a genetic component plays a role in the development of these disorders. For instance, Scott and Fuller (1965) found that all basenji puppies showed some fear response during a handling test compared to only 38% of cocker spaniel puppies. Another example is the work with nervous pointer dogs involving two collaborating research groups in Arkansas, USA. They established two breeding lines of pointers that were maintained for decades (Dykman *et al.*, 1966). One line showed extreme fearfulness and avoidance of novel stimuli. The other was a stable control population. The nervous pointer dogs are considered a genetic animal model of severe anxiety. Goddard & Beilharz (1982; 1983) published papers on the heritability of traits that determine the suitability of dogs as guide dogs for the blind. Fearfulness was the most frequent cause of failure of potential guide dogs. It was measured with a behavioral test, scoring nervousness, suspicion, sound shyness, and anxiety. Fearfulness was estimated to have a heritability of 0.46–0.5 in this population of dogs (Goddard and Beilharz, 1982; 1983).

Aggressive behavior is also related to guide dog failure (Takeuchi *et al.*, 2009a). Aggression is relatively well studied in dogs because of its serious implications for the bond between dog and owner (De Keuster *et al.*, 2006; Landsberg, 2004; Mikkelsen & Lund, 2000). Like fearfulness, canine aggression is usually normal behavior (Borchelt and Voith, 1996; Mills, 2003; Mugford, 1984; Reisner, 1997). Wolves use aggression to defend themselves from predators and to compete for food, territory, social status, or reproductive opportunities. Situations that elicit aggressive behavior in wolves can also elicit aggression in dogs. There are several kinds of aggression and the subtypes seem to have a distinct genetic basis (Lesch and Merschdorf, 2000; Popova *et al.*, 1993; Yeh *et al.*, 2010). Some breeds have intentionally been selected for aggressiveness. For instance, Rottweilers, Dobermans, and German shepherds have been selected for stranger-directed aggression and American pit bull terriers have been selected for fighting purposes (Lockwood and Rindy, 1987; see also Lockwood, Chapter 9). There is substantial scientific evidence for breed differences in aggressiveness (e.g. Beaver, 1993; Blackshaw, 1991; Borchelt, 1983; Bradshaw *et al.*, 1996; Duffy *et al.*, 2008; Hart & Miller, 1985; Landsberg, 1991; Wilsson & Sundgren, 1997b). Some early studies of aggression-related traits in police or military dogs failed to produce h^2 estimates higher than zero (Reuterwall & Ryman, 1973; Willis, 1976). However, this is probably due to methodological problems (Houpt & Willis, 2001; Mackenzie *et al.*, 1986). Heritabilities of aggression in the DMA were low but significant: between 0.06 and 0.12 (Saetre *et al.*, 2006). Courreau & Langlois (2005) reported heritabilities of 0.14–0.16 for aggressive behavior in defense competitions of Belgian shepherd dogs. Pérez-Guisado *et al.* (2006) obtained an h^2 estimate of 0.33 for dominant-aggressive behavior in the Campbell test. It thus seems that the heritability of aggression is low but significant in the general dog population, although it may be much higher in specific dog populations (e.g. Liinamo *et al.*, 2007).

5.3   Finding the underlying genes: Behavioral gene mapping

5.3.1   Principles of gene mapping

People are also interested in pinpointing the genetic variants that explain the inheritance of behavioral traits, i.e. gene mapping. Such molecular genetic information may facilitate the development of genetic tests that can be applied in dog breeding. Gene mapping is based on the assumption that a mutation that affects protein structure or level occurred in the germline of an ancestral dog. Such a mutation is referred to as the causative (or causal or functional) variant. Scientists use flanking polymorphisms[9] to determine the position of the causative variant in the genome. Examples of such polymorphisms are single nucleotide polymorphisms (SNPs[10]), variable number of tandem repeats (VNTRs[11]), and short interspersed nuclear elements (SINEs[12]). The polymorphisms are referred to as polymorphic markers in this context.

If the trait of interest is monogenic (i.e. variation in the trait is influenced by variation in a single gene), we expect a simple relationship between causative variant and trait, e.g. all Labrador and golden retrievers with a premature stop codon in the melanocyte-stimulating hormone receptor gene have a yellow coat (Everts et al., 2000). Such variants can be mapped using linkage analysis in dog pedigrees (e.g. Acland et al., 1998). In complex traits such as behavior, a single mutation is likely to have only a small effect on the trait (see Box 5.1). The relationship between causal variant and trait is then diluted by variation in other genetic factors and the environment. Linkage analysis is less suitable in this situation. Association studies are used for mapping the polygenes involved in complex traits. In association studies, genotypes are correlated with a quantitative trait (quantitative trait association study) or allele frequencies are compared between cases and controls (case-control study design).

Association studies can focus on candidate genes or apply a genome-wide approach. Candidate genes are chosen based on pre-existing data derived from pharmacological, physiological, biochemical, anatomical, or knockout mouse studies. In behavioral genetic studies they often involve brain neurotransmitter systems. The selection of candidate genes is necessarily based on limited understanding of the biological pathways involved in the trait. Further progress in behavioral trait mapping is expected with genome wide association studies (GWAS). In a GWAS, the complete genome is scanned for association with a trait in multiple unrelated individuals using a large number of SNPs. Here, there is no a priori assumption about which genes are involved in the phenotype. This opens the opportunity for finding genes that have not been associated with behavior to date. Such analyses have only recently become possible because of the sophisticated genomic resources and the large number of subjects required.

[9] A polymorphism is the occurrence of two or more versions of the same DNA fragment in a population. In other words, a polymorphism is a variation in DNA sequence from a reference sequence. A polymorphism is the result of a single random mutation which has spread through the population by inheritance. Note that the difference between a mutation and a polymorphism is their population frequency: when the frequency of a mutation rises above 1%, it is referred to as a polymorphism. The general term "genetic variant" refers to both mutations and polymorphisms. A polymorphism can be neutral or it can affect protein structure or level.

[10] A SNP is a DNA sequence variation where a single nucleotide differs between individuals. Millions of SNPs have been identified in the genome of the dog: about one nucleotide position in every 900 is variable. The dog genome project resulted in a catalogue of the positions of more than two million SNPs.

[11] A VNTR is a short nucleotide sequence that is organized as a tandem repeat. The length of VNTRs varies between individuals, i.e. multiple alleles exist in the population.

[12] A SINE is a stretch of DNA of less than 500 nucleotides in length. SINES are able to replicate and re-insert themselves into the genome to produce mutations by inserting near or within genes. SINEs represent about 7% of the dog genome sequence (Kirkness et al., 2003).

Box 5.1 Genetic architecture of behavior: Lessons from human genetics

Behavior is produced by intricate neural networks that are developed and maintained under influence of a variety of genes and environmental factors (Hamer, 2002; Robinson, 2004). Some of the genes involved in the regulation of behavior may have the same DNA sequence in all individuals, i.e. they are monomorphic. Such genes are important for the regulation of behavior, but they do not contribute to individual *variation* in behavior. Other genes are polymorphic, i.e. different versions of the gene exist in the general population. A genetic polymorphism may affect the structure of the protein encoded by the gene or the level, timing, or tissue-specific expression of certain proteins. Selection – natural or artificial – alters the frequency of genetic polymorphisms and in this way eventually leads to phenotypic changes at the population level.

An illustrative example of a gene involved in the regulation of behavior in humans is the gene encoding monoamine oxidase A (*MAOA*). The MAOA enzyme catalyzes the degradation of the neurotransmitters serotonin, dopamine, and norepinephrine in the brain. These neurotransmitters are involved in the regulation of mood (Fan *et al.*, 2010). Brunner *et al.* (1993) described a Dutch family with a point mutation[13] in *MAOA*. Male members of this family produced no MAOA enzyme because the mutation caused a premature stop codon.[14] These males were mentally retarded and showed impulsive violent behavior, including arson, rape, and murder. The researchers hypothesized that accumulation of the neurotransmitters that are normally degraded by the MAOA enzyme lowered the threshold for aggression in these men when under stress (Brunner *et al.*, 1993).

The Dutch family had a rare mutation that completely destroyed the function of the *MAOA* gene. The normal range of behavioral variation in humans is the result of many genetic variants with a small effect in combination with environmental influences (Plomin, 1990). In other words, behavior is a complex trait. This is also illustrated by the gene *MAOA*. In the general human population, there are two forms of the *MAOA* gene: a form that is highly expressed and gives rise to high levels of MAOA enzyme, and a low-expressed form. Caspi *et al.* (2002) studied this polymorphism in a large cohort of male subjects that had been followed from birth to adulthood. The aim of the study was to determine why some children who are maltreated grow up to develop antisocial behavior, whereas others do not. Animal studies suggest that maltreatment alters serotonin, dopamine, and norepinephrine neurotransmitter systems in the brain in ways that can influence behavior later in life. Caspi *et al.* (2002) found that childhood maltreatment was a much stronger predictor of adult antisocial behavior in children with a genotype conferring low levels of MAOA expression (Figure 5.2). This suggests that MAOA levels in these children are insufficient to constrain maltreatment-induced changes to neurotransmitter systems. We can conclude that behavior in the general human population is a complex polygenic trait, but that a disruption (e.g. a mutation that causes a premature stop codon) of one of these polygenes can result in a severe deregulation of development.

As in humans, the normal range of behavioral variation in dogs is probably regulated by multiple genetic variants (rare or common) and environmental influences. However, it has been argued that the genetic regulation of complex traits may be simpler in dogs than in humans and that the genetic variants involved have larger effects (Lindblad-Toh *et al.*, 2005). For instance, Boyko *et al.* (2010) needed only two to six genetic loci[15] to explain a large

---

[13] A single DNA nucleotide is altered in a point mutation.

[14] Only males were affected because *MAOA* is located on the X chromosome.

[15] The term "locus" is used to denote a specified position in the genome.

proportion (~70%) of the variation in canine morphological traits such as body size and bone shape. Similar traits in humans are governed by hundreds of loci with small effects (Manolio *et al.*, 2009). Boyko *et al.* (2010) explain their finding by the unique population history of the domestic dog, in which novel variants with large effects were preserved by artificial selection for fancy traits, especially during the Victorian era. Lequarré *et al.* (2011) suggest that the small effective population size within many dog breeds has resulted in larger gene effects because these are less effectively counter-selected in smaller populations. It is at this point unclear if this also applies to genes involved in dog behavior, because the theories rely on the assumption that there have been mutations with large effects on the phenotype in the past. Mutations with a large effect on behavior such as the *MAOA* null mutation are very rare (Brunner *et al.*, 1993). In addition, behavior was probably never the only parameter that was selected for by dog breeders. Selection for canine behavior may have been more similar to traditional selection for quantitative production traits in livestock. In farm animals, the population averages for economically useful quantitative traits such as milk production, fecundity, and meat quality have been altered by progressive directional selection over many generations. This selection acted on small individual differences in the traits. The genetic architecture of behavior in dogs may, however, be simpler than in livestock because some genetic variants may have been removed from certain breeds by drift or by selection for linked traits. In conclusion, canine behavior is probably controlled by a smaller number of loci than human behavior, but it is still a complex trait involving many genes and gene–gene or gene–environment interactions.

5.3.2   Human behavioral gene mapping

Several reviews of candidate gene studies of human behavioral traits are available in the literature (Burmeister *et al.*, 2008, Hill, 2010, Li & Burmeister, 2009). Candidate gene associations have proven difficult to replicate (Hirschhorn *et al.*, 2002; Todd, 2006). Possible reasons include inadequate sample sizes leading to spurious associations, differences in the study populations, differences in phenotype definitions, and publication bias (Colhoun *et al.*, 2003). This has led to increasing skepticism about the value of candidate gene association studies for detecting genetic variants contributing to complex traits. Meta-analyses are now considered necessary to firmly establish candidate gene associations in human genetics (e.g. Stutzmann *et al.*, 2007).

GWAS studies in humans have firmly established associations of genetic variants with a variety of complex diseases (McCarthy *et al.*, 2008). GWAS of human behavioral traits have lagged behind those of somatic diseases. In 2011, the catalog of published GWAS of the National Human Genome Research Institute contained 14 papers on schizophrenia, 14 on bipolar disorder, and two on depression (www .genome.gov/GWAStudies/; Liu, 2011). The strongest evidence for a mental disease gene so far comes from an aggregation of GWASs (International Schizophrenia Consortium *et al.*, 2009). This study implicated the major histocompatibility complex in schizophrenia. The Psychiatric GWAS Consortium plans to combine psychiatric GWASs to create a data set of 59 000 independent cases and controls and 7700 family trios for use in meta- and mega-analyses (Psychiatric GWAS Consortium Steering Committee, 2009).

5.3.3   Candidate gene association studies of dog behavior

Most candidate gene studies of canine behavior are focused on genes that play a role in personality traits or mental disorders in humans. The candidate genes usually code for aspects of brain neurotransmission systems. An example is the serotonergic system, which plays a key role in the modulation of behavioral traits in various species (Lesch & Merschdorf, 2000). Serotonergic drugs, for example, are successfully applied in the treatment of impulsive and anxious behavior in humans (Fernandez *et al.*, 2001; Messa *et al.*, 2003). Biochemical and neuroimaging studies suggest that the serotonergic system modulates behavior in dogs as well (Badino *et al.*, 2004; Reisner *et al.*, 1996; Vermeire *et al.*, 2011; Wright *et al.*, 2012).

The majority of studies that have attempted to associate candidate gene polymorphisms with canine behavioral traits focused on aggressive behavior or impulsivity/activity-related behaviors. The behavior of the dogs was measured using owner-report questionnaires, owner reports, or trainer ratings in these studies. Significant associations with measures of aggression were reported for the genes encoding the androgen receptor (Konno *et al.*, 2011), the dopamine D1 receptor (Våge *et al.* 2010a), the serotonin receptors 1D and 2C (Våge *et al.*, 2010a), solute carrier family 6 (neurotransmitter transporter, gamma-aminobutyric acid) member 1 (Våge *et al.*, 2010a), and solute carrier family 1 (neuronal/epithelial high affinity glutamate transporter), member 2 (Takeuchi *et al.*, 2009b). The phenotype "impulsivity" is related to inhibitory control (Wright *et al.*, 2012). Impulsivity can influence responsiveness to training and the dog's reactions to its environment (Wright *et al.*, 2012). "Activity" refers to self-initiated movement (Kubinyi *et al.*, 2012). For the activity-impulsivity phenotype, significant associations were reported with polymorphisms in the catechol-O-methyltransferase gene (Takeuchi *et al.*, 2009a), the dopamine D4 receptor gene (Hejjas *et al.*, 2009), the solute carrier family 1 (neuronal/epithelial high affinity glutamate transporter) member 2 gene (Takeuchi *et al.*, 2009a), and the tyrosine hydroxylase gene (Kubinyi *et al.*, 2012).

Candidate gene studies illustrate that behavior is not only a product of genes, but also of other factors, including sex and training. An example is the work of Hejjas *et al.* (2007a, 2007b) on the association of polymorphisms in the dopamine D4 receptor gene (*drd4*) with activity-impulsivity in German shepherd dogs. The dopamine D4 receptor is abundant in the limbic system of the brain, a region that is involved in emotion and cognitive function. A polymorphism in the human ortholog of *drd4* may be associated with human personality traits and mental disorders including attention deficit hyperactivity disorder (ADHD) (Benjamin *et al.*, 1996; Ebstein *et al.*, 1997). A VNTR in exon 3 of *drd4* was studied in German shepherd dogs using a questionnaire measure of activity-impulsivity (Hejjas *et al.*, 2007b). The VNTR was significantly associated with the personality measure in police dogs (n = 87), but not in pet dogs (n = 102), suggesting a gene–environment interaction (Hejjas *et al.*, 2007b). Environment may include responder variation in this study: there may be a difference in the way those who work with police dogs and those who keep German shepherd dogs as pets answer the questions about dog behavior. Another example is the work of Konno *et al.* (2011), who studied an androgen receptor gene (*ar*) VNTR in Japanese akita inu dogs. Androgens play a key role in modulating behavior. A similar polymorphism in the human androgen receptor gene affects the level of expression of the gene (Chamberlain *et al.*, 1994). Questionnaire scores of aggression differed significantly between 30 male dogs with a short version of the VNTR and 24 male dogs with a long repeat. In female dogs, no association between aggression scores and genotype was found, so the association was sex-specific.

The results of the candidate gene association studies described above should be interpreted with caution for several reasons. First, familial relationships between the dogs were not fully taken into account in most studies. This may give rise to spurious associations. Second, candidate gene associations in human genetics have proven difficult to replicate. As was discussed in the section about human behavioral gene mapping, possible reasons include differences in the study populations, differences in phenotype definitions, small sample sizes leading to spurious associations, and publication bias. The same problems can be recognized in the dog candidate gene studies. For instance, results of association studies of the *drd4* exon 3 VNTR with impulsivity-related pheno-types depended on breed and phenotype definitions. In addition, sample sizes of the dog studies are typically small. It has been suggested that genetic association studies of complex traits require smaller sample sizes in dogs than in humans because of the simpler architecture of the canine genome (see Box 5.1). Simulations estimated that only 100 cases and 100 controls are required to map a complex trait that confers a five-fold increased risk in dogs (Karlsson *et al.*, 2007). However, it is still unclear whether this is also true for behavioral traits. Finally, most of the dog studies used a limited number of markers to study the genes of interest. As a result, the studies may not have captured all variation in the candidate gene regions and may thus have missed associations. In conclusion, candidate gene studies of dog behavior are still in their infancy and replication studies are required.

5.3.4   Genome-wide association studies of dog behavior

Canine GWAS became possible with the release of the assembled DNA sequence of the genome of a Boxer named Tasha in 2005 (Lindblad-Toh *et al.*, 2005). Tasha's genome revealed the unique archi-tecture of the canine genome. The initial domestication of dogs from wolves, and the later formation of the variety of breeds that exist today, have left indelible marks on the canine genome (Parker *et al.*, 2010). The unique structure of the canine genome is expected to facilitate the detection of genetic variants that influence complex traits such as behavior using the dog. Indeed, quantitative trait loci (QTLs[16]) for several breed-defining complex traits have been identified using genome-wide methods in the past few years, e.g. skeletal traits (Parker *et al.*, 2009; Sutter *et al.*, 2007), hair char-acteristics (Cadieu *et al.*, 2009; Drögemüller *et al.*, 2008; Salmon Hillbertz *et al.*, 2007), coat color (Candille *et al.*, 2007; Karlsson *et al.*, 2007), and wrinkled skin (Akey *et al.*, 2010). For several of these traits, the causal genetic variant has been identified. An example is the short-legged phenotype of dog breeds such as dachshund, corgi, and basset hound. The short legs seem to be caused by the expression of a retrogene[17] encoding fibroblast growth factor 4 (Parker *et al.*, 2009; vonHoldt & Driscoll, Chapter 3).

As in humans, GWAS of canine behavioral traits have lagged behind those of traits related to physical appearance and somatic disease. In 2010, the first GWAS for a behavioral trait in dogs was reported (Dodman *et al.*, 2010). The study concerned flank and blanket sucking obsessive-compulsive behavior (OCD) in Doberman pinschers. Canine OCD can manifest as obsessive predatory behaviors (e.g. fly snapping, tail chasing), obsessive oral behaviors (e.g. acral lick der-matitis, flank sucking, blanket sucking) or obsessive locomotion (Brown *et al.*, 1987; Dodman *et al.*, 1993, 2010; Heywood, 1977; Overall, 2000; Rapoport *et al.*, 1992; Schwartz, 1993). OCD is normal behavior manifested in extreme or inappropriate ways (Overall, 2000), and it usually appears first between pre-pubescence and early social maturity. At first, the behavior is triggered by

---

[16]A quantitative trait is continuously varying in the sense that individuals cannot be readily classified into distinct classes. Many traits of interest in animal breeding, including behavior, are considered quantitative traits. The term "locus" is used to denote a specified position in the genome. A QTL is a stretch of DNA that contains one or more genetic variants that affect a quantitative trait.

[17]A retrogene arises when RNA is copied to DNA and then incorporated into the genome. This process (called reverse transcription) is a common source of novel DNA sequence acquired during the evolution of species. The majority of retrogenes rapidly accumulate mutations that disrupt the reading frame of the gene and thus become inactive. A small percentage become new genes that encode functional proteins.

environmental stressors. Soon it becomes fixed and is displayed in the absence of obvious stressors (Overall & Dunham, 2002). OCD may be improved with treatment, but is generally regarded as incurable and has disastrous consequences for animal welfare. Certain breeds seem predisposed to the disorders. For example, bull terriers frequently exhibit tail chasing, while Doberman pinschers are prone to acral licking. This breed-specific prevalence is suggestive of a genetic origin.

Dodman *et al.* (2010) analyzed 14 700 SNPs in the genomes of around 90 Doberman OCD cases and 70 controls. OCD diagnoses were obtained from veterinarians. They found an association with a SNP on dog chromosome 7. Sixty percent of the Dobermans that showed multiple compulsive behaviors (chewed their flanks, blankets, etc.) had the risk allele, compared with 43% of the dogs with a less severe phenotype and 22% of those without OCD (Dodman *et al.*, 2010). The SNP is located in a gene called cadherin 2 (*chd2*). Cadherin 2 is involved in forming connections between neural cells and it is widely expressed. Tiira *et al.* (2011, 2012) subsequently tested the association of the *chd2* SNP with compulsive tail-chasing in bull terriers and German shepherds. They failed to find an association, but these studies may have been underpowered. It is therefore at this point unclear in which breeds and in which types of compulsive behavior the *chd2* gene plays a role. The GWAS study of Dodman *et al.* (2010) found several additional SNPs associated with flank and blanket sucking, suggesting that in addition to *chd2*, other genes contribute to OCD in Dobermans. These may include serotonergic and dopaminergic genes because a neuro-imaging study of Vermeire *et al.* (2012) provided preliminary evidence for imbalances in these neurotransmitter systems in dogs with OCD.

5.3.5   Across-breed genome-wide association studies of dog behavior

An alternative to within-breed GWAS is across-breed genome-wide association mapping (Boyko *et al.*, 2010; Chase *et al.*, 2009; Karlsson & Lindblad-Toh, 2008). In this method, breed-average phenotypes are used. The breed-average phenotype is associated with the breed allele frequency of a genome-wide set of SNPs that have been genotyped in a large number of breeds. Jones *et al.* (2008) used this method to identify QTLs for several breed stereotypes, including the behavioral traits boldness, pointing, herding, trainability, and excitability. An experienced dog trainer scored the average breed phenotypes for boldness, pointing, herding and trainability as dichotomous variables, e.g. bold or non-bold. Breed phenotypes for excitability were quantitative rates (1–10) derived from the studies of Hart & Miller (1985).[18] Genotypes of 1536 SNPs from 2801 dogs of 147 breeds were used in the study. The majority of breeds were represented by at least 10 dogs. They used 147 (=number of breeds) combinations of breed-specific phenotype (e.g. bold or non-bold) with breed-specific allele frequency of a SNP (=value between 0 and 1) to calculate a Pearson product correlation between phenotype and SNP, weighted for the number of dogs per breed. Twelve loci were identified; five of these contained interesting genes. A herding QTL on canine chromosome 1 contains the genes *mc2r* and *c18orf1*. The former is a melanocortin receptor; the latter has been implicated in schizophrenia. The pointing locus on canine chromosome 8 contains the gene *cnih*, which has been implicated in cranial nerve development. A locus on canine chromosome 22 was identified for boldness. This genomic region contains the *pcdh9* gene, which encodes a protein involved in specific neural connections and signal transduction. Two other loci

---

[18] Hart & Miller (1985) asked a group of randomly selected veterinarians and dog obedience judges to rank breeds for several behavioral traits (see also Hart & Hart, Chapter 7).

for boldness included the *igf1* gene and the gene encoding the dopamine receptor 1 (*drd1*) (Chase *et al.*, 2009). The association of *drd1* and *igf1* with dog behavior is supported by other studies: *drd1* was associated with English Cocker Spaniel aggression in the candidate gene study of Våge *et al.* (2010a). IGF-1 has been implicated in anxiety: nervous pointer dogs have lower serum IGF-1 levels than normal pointers (Uhde *et al.*, 1992).

Vaysse *et al.* (2011) also used across-breed mapping to search for genomic regions affecting boldness. They used the same phenotypic definitions as Jones *et al.* (2008), but a different statistical approach in which they assigned each individual dog its breed-specific phenotype and then performed a "normal" GWAS. They examined the dog genome at a higher resolution than Jones *et al.* (2008) because they used more SNPs. When 18 bold and 19 non-bold breeds were compared, a highly significant association was found on chromosome 10, near the gene *hmga2* (high mobility group at-hook 2). This gene is involved in transcriptional activation of genes involved in cell proliferation (Pfannkuche *et al.*, 2009). The region was not detected in the study of Jones *et al.* (2008), which is probably due to methodological differences between the studies, e.g. different breeds, different lineages within a breed, different numbers from each breed, and different SNP sets. Vaysse *et al.* (2011) also used DMA data about sociability, curiosity, playfulness, chase-proneness, and aggressiveness for 509 dogs from 46 diverse breeds for across-breed GWAS. A genome-wide significant association for the sociability trait was found on the X chromosome (Vaysse *et al.*, 2011). No significant associations were detected for the other DMA traits.

The results of the across-breed studies are very interesting, but they should be treated with caution. The across-breed mapping strategy is sensitive to false positive results due to complex unequal relatedness between breeds (Jones *et al.*, 2008). In addition, other complex effects such as interactions between genes or co-selection of loci[19] during breed formation may confound the results (Jones *et al.*, 2008). The use of breed-average phenotypes is obviously a simplification of reality. The behavioral phenotypes may vary as much within breeds as across breeds (Figure 5.1). Validation of the loci using within-breed segregation analysis is thus required.

5.3.6   Genome-wide comparisons with other canid species

vonHoldt *et al.* (2010) compared genotypes of more than 48 000 SNPs in 912 dogs and 225 grey wolves. They searched for genomic regions that showed signs of positive selection during early dog domestication (see also vonHoldt & Driscoll, Chapter 3). Two out of three genomic regions that were identified have been implicated in memory formation and/or behavioral sensitization in mice or humans (ryanodine receptor 3 and adenylate cyclase 8). They also found evidence for positive selection for a SNP near the *wbscr17* gene. Mutations in this gene result in Williams-Beuren syndrome in humans, which is characterized by social traits such as exceptional gregariousness. Another genomic region, on dog chromosome 5, is orthologous to a region associated with tame behavior in the farm fox experiment (Kukekova *et al.*, 2011a). This makes it plausible that this region is indeed involved in domestication of dogs.

[19] When the frequency of a certain DNA fragment in a breed increases due to selection, the DNA flanking this fragment is also increasing in frequency. This is referred to as co-selection. The flanking regions may contain genetic variants that affect disease risk or behavior. In this way, selection for physical appearance can result in an increased disease allele frequency or in an increase of a genetic variant affecting behavior.

5.4   Discussion

5.4.1   What's in a name: Phenotype

One of the reasons for the slow progress of the field of canine behavioral genetics is the difficulty of measuring behavior (Bearden *et al.*, 2004; Mills, 2003; Smoller and Tsuang, 1998). As Felix Brown stated in 1942, "The chief difficulty is to define the condition the heredity of which one is attempting to trace." Early behavioral genetics research in fruit flies and rodents used objective metrics such as timed latencies or frequencies of a behavior. Scott and Fuller also used very specific measures in their classic work, e.g. "barks in a specified time frame." The recent work of Kukekova *et al.* (2011a) also applied objective metrics to fox behavioral genetics. The fox researchers developed a behavioral test in which an investigator approached the caged fox and tried to open the cage and touch the animal. Reactions of the foxes were videotaped and evaluated in a binary manner (yes/ no) for a set of traits that involved the fox's body language, actions and position with respect to the investigator. Factor analysis was used to group the behavioral elements into a quantitative measure of tame versus aggressive behavior. These factors were then used as phenotypes for gene mapping (see Section 5.4.4 below).

The dog genetic studies reviewed in this chapter used more subjective phenotypic measures. Most heritability studies used phenotypes based on the behavior of dogs in test batteries. Jones and Gosling (2005) have reviewed studies of canine personality and noted that, "In theory, test batteries were the closest to achieving objectivity, but in practice the levels of objectivity actually attained varied substantially." The molecular genetic studies mostly used even more subjective measures such as owner-report questionnaires and expert ratings (experts being veterinarians, trainers, or dog obedience judges). Owner and expert ratings may be influenced by a variety of factors other than the behavior of the dog, e.g. owner personality and expectations of typical dog behavior. Intuitively, the use of specific and objective metrics in genetic studies seems preferable. However, behavior of dogs in a test battery may not be representative of their behavior in everyday life and it is often unclear what exactly is being measured. Van den Berg and colleagues used three methods for measuring canine aggressive behavior: a behavioral test of the dog (van den Berg *et al.*, 2003), a questionnaire for the dog owner (van den Berg *et al.*, 2006), and a personal interview with the dog owner (van den Berg *et al.*, 2003, 2006). The most promising heritability estimates (i.e. high heritability with low standard errors) were obtained for the owner impressions collected during the personal interview (Liinamo *et al.*, 2007). This is rather surprising because of the subjectivity of these phenotypes. Large coordinated projects, such as the European LUPA consortium, make an effort to clarify dog behavioral phenotypes by following standard procedures to describe dog behavior (Lequarré *et al.*, 2011). This is of great value for progress in canine behavioral genetics.

5.4.2   Between genes and behavior: Endophenotypes

One potential approach to attack the complexity of behavior is to focus on less complex phenotypic variation, i.e. endophenotypes (Doyle *et al.*, 2005). Endophenotypes are closer to the biological basis of a complex trait, e.g. metabolites in urine or blood. Endophenotypes are assumed to be influenced by a subset of the genes that influence the complex trait. This reduced genetic complexity is the result of: (1) the relative proximity of the endophenotype to genes in the chain of events leading from gene to behavior, and (2) its potential to target one of several pathways that combine to create the trait. The reduced genetic complexity is expected to result in greater statistical power to detect the effects of individual genes. The endophenotype approach is popular in human psychiatric genetics (Robbins *et al.*, 2012). Endophenotypes have not been used in canine behavioral genetic studies as yet, but they could include neuroimaging data (e.g. Vermeire *et al.*, 2011, 2012), levels of metabolites in blood, urine or saliva (Wright *et al.*, 2012), or gene expression data (Våge *et al.*, 2010b).

5.4.3   Brain gene expression studies

Gene expression in the brain also occurs in between gene and behavioral phenotype. Large-scale analysis of gene expression has become feasible with massive parallel sequencing technologies. Such techniques sample all transcripts in a tissue, including noncoding sequences (Liu, 2011; Mattick *et al.*, 2010). Saetre *et al.* (2004) compared gene expression in brains of wolves and dogs. They suggest that domestication of dogs has resulted in changes in expression patterns of several hypothalamic genes with multiple functions, e.g. the neuropeptides, *calcb* and *npy*. Kukekova *et al.* (2011b) compared the prefrontal cortical brain transcriptome[20] from a tame and an aggressive silver fox. Many of the genes that were overexpressed in the tame fox compared to the aggressive fox were involved in neurological diseases in humans (Kukekova *et al.*, 2011b). One of these genes encodes the serotonin receptor 2C (*htr2c*), which has also been reported as being overexpressed in tame compared to aggressive rats (Popova *et al.*, 2010). A non-coding SNP in this gene was associated with aggressive behavior in English cocker spaniel dogs in a candidate gene association study of Våge *et al.* (2010a). In the aggressive fox, several genes involved in cardiovascular disease were overexpressed. None of the genes that was differentially expressed in the dog/wolf study of Saetre *et al.* (2004) was differently expressed between the fox samples.

Våge *et al.* (2010b) studied the expression of nine genes in the brains of 11 dogs that were euthanized because of aggressive behavior, and nine non-aggressive dogs euthanized for unrelated reasons. The candidate genes were identified in an initial screening. The studied brain regions were amygdala, frontal cortex, hypothalamus and parietal cortex. These brain areas are involved in emotion. Two of the nine genes, *ube2v2* and zinc finger protein227 (*znf*227) were differentially expressed in brains of aggressive and non-aggressive dogs. The *ube2v2* gene participates in a variety of cellular biochemical processes, including cell proliferation, regulation of DNA repair, regulation of progression through cell cycles, and protein modification. *znf*227 is likely to be a transcriptional regulator, i.e. it affects the expression of various genes. However, the expression differences were very small and formally not statistically significant. Further work, including testing the results in additional individuals, is needed to confirm the results of the gene expression studies discussed here.

5.4.4   Behavior is a complex trait: Epigenetics and epistasis

The slow progress in behavioral genetics is also caused by the fact that behavior is such a complex trait. Gene–environment and gene–gene interactions play a role in behavioral regulation. The study of Caspi *et al.* (2002) is an example of how genes (*MAOA*) interact with the environment (*maltreatment*) to determine biological processes in the brain, and as a result, behavior (*antisocial behavior*) (Figure 5.2). It is becoming increasingly clear that epigenetics may provide an explanation at

---

[20] The term "transcriptome" is used to denote all transcribed DNA sequence in a certain tissue.

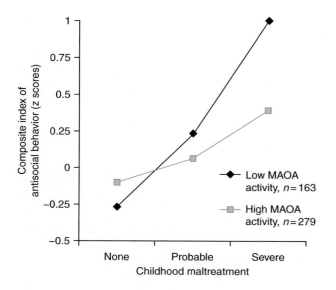

Figure 5.2 Mean antisocial behavior scores as a function of childhood history of maltreatment and MAOA activity in the study of Caspi *et al.* (2002). Subjects were males that were studied from birth to adulthood. Childhood maltreatment is grouped into three categories on the horizontal axis. The vertical axis represents an antisocial behavior composite score, which was standardized to a mean of 0 and SD of 1. MAOA activity (grouped into low and high) is the gene expression level associated with allelic variants of the *MAOA* gene polymorphism. (From Caspi, A. *et al.* (2002). Science, 297, 851–854. Reprinted with permission from AAAS.)

the molecular level for such gene–environment interactions (Hoffmann & Spengler, 2012; Hunter, 2012). Epigenetics refers to mitotically stable changes in gene expression potential that are not caused by changes in DNA sequence. Epigenetic modifications enable the same genotype to produce different cellular phenotypes. Histone modifications and DNA methylation are examples of epigenetic changes. These modifications affect gene expression potential through altered accessibility of the DNA to transcription factors. For instance, dense methylation of CG dinucleotides in a gene promoter results in transcriptional silence. Such changes may even be stable across multiple generations (Stöger, 2008; Waterland *et al.*, 2008). Early embryogenesis is a critical period for the establishment of epigenetic patterns (Gluckman *et al.*, 2009). For instance, a maternal diet deficient in methyl donors and cofactors results in hypomethylation of the promoter of the agouti gene in mice (Waterland & Jirtle, 2003). The agouti protein induces yellow pigmentation in hair follicles and antagonizes satiety signaling in the hypothalamus. Hypomethylation of the agouti promoter results in yellow coat color and increased prevalence of obesity in the mice offspring. A similar relationship has been observed in humans: prenatal famine exposure during the Dutch Hunger Winter was associated with persistent changes in DNA methylation of genes involved in growth and metabolic disease (Heijmans *et al.*, 2008; Tobi *et al.*, 2009). No epigenetic studies of dog behavior have been performed yet (although see Koch *et al.*, 2016), but it is expected that similar mechanisms are at work.

In addition to gene-environment interactions, gene-gene interactions (termed epistasis) play a role in behavioral variation. Albert *et al.* (2009) showed that a five locus epistatic network influences tameness in rats. An interesting study of Kukekova *et al.* (2011a) suggests that a similar mechanism may be operating in silver foxes. As was described above, the fox researchers developed a behavioral test that resulted in a quantitative measure of tame versus aggressive behavior. The test was applied to several fox populations, including a tame population that was selected for tameness for many generations, an aggressive population that was selected for aggressive behavior for many generations, and their crosses, intercrosses and backcrosses. Mean scores on the tameness factor differed between the populations, showing a linear gradient from tame to aggressive, which is consistent with its heritability (Figure 5.3). The tameness factor mapped to fox chromosome 12, in a region orthologous to the region on dog chromosome 5 that was associated with dog domestication

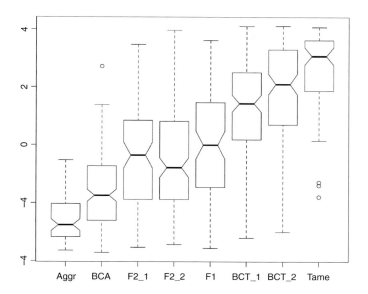

Figure 5.3 Tameness scores of silver fox populations in the study of Kukekova *et al.* (2011a). Tameness scores were derived from a standardized videotaped test in which an investigator approached the caged fox and tried to open the cage and touch the animal. Each fox was evaluated in a binary (yes/no) manner for a set of traits, e.g. wagging the tail, coming to the front of the cage, allowing head to be touched, holding observer's hand with its mouth. Factor analysis was used to detect underlying behavioral patterns in the dataset. The vertical axis in this figure represents scores on a factor that distinguishes between the tame and aggressive fox populations. Aggr = "aggressive" founder population; BCA = backcross-to-aggressive; F2_1 and F2_2 = two different F2 populations (F1 x F1); F1 = F1 population ("tame" x "aggressive"); BCT_1 and BCT_2 = two different backcross-to-tame populations; Tame = "tame" founder population. Horizontal bars within each box represent the population median. Confidence intervals for the medians are shown as notches such that two distributions with non-overlapping notches are significantly different. The bottom and top edges of the boxes indicate the 25 and 75 percentiles. The whiskers indicate the range of data up to 1.5 times the interquartile range. Outliers are shown as individual circles. (Figure reprinted from Kukekova *et al.*, 2011a with permission from Springer.)

in the study of vonHoldt *et al.* (2010; see Section 5.3.6). However, the exact region of association within fox chromosome 12 differed between populations, i.e. it depended on genomic context. This suggests that epistasis is involved.

5.4.5 Importance of behavioral genetic studies in the dog

Dogs fulfill important functions in our society as working partners in military and police organizations, as farm dogs, assistance dogs, and guide dogs for the blind. In addition, dogs provide much-valued companionship to humans. Behavioral considerations are important in dog breeding programs because breeding can create better working dogs and better companions. Rapid changes in canine behavioral traits are possible in just a few generations (Svartberg, 2006; Trut *et al.*, 2009).

Genomic selection has recently expanded the repertoire of tools available to the breeder to initiate genetic change. Genomic selection calculates a genetic score based on the proportion of favorable genetic markers from a genome-wide set associated with a complex trait of interest. This technique is already applied in livestock species (Goddard & Hayes, 2009). In dog breeding, the application of genomic selection would require a coordinated effort on a national or international scale (Wilson & Wade, 2012). This might be difficult to achieve because most countries hold many dispersed small dog breeding enterprises. Such small populations, each with different breeding objectives, are probably altered more by genetic drift than by the intended selective pressure applied by the breeder (Bulmer, 1972). Breed registries are also often averse to accepting outcrosses to introduce additional genetic variation to a breed.

Molecular genetic tests could also be used to predict individual risk of problem behavior in the future. This may be very useful in the debate about "breed *versus* deed." Ownership of dog breeds that are considered to be dangerous is restricted in many countries (Overall, 2010; Lockwood, Chapter 9). Breed-specific legislation has also created pressure on animal shelters to employ pre-dictors of aggression risk in dogs. However, the heritability of the behavioral traits presented in this chapter shows that behavior in any individual dog is a product not only of its genes, but also its environment, including access to socialization, training, and exercise (Serpell *et al.*, Chapter 6). It is thus uncertain whether a reliable molecular test can be developed, even when complete knowledge of the genetics of canine antisocial behavior would be available. Genetic profiling for personalized medicine has also met criticism in human complex disease genetics (Janssens & van Duijn, 2008). The same is true for gene expression patterns as predictors for problem behavior. Measuring gene expression patterns associated with antisocial behavior may also be difficult to apply in practice due to limited access to the tissues of expression in living animals. A more feasible application of the knowledge of the genes and pathways involved in dog behavior might be the elucidation of drug targets. This may lead to better treatment or prediction of drug efficacy in dogs showing problem behavior.

Studying the genetics of behavior in dogs may also prove important to our scientific understanding of human psychology (Cyranoski, 2010). Evidence for causal associations between specific genetic variants and behavioral traits in humans is often inconclusive (Bearden *et al.*, 2004; Colhoun *et al.*, 2003; Hamer, 2002; Inoue & Lupski, 2003). Both humans and dogs descend from social species that show cooperative and altruistic behaviors. Many canine behavioral disorders resemble human mental problems that are treated with the same medications (Dodman & Shuster, 1998; Overall, 2000). The genome of purebred dogs has characteristics that are favorable for molecular genetic studies of complex traits (Lindblad-Toh *et al.*, 2005). Localizing behavioral genes is thus expected to be substantially easier in dogs than in humans. As soon as causal mutations in canine genes have been found, it will be interesting to study the involvement of the corresponding genes and proteins in human behavior.

This has already proven to be a successful approach for the study of narcolepsy (Chen *et al.*, 2009). This disease is characterized by excess daytime sleepiness, striking transitions from wakefulness into rapid eye movement (REM) sleep, and cataplexy triggered by positive emotions. It affects 0.02 to 0.18% of the general human population and is a key to understanding other, more common sleep disorders. Familial cases have been reported, but most cases are sporadic. It is considered a com-plex trait in humans. Some dog breeds also suffer from narcolepsy. The dogs experience cataplexy during vigorous play or when they are excited by being offered their favorite foods (http://med.stan-ford.edu/school/Psychiatry/narcolepsy/moviedog.html). As in humans, both sporadic and familial cases are observed. Researchers at Stanford University studied a purpose-bred colony of narcoleptic Dobermans and Labrador retrievers (Lin *et al.*, 1999). Linkage analysis and fine-mapping resulted in the identification of mutations in the hypocretin-2-receptor gene (*hcrtr2*) as causal to the canine disease. Subsequent studies in humans showed that the number of hypocretin-containing neurons in post-mortem samples of the hypothalamus of narcoleptic patients was reduced by 90% (Thannickal *et al.*, 2000). Hypocretin was found to play a role in circadian clock-dependent alertness. The hypocretin system might therefore be a therapeutic target for more common sleep disturbances in humans.

5.5   Conclusion

This review tells us that variation in canine behavior is substantially correlated with underlying genetic variation. Breed differences in behavior exist and behavioral dispositions can be selected for. The relative importance of genetic and environmental influences on dog behavior can be estimated by calculating the heritability. Heritability estimates for canine behavioral traits are mostly low to medium, with an average of 0.20. Researchers have pinpointed some genetic variants involved in dog behavior using candidate gene association studies, within-breed genome-wide association studies, across-breed genome-wide association studies, and by comparisons of the dog genome with those of the wolf and fox. Some of the reported genetic associations seem plausible because they are supported by several studies using different methodologies. However, the majority of results of molecular genetic studies are tentative and require future replication. The identification of genetic variants that affect canine behavior has progressed more slowly than the identification of genetic variants for morphological traits and somatic diseases. Reasons for the slow progress of the field include the difficulty of measuring behavior, and the fact that behavior is a complex trait involving many genes with small effects. Nevertheless, the field of canine behavioral genetics has led to breakthroughs that have informed research on neuropsychiatric disorders in humans. Behavioral considerations are important in dog breeding programs. Programs directed toward changes at the breed level will likely require coordinated national or international efforts.

Acknowledgements

The author would like to thank James Serpell for the invitation to write this chapter. In addition, Peter Leegwater, Eldin Leighton, Diane van Rooy, and Claire Wade are thanked for critical review of parts of the manuscript. Anna Kukekova, Gordon Lark and Matt Webster are thanked for fruitful e-mail discussions.

References

Acland, G. M., Ray, K., Mellersh, C. S. *et al.* (1998). Linkage analysis and comparative mapping of canine progressive rod-cone degeneration (prcd) establishes potential locus homology with retinitis pigmentosa (RP17) in humans. *Proceedings of the National Academy of Sciences USA*, 95: 3048–53.

Akey, J. M., Ruhe, A. L., Akey, D. T. *et al.* (2010). Tracking footprints of artificial selection in the dog genome. *Proceedings of the National Academy of Sciences USA*, 107: 1160–5.

Albert, F. W., Carlborg, O., Plyusnina, I. *et al.* (2009). Genetic architecture of tameness in a rat model of animal domestication. *Genetics*, 182: 541–54.

Appleby, D. L., Bradshaw, J. W. & Casey, R. A. (2002). Relationship between aggressive and avoidance behavior by dogs and their experience in the first six months of life. *Veterinary Record*, 150: 434–8.

Arvelius, P., Malm, S., Svartberg, K. & Strandberg, E. (2009). Genetic analysis of herding behavior in Swedish Border Collie dogs. *Journal of Veterinary Behavior*, 4: 237–57.

Badino, P., Odore, R., Osella, M. C. *et al.* (2004). Modifications of serotonergic and adrenergic receptor concentrations in the brain of aggressive *Canis familiaris*. *Comparative Biochemistry and Physiology Part A: Molecular & Integrative Physiology*, 139: 343–50.

Bamberger, M. & Houpt, K. A. (2006). Signalment factors, comorbidity, and trends in behavior diagnoses in dogs: 1,644 cases (1991–2001). *Journal of the American Veterinary Medical Association*, 229: 1591–601.

Bearden, C. E., Reus, V. I. & Freimer, N. B. (2004). Why genetic investigation of psychiatric disorders is so difficult. *Current Opinion in Genetics & Development*, 14: 280–6.

Beaver, B. V. (1993). Profiles of dogs presented for aggression. *Journal of the American Animal Hospital Association*, 29: 564–9.

Benjamin, J., Li, L., Patterson, C. *et al.* (1996). Population and familial association between the D4 dopamine receptor gene and measures of novelty seeking. *Nature Genetics*, 12: 81–4.

Blackshaw, J. K. (1991). An overview of types of aggressive behavior in dogs and methods of treatment. *Applied Animal Behaviour Science*, 30: 351–61.

Boomsma, D., Busjahn, A. & Peltonen, L. (2002). Classical twin studies and beyond. *Nature Reviews Genetics*, 3: 872–82.

Borchelt, P. L. (1983). Aggressive behavior of dogs kept as companion animals: classification and influence of sex, reproductive status and breed. *Applied Animal Ethology*, 10: 45–61.

Borchelt, P. L. & Voith, V. L. (1996). Aggressive behavior in dogs and cats. In *Readings in Companion Animal Behavior*, eds. V. L. Voith & P. L. Borchelt. Trenton, NJ: Veterinary Learning Systems, pp. 217–29.

Bourdon, R. M. (1997). Heritability and repeatability. In *Understanding Animal Breeding*, ed. R. M. Bourdon. Upper Saddle River, NJ: Prentice Hall, pp. 149–84.

Boyko, A. R., Quignon, P., Li, L. *et al.* (2010). A simple genetic architecture underlies morphological variation in dogs. *PLoS Biology*, 8: e1000451.

Bradshaw, J. W., Goodwin, D., Lea, A. M. & Whitehead, S. L. (1996). A survey of the behavioral characteristics of pure-bred dogs in the United Kingdom. *Veterinary Record*, 138: 465–8.

Brown, S. A., Crowell-Davis, S., Malcolm, T. & Edwards, P. (1987). Naloxone-responsive compulsive tail chasing in a dog. *Journal of the American Veterinary Medical Association*, 190: 884–6.

Brunner, H. G., Nelen, M., Breakefield, X. O., Ropers, H. H. & van Oost, B. A. (1993). Abnormal behavior associated with a point mutation in the structural gene for monoamine oxidase A. *Science*, 262: 578–80.

Bulmer, M. G. (1972). The genetic variability of polygenic characters under optimizing selection, mutation and drift. *Genetics Research*, 19: 17–25.

Burmeister, M., McInnis, M. G. & Zöllner, S. (2008). Psychiatric genetics: progress amid controversy. *Nature Reviews Genetics*, 9, 527–40.

Cadieu, E., Neff, M. W., Quignon, P. *et al.* (2009). Coat variation in the domestic dog is governed by variants in three genes. *Science*, 326: 150–3.

Candille, S. I., Kaelin, C. B., Cattanach, B. M. *et al.* (2007). A bdefensin mutation causes black coat color in domestic dogs. *Science*, 318: 1418–23.

Caspi, A., McClay, J., Moffitt, T. E. *et al.* (2002). Role of genotype in the cycle of violence in maltreated children. *Science*, 297: 851–4.

Chamberlain, N. L., Driver, E. D. & Miesfeld, R. L. (1994). The length and location of CAG trinucleotide repeats in the androgen receptor N-terminal domain affect transactivation function. *Nucleic Acids Research*, 22: 3181–6.

Chase, K., Jones, P., Martin, A., Ostrander, E. A. & Lark, K. G. (2009). Genetic mapping of fixed phenotypes: disease frequency as a breed characteristic. *Journal of Heredity*, 100(Suppl 1): S37–41.

Chen, L., Brown, R. E., McKenna, J. T. & McCarley, R. W. (2009). Animal models of narcolepsy. *CNS & Neurological Disorders – Drug Targets*, 8: 296–308.

Colhoun, H. M., McKeigue, P. M. & Davey Smith, G. (2003). Problems of reporting genetic associations with complex outcomes. *Lancet*, 361: 865–72.

Courreau, J.-F. & Langlois, B. (2005). Genetic parameters and environmental effects which characterise the defence ability of the Belgian shepherd dog. *Applied Animal Behaviour Science*, 91: 233–45.

Cyranoski, D. (2010). Genetics: pet project. *Nature*, 466: 1036–8.

De Keuster, T., Lamoureux, J. & Kahn, A. (2006). Epidemiology of dog bites: a Belgian experience of canine behavior and public health concerns. *Veterinary Journal*, 172: 482–7.

Dodman, N. H., Bronson, R. & Gliatto, J. (1993). Tail chasing in a bull terrier. *Journal of the American Veterinary Medical Association*, 202, 758–60.

Dodman, N. H., Karlsson, E. K., Moon-Fanelli, A. *et al.* (2010). A canine chromosome 7 locus confers compulsive disorder susceptibility. *Molecular Psychiatry*, 15: 8–10.

Dodman, N. H. & Shuster, L. (1998). *Psychopharmacology of Animal Behavior Disorders*. London: Blackwell Science.

Doyle, A. E., Faraone, S. V., Seidman, L. J. *et al.* (2005). Are endophenotypes based on measures of executive functions useful for molecular genetic studies of ADHD? *Journal of Child Psychology & Psychiatry*, 46: 774–803.

Drögemüller, C., Karlsson, E. K., Hytönen, M. K. *et al.* (2008). A mutation in hairless dogs implicates FOXI3 in ectodermal development. *Science*, 321: 1462.

Duffy, D. L., Hsu, Y. & Serpell, J. A. (2008). Breed differences in canine aggression. *Applied Animal Behavior Science*, 114: 441–60.

Dykman, R. A., Murphree, O. D. & Ackerman, P. T. (1966). Litter patterns in the offspring of nervous and stable dogs: II. autonomic and motor conditioning. *The Journal of Nervous and Mental Disease*, 141: 419–32.

Ebstein, R. P., Segman, R., Benjamin, J. *et al.* (1997). 5-HT2C (HTR2C) serotonin receptor gene polymorphism associated with the human personality trait of reward dependence: interaction with dopamine D4 receptor (D4DR) and dopamine D3 receptor (D3DR) polymorphisms. *American Journal of Medical Genetetics*, 74: 65–72.

Everts, R. E., Rothuizen, J. & van Oost, B. A. (2000). Identification of a premature stop codon in the melanocyte-stimulating hormone receptor gene (MC1R) in Labrador and Golden retrievers with yellow coat colour. *Animal Genetics*, 31: 194–9.

Fan, M., Liu, B., Jiang, T. *et al.* (2010). Meta-analysis of the association between the monoamine oxidase-A gene and mood disorders. *Psychiatric Genetics*, 20: 1–7.

Fernandez, M., Pissiota, A., Frans, O. *et al.* (2001). Brain function in a patient with torture related post-traumatic stress disorder before and after fluoxetine treatment: a positron emission tomography provocation study. *Neuroscience Letters*, 297: 101–4.

Fisher, R. A. (1930). *The Genetical Theory of Natural Selection*. Oxford: Clarendon Press.

Gluckman, P. D., Hanson, M. A., Buklijas, T., Low, F. M. & Beedle, A. S. (2009). Epigenetic mechanisms that underpin metabolic and cardiovascular diseases. *Nature Reviews Endocrinology*, 5: 401–8.

Goddard, M. E. & Hayes, B. J. (2009). Mapping genes for complex traits in domestic animals and their use in breeding programmes. *Nature Reviews Genetics*, 10: 381–91.

Goddard, M. E. & Beilharz, R. G. (1983). Genetics of traits which determine the suitability of dogs as guide-dogs for the blind. *Applied Animal Ethology*, 9: 299–315.

Goddard, M. E. & Beilharz, R. G. (1982). Genetic and environmental factors affecting the suitability of dogs as guide dogs for the blind. *Theoretical and Applied Genetics*, 62: 97–102.

Hall, N. J. & Wynne, C. D. (2012). The canid genome: behavioral geneticists' best friend? *Genes, Brain and Behavior*, 11: 889–902.

Hamer, D. (2002). Genetics. Rethinking behavior genetics. *Science*, 298: 71–2.

Hart, B. L. & Miller, M. F. (1985). Behavioral profiles of dog breeds. *Journal of the American Veterinary Medical Association*, 186: 1175–80.

Henderson, C. R. (1975). Best linear unbiased estimation and prediction under a selection model. *Biometrics*, 31: 423–47.

Hejjas, K., Kubinyi, E., Ronai, Z. *et al.* (2009). Molecular and behavioral analysis of the intron 2 repeat polymorphism in the canine dopamine D4 receptor gene. *Genes Brain and Behavior*, 8: 330–6.

Hejjas, K., Vas, J., Kubinyi, E., *et al.* (2007a). Novel repeat polymorphisms of the dopaminergic neurotransmitter genes among dogs and wolves. *Mammalian Genome*, 18, 871–879.

Hejjas, K., Vas, J., Topal, J. *et al.* (2007b). Association of polymorphisms in the dopamine D4 receptor gene and the activity-impulsivity endophenotype in dogs. *Animal Genetics*, 38: 629–33.

Heijmans, B. T., Tobi, E. W., Stein, A. D. *et al.* (2008). Persistent epigenetic differences associated with prenatal exposure to famine in humans. *Proceedings of the National Academy of Sciences USA*, 105: 17046–9.

Heywood, S. (1977). Chasing one's own tail? An example of self-pursuit in a red setter. *Perception*, 6: 483.

Hill, S. Y. (2010). Neural plasticity, human genetics, and risk for alcohol dependence. *International Review of Neurobiology*, 91: 53–94.

Hirschhorn, J. N., Lohmueller, K., Byrne, E. & Hirschhorn, K. (2002). A comprehensive review of genetic association studies. *Genetics in Medicine*, 4: 45–61.

Hoffmann, A. & Spengler, D. (2014). DNA memories of early social life. *Neuroscience*, 264: 64–75.

Houpt, K. A. & Willis, M. B. (2001). Genetics of behavior. In *The Genetics of the Dog*, eds. A. Ruvinsky & J. Sampson. Oxon, New York: CABI Publishing, pp. 371–400.

Hradecká, L., Bartoš, L., Svobodová, I. & Sales, J. (2015). Heritability of behavioural traits in domestic dogs: a meta-analysis. *Applied Animal Behaviour Science*, 170: 1–13.

Hunter, R. G. (2012). Epigenetic effects of stress and corticosteroids in the brain. *Frontiers in Cellular Neuroscience*, 6: 18.

Huson, H. J., Parker, H. G., Runstadler, J. & Ostrander, E. A. (2010). A genetic dissection of breed composition and performance enhancement in the Alaskan sled dog. *BMC Genetics*, 11: 71.

Inoue, K. & Lupski, J. R. (2003). Genetics and genomics of behavioral and psychiatric disorders. *Current Opinion in Genetics & Development*, 13: 303–9.

International Schizophrenia Consortium, Purcell, S. M., Wray, N. R. *et al.* (2009). Common polygenic variation contributes to risk of schizophrenia and bipolar disorder. *Nature*, 460: 748–52.

Janssens, A. C. & van Duijn, C. M. (2008). Genome-based prediction of common diseases: advances and prospects. *Human Molecular Genetics*, 17(R2): R166–73.

Jones, A. C. & Gosling, S. D. (2005). Temperament and personality in dogs (*Canis familiaris*): a review and evaluation of past research. *Applied Animal Behaviour Science*, 95: 1–53.

Jones, P., Chase, K., Martin, A. *et al.* (2008). Single-nucleotide-polymorphism-based association mapping of dog stereotypes. *Genetics*, 179: 1033–44.

Karlsson, E. K., Baranowska, I., Wade, C. M. *et al.* (2007). Efficient mapping of mendelian traits in dogs through genome-wide association. *Nature Genetics*, 39: 1321–8.

Karlsson, E. K. & Lindblad-Toh, K. (2008). Leader of the pack: gene mapping in dogs and other model organisms. *Nature Reviews Genetics*, 9: 713–25.

Kirkness, E. F., Bafna, V., Halpern, A. L. *et al.* (2003). The dog genome: survey sequencing and comparative analysis. *Science*, 301: 1898–903.

Koch, I. J., Clark, M. M., Thompson, M. J., Deere-Machemer, K. A., Wang, J., Duarte, L., *et al.* (2016)

The concerted impact of domestication and transposon insertions on methylation patterns between dogs and grey wolves. *Molecular Ecology*, 25: 1838–855. http://doi: 10.1111/mec.13480

Konno, A., Inoue-Murayama, M. & Hasegawa, T. (2011). Androgen receptor gene polymorphisms are associated with aggression in Japanese Akita Inu. *Biology Letters*, 7: 658–60.

Kubinyi, E., Vas, J., Hejjas, K. *et al.* (2012). Polymorphism in the tyrosine hydroxylase (TH) gene is associated with activity-impulsivity in German shepherd dogs. *PLoS One*, 7: e30271.

Kukekova, A. V., Trut, L. N., Chase, K. *et al.* (2011a). Mapping loci for fox domestication: deconstruction/reconstruction of a behavioral phenotype. *Behavior Genetics*, 41: 593–606.

Kukekova, A. V., Johnson, J. L., Teiling, C. *et al.* (2011b). Sequence comparison of prefrontal cortical brain transcriptome from a tame and an aggressive silver fox (*Vulpes vulpes*). *BMC Genomics*, 12: 482.

Landsberg, G. (2004). Canine aggression. In *Handbook of Behavior Problems of the Dog and Cat*, eds. G. Landsberg, W. Hunthausen & L. Ackerman. Edinburgh: Saunders, pp. 385–426.

Landsberg, G. (1991). The distribution of canine behavior cases at three behavior referral practices. *Veterinary Medicine*, 1011–17.

Lequarré, A. S., Andersson, L., André, C. *et al.* (2011). LUPA: a European initiative taking advantage of the canine genome architecture for unravelling complex disorders in both human and dogs. *Veterinary Journal*, 189: 155–9.

Lesch, K. P. & Merschdorf, U. (2000). Impulsivity, aggression, and serotonin: a molecular psychobiological perspective. *Behavioral Sciences & the Law*, 18: 581–604.

Li, M. D. & Burmeister, M. (2009). New insights into the genetics of addiction. *Nature Reviews Genetics*. 10: 225–31.

Liinamo, A.-E., van den Berg, L., Leegwater, P. A. J. *et al.* (2007). Genetic variation in aggression-related traits in golden retriever dogs. *Applied Animal Behavior Science*, 104: 95–106.

Lin, L., Faraco, J., Li, R. *et al.* (1999). The sleep disorder canine narcolepsy is caused by a mutation in the hypocretin (orexin) receptor 2 gene. *Cell*, 98: 365–76.

Lindberg, S., Strandberg, E. & Swenson, L. (2004). Genetic analysis of hunting behavior in Swedish Flatcoated Retrievers. *Applied Animal Behavior Science*, 88: 289–98.

Lindblad-Toh, K., Wade, C. M., Mikkelsen, T. S. *et al.* (2005). Genome sequence, comparative analysis and haplotype structure of the domestic dog. *Nature*, 438: 803–19.

Liu, C. (2011). Brain expression quantitative trait locus mapping informs genetic studies of psychiatric diseases. *Neuroscience Bulletin*, 27: 123–33.

Lockwood, R. & Rindy, K. (1987). Are "pit bulls" different? An analysis of the pit bull terrier controversy. *Anthrozoos*, 1: 2–8.

Mackenzie, S. A., Oltenacu, E. A. B. & Houpt, K. A. (1986). Canine behavioral genetics – a review. *Applied Animal Behaviour Science*, 15: 365–93.

Manolio, T. A., Collins, F. S, Cox, N. J. *et al.* (2009). Finding the missing heritability of complex diseases. *Nature*, 461: 747–53.

Mattick, J. S., Taft, R. J. & Faulkner, G. J. (2010). A global view of genomic information-moving beyond the gene and the master regulator. *Trends in Genetics*, 26: 21–8.

McCarthy, M. I., Abecasis, G. R., Cardon, L. R. *et al.* (2008). Genome-wide association studies for complex traits: consensus, uncertainty and challenges. *Nature Reviews Genetics*, 9, 356–69.

Messa, C., Colombo, C., Moresco, R. M. *et al.* (2003). 5-HT(2A) receptor binding is reduced in drug-naive and unchanged in SSRI-responder depressed patients compared to healthy controls: a PET study. *Psychopharmacology (Berl)*, 167: 72–8.

Mikkelsen, J. & Lund, J. D. (2000). Euthanasia of dogs due to behavioral problems: an epidemiological study of euthanasia of dogs in Denmark, with a special focus on problems of aggression. *The European Journal of Companion Animal Practice*, 10: 143–50.

Mills, D. S. (2003). Medical paradigms for the study of problem behavior: a critical review. *Applied Animal Behaviour Science*, 81: 265–77.

Mugford, R. A. (1984). Behavior problems in the dog. In *Nutrition and Behavior in Dogs and Cats*, ed. R. S. Anderson. Oxford: Pergamon Press, pp. 207–15.

Nicholas, F. W. (2003). Quantitative variation. In *Introduction to Veterinary Genetics*, ed. F.W. Nicholas, Oxford: Blackwell Publishing, pp. 191–201.

Overall, K. L. (2000). Natural animal models of human psychiatric conditions: assessment of mechanism and validity. *Progress in Neuro-Psychopharmacology & Biological Psychiatry*, 24: 727–76.

Overall, K. L. (2010). Breed specific legislation: how data can spare breeds and reduce dog bites. *The Veterinary Journal*, 186: 277–9.

Overall, K. L. & Dunham, A. E. (2002). Clinical features and outcome in dogs and cats with obsessive-compulsive disorder: 126 cases (1989–2000). *Journal of the American Veterinary Medical Association*, 221: 1445–52.

Parker, H. G., Shearin, A. L. & Ostrander, E. A. (2010). Man's best friend becomes biology's best in show: genome analyses in the domestic dog. *Annual Reviews of Genetics*, 44: 309–36.

Parker, H. G., vonHoldt, B. M., Quignon, P. *et al.* (2009). An expressed fgf4 retrogene is associated with breed-defining chondrodysplasia in domestic dogs. *Science*, 325: 995–8.

Pérez-Guisado, J., Lopez-Rodríguez, R. & Muñoz-Serrano, A. (2006). Heritability of dominant–aggressive behavior in English cocker spaniels. *Applied Animal Behaviour Science*, 100: 219–27.

Pfannkuche, K., Summer, H., Li, O., Hescheler, J. & Dröge, P. (2009). The high mobility group protein HMGA2: a co-regulator of chromatin structure and pluripotency in stem cells? *Stem Cell Reviews*, 5: 224–30.

Plomin, R. (1990). *Nature and Nurture: An Introduction to Human Behavioral Genetics*. Pacific Grove, CA: Brooks/Cole.

Podberscek, A. L & Serpell, J. A. (1997). Environmental influences on the expression of aggressive behavior in English cocker spaniels. *Applied Animal Behaviour Science*, 52: 215–27.

Popova, N. K., Naumenko, V. S., Kozhemyakina, R. V. & Plyusnina, I. Z. (2010). Functional characteristics of serotonin 5-HT2A and 5-HT2C receptors in the brain and the expression of the 5-HT2A and 5-HT2C receptor genes in aggressive and non-aggressive rats. *Neuroscience and Behavioral Physiology*, 40: 357–61.

Popova, N. K., Nikulina, E. M. & Kulikov, A. V. (1993). Genetic analysis of different kinds of aggressive behavior. *Behavior Genetics*, 23: 491–7.

Psychiatric GWAS Consortium Steering Committee (2009). A framework for interpreting genome-wide association studies of psychiatric disorders. *Molecular Psychiatry*, 14: 10–17.

Rapoport, J. L, Ryland, D. H. & Kriete, M. (1992). Drug treatment of canine acral lick. An animal model of obsessive-compulsive disorder. *Archives of General Psychiatry*, 49, 517–21.

Reisner, I. R. (1997). Assessment, management, and prognosis of canine dominance-related aggression. *Veterinary Clinics of North America Small Animal Practice*, 27: 479–95.

Reisner, I. R., Mann, J. J., Stanley, M., Huang, Y. Y. & Houpt, K. A. (1996). Comparison of cerebrospinal fluid monoamine metabolite levels in dominant-aggressive and non-aggressive dogs. *Brain Research*, 714: 57–64.

Reuterwall, C. & Ryman, N. (1973). An estimate of the magnitude of additive genetic variation of some mental characters in Alsatian dogs. *Hereditas*, 73: 277–84.

Robbins, T. W., Gillan, C. M., Smith, D. G., de Wit, S. & Ersche, K. D. (2012). Neurocognitive endophenotypes of impulsivity and compulsivity: towards dimensional psychiatry. *Trends in Cognitive Sciences*, 16: 81–91.

Robinson, G. E. (2004). Genomics. Beyond nature and nurture. *Science*, 304: 397–9.

Ruefenacht, S., Gebhardt-Henrich, S., Miyake, T. & Gaillard, C. (2002). A behavior test on German shepherd dogs: heritability of seven different traits. *Applied Animal Behavior Science*, 79: 113–32.

Saetre, P., Lindberg, J., Leonard, J. A. *et al.* (2004). From wild wolf to domestic dog: gene expression changes in the brain. *Brain Research and Molecular Brain Research*, 126: 198–206.

Saetre, P., Strandberg, E., Sundgren, P. E. *et al.* (2006). The genetic contribution to canine personality. *Genes Brain and Behavior*, 5: 240–8.

Salmon Hillbertz, N. H., Isaksson, M., Karlsson, E. K. *et al.* (2007). Duplication of FGF3, FGF4, FGF19 and ORAOV1 causes hair ridge and predisposition to dermoid sinus in ridgeback dogs. *Nature Genetics*, 39: 1318–20.

Schwartz, S. (1993). Naltrexone-induced pruritus in a dog with tail-chasing behavior. *Journal of the American Veterinary Medical Association*, 202: 278–80.

Scott, J. P. & Fuller, J. L. (1965). *Genetics and the Social Behavior of the Dog*. Chicago, IL: The University of Chicago Press.

Smoller, J. W. & Tsuang, M. T. (1998). Panic and phobic anxiety: defining phenotypes for genetic studies. *American Journal of Psychiatry*, 155: 1152–62.

Stamps, J. & Groothuis, T. G. G. (2010). The development of animal personality: relevance, concepts and perspectives. *Biological Reviews*, 85: 301–25.

Stöger, R. (2008). The thrifty epigenotype: an acquired and heritable predisposition for obesity and diabetes? *Bioessays*, 30, 156–66.

Stutzmann, F., Vatin, V., Cauchi, S. *et al.* (2007). Non-synonymous polymorphisms in melanocortin-4 receptor protect against obesity: the two facets of a Janus obesity gene. *Human Molecular Genetics*, 16: 1837–44.

Sutter, N. B., Bustamante, C. D., Chase, K. *et al.* (2007). A single IGF1 allele is a major determinant of small size in dogs. *Science*, 316: 112–15.

Sutter, N. B. & Ostrander, E. A. (2004). Dog star rising: the canine genetic system. *Nature Reviews Genetics*, 5: 900–10.

Svartberg, K. (2002). Shyness-boldness predicts performance in working dogs. *Applied Animal Behaviour Science*, 79: 157–74.

Svartberg, K. (2006). Breed-typical behavior in dogs – historical remnants or recent constructs? *Applied Animal Behaviour Science*, 96: 293–313.

Svartberg, K. & Forkman, B. (2002). Personality traits in the domestic dog (*Canis familiaris*). *Applied Animal Behaviour Science*, 79: 133–155.

Takeuchi, Y., Hashizume, C., Arata, S. *et al.* (2009a). An approach to canine behavioral genetics employing guide dogs for the blind. *Animal Genetics*, 40: 217–24.

Takeuchi, Y., Kaneko, F., Hashizume, C. *et al.* (2009b). Association analysis between canine behavioral traits and genetic polymorphisms in the shiba inu breed. *Animal Genetics*, 40: 616–22.

Thannickal, T. C., Moore, R. Y., Nienhuis, R. *et al.* (2000). Reduced number of hypocretin neurons in human narcolepsy. *Neuron*, 27: 469–74.

Tiira, K., Escriou, C., Thomas, A. *et al.* (2011). Phenotypic and genetic characterization of tail chasing in bull terriers. *Journal of Veterinary Behavior: Clinical Applied Research*, 6: 83.

Tiira, K., Hakosalo, O., Kareinen, L. *et al.* (2012). Environmental effects on compulsive tail chasing in dogs. *PLoS One*, 7: e41684.

Tobi, E. W., Lumey, L. H., Talens, R. P. *et al.* (2009). DNA methylation differences after exposure to prenatal famine are common and timing- and sex-specific. *Human Molecular Genetics*, 18: 4046–53.

Todd, J. A. (2006). Statistical false positive or true disease pathway? *Nature Genetics*, 38: 731–3.

Trut, L., Oskina, I. & Kharlamova, A. (2009). Animal evolution during domestication: the domesticated fox as a model. *Bioessays*, 31: 349–60.

Uhde, T. W., Malloy, L. C. & Slate, S. O. (1992). Fearful behavior, body size, and serum IGF-I levels in nervous and normal pointer dogs. *Pharmacology, Biochemistry and Behavior*, 43: 263–9.

Våge, J., Wade, C., Biagi, T. *et al.* (2010a). Association of dopamine- and serotonin-related genes with canine aggression. *Genes Brain and Behavior*, 9: 372–8.

Våge, J., Bønsdorff, T. B., Arnet, E., Tverdal, A. & Lingaas, F. (2010b). Differential gene expression in brain tissues of aggressive and non-aggressive dogs. *BMC Veterinary Research*, 6: 34.

Van den Berg, L., Schilder, M. B., de Vries, H., Leegwater, P. A. & van Oost, B. A. (2006). Phenotyping of aggressive behavior in golden retriever dogs with a questionnaire. *Behavior Genetics*, 36: 882–902.

Van den Berg, L., Schilder, M. B. H. & Knol, B. W. (2003). Behavior genetics of canine aggression: behavioral phenotyping of golden retrievers by means of an aggression test. *Behavior Genetics*, 33: 469–83.

Vaysse, A., Ratnakumar, A., Derrien, T. *et al.* (2011). Identification of genomic regions associated with phenotypic variation between dog breeds using selection mapping. *PLoS Genetics*, 7: e1002316.

Vermeire, S., Audenaert, K., De Meester, R. *et al.* (2012). Serotonin 2A receptor, serotonin transporter and dopamine transporter alterations in dogs with compulsive behavior as a promising model for human obsessive-compulsive disorder. *Psychiatry Research*, 201: 78–87.

Vermeire, S. T., Audenaert, K. R., De Meester, R. H. *et al.* (2011). Neuro-imaging the serotonin 2A receptor as a valid biomarker for canine behavioral disorders. *Research in Veterinary Science*, 91: 465–72.

Vonholdt, B. M., Pollinger, J. P., Lohmueller, K. E. *et al.* (2010). Genome-wide SNP and haplotype analyses reveal a rich history underlying dog domestication. *Nature*, 464: 898–902.

Waterland, R. A. & Jirtle, R. L. (2003). Transposable elements: targets for early nutritional effects on epigenetic gene regulation. *Molecular and Cellular Biology*, 23: 5293–300.

Waterland, R. A., Travisano, M., Tahiliani, K. G., Rached, M. T. & Mirza, S. (2008). Methyl donor supplementation prevents transgenerational amplification of obesity. *International Journal of Obesity (Lond)*, 32: 1373–9.

Willis, M. B. (1976). *The German Shepherd Dog: Its History, Development and Genetics*. Leicester, UK: K.&R. Books.

Wilson, B. J. & Wade, C. M. (2012). Empowering international canine inherited disorder management. *Mammalian Genome*, 23: 195–202.

Wilson, D., Clark, A., Coleman, K. & Dearstyne, T. (1994). Shyness and boldness in humans and other animals. *Trends in Ecology & Evolution*, 9: 442–6.

Wilsson, E. & Sundgren, P.-E. (1997a). The use of a behavior test for the selection of dogs for service and breeding, II: heritability for tested parameters and effect of selection based on service dog characteristics. *Applied Animal Behaviour Science*, 54: 235–41.

Wilsson, E. & Sundgren, P.-E. (1997b). The use of a behavior test for the selection of dogs for service and breeding, I: method of testing and evaluating test results in the adult dog, demands on different kinds of service dogs, sex and breed differences. *Applied Animal Behaviour Science*, 53: 279–95.

Wright, H. F., Mills, D. S. & Pollux, P. M. (2012). Behavioral and physiological correlates of impulsivity in the domestic dog (*Canis familiaris*). *Physiology & Behavior*, 105: 676–82.

Yeh, M. T., Coccaro. E. F. & Jacobson, K. C. (2010). Multivariate behavior genetic analyses of aggressive behavior subtypes. *Behavior Genetics*, 40: 603–61

6

Becoming a dog: Early experience and the development of behavior

JAMES SERPELL, DEBORAH L. DUFFY AND J. ANDREW JAGOE

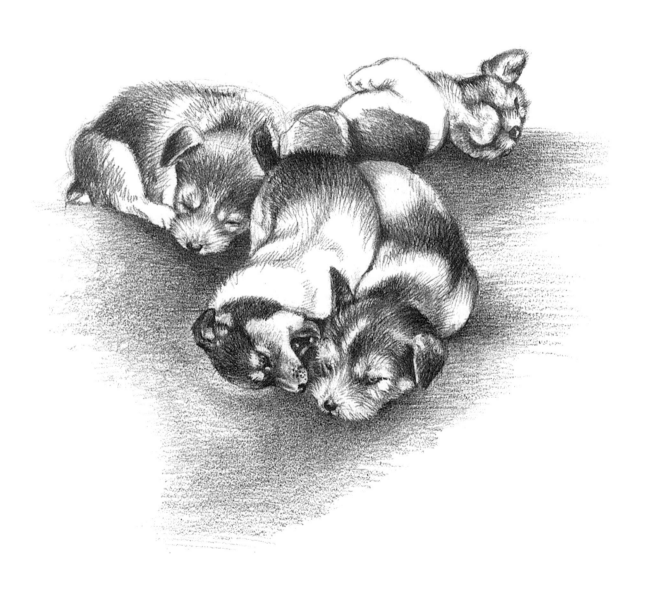

6.1 Introduction

Early life experiences[1] are known to have more profound and persistent effects on behavioral development than those occurring at other stages of the life cycle (see Bale *et al.*, 2010; Bateson, 1981; Crews, 2011; Levine, 1962; Simmel & Baker, 1980). Pioneering studies of the domestic dog have contributed significantly to our current understanding of these effects of early experience. In 1945 an extensive program of research was initiated at the Roscoe B. Jackson Memorial Laboratory at Bar Harbor, Maine, on the relationship between heredity and social behavior in dogs. This work, which included detailed descriptive and experimental studies of behavioral genetics and ontogeny, led to the conclusion that there are particular "critical" periods in early development when puppies are unusually sensitive to environmental influences and, therefore, especially susceptible to the effects of early experience (see Elliot & Scott, 1961; Freedman *et al.*, 1961; Fuller, 1967; Scott, 1962, 1963; Scott & Fuller, 1965; Scott & Marston, 1950; Scott *et al.*, 1974).

In the last 10–15 years, the emerging field of behavioral epigenetics has revolutionized our understanding of the ways in which genes and experience – nature and nurture – interact during development to produce such effects. It is now known, for example, that a wide variety of environmental factors, including maternal behavior, physical and emotional stress, and exposure to toxins, drugs and hormones – especially during the early part of life – can modify the expression of the genes that regulate the central nervous system without altering the DNA sequence. This essentially means that, while the genome still provides the design blueprint for the developing brain and nervous system, it is an adjustable blueprint that can respond dynamically to information and experience coming from the environment, and thereby alter the course of behavioral development in adaptive ways (Bale *et al.*, 2010; Berger *et al.*, 2009; Cardoso *et al.*, 2015; Heim & Binder, 2012; Sweatt, 2013; van den Berg, Chapter 5). Furthermore, at least some of these changes in gene expression appear to be heritable in the sense that they can be propagated, either through germ cells or via the quality of parental behavior, to affect later generations (Crews, 2011; Curley *et al.*, 2011a, 2011b; Dunn *et al.*, 2011; Lynch & Kemp, 2014; Patchev *et al.*, 2014).

It is important to stress that these changes in gene expression occur more readily at certain stages of brain development. The early growth and development of the brain is punctuated by periods of increased plasticity during which it is more susceptible to remodeling and reorganization in response to environmental triggers (Meredith, 2014). These episodes of sensitivity tend to occur in a similar sequence across mammal species, but the time scales involved may differ considerably from one species to another (Heim & Binder, 2012). It is therefore important to specify the key stages of development that are characteristic of the domestic dog and its nearest relatives.

This chapter reviews our current understanding of the major milestones in canine behavioral development, and examines the evidence linking adult behavior and temperament with the effects of early experience, particularly with regard to the development of so-called behavior problems.

6.2 Stages of development

According to the findings of the Bar Harbor studies, the early development of the dog can be divided into a series of four "natural" stages or periods: (1) the *neonatal period*; (2) the *transition period*; (3) the *socialization period*; and (4) the *juvenile period* (see Scott & Fuller, 1965; Scott *et al.*, 1974).

[1]For the purposes of this review, the term "early life" in dogs will refer to the first few months of life, up to and including puberty.

To these should be added the *prenatal* and *pubertal periods*, since it is now known that long-term effects on behavioral development can also be produced in mammals by events and exposures occurring both *in utero* and during the transition to sexual maturity (see Champagne, 2008; Heim & Binder, 2012; Joffe, 1969).

6.2.1   The prenatal period

The prenatal period has been largely ignored as a developmental stage in the ontogenesis of canid behavior and temperament. Nevertheless, numerous studies of rodents and both human and non-human primates indicate that transplacental maternal influences can exert significant long-term effects on the subsequent behavior of the offspring. Subjecting female rats to stressful experiences during pregnancy activates the maternal hypothalamic–pituitary–adrenal (HPA) axis, resulting in the release of glucocorticoid (stress) hormones. Offspring exposed to sufficiently high levels of these maternal hormones *in utero* display enhanced stress sensitivity when tested later in life, and more emotional females tend to give birth to more emotional offspring independent of genetic influences (Champagne, 2008; DeFries *et al.*, 1967; Denenberg & Morton, 1962; Weinstock, 2008). Similar effects have yet to be investigated in dogs, and it should be emphasized that such influences may not be generalizable across mammal species due to differences in placentation patterns. However, female cubs of a related canid, the blue fox (*Alopex lagopus*), whose mothers were subjected to stressful handling during the last third of pregnancy, were found to display higher behavioral reactivity in novel test situations at 35 days post-partum than those of unhandled females (Braastad *et al.*, 1998).

Androgens derived either from maternal circulation or from the proximity and preponderance of male littermates have also been shown to exert a prepartum "masculinizing" influence on the subsequent behavior of female rat and mouse pups (see Hart *et al.*, 2006). Whether similar effects exist in canids is at present unknown, and again, differences in placentation may limit such influences in dogs compared with rodents. One recent study, for example, failed to detect any convincing long-term effects of litter sex ratio on the behavior of military working dogs (Foyer *et al.*, 2013). Various preferences and species recognition patterns may also be influenced prenatally (see Gottlieb, 1976; Joffe, 1969). For instance, Wells & Hepper (2006) demonstrated that puppies *in utero* are able to "learn" and subsequently recognize distinctive odors added to the mother's diet during the final weeks of pregnancy.

6.2.2   The neonatal period

During the *neonatal period* the puppy is still comparatively helpless and dependent on the mother, and adapted to a life of suckling and care-soliciting. At this age, from birth to approximately two weeks, puppies are sensitive to tactile stimuli and certain tastes and odors, but their motor abilities are limited, and neither their eyes nor their ear canals are open or functional (Pal, 2008; Scott & Fuller, 1965). Because of the immature state of their neurosensory systems, it was originally assumed that canine neonates were largely incapable of associative learning (Scott & Marston, 1950). Subsequently, it has been shown that neonatal puppies can learn simple associations, although slowly compared with older pups, and only within the limits of their own rather specialized sensory and behavioral capacities (see Cornwell & Fuller, 1960; Stanley, 1970, 1972). Both Fox (1971) and Zimen (1987) reported that wolves hand-reared from birth or six days of age are more reliable and friendlier towards humans than those hand-reared from 15 days or subsequently. The mechanism for this effect is unknown but it is likely to involve some form of olfactory imprinting during the neonatal period (see e.g. Leon, 1992; Lord, 2013).

Despite their cognitive limitations, it is well established that mammalian neonates are acutely sensitive to some aspects of their early environment, and that these influences can have long-term effects on their behavior. Studies in primates and rodents have demonstrated, for example, that gluco-corticoid levels in the mother's milk can affect the development of temperamental characteristics in her offspring, although the direction of these effects may differ between species. In rats, high levels of glucocorticoids in milk during lactation were associated with greater "confidence" in offspring, whereas in rhesus macaques, high levels of cortisol in milk were linked to increased nervousness and reduced confidence. Furthermore, male and female macaque infants reacted differently depending on the concentrations of cortisol at different time points in the lactation cycle (Hinde et al., 2014). Equivalent studies have not been performed in dogs, although this represents a potentially fruitful topic for future research.

Episodes of early life stress (ELS) can also have marked, long-term effects on the behavioral and physical development of mammalian neonates, including puppies. In rodents, intense or pro-longed stress, such as two or more hours of separation from the mother, seems to intensify neonatal sensitivity to stressful or anxiety-provoking situations later in life. In contrast, mild to moderate stressors, such as brief periods of separation from the mother and litter, or daily handling, appear to have a positive impact on stress resilience, as well as producing accelerated maturation of the nerv-ous system, more rapid hair growth and weight gain, enhanced development of motor and problem solving skills, and earlier opening of the eyes (Curley et al., 2011a; Denenberg, 1968; Fox, 1978; Gazzano et al., 2008; Levine, 1962; Lupien et al., 2009; Lyons et al., 2010; Macri et al., 2011; Whimbey & Denenberg, 1967). Some canine studies have found similar effects. For example, pup-pies exposed to varied stimulation from birth to five weeks of age were found to be more confident, exploratory and socially dominant when tested later in strange situations than unstimulated controls (Fox, 1978), and puppies handled gently on a daily basis from 3 to 21 days after birth were calmer, more exploratory, and gave fewer distress calls in 8-week puppy isolation tests than littermates who were not handled (Gazzano et al., 2008). In contrast, a study of puppies receiving early stimulation from 3 to 16 days post-partum showed no differences in behavior at 10 weeks from unstimulated controls, perhaps due to their younger age at the time of stimulation, or because the effects were masked by the influence of extensive human socialization during subsequent weeks (Schoon & Berntsen, 2011).

To account for these effects of early life stress, Levine (1967) originally proposed that early handling and mild stress produce an adaptive change in the animal's HPA system that enables it to cope more effectively with stressful situations in adulthood. More recent work indicates that the effects of these mild-moderate stressors are probably mediated through the changes they induce in maternal behavior when the pups are returned to the nest.

Variation in maternal behavior toward offspring during the neonatal period is now known to have profound and lasting effects on the development of their physiological and behavioral responses to stress (Champagne, 2008; Champagne et al., 2003; Curley et al., 2011a; Meaney, 2001; Sapolsky, 2004; Weaver et al., 2004). These effects appear to be mediated by four key hormones – corticotrophin releasing hormone, arginine vasopressin, oxytocin, and prolactin – all of which contribute in different way to changes in the developing brain's responsiveness to stress hormones (Bales et al., 2011; Kappeler & Meaney, 2010; Nephew & Murgatroyd, 2013). Female rodents whose pups are subjected to experimental stressors tend to lick and groom them more than the mothers of unstressed pups, and this extra attention suppresses the pups' hypothalamo–pituitary–adrenal (HPA) responsiveness. Conversely, stressed mother rodents tend to engage in reduced levels of licking and grooming of their offspring who respond to this by developing higher reactivity to stress and a lower propensity to engage in parental behavior as adults, thereby perpetuating the stress-sensitive phenotype across generations (Champagne, 2008; Champagne *et al.*, 2003; Curley *et al.*, 2011a; Meaney, 2001; Sapolsky, 2004; Smotherman *et al.*, 1977; Weaver *et al.*, 2004). To date, no studies have investigated the existence of these phenomena in dogs, although recent work with military working dogs has demonstrated a positive association between a female's maternal parity (and assumed experience) and the later confidence of her offspring (Foyer *et al.*, 2013).

Referring to humans, one expert has recently described early life stress as, "one of the most explicit and undisputed environmental risk factors for disease in later life, including metabolic and psychiatric disease" (Schmidt, 2010). Despite this, surprisingly little is currently known about the extent to which ELS during the neonatal or subsequent periods either prevents or contributes to the development of behavior and behavior problems in domestic dogs. This is an area that would be likely to repay further investigation.

6.2.3   The transition period

As its name suggests, the *transition period* is marked by a period of rapid transition or metamorphosis during which the patterns of behavior associated with neonatal existence disappear and are replaced by those more typical of later puppyhood and adult life. The whole process takes about a week, beginning with the opening of the eyes at around 13 (±3) days, and ending at approximately 18–20 days with the opening of the ear canals and the first appearance of the auditory "startle" response to sudden, loud noises. Electroencephalogram (EEG) readings of visual cortex activity also indicate a sudden increase in alpha waves at about three weeks of age, although brain wave patterns and visual and auditory acuity do not attain adult levels until about 6–8 weeks. Puppies also exhibit a number of changes in behavior during this transitional phase. They show an ability to crawl backwards as well as forwards, and begin to stand and walk, albeit clumsily. They start to defecate and urinate outside the nest, and anogenital licking by the mother is no longer required to stimulate elimination. Puppies begin showing an interest in solid food at this time. They also start to engage in social play with littermates and display social signals such as growling and tail wagging. Patterns of distress vocalization also change. Whereas neonatal puppies yelp primarily in response to cold or hunger, a three-week-old puppy will also yelp if it finds itself outside the nest in an unfamiliar environment, even if it is otherwise warm and well-fed (Fox, 1971; Lord, 2013; Pal, 2008; Schoon & Berntsen, 2011; Scott & Fuller, 1965).

Most of these behavioral changes make sense when considered in the context of development under non-domestic conditions. Among wolf pups living in the wild, 2–3 weeks represents the age at which they first emerge from the dark interior of the breeding den. Evidence from comparative studies suggests, however, that this period of transition begins slightly earlier and is completed more rapidly in wolves than in domestic dogs (Frank & Frank, 1982, 1985; Lord, 2013; Schoon & Berntsen, 2011; Zimen, 1987).

In terms of learning and the effects of early experience, the transition period more or less resembles a continuation of the neonatal stage. Puppies' performances on both classical and operant conditioning tasks show a steady improvement at this age, although rates of learning and the stability of conditioned responses do not reach adult levels until 4–5 weeks (Scott & Fuller, 1965).

6.2.4   The socialization period

The socialization period in puppies was first described as a "critical period" for the formation of primary social relationships or social attachments (Scott, 1962; Scott et al., 1974). The concept of the "critical period" was borrowed originally from embryology by Konrad Lorenz (1935), who used it to account for the phenomena of filial and sexual imprinting in precocial birds (i.e. those that are able to move about and feed themselves immediately after hatching). In this context, the *critical* period was seen as a narrow and clearly defined developmental window during which specific stimuli produced long-term and irreversible effects on subsequent behavior. According to some interpretations, appropriate stimulation within the critical period was also necessary for normal development to proceed (e.g. Fox, 1978). Later evidence, however, suggested that the boundaries of such periods are not always as rigid as originally conceived, and that behavior or preferences acquired within them can often be modified or reversed at later stages, albeit with varying degrees of difficulty. As a result, most authorities now favor the term "sensitive periods" to describe these phases in development when particular responses or preferences are acquired more readily than at other times (see Bateson 1979, 1981; Heim & Binder, 2012; Hinde, 1970; Immelmann & Soumi, 1981; Meredith, 2014).

Primary socialization in puppies has been found to be largely independent of associated rewards or punishments, although emotionally arousing stimuli – both positive and negative – seem to accelerate the process (Scott, 1963; Scott & Fuller, 1965; Scott et al., 1974). Among wolf pups reared under natural conditions, the process of socialization ensures that the young animals form their primary social attachments for their littermates, parents and other pack members. In the case of the domestic dog, it enables puppies to form non-conspecific attachments for humans or other animals encountered socially during the same period. For example, puppies are capable of recognizing their littermates at 4–5 weeks (Hepper, 1985), and cross-fostered puppies raised throughout the socialization period (3–16 weeks) with only kitten littermates tend to avoid interacting with strange puppies when first exposed to them. This is in contrast to their kitten foster siblings who will interact playfully with strange puppies on a first encounter (Fox, 1969). Such experiments demonstrate that the character of the socialization experience not only determines the young animal's choice of future social partners but also, to some extent, defines the species to which it belongs. It has also been shown that early, non-conspecific encounters do not need to be particularly frequent or protracted for socialization to occur. Fuller (1967) found that puppies could be socialized to humans during this period with as little as two 20-minute sessions of exposure per week, and Wolfle (1990) described a program that achieved "adequate socialization" of laboratory beagles with less than five minutes of human social contact per pup per week.

The ease with which most domestic dog puppies are able to establish non-conspecific social attachments is presumably a product of selection under domestication. Experimental studies have demonstrated that young wolves need to be hand-reared from at least 2–3 weeks of age in order to develop reliable and positive social bonds with humans, and by 6 weeks their fearful/avoidant responses to strangers are strong enough to effectively prevent further socialization of naïve animals. Domestic dog puppies, in contrast, readily form such attachments as long as they have some human exposure before 7–8 weeks of age, and their socialization "window" seems to remain open until around 12–14 weeks or even longer in some individuals (Fentress, 1967; Fox, 1971; Frank & Frank, 1982, 1985; Lord, 2013; Miklósi, 2007; Zimen, 1987). Belyaev et al. (1985) proposed that this difference between dogs and wolves was due primarily to delayed maturation of the HPA axis in dogs resulting in retarded onset of the normal or "wild-type" fearful/avoidant response to unfamiliar individuals and situations. Confirming this idea, recent work by Morrow et al. (2015) detected significant breed differences in the age of onset of fearful/avoidant responses in puppies, as well as correlated differences in stress responses as measured by salivary cortisol. Socialization also appears to involve a strong prosocial element – i.e. the desire to approach and make contact with strangers – in addition to a reduction in fear, and this also seems to have been accentuated in the dog relative to the wolf. Results from recent studies in dogs and other animals indicate that genetic polymorphisms in the oxytocin receptor gene (OXTR) may account for some these differences in prosocial tendencies among dogs, and between dogs and wolves (Arueti et al., 2014; Chen et al., 2011; Kis et al., 2014). Both traits – reduction in fear/avoidance and enhanced prosocial tendencies – are presumably the outcome of selection for extreme *socializeability* early in the domestication process (Lord et al., Chapter 4; Trut et al., 2004).

During the sensitive period for socialization, puppies may also form attachments for particular places, a phenomenon referred to as "localization" by Scott & Fuller (1965). According to these authors, the consequences of socialization and localization are so similar that they may represent the same process applied to different objects: "this would mean that the puppy becomes attached to both the living and non-living parts of its environment at this age" (1965, p. 112).

Puppies' cognitive abilities develop rapidly during this period. It has been shown, for example, that 3–5-week-old puppies can learn to recognize novel objects they have viewed previously only on video, and will subsequently exhibit less fear of the actual objects when tested with them at 7–8 weeks (Pluijmakers et al., 2010). Between 5 and 8 weeks of age, puppies also develop so-called "object permanence" (the ability to understand the visible displacement of an object from one concealed position to another) (Gagnon & Doré, 1994) and, according to some studies, puppies as young as 6–9 weeks can recognize and follow human communication signals such as pointing in order to find hidden food (Gácsi et al., 2009; Riedel et al., 2008). This latter claim, however, has been challenged by other researchers who suggest that this ability may not emerge consistently until 5–6 months of age (Dorey et al., 2010; Wynne et al., 2008).

The upper and lower boundaries of the socialization period have been determined by laboratory experiments in which puppies' social contacts have been observed and manipulated at different points and for different periods in early development. In what is often regarded as the definitive study, Freedman et al. (1961) reared eight litters of cocker spaniel and beagle pups in isolation (from humans, but not from their mothers or littermates) until 14 weeks of age, during which time each pup received one week of moderately intensive human testing and handling before being returned to the litter. Some pups received this week of human socialization at two weeks, others at three, five, seven or nine weeks of age. Five "control" pups remained unsocialized until 14 weeks of age. At 14 weeks, all the pups were tested (or retested) for their responses to a "passive" human handler, to being walked on a leash, and to being strapped into a physiological harness and subjected to various arousing or unpleasant stimuli. Those pups socialized between five and nine weeks approached a passive handler most readily, and were more easily trained to walk on a leash. Those socialized at seven weeks obtained the most favorable scores in terms of their reactions to being tested in harness. Control pups remained uniformly fearful and intractable even after many weeks of careful handling and petting. Based on these findings, the authors concluded that, "2½ to 9–13 weeks of age approximates a critical period for socialization" (Freedman et al., 1961, p. 1017).

Behavioral observations of naive puppies' responses to human handlers at different ages have tended to confirm these findings. Although initially fearful in the presence of an "active" human handler, young puppies show a rapid increase in their tendency to approach and make social contact with an unfamiliar person between the ages of three and five weeks. Thereafter, this tendency declines. Conversely, from three to five weeks most pups show little or no fear of a "passive" handler, but they then become increasingly wary or fearful of strange individuals or situations beyond this age. On the basis of this kind of evidence, Scott & Fuller (1965) concluded that the primary socialization period ran from about the third to the twelfth week after birth, with a peak of sensitivity between six and eight weeks. Below three weeks of age, they argued, a puppy's neurosensory systems are too underdeveloped to permit socialization, and beyond 12 weeks its growing tendency to react fearfully to novel persons or situations puts an effective upper limit on further socialization. Between six and eight weeks, however, a pup's social motivation to approach and make contact with a stranger outweighs its natural wariness, hence the view that this period represents the optimum time for socialization.

Based on the results of conditioned aversion experiments with beagle pups, Fox & Stelzner (1966) identified a period at around eight weeks when pups are hypersensitive to distressing psychological or physical stimuli. Puppies' heart rates and rates of distress vocalization in strange situations also tend to show developmental peaks during this 6th–8th week period (Elliot & Scott, 1961; Scott & Fuller, 1965). On the other hand, naturalistic observations of free-roaming dog litters have revealed that puppies also exhibit a peak in social play at around 7–8 weeks of age (Pal, 2008), which would suggest that the heightened sensitivity displayed by pups at this age may be related to the rapid acquisition of social skills.

Other studies and observations suggest that the upper boundary of the socialization period may be less clearly defined than previously supposed. Good evidence exists that young wolves and dogs that are well socialized at three months will, nevertheless, regress and become fearful again in the absence of periodic social reinforcement until the age of 6–8 months (Fox, 1971, 1978; Woolpy & Ginsberg, 1967; Woolpy, 1968). Once properly socialized, however, adult wolves appear to remain so despite long periods of isolation from human contact (Woolpy & Ginsberg, 1967). Anecdotal evidence that young wolves experience a second, sudden-onset phase of heightened sensitivity to threatening stimuli at around 4–6 months of age may help to account for these phenomena (see Fentress, 1967; Fox, 1971; Mech, 1970). Conversely, it has also been established that adult, untamed wolves and inadequately socialized dogs can still be socialized to humans, although the process requires considerable patience and, in the case of wolves, involves isolating the animal from everything but human contact for periods of 6–7 months (Woolpy & Ginsberg, 1967; Niebuhr et al., 1980). Finally, most authorities agree that substantial individual and breed differences exist in the precise timing and quality of the socialization process (see e.g. Lord, 2013). Zimen (1987, p. 290) attributed some of this variation to the variable and conflicting expression of, "two genetically independent motivational systems," the motivation to make social approaches to strangers and the motivation to avoid novel stimuli. In a study of social development in wolves, poodles and their hybrids, he found that these approach–avoidance tendencies tended to segregate out among the F_2 backcrosses (Zimen, 1987). Other work on wolves and foxes (*Vulpes vulpes*) suggests that differences in developing aggressive tendencies may also affect the upper age limit for socialization (Plyusnina et al., 1991; Woolpy & Ginsberg, 1967).

The results of the Bar Harbor studies, and subsequent, related investigations by Guide Dogs for the Blind, USA (see Pfaffenberger et al., 1976), gave rise to various practical recommendations regarding the husbandry and training of domestic dogs. In particular, two basic rules for producing a well-balanced and well-adjusted dog were proposed. First, that the ideal time to produce a close social relationship between a young dog and its human owner is between six and eight weeks of age, and that this is, therefore, "the optimal time to remove a puppy from the litter and make it into a house pet" (Scott & Fuller, 1965, p. 385). Second, that puppies should be introduced, at least in a preliminary way, to the circumstances and conditions they are likely to encounter as adults, preferably by eight weeks, and certainly no later than 12 weeks of age (Scott & Fuller, 1965; Pfaffenberger & Scott, 1976). Slabbert & Rasa (1993) later criticized the recommended practice of removing pups from their maternal environment as early as six weeks of age. In a study of socialization and development in German shepherd puppies, these authors found that pups separated from their mothers and litter sites (but not their littermates) at six weeks exhibited loss of appetite and weight, and increased distress, mortality and susceptibility to disease compared with pups that remained at home with their mothers until 12 weeks of age. Both groups, however, showed the same degree of socialization towards their human handlers. Although the rates of morbidity and mortality observed in this study appear to be abnormally high, Slabbert & Rasa (1993, p. 7) nevertheless concluded that conventional rehoming procedures for puppies are deleterious to the animals' welfare, and that the early evidence on primary socialization in dogs has been wrongly interpreted to mean that "exclusive access to the desired bonding partner" is actually *necessary* at this time in order to achieve correct socialization.

Some support for the validity of Slabbert & Rasa's (1993) contention that puppies should be rehomed after six weeks of age comes from two more recent studies. Pierantoni *et al.* (2011) investigated the prevalence of behavioral problems in adult dogs separated from their litters between 30 and 40 days (≤ 6 weeks) after birth *versus* those separated at 60 days (8 weeks). According to their owners' responses to a questionnaire survey, the dogs in the early separation group displayed a significantly greater prevalence of destructiveness, excessive barking, fearfulness and reactivity to noises, resource guarding, and attention seeking than those separated later (Pierantoni *et al.*, 2011). These findings should be interpreted with caution, however, since the authors did not correct statistically for multiple comparisons, and a significantly higher proportion of the early separated dogs were obtained from pet stores. A second study of stereotypic tail-chasing in a Finnish sample of bull terriers, Staffordshire bull terriers and German shepherds found that tail-chasers had been separated from their mothers at a significantly younger age (average 7 weeks) than the dogs that did not chase their tails (average 8 weeks) (Tiira *et al.*, 2012).

Such findings are at least partly consistent with those of prolonged maternal separation experiments in rodents in which epigenetic changes resulted in long-term heightened responsiveness to stressful situations (Curley *et al.*, 2011a). It is also possible that the observed effects are a consequence of the acute stress of early weaning. Although some variation is reported, most wolves and dogs wean their pups naturally between 5 and 10 weeks of age, and the process is usually accomplished gradually over a period of weeks (Lord, 2013; Malm, 1995; Mech, 1970; Pal, 2005). Abruptly removing a puppy from its mother at 6 weeks or earlier may therefore represent a significant stressor. Certainly, experimental studies in mice and rats have confirmed that early weaned individuals show higher rates of anxiety-related and aggressive behavior later in life than those weaned normally, suggesting that the stress of early weaning may have persistent effects on the HPA axis (Ito *et al.*, 2006; Kikusui *et al.*, 2006). Surprisingly, given its likely effects on later behavior, the timing of weaning has received very little attention in the literature on canine behavioral development.

6.2.5 The juvenile and pubertal periods

According to Scott & Fuller (1965), the juvenile period runs from approximately 12 weeks (the putative end of the socialization period) until 6 months of age or later, corresponding to the onset of sexual development (i.e. puberty). The timing of this transition from pre-adolescence to adolescence varies greatly according to breed. Some small or miniature breeds may be sexually mature at 6–7 months while some large or giant breeds may not reach this stage until they are 18–24 months old. It is commonly reported that domestic dogs achieve sexual maturity earlier than wolves (e.g. Hayssen *et al.*, 1993; Price, 1984), although at least one study found that male poodles and wolves living under similar conditions in captivity reached physiological sexual maturity at almost the same ages (Haase, 2000).

This period of the young dog's life is probably the most poorly studied in terms of its effects on adult behavior (Miklósi, 2007), despite the fact that gonadal hormones are known to modulate adolescent brain plasticity (Heim & Binder, 2012). Anecdotal evidence certainly suggests that experiences during the pre-adolescent and adolescent periods can exert long-term effects on behavior (Dehasse, 1994; Fentress, 1967; Fox, 1971; Mech, 1970), and recent studies of working dogs have found associations between dogs' experiences during this period and long-term changes in adult behaviour (Foyer *et al.*, 2014; Harvey *et al.*, 2016; Serpell & Duffy, 2016). In rats, environmental enrichment around puberty was found to completely erase the negative effects of early life stress on the HPA axis (Francis *et al.*, 2002).

6.3   Development of major behavior problems

Behavioral problems are probably the leading risk factor for relinquishment of dogs to animal shelters, with approximately 40% of relinquishing owners citing behavioral problems as a contributory factor, and roughly a quarter citing them as the primary reason for relinquishment (Herron *et al.*, 2007; Miller *et al.*, 1996; Patronek *et al.*, 1996; Reisner, Chapter 11; Salman *et al.*, 1998; Zawistowski & Reid, Chapter 12). Behavior problems can also lead dog owners to request elective euthanasia for their pets, as well as inducing them to abandon them or subject them to physical abuse. Some behavior problems, particularly aggression, also represent a significant public health concern (Lockwood, Chapter 9). Additionally, a large proportion of valuable working dogs are released from training programs due to the development of problematical behavior that interferes with their working ability (Duffy & Serpell, 2012). For these and other reasons, it is important to understand the influence of development on the expression of canine behavior problems, particularly the "major" problems associated with aggression and fear/anxiety.

6.4.1   Aggression

Aggression is the most commonly reported category of behavior problems in domestic dogs (Hart *et al.*, 2006; Lindsay, 2001; Overall, 1997), and one that has received an inordinate amount of public and media attention in recent years (see Lockwood, Chapter 9; Serpell, Chapter 15). Despite the popular idea of aggressiveness being a single temperament trait (Lorenz, 1966), most modern ethologists would accept that dog aggression, like aggression in other species, is likely to be context dependent, and that a dog that responds aggressively in one situation is not necessarily likely to do so in others. Unfortunately, wide disparities in methods of classifying aggressive behavior problems now exist in the relevant literature (see e.g. Borchelt, 1983a; Borchelt & Voith, 1982a; Lindsay, 2001; Moyer, 1968; Overall, 1997), and this has tended to hamper efforts to understand the ontogeny of this important category of problems (Jagoe, 1994). In this section we consider just two forms of aggressive behavior problem: aggression directed toward unfamiliar individuals particularly within the dog's home range or territory, and aggression directed toward familiar individuals living in the same household as the dog.

Aggression towards strangers
Like wolves, many dogs display a tendency to react aggressively to unfamiliar individuals (human and canine), especially within their home ranges. In practice, this home range or territory usually

comprises the immediate vicinity of the owner's home, but may also include other areas where the dog is regularly walked or confined. As with most traits, there are marked individual and breed differences in the tendency to display this type of behavior, and it would appear that elements have been amplified by human selection, particularly in certain guarding breeds (Adams & Johnson, 1993; Duffy *et al.*, 2008; Hart & Hart, Chapter 7; Hart *et al.*, 2006; Serpell & Duffy, 2014). Extreme territorial aggression is also one of the more common forms of behavior problem in dogs. One large North American survey reported that over 18% of owners classified their dogs as being "overprotective" in a territorial sense (Campbell, 1986).

There have been surprisingly few studies of the development of stranger-directed aggression in either domestic dogs or wild canids. According to Borchelt & Voith (1982a), dogs with this behavior problem are usually from 1 to 3 years of age, although this presumably reflects the age when the behavior became a problem rather than the age when it first developed. Anecdotally, a number of authors describe the first appearance of overt hostility towards unfamiliar intruders in wolf pups at around 16–20 weeks, coinciding with a sudden phase of heightened sensitivity to novel or threatening stimuli (Fentress, 1967; Fox, 1971; Mech, 1970). Whether this represents some sort of sensitive period for the acquisition of this type of defensive aggression is not known, although Mech (1970) pointed out that this is about the age when young wolves start moving away from the familiar den and rendezvous sites, and when they are therefore more likely to encounter strange or hostile territorial intruders. Recent evidence suggests that some dog breeds show a similar increase in aggressive responses to strangers at this age (Serpell & Duffy 2016).

Other evidence suggests that various aspects of the early rearing environment can influence the development of aggression toward strangers in dogs. For example, in their survey of owners of dogs involved in fights with other unfamiliar dogs, Roll & Unshelm (1997) reported that a high percentage (44%) had experienced few interactions with conspecifics between the ages of 5 weeks and 5 months. Serpell & Jagoe (1995) also found higher rates of aggression toward strangers among pet dogs that had been ill as puppies (0–16 weeks), and reported a linear relationship between the prevalence of "territorial-type aggression" and age at first vaccination (at least up to the age of 20 weeks). Similarly, Appleby *et al.* (2002) found highest rates of aggression toward unfamiliar people among dogs born and reared in kennel environments, and among those with no experience of urban environments between 3 and 6 months of age. Most of these findings can be interpreted as effects of inadequate early socialization. McMillan *et al.* (2013) found that dogs acquired as puppies from pet stores were more likely to develop stranger-directed aggression than those acquired from non-commercial breeders, but they were unable to specify the precise cause of this effect.

Owner-directed aggression

Owner-directed aggression, as its name suggests, is characterized by threats or attacks directed at the owner or a member of the owner's household (including other dogs) rather than at strangers. It is another commonly reported behavior problem seen by behavior counselors and trainers that is rarely reported before 1 year of age, and seems to occur more frequently among intact males and neutered females (see Borchelt, 1983a; Campbell, 1975; Hart *et al.*, 2006; Lindsay, 2001; Line & Voith, 1986; O'Farrell, 1986; Overall, 1997; Voith & Borchelt, 1982; Wright & Nesselrote, 1987). The motivation(s) underlying this form of canine aggression is hotly debated in the literature. Earlier works on canine behavior problems tended to use labels such as "dominance aggression" and "dominance-related aggression" to describe owner-directed aggression based on the perception (or assumption) that these dogs were either "pulling rank" or reacting aggressively to apparent challenges to their positions within existing social hierarchies: for example, in situations in which the owner was treated as a competitor for resources – e.g. food, space, resting location, etc. – or in response to supposedly "dominant" gestures by the owner, such as holding, petting, grooming, restraining, punishing or pushing past the animal, staring or yelling at it, or even leaning over it. In more recent literature, the term "dominance" is increasingly eschewed, partly to avoid making unwarranted assumptions regarding the dogs' true motivations for displaying this type of aggression, and partly to discourage owners from trying to assert their "dominant" status by using punitive, coercive or intimidating training techniques that are generally considered ineffective, inhumane and potentially dangerous (Bradshaw & Rooney, Chapter 8; Reisner, Chapter 11; Zawistowski & Reid, Chapter 12).

Displays of dominance nevertheless appear to be an important and pervasive behavior in groups of wild canids, such as wolves and coyotes (Bekoff, 2012; Mech & Cluff, 2010), and stable dominance hierarchies have also been observed in communities of free-roaming domestic dogs (Cafazzo *et al.*, 2010). In naturally occurring (as opposed to captive) groups, dominance rank tends to be positively correlated with age/seniority, so it may be more appropriate to describe these as *senior–junior* rather than *dominance–subordinance* relationships. There is also little evidence that individuals are constantly jockeying for "top dog" or *alpha* positions within such hierarchies (Cafazzo *et al.*, 2010; Mech, 2008), so the idea that the dog has some sort of innate predisposition to compete for social status is probably erroneous. Indeed, it is not even known whether dogs are aware of relative differences in social rank between group members, as has been demonstrated in some non-human primates (Range & Viranyi, Chapter 10). Some authorities have further suggested that the terms *dominant* and *dominance* should be confined to describing dyadic relationships, and that a term such as "assertiveness" should be used to describe an individual's propensity to strive for a dominant position within such relationships (Lockwood, 1979; van Hooff & Wensing, 1987).

Experimental studies of the development of so-called "dominance" behavior in canids have been fraught with methodological problems. Despite strong theoretical reasons for rejecting this approach, social dominance has usually been assessed experimentally in young in canids by placing two (or more) littermates together in an artificial competitive situation – the so-called *bone-in-pen test* – and ranking them according to their ability to gain and keep possession of some desired object, such as a bone or toy, for a fixed period of time (see Fox, 1972; Scott & Fuller, 1965). This technique ignores the possible effects of transient motivational differences between individuals at the time of testing, or the influence of individual temperamental factors, such as overall persistence or confidence, which may or may not be related to social dominance (see e.g. Hinde, 1974).

In wolf pups, both Fox (1972) and MacDonald (1987) found that paired contests were unreliable as a means of assessing dominance. In this context, pups tended to share the bone rather than compete for it. When littermates were tested *en masse*, however, both authors regarded the outcome of such contests as a reliable indicator of the most socially dominant individual(s) within each litter. According to Fox (1972) the highest ranking individuals in this test also tended to be more active and exploratory when confronted by novel objects, and were more adept at killing prey (live rats) than low ranking pups. He also found that test results obtained at eight weeks of age correlated reasonably well with dominance ratings 10 months later. MacDonald (1987) tested a litter of five male wolf pups *en masse* at frequent intervals between the ages of 17 and 180 days, and found that by the fifth week one pup was consistently outcompeting the others for possession of the bone. Between 15 and 20 weeks, this same pup was beaten sporadically by some of his littermates, but thereafter he won consistently until the end of the study. By about six weeks, this pup also ranked consistently highest in tests of boldness or "leadership" in unfamiliar situations. These findings led the author to conclude that the tendency to become socially dominant in wolves is one aspect of a relatively stable personality trait that can be detected as early as six or seven weeks of age (MacDonald, 1987).

The picture for domestic dog puppies is more confusing, and is characterized by marked breed and population differences. In a study of free-roaming dog puppies in India, Pal (2008) reported that agonistic play within the six litters he observed reached a peak at around 8 weeks of age before declining sharply in frequency. Males engaged in aggressive play more frequently than females, and one male puppy in each litter was responsible for the majority of these interactions. He concluded that stable dominance relationships within these litters were established by approximately 7 weeks of age. Scott & Fuller (1965) based their assessments of dominance on standard, paired bone-in-pen style contests conducted at 5, 11, 15 and 52 weeks of age. They also allowed their puppies weekly "training periods" with the bone between the ages of 2 and 10 weeks. At five weeks they found little evidence of consistent dominance (defined as the ability to possess the bone for more than 80% of a 10-minute test period) in any of the five breeds they studied. By 11 weeks, all breeds showed a large increase in the number of completely dominant relationships. Beyond this point, however, wire-haired fox terriers, Shetland sheepdogs, and basenjis showed a continuing increase until 52 weeks – though at different rates – while dominant relationships among beagles and cocker spaniels tended to decrease.

Breeds also differed in their tendency to threaten or attack each other in the test situation. Beagles and cocker spaniels almost never fought for possession of the bone and appeared to show very low levels of aggression at any age. Fox terriers also hardly ever fought in dyadic encounters, not because they were unaggressive (at around 7 weeks, aggression became such a problem in some litters that the pups needed to be separated) but because dominance relationships were apparently established at an early age in this breed. In contrast, shelties fought or attacked each other quite frequently at five weeks, but almost never after this, while basenjis continued to fight in competitive situations until they were a year old. The different breeds also showed sex differences in their tendency to establish dominance relationships. In the more aggressive breeds, such as fox terriers and basenjis, males tended to become completely dominant over females by 15 weeks or even earlier. In beagles and cocker spaniels there was no discernible tendency for males to be dominant over females at any age and, while male shelties showed no particular tendency to be dominant over females in competition for bones, other observations suggested that they were completely dominant in contexts unrelated to food competition. On the basis of these findings, Scott & Fuller (1965) concluded that the capacity to establish stable dominance relationships is ultimately a product of inherited aggressive tendencies, and that an individual's likelihood of becoming socially dominant is strongly dependent on previous experience of interactions with other members of the litter or social group.

Subsequently, Wright (1980) challenged the view that bone competition tests provide a reliable measure of social dominance in puppies. He investigated dyadic bone-in-pen test outcomes, neophobic responses in a modified "open field test," and social interactions in the rearing environment in a litter of five German shepherd puppies at 5½, 8½ and 11½ weeks, and found that puppies' apparent social ranks within the litter environment bore little or no relation to their likelihood of monopolizing a bone in a test situation. As in the studies of wolf litters described above, however, competitive ability in the bone-in-pen tests was correlated with confidence and exploratory behavior in the unfamiliar open field. Wright (1980) concluded that neophobic responses to the unfamiliar test situation prevented otherwise socially dominant pups from competing successfully in the bone-in-pen test, and that these tests actually measure competitive tendencies rather than social dominance. He also suggested that the social dominance hierarchy within the litter did not appear to stabilize until 11½ weeks.

The results of all these various studies suggest that human selection under domestication has had marked effects on the expression of social aggression or assertiveness in *Canis familiaris*. Evidence from wolves and free-roaming village dogs indicates that dominance relationships within litters of pups tend to become established between four and eight weeks of age, at least as far as the highest ranking or most assertive individuals are concerned (Bekoff, 1974; Fox, 1972; Fox et al., 1976;

MacDonald, 1987; Mech, 1970; Pal, 2008). However, in domestic dogs different breeds vary substantially with respect to the developmental onset of this type of aggression and the contexts in which it is exhibited. In some it may be obvious in relation to food competition, while in others it may only be expressed during conflicts over space or the attentions of the owner. Some dog breeds, particularly certain terriers, appear to establish dominance relationships as early as wolf pups, while others, such as cocker spaniels and beagles, may never develop stable dominance relationships regardless of circumstances (Duffy *et al.*, 2008; Fox, 1972; Bradshow & Nott, 1995; Scott & Fuller, 1965; Serpell & Duffy, 2014). Even in beagles, however, postures associated with assertiveness, such as *standing over*, first start appearing in the behavioral repertoire at around four weeks of age during bouts of social play (Fox *et al.*, 1976). This would suggest that, if there is a sensitive period for the acquisition of this type of behavior in dogs, it is likely to peak during the first few weeks of the socialization period.

Regarding the possible effects of early experience on the development of this type of aggression, the evidence is sparse and complicated by the current level of uncertainty about the motivational basis for the behavior – i.e. whether it is primarily motivated by possessiveness with respect to particular resources (resource guarding), assertiveness in relation to the acquisition of social rank, or simply an acquired defensive response to punishment by the owner. At least two studies report significantly higher rates of owner-directed aggression among puppies acquired from pet stores compared with those obtained from either non-commercial breeders (McMillan *et al.*, 2013) or other sources in general (Serpell & Jagoe, 1995). These authors also reported a higher incidence of what they called "dominance-related aggression" in dogs that had been ill as puppies (0–16 weeks). While the particular causative factor(s) responsible for these findings are unknown, both pre- and post-natal maternal stress, and early life stress would appear to be plausible candidates. Common sense would suggest that early handling effects, early interactions and experience with the mother, littermates and human caregivers, and/or inappropriate socialization could also exert a modifying influence on the development of this behavior.

6.4.2   Fears and phobias

Nervous or fearful responses to strangers and unfamiliar situations are another common source of behavior problems in dogs. Analysis of reasons for rejecting dogs from the US Guide Dogs for the Blind program revealed that, out of 600 animals, 19% were frightened of loud noises, 15% were afraid of cars or farm machinery and 12% evinced fear of other animals. Eighteen percent also displayed fear in a range of miscellaneous or unspecified situations (Tuber *et al.*, 1982). Fearfulness is also cited as the most common reason for rejecting potential guide dogs by Goddard & Beilharz (1982, 1984). Campbell (1986) reported a 20% incidence of "fear of noises" in his survey of 1422 American dog owners, while a more recent survey of owners in the UK gave a figure of 25% (Blackwell *et al.*, 2013). Data from one behavior problem referral clinic suggested that roughly one-third of all behavior consultations involved fear-related behavior problems, although it is not clear whether this figure included separation-related anxieties (Shull-Selcer & Stagg, 1991). Population-based surveys of dog owners have also detected breed differences in fearfulness, with mixed breed dogs tending to exhibit more fearfulness than purebreds, and small breed dogs typically displaying higher rates of fearfulness compared with medium and large breeds (Blackwell *et al.*, 2013; McGreevy *et al.*, 2013; Serpell & Duffy, 2014).

Interpreting the available information on the development of canine fearfulness is rendered more difficult by the use of widely varying systems of classifying aversive or fearful behavior. On the one hand, different fears or phobias are sometimes regarded as being more or less distinct (Hart *et al.*, 2006; Serpell & Duffy, 2014), while on the other they may be lumped together with more generalized anxieties (Tuber *et al.*, 1982), or treated as symptomatic of some global temperament trait, such as "emotionality" (Scott & Bielfelt, 1976; Scott & Fuller, 1965) or "stimulus reactivity" (Wright & Nesselrote, 1987). Regardless of how it is classified, it is apparent that there is a genetic basis to fearful behavior (see Serpell, 1987; van den Berg, Chapter 5). In 1944, investigations into the high prevalence of abnormally shy or fearful dogs in one laboratory colony revealed that 52% of the nervous animals were directly descended from a single female basset hound who was a notorious fear-biter. It was concluded that "shyness" is a dominant trait in dogs that is normally strongly selected against in the pet dog population (Thorne, 1944). Scott & Fuller's (1965) Bar Harbor studies seemed to confirm this assessment. Their findings with regard to puppies' fearful responses to being approached and handled by humans among basenjis, cocker spaniels and their various hybrids and backcrosses were, in their own words, consistent with the action of, "a single dominant gene causing wildness in the basenji … and a contrasting [recessive] gene for tameness in the cockers" (1965, p. 268). More recent evidence from guide dog breeding programs demonstrates that the "fearfulness" trait is moderately heritable (Goddard & Beilharz, 1982), and efforts to breed strains of abnormally fearful or "nervous" pointer dogs, to serve as research models of human anxiety disorders, have also been highly successful (see Dykman *et al.*, 1965, 1966, 1979; Murphree, 1973; Murphree & Dykman, 1965; Murphree *et al.*, 1977; Newton & Lucas, 1982).

In addition to genetic factors, it is likely that both prenatal and neonatal environment and experiences can influence puppies' subsequent reactions to stressful or frightening situations through their effects on the development of hypothalamo-pituitary-adrenocortical responsiveness (Denenberg, 1968; Fox, 1978; Levine, 1962; Whimbey & Denenberg, 1967). Evidence from studies of rodents and foxes suggests that the offspring of female dogs stressed during pregnancy would be more nervous in strange situations than normal puppies (Braastad *et al.*, 1998; Hinde, 1970). In contrast, exposing puppies or fox cubs to handling or other mild stressors during the neonatal period tends to produce more phlegmatic and less easily stressed or frightened individuals (Fox, 1978; Fox & Stelzner, 1966; Gazzano *et al.*, 2008; Pedersen & Jeppesen, 1990; Pluijmakers *et al.*, 2010). Other, as yet unidentified, aspects of maternal style and behavior may also affect puppies' confidence in stressful situations (see Scott & Bielfelt, 1976; Wilsson 1984). Abundant evidence also exists for the learned acquisition of fearful and phobic behavior (Lindsay, 2001; Overall, 1997; Serpell & Duffy, 2016).

Various early isolation experiments demonstrated that puppies reared in restricted, visually isolated or environmentally impoverished conditions from weaning until around 12–14 weeks of age or later exhibit varying degrees of neophobia when placed in unfamiliar situations (Clarke *et al.*, 1951; Fuller, 1967; Melzack & Thompson, 1956). For instance, pups reared with little or no human contact for the duration of the socialization period tend to develop a generalized fear of humans that is difficult, if not entirely impossible, to overcome subsequently (Elliot & Scott, 1961; Freedman *et al.*, 1961; Scott & Fuller, 1965). Isolation effects are also thought to account for so-called "kennel dog syndrome" – that is, the effect of leaving dogs in relatively restricted breeding kennels beyond 12 weeks of age, resulting in animals that exhibit abnormal levels of timidity toward novel people and situations (Appleby *et al.*, 2002; Serpell & Jagoe, 1995; Pfaffenburger & Scott, 1976). Conversely, pups exposed to audiovisual simulations of novel objects from 3 to 5 weeks of age were significantly less fearful toward the actual objects when tested at 8 weeks compared to unexposed pups (Pluijmakers *et al.*, 2010). Such findings are consistent with the idea that young dogs preferentially "imprint" on, or habituate to, certain biologically important aspects of their environment during the early weeks of life, and that once these preferences and associations are formed they are reinforced by the subsequent development of increasingly fearful and avoidant responses to anything novel or unfamiliar (see Bateson, 1979).

The results of conditioned aversion experiments further suggest that there may be relatively narrow periods of maximum sensitivity to frightening stimuli within the socialization period. By training beagle pups to associate human contact with electric shocks at 5, 8 and 12 weeks of age, Fox & Stelzner (1966) were able to demonstrate a short period at approximately eight weeks when pups were hypersensitive to distressing psychological or physical stimuli, and during which a single unpleasant experience could produce long-term aversive or abnormal effects. They concluded from this that, below five weeks of age, the effects of conditioning were unstable and quickly "forgotten," while at 12 weeks the aversive effects were completely over-ridden by positive affiliative tendencies towards humans established during the socialization period. At around eight weeks, however, conditioning is stable and effective but strong social bonds are not yet fully established, hence the vulnerability of these puppies to psychological trauma at this time (Fox & Stelzner, 1966). This stress-sensitive peak occurs at precisely the recommended time for rehoming puppies, and suggests that the overall level of stress or trauma experienced during the rehoming process may be an important predictor of later behavior problems. This might help to explain why dogs acquired from pet stores as puppies are reported to display more behavior problems (including fear and anxiety) than those acquired at a similar age from non-commercial breeders (McMillan et al., 2013).

Anecdotal evidence from observations of tame or captive wolves indicate that at least some individuals go through a second period of sensitivity to threatening situations at around 4–5 months of age (see Fentress, 1967; Fox, 1971; MacDonald, 1983; Mech, 1970). It is not known if an equivalent period exists in dogs or whether frightening events occurring at this age have stronger or more durable effects on subsequent behavior.

Fearful behavior in dogs may be relatively stimulus-specific. For example, although most dogs are wary of unfamiliar objects in their home environment, particularly if the object is large or moves suddenly, it is apparent that some animals are far more aversive in these contexts than others (Melzack, 1954; Serpell & Duffy, 2014; Voith & Borchelt, 1985a). Similarly, noise phobic or "gun-shy" dogs are a well-established category of problem animals (Blackwell et al., 2013; Hart et al., 2006; Shull-Selcer & Stagg, 1991; Stur, 1987), and specific "anthropophobic" responses have been described in inbred strains of "nervous" pointers (Dykman et al., 1979). Individual differences in response to specific fear-evoking stimuli may also exist in wild canids, such as wolves. MacDonald (1983), for example, detected an inverse relationship between fear of strange people and fear of unfamiliar objects in a sample of five wolf pups. The most plausible explanation for all of these observations would be that most dogs (and wolves) are born with a "biological 'preparedness' to learn to fear certain evolutionarily relevant or prepotent stimuli" (Shull-Selcer & Stagg, 1991, p. 355), but that early experience plays a major part in determining which fears are acquired and how strongly they are expressed in adult life.

6.4.3   Separation-related behavior problems

'Separation-related behavior" and "separation anxiety" are terms commonly used in the behavior problem literature to describe a particular class of problematical behavior patterns in dogs that occur only in response to separation from the owner. Such problems include: *separation-related destructiveness* – biting, chewing and scratching household furniture and fittings, often near the site of the owner's most recent departure; *separation-related vocalizing* – barking, whining or howling; and *separation-related defecation* and *urination* (Podberscek et al., 1999; Sherman & Mills, 2008).

The latter may be symptomatic of generalized anxiety (although house-training problems, marking behavior and pathophysiological disorders cannot be excluded), while the two former behavior problems are most easily interpreted as attempts by the dog to restore contact with the owner, either by escaping from confinement and following him/her, or by maintaining vocal contact (Borchelt & Voith, 1982b; McCrave, 1991; Voith & Borchelt, 1985b).

Separation-related behavior problems have a high prevalence in the pet dog population. According to McCrave (1991) such problems represent roughly 20% of the caseloads of behavior consultants in the United States, although some report much higher figures (see e.g. Borchelt, 1983b). Marked breed differences in prevalence have also been reported. Mugford (1985) mentions unusually high prevalence in Labrador retrievers, German shepherd dogs and English cocker spaniels, but also states that mixed breed dogs are far more prone to these problems than any pure breed. This statement is confirmed by the findings of McCrave (1991), who attributed the bias entirely to the fact that mixed breed dogs are significantly more likely to be obtained from animal shelters. More recent population-based surveys of behavior problem prevalence have found significantly higher rates of separation-related behavior problems among small breed dogs compared to medium or large breeds (McGreevy et al., 2013; Serpell & Duffy, 2014).

Theories concerning the development of separation-related problems in dogs have been influenced by the extensive psychological literature on the effects of attachment and separation in human and non-human primates (e.g. Ainsworth et al., 1978; Bowlby, 1973; Harlow & Harlow, 1966). According to the primate model of secure attachment, the mother or primary caregiver provides the "secure base" from which the infant learns to explore its world and acquire confidence and stability in its relationships with others. Mothers who are anxious or ambivalent, however, disrupt the normal attachment process and tend to give rise to clingy, over-dependent infants who are abnormally distressed by separation.

These ideas find parallels in the dog behavior problem literature. For instance, the most commonly reported predisposing factor in the etiology of separation-related problems in dogs is said to be a sudden episode of enforced separation from the owner *preceded* by a period of prolonged and relatively constant and/or exclusive contact. The theory is that such dogs have either never learned to cope with separation from the primary attachment figure, and/or have developed an overly intense attachment as a result of experiencing a long phase of constant and, presumably, highly rewarding companionship. Some support for this idea comes from a study by Flannigan & Dodman (2001), who found that having a single adult owner was a predisposing factor for the development of separation-related behavior problems in dogs. It has also been suggested that dogs who experience the loss of a primary attachment figure are more likely to develop insecure attachments to subsequent owners (Borchelt & Voith, 1982b; McCrave, 1991; Voith & Borchelt, 1985b), and this has been proposed as an explanation for the unusually high incidence of separation-related problems in animals adopted from animal shelters (McCrave, 1991). In some cases, this tendency of some dogs to react badly to separation from the owner has been interpreted as a side effect of unconscious human selection for increasingly affectionate, socially dependent and infantilized pets (see Fox, 1978; Mugford, 1985; Serpell, 1983, 2003; Topál et al., 2005). In practice, however, it may be difficult to distinguish the genetic effects of human selection from learned patterns of behavior acquired in response to the unusually dependent, childlike roles that many dogs are expected to play.

Regarding the possible impact of early experience on the development of separation-related behavior, there has been surprisingly little research, although Borchelt (1984) stressed the importance of gradually introducing young puppies to separation in their new homes. Experiments at Bar Harbor revealed that, from about three weeks of age, puppies become extremely distressed if placed alone in a strange situation, away from the mother, littermates and nest sites (Elliot & Scott, 1961; Scott, 1962). The level of distress, as measured by frequency of distress vocalizations, rises to a peak at around 6–7 weeks of age after which it steadily declines, although animals which have experienced no separations until 9 or 12 weeks exhibit more distress when first tested than previously tested puppies of the same age (Elliot & Scott, 1961).

In their work with German shepherd puppies, Slabbert & Rasa (1993) argued that separation from the *mother* at six weeks of age has adverse effects on puppies' overall health and welfare, although it is not clear from their data whether the pups reacted specifically to separation from the mother or from the nest site. Pierantoni *et al.* (2011) reported that puppies rehomed between 30 and 40 days postpartum were more likely to display a wide range of behavior problems as adults than puppies rehomed at 60 days, but unfortunately did not include separation-related behavior among the problems they investigated. In contrast, Flannigan & Dodman (2001) found that separation-related problems were not more common among dogs separated from their dams and littermates at an early age, and Serpell & Jagoe (1995) found no association between age of acquisition and separation-related problems in their retrospective study. McMillan *et al.* (2013) found higher rates of separation-related behavior problems among dogs acquired as puppies from pet stores compared with those acquired from non-commercial breeders, but were not able to determine whether these pups were separated from the mothers or litters at an earlier age.

From a purely biological standpoint, it would be maladaptive for puppies beyond the age of 3–4 weeks to be greatly distressed by periodic separation from their mothers, at least under natural conditions. Unlike primate infants who rely on their mothers (or other care-givers) for constant care and protection, young wild canids remain in one location while their parents are foraging, and can retreat to the safety of the den when danger threatens. Field observations of wolves have shown that, when pups are about 3–4 weeks old, the mother begins leaving them at the den site for periods of 2–18 hours daily (Ballard *et al.*, 1991). Pups remain at the den continuously and do not begin to follow the adult members of the pack until they are at least 10–12 weeks old, and usually somewhat older (Gray, 1993). Evidence from wild canids would therefore suggest that removal from the familiar nest location is the most probable cause of the distress that accompanies rehoming in domestic dog puppies, rather than separation from the mother *per se*. This distress may, however, have the effect of accelerating and intensifying the bond that is concurrently established with the new owner (see e.g. Scott *et al.*, 1974), and this may in turn exacerbate the effects of subsequent separations. It is also possible that under the effects of human selection, domestic dogs have evolved a capacity for attachments to humans that is functionally unique and unlike anything that exists in wild canids (see Topál *et al.*, 2005).

6.5   Conclusions

A number of important questions and issues concerning the development of behavior have been highlighted by this review. First, there appear to be substantial individual and breed differences in the propensity to develop particular behavior problems. While it is sometimes convenient to explain all canine behavior in terms of supposedly ancestral lupine patterns, or to lump dog breeds together as if the processes underlying their development were identical, the reality is that each breed is behaviorally different, and that a pattern or process that appears to hold true for one breed may not apply to the same extent in others. Furthermore, as Lord *et al.* (Chapter 4) point out, the investigation of breed differences in the timing of behavioral development in dogs represents a potentially powerful biological model for understanding the mechanisms of rapid evolutionary changes in behavior and morphology.

In view of their potential importance with regard to puppies' initial responses to stressful or alarming situations, there has been a surprising dearth of research into the long-term epigenetic effects of variation in prenatal and neonatal environment. At present, the possible long-term behavioral consequences for the developing puppy of maternal stress, either during pregnancy or the neonatal period, have not been investigated. Similarly, the ways in which mother–neonate and owner–neonate interactions can affect puppies' subsequent resilience to stress remain under-explored. All of these areas deserve more detailed study.

Lastly, it may be time to revise or review the established belief that correct socialization necessarily requires removing a puppy to its new home during the peak of the sensitive period for socialization. This idea is based on a misinterpretation of the available evidence, and it is one that may have adverse effects on puppy welfare and development. Abruptly separating puppies from their mothers and littermates before 7–8 weeks of age interrupts the natural process of weaning and may inflict acute and/or chronic stress. Separation from the natal environment at this vulnerable age is known to cause considerable distress in some puppies (see Elliot & Scott, 1961; Slabbert & Rasa, 1993), and seems to contribute to the development of adult behavior problems (Pierantoni *et al.*, 2011; Serpell & Jagoe, 1995). More effort should be given to exploring methods of adequately socializing puppies during this period without necessarily subjecting them to the trauma of rehoming until they are old enough to cope more easily with this difficult transition.

Perhaps the strongest conclusion to be drawn from this review is how little we still know about the development of behavior and temperament in dogs, despite the obvious value of such knowledge in the production of well-balanced pets and effective working animals, and in the struggle to reduce or eliminate behavior problems in the dog population as a whole. For both ethical and economic reasons, it may be difficult to study the effects of phenomena such as early life stress in dogs experimentally, but there are numerous potential opportunities to explore such questions using the naturally occurring variation that exists in current breeding and husbandry practices. The systematic collection of information on the behavior and individual life histories of both companion and working dogs by veterinarians, behavioral counselors, and breeders could also contribute substantially to current knowledge in this important area.

References

Adams, G. J. & Johnson, K. G. (1993). Sleep-wake cycles and other night-time behaviors of the domestic dog, *Canis familiaris. Applied Animal Behavior Science*, 36: 233–48.

Ainsworth, M. D. S., Blehar, C. S., Waters, E. & Wall, S. (1978). *Patterns of Attachment: A Psychological Study of the Strange Situation*. Hillsdale, NJ: Erlbaum.

Appleby, D. L., Bradshaw, J. W. S. & Casey, R. A. (2002). Relationship between aggressive and avoidance behavior by dogs and their experience in the first six months of life. *Veterinary Record*, 150: 434–8.

Arueti, M., Perach-Barzilay, N., Tsoory, M. M., Berger, B., Getter, N. & Shamay-Tsoory, S. G. (2014) When two become one: the role of oxytocin in interpersonal coordination and cooperation. *Journal of Cognitive Neuroscience*, 25: 1418–27.

Bale, T. L., Baram, T. Z., Brown, A. S. *et al.* (2010). Early life programming and neurodevelopmental disorders. *Biological Psychiatry*, 68: 314–19.

Bales, K. L., Boone, E., Epperson, P., Hoffman, G. & Carter, C. S. (2011). Are behavioral effects of early experience mediated by oxytocin? *Frontiers in Psychiatry*, 2: article 24.

Ballard, W. B., Ayres, L. A., Gardner, C. L. & Foster, J. W. (1991). Den site activity patterns of grey wolves, *Canis lupus*, in southcentral Alaska. *Canadian Field-Naturalist*, 105, 497–504.

Bateson, P. (1979). How do sensitive periods arise and what are they for? *Animal Behavior*, 27: 470–86.

Bateson, P. (1981). Control of sensitivity to the environment during development. In *Behavioral Development*, ed. K. Immelmann, G. W. Barlow, L. Petrovich & M. Main. Cambridge: Cambridge University Press, pp. 433–53.

Bekoff, M. (1974). Social play and play-soliciting by infant canids. *American Zoologist*, 14, 323–40.

Bekoff, M. (2012). Social dominance is not a myth: wolves, dogs, and other animals. *Psychology Today*, February 15. [Online]. Available: www.psychologytoday.com/blog/animal-emotions/201202/social-dominance-is-not-myth-wolves-dogs-and-other-animals

Belyaev, D. K., Plyusnina, I. Z. & Trut, L. N. (1985). Domestication in the silver fox (*Vulpes vulpes*): changes in physiological boundaries of the sensitive period of primary socialization. *Applied Animal Behaviour Science*, 32: 253–68.

Berger, S. L., Kouzarides, T., Shiekhattar, R. & Shilatifard, A. (2009). An operational definition of epigenetics. *Genes and Development*, 23: 781–3.

Blackwell, E. J., Bradshaw, J. W. S. & Casey, R. A. (2013). Fear responses to noises in domestic dogs: prevalence, risk factors and co-occurrence with other fear related behavior. *Applied Animal Behaviour Science*, 145: 15–25.

Borchelt, P. L. (1983a). Aggressive behavior of dogs kept as companion animals: classification and influence of sex, reproductive status and breed. *Applied Animal Ethology*, 10, 45–61.

Borchelt, P. L. (1983b). Separation-elicited behavior problems in dogs. In *New Perspectives on Our Lives with Companion Animals*, eds. A. H. Katcher & A. M. Beck. Philadelphia, PA: University of Pennsylvania Press, pp. 187–96.

Borchelt, P. L. (1984). Behavioral development of the puppy. In *Nutrition and Behavior in Dogs and Cats*, ed. R. S. Anderson. Oxford: Pergamon Press, pp. 165–74.

Borchelt, P. L. & Voith, V. L. (1982a). Classification of animal behavior problems. *Veterinary Clinics of North America: Small Animal Practice*, 12, 571–85.

Borchelt, P. L. & Voith, V. L. (1982b). Diagnosis and treatment of separation-related behavior problems in dogs. *Veterinary Clinics of North America: Small Animal Practice*, 12, 625–35.

Bowlby, J. (1973). *Attachment and Loss, Vol. 2: Separation*. New York: Basic Books.

Braastad, B.O., Osadchuk, L. V., Lund, G. & Bakken, M. (1998). Effects of prenatal handling stress on adrenal weight and behavior in novel situations in blue fox cubs (*Alopex lagopus*). *Applied Animal Behaviour Science*, 57: 157–69.

Bradshaw, J. W. S. & Nott, H. M. R. (1995). Social and communication behaviour of companion dogs. In *The Domestic Dog: Its Evolution, Behaviour and Interactions with People*, ed. J. A. Serpell. Cambridge: Cambridge University Press.

Cafazzo, S., Valsecchi, P., Bonanni, R. & Natoli, E. (2010). Dominance in relation to age, sex, and competitive contexts in a group of free-ranging domestic dogs. *Behavioral Ecology*, http://doi:10.1093/beheco/arq001

Campbell, W. E. (1975). *Behavior Problems in Dogs*. Santa Barbara, CA: American Veterinary Publications.

Campbell, W. E. (1986). The prevalence of behavioral problems in American dogs. *Modern Veterinary Practice*, 67: 28–31.

Cardoso, S. D., Teles, M. C. & Oliveira, R. F. (2015). Neurogenomic mechanisms of social plasticity. *Journal of Experimental Biology*, 218: 140–9.

Champagne, F. A. (2008). Epigenetic mechanisms and the transgenerational effects of maternal care. *Frontiers in Neuroendocrinology*, 29: 386–97.

Champagne, F. A., Francis, D. D., Mar, A., Meaney, M. J. (2003). Variations in maternal care in the rat as a mediating influence for the effects of environment on development. *Physiology and Behavior*, 79: 359–71.

Chen, F. S., Barth, M. E., Johnson, S. L., Gotlib, I. H. & Johnson, S. C. (2011). Oxytocin receptor polymorphisms and attachment in human infants. *Frontiers in Psychology*, 2. http://doi:10.3389/fpsyg.2011.00200

Clarke, R. S., Heron, W., Fetherstonhaugh, M. L., Forgays, D. G. & Hebb, D. O. (1951). Individual differences in dogs: preliminary report on the effects of early experience. *Canadian Journal of Psychology*, 5: 150–6.

Cornwell, A. C. & Fuller, J. L. (1960). Conditioned responses in young puppies. *Journal of Comparative and Physiological Psychology*, 54: 13–15.

Crews, D. (2011). Epigenetic modifications of brain and behavior: theory and practice. *Hormones and Behavior*, 59: 393–8.

Curley, J. P., Jensen, C. L., Mashoodh, R. & Champagne, F. A. (2011a). Social influences on neurobiology and behavior: epigenetic effects during development. *Psychoneuroendocrinology*, 36: 352–71.

Curley, J. P., Mashoodh, R. & Champagne, F. A. (2011b). Epigenetics and the origins of paternal effects. *Hormones and Behavior*, 59: 306–14.

DeFries, J. C., Weir, M. W. & Hegmann, J. P. (1967). Differential effects of prenatal maternal stress on offspring behavior in mice as a function of genotype and stress. *Journal of Comparative and Physiological Psychology*, 63: 332–4.

Dehasse, J. (1994). Sensory, emotional and social development of the young dog. *Bulletin for Veterinary Clinical Ethology*, 2: 6–29.

Denenberg, V. H. (1968). A consideration of the usefulness of the critical period hypothesis as applied to the stimulation of rodents in infancy. In *Early Experience and Behavior*, eds. G. Newton & S. Levine. Springfield, IL: Charles Thomas., pp. 142–67.

Denenberg, V. H. & Morton, J. R. C. (1962). Effects of environmental complexity and social groupings upon modification of emotional behavior. *Journal of Comparative and Physiological Psychology*, 55: 242–6.

Dorey, N. R., Udell, M. A. R. & Wynne, C. D. L. (2010). When do domestic dogs, *Canis familiaris*, start to understand human pointing? The role of ontogeny in the development of interspecies communication. *Animal Behaviour*, 79: 37–41.

Duffy, D. L., Hsu, Y. & Serpell, J. A. (2008). Breed differences in canine aggression. *Applied Animal Behaviour Science*, 114: 441–60.

Duffy, D. L. & Serpell, J. A. (2012). Predictive validity of a method for evaluating temperament in young guide and service dogs. *Applied Animal Behaviour Science*, 138: 99–109.

Dunn, G. A., Morgan, C. P. & Bale, T. L. (2011). Sex-specificity in transgenerational epigenetic programming. *Hormones and Behavior*, 59: 290–6.

Dykman, R. A., Mack, R. L. & Ackerman, P. T. (1965). The evaluation of autonomic and motor components of the nonavoidance conditioned response in the dog. *Psychophysiology*, 1, 209–30.

Dykman, R. A., Murphree, O. D. & Ackerman, P. T. (1966). Litter patterns in the offspring of nervous and stable dogs. II. Autonomic and motor conditioning. *Journal of Nervous and Mental Disease*, 141: 419–31.

Dykman, R. A., Murphree, O. D. & Reese, W. G. (1979). Familial anthropophobia in pointer dogs? *Archives of General Psychiatry*, 36: 988–93.

Elliot, O. & Scott, J. P. (1961). The development of emotional distress reactions to separation in puppies. *Journal of Genetic Psychology*, 99: 3–22.

Fentress, J. C. (1967). Observations on the behavioral development of a hand-reared male timber wolf. *American Zoologist*, 7, 339–51.

Flannigan, G. & Dodman, N. H. (2001). Risk factors and behaviors associated with separation anxiety in dogs. *Journal of the American Veterinary Medical Association*, 219: 460–466.

Fox, M. W. (1969). Behavioral effects of rearing dogs with cats during the "critical period of socialization". *Behavior*, 35: 273–80.

Fox, M. W. (1971). *Behavior of Wolves, Dogs and Related Canids*. New York: Harper and Row.

Fox, M. W. (1972). Socio-ecological implications of individual differences in wolf litters: a developmental and evolutionary perspective. *Behavior*, 41: 298–313.

Fox, M. W. (1978). *The Dog: Its Domestication and Behavior*. New York: Garland STPM Press.

Fox, M. W., Halperin, S., Wise, A. & Kohn, E. (1976). Species and hybrid differences in frequencies of play and agonistic actions in canids. *Zeitschrift für Tierpsychologie*, 40: 194–209.

Fox, M. W. & Stelzner, D. (1966). Behavioral effects of differential early experience in the dog. *Animal Behavior*, 14: 273–81.

Foyer, P., Bjällerhag, N., Wilsson, W. & Jensen, P. (2014). Behaviour and experiences of dogs during the first year of life predict the outcome in a later temperament test. *Applied Animal Behaviour Science*, 155: 93–100.

Foyer, P., Wilsson, E., Wright, D. & Jensen, P. (2013). Early experiences modulate stress coping in a population of German shepherd dogs. *Applied Animal Behaviour Science*, 146: 79–87.

Francis, D. D., Diorio, J., Plotsky, P. M. & Meaney, M. J. (2002). Environmental enrichment reverses the effects of maternal separation on stress reactivity. *Journal of Neuroscience*, 22: 7840–3.

Frank, H. & Frank, M. G. (1982). On the effects of domestication on canine social development and behavior. *Applied Animal Ethology*, 8: 507–25.

Frank, H. & Frank, M. G. (1985). Comparative manipulation-test performance in ten-week-old wolves (*Canis lupus*) and Alaskan malamutes (*Canis familiaris*): a Piagetian interpretation. *Journal of Comparative Psychology*, 99: 266–74.

Freedman, D. G., King, J. A. & Elliot, O. (1961). Critical periods in the social development of dogs. *Science*, 133: 1016–17.

Fuller, J. L. (1967). Experiential deprivation and later behavior. *Science*, 158: 1645–52.

Gácsi, M., Kara, E., Belényi, B. & Topál, J. (2009). The effect of development and individual differences in pointing comprehension of dogs. *Animal Cognition*, 12: 471–9.

Gagnon, S. & Doré, F. Y. (1994). Cross-sectional study of object permanence in domestic puppies (*Canis familiaris*). *Journal of Comparative Psychology*, 108: 226–32.

Gazzano, A., Mariti, C., Notari, L., Sighieri, C. & McBride, E. A. (2008). Effects of early gentling and early environment on emotional development of puppies. *Applied Animal Behaviour Science*, 110: 294–304.

Goddard, M. E. & Beilharz, R. G. (1982). Genetic and environmental factors affecting the suitability of dogs as guide dogs for the blind. *Theoretical and Applied Genetics*, 62, 97–102.

Goddard, M. E. & Beilharz, R. G. (1984). Factor analysis of fearfulness in potential guide dogs. *Applied Animal Behavior Science*, 12, 253–65.

Gottlieb, G. (1976). The roles of experience in the development of behavior and the nervous system. In *Neural and Behavioral Specificity*, ed. J. P. Scott. New York: Academic Press, pp. 25–54.

Gray, D. R. (1993). The use of muskox kill sites as temporary rendezvous sites by arctic wolves with pups in early winter. *Arctic*, 46: 324–30.

Haase, E. (2000). Comparison of reproductive biological parameters in male wolves and domestic dogs. *Zeitschrift fur Saugetierkunde*, 65: 257–70.

Harlow, H. F. & Harlow, M. K. (1966). Learning to love. *American Scientist*, 54: 244–72.

Hart, B. L., Hart, L. A. & Bain, M. J. (2006). *Canine and Feline Behavioral Therapy*; 2nd edition. Oxford: Blackwell.

Harvey, N. D., Craigon, P. J., Blythe, S. A., England, G. C. W. & Asher, L. (2016). Social rearing environment influences dog behavioral development. *Journal of Veterinary Behavior*, doi: 10.1016/j.jveb.2016.03.004.

Hayssen, V., van Tienhoven, A. & van Tienhoven, A. (1993). *Asdell's Patterns of Mammalian Reproduction*. Ithaca, NY: Cornell University Press.

Heim, C. & Binder, E. B. (2012) Current research trends in early life stress and depression: Review of human studies on sensitive periods, gene-environment interactions, and epigenetics. *Experimental Neurology*, 233: 102–11.

Hepper, P. G. (1985). Sibling recognition in the domestic dog. *Animal Behaviour*, 34: 288–9.

Herron, M. E., Lord, L. K., Hill, L. N. & Reisner, I. R. (2007). Effects of preadoption counseling for owners on house-training success among dogs acquired from shelters. *Journal of the American Veterinary Medical Association*, 231: 558–62.

Hinde, K., Skibiel, A. L., Foster, A. B. *et al.* (2014). Cortisol in mother's milk across lactation reflects maternal life history and predicts infant temperament. *Behavioral Ecology*: http://doi:10.1093/beheco/aru186

Hinde, R. A. (1970). *Animal Behavior*, 2nd edition. New York: McGraw-Hill.

Hinde, R. A. (1974). *Biological Bases of Human Social Behavior*. New York: McGraw-Hill.

Immelmann, K. and Soumi, S. J. (1981). Sensitive phases in development. In *Behavioral Development*, eds. K. Immelmann, G. W. Barlow, L. Petrovich & M. Main. Cambridge: Cambridge University Press, pp. 395–431.

Ito, A., Kikusui, T., Takeuchi, Y. & Mori, Y. (2006), Effects of early weaning on anxiety and autonomic responses to stress in rats. *Behavioural Brain Research*, 171: 87–93.

Jagoe, J. A. (1994). Behavior problems in the domestic dog: a retrospective and prospective study to identify factors influencing their development. Unpublished Ph.D. thesis, University of Cambridge.

Joffe, J. M. (1969). *Prenatal Determinants of Behavior*. New York: Pergamon Press.

Kappeler, L. & Meaney, M. J. (2010). Epigenetics and parental effects. *Bioessays* 32: 818–27.

Kikusui, T., Nakamura, K., Kakuma, Y. & Mori, Y. (2006). Early weaning augments neuroendocrine stress responses in mice. *Behavioural Brain Research*, 175: 96–103.

Kis, A., Bence, M., Lakatos, G. *et al*. (2014). Oxytocin gene receptor polymorphisms are associated with human directed social behavior in dogs (*Canis familiaris*). *PloS One*, 9: e83993. http://doi:10.1371/journal.pone.0083993

Leon, M. (1992). Neuroethology of olfactory preference development. *Journal of Neurobiology*, 23: 1557–73.

Levine, S. (1962). Plasma free corticosteroid response to electric shock in rats stimulated in infancy. *Science*, 135: 795–6.

Levine, S. (1967). Maternal and environmental influences on the adrenocortical response to stress in weanling rats. *Science*, 156; 258–60.

Lindsay, S. R. (2001). *Handbook of Applied Dog Behavior and Training, Vol. 2: Etiology and Assessment of Behavior Problems*. Ames, IA: Iowa State University Press.

Line, S. & Voith, V. L. (1986). Dominance aggression of dogs towards people: behavior profile and response to treatment. *Applied Animal Behavior Science*, 16: 77–83.

Lockwood, R. (1979). Dominance in wolves: useful construct or bad habit? In *The Behavior and Ecology of Wolves*, ed. E. Klinghammer. New York: Garland STPM Press, pp. 225–44.

Lord, K. (2013). Comparison of the sensory development of wolves (*Canis lupus*) and dogs (*Canis lupus familiaris*). *Ethology*, 119: 110–20.

Lorenz, K. (1935). Der Kumpan in der Umwelt des Vogels. *Journal für Ornithologie*, 83: 137–213, 289–413.

Lorenz, K. (1966). *On Aggression*. London: Methuen.

Lupien, S. J., McEwen, B. S., Gunnar, M. R. & Heim, C. (2009). Effects of stress throughout the lifespan on the brain, behavior and cognition. *Nature Reviews Neuroscience*, 10: 434–45.

Lynch, K. E. & Kemp, D. J. (2014). Nature-via-nurture and unraveling causality in evolutionary genetics. *Trends in Ecology & Evolution*, 29. http://dx.doi.org/10.1016/j.tree.2013.10.005

Lyons, D. M., Parker, K. J. & Schatzberg, A. F. (2010). Animal models of early life stress: implications for understanding resilience. *Developmental Psychobiology*, 52: 616–24.

MacDonald, K. B. (1983). Stability of individual differences in behavior in a litter of wolf, cubs (*Canis lupus*). *Journal of Comparative Psychology*, 97: 99–106.

MacDonald, K. B. (1987). Development and stability of personality characteristics in pre-pubertal wolves: implications for pack organization and behavior. In *Man and Wolf*, ed. H. Frank. Dordrecht, The Netherlands: Dr W. Junk Publishers, pp. 293–312.

Macrì, S., Zoratto, F. & Laviola, G. (2011). Early-stress regulates resilience, vulnerability and experimental validity in laboratory rodents through mother-offspring hormonal transfer. *Neuroscience and Biobehavioral Reviews*, 35: 1534–43.

Malm, K. (1995). Behaviour of parents and offspring in two canids. Unpublished Ph.D., Skara, Sweden: Sveriges Lantbruksuniversitet.

McCrave, E. A. (1991). Diagnostic criteria for separation anxiety in the dog. *Veterinary Clinics of North America: Small Animal Practice*, 21: 247–55.

McGreevy, P. D., Georgevsky, D., Carrasco, J., Valenzuela, M., Duffy, D. L. & Serpell, J. A. (2013). Dog behavior co-varies with height, bodyweight and skull shape. *PLoS ONE* 8: e80529. http://doi:10.1371/journal.pone.0080529

McMillan, F. D., Serpell, J. A., Duffy, D. L., Masaoud, E. & Dohoo, I. R. (2013). Differences in behavioral and psychological characteristics between dogs obtained as puppies from pet stores and those obtained from noncommercial breeders. *Journal of the American Veterinary Medical Association*, 242: 1359–63.

Meaney, M. J. (2001). Maternal care, gene expression, and the transmission of individual differences in stress reactivity across generations. *Annual Review of Neuroscience*, 24: 1161–92.

Mech, L. D. (1970). *The Wolf: the Ecology and Behavior of an Endangered Species*. New York: Natural History Press.

Mech, L. D. (2008). Whatever happened to the term "alpha wolf"? *International Wolf*, Winter: 4–8: www.wolf.org/

Mech, L. D. & Cluff, H. D. (2010). Prolonged intensive dominance behavior between grey wolves, *Canis lupus. Canadian Field-Naturalist*, 124: 215–18.

Melzack, R. (1954). The genesis of emotional behavior: an experimental study of the dog. *Journal of Comparative and Physiological Psychology*, 47; 166–8.

Melzack, R. & Thompson, W. R. (1956). Effects of early experience on social behavior. *Canadian Journal of Psychology*, 10: 82–92.

Meredith, R. M. (2014). Sensitive and critical periods during neurotypical and aberrant neurodevelopment: a framework for neurodevelopmental disorders.

Neuroscience and Biobehavioral Reviews. http://dx.doi.org/10.1016/j.neubiorev.2014.12.001

Miklósi, A. (2007). *Dog Behaviour. Evolution, and Cognition*. Oxford: Oxford University Press.

Miller D. M., Stats, S. R., Partlo, B. S. & Rada, K. (1996). Factors associated with the decision to surrender a pet to an animal shelter. *Journal of the American Veterinary Medical Association*, 209: 738–42.

Morrow, M., Ottobre, J., Ottobre, A. *et al.* (2015). Breed-dependent differences in the onset of fear-related avoidance behavior in puppies. *Journal of Veterinary Behavior*. http://doi:10.1016/j.jveb.2015.03.002

Moyer, K. E. (1968). Kinds of aggression and their physiological basis. *Communications in Behavioral Biology. Part A*, 2, 65–87.

Mugford, R. A. (1985). Attachment versus dominance: an alternative view of the man-dog relationship. In *The Human-Pet Relationship*. Vienna: IEMT (Institute for Interdisciplinary Research on the Human-Pet Relationship), pp. 157–65.

Murphree, O. D. (1973). Inheritance of human aversion and inactivity in two strains of the pointer dog. *Biological Psychiatry*, 7: 23–9.

Murphree, O. D., Angel, C, DeLuca, D. C. & Newton, J. E. O. (1977). Longitudinal studies of genetically nervous dogs. *Biological Psychiatry*, 12: 573–6.

Murphree, O. D. & Dykman, R. A. (1965). Litter patterns in the offspring of nervous and stable dogs. I. Behavioral tests. *Journal of Nervous and Mental Disease*, 141: 321–32.

Nephew, B. & Murgatroyd, C. (2013). The role of maternal care in shaping CNS function. *Neuropeptides*, 47: 371–8.

Newton, J. E. O. & Lucas, L. A. (1982). Differential heart-rate responses to person in nervous and normal pointer dogs. *Behavioral Genetics*, 12, 379–93.

Niebuhr, B. R., Levinson, M., Nobbe, D. E. & Tiller, J. E. (1980). Treatment of an incompletely socialized dog. In *Canine Behavior*, ed. B. L. Hart. Santa Barbara, CA: Veterinary Practice Publishing Co., p. 83.

O'Farrell, V. (1986). *Manual of Canine Behavior*. Cheltenham: BSAVA Publications.

Overall, K. L. (1997). *Clinical Behavioral Medicine for Small Animals*. St. Louis, MO: Mosby-Year Book, Inc.

Pal, S. K. (2005) Parental care in free-ranging dogs, *Canis familiaris. Applied Animal Behaviour Science*, 90: 31–47.

Pal, S. K. (2008). Maturation and development of social behavior during early ontogeny in free-ranging dog puppies in West Bengal, India. *Applied Animal Behaviour Science*, 111: 95–107.

Patchev, A. V., Rodrigues, A. J., Sousa, N., Spengler, D. & Almeida, O. F. X. (2014). The future is now: Early life events preset adult behaviour. *Acta Physiologica*, 210: 46–57.

Patronek G. J., Glickman L. T., Beck A. M., McCabe G. P. & Ecker C. (1996). Risk factors for relinquishment of dogs to an animal shelter. *Journal of the American Veterinary Medical Association*, 209: 572–81.

Pedersen, V. & Jeppesen, L. L. (1990). Effects of early handling on later behavior and stress responses in the Silver Fox (*Vulpes vulpes*). *Applied Animal Behavior Science*, 26: 383–93.

Pfaffenberger, C. J. & Scott, J. P. (1976). Early rearing and testing. In *Guide Dogs for the Blind: Their Selection, Development and Training*, eds. C. J. Pfaffenberger, J. P. Scott, J. L. Fuller, B. E. Ginsburg & S. W. Bielfelt. Amsterdam: Elsevier, pp. 13–37.

Pfaffenberger, C. J., Scott, J. P., Fuller, J. L., Ginsburg, B. E. & Bielfelt, S. W. (1976). *Guide Dogs for the Blind: Their Selection, Development and Training*. Amsterdam: Elsevier.

Pierantoni, L., Albertini, M. and Pirrone, F. (2011). Prevalence of owner-reported behaviours in dogs separated from the litter at two different ages. *Veterinary Record*, 169: 648

Pluijmakers, J. J. T. M., Appleby, D. L. & Bradshaw, J. W. S. (2010). Exposure to video images between 3 and 5 weeks of age decreases neophobia in domestic dogs. *Applied Animal Behaviour Science*, 126: 51–58.

Plyusnina, I. Z., Oskina, I. N. & Trut, L. N. (1991). An analysis of fear and aggression during early development of behavior in silver foxes (*Vulpes vulpes*). *Applied Animal Behavior Science*, 32: 253–68.

Podberscek, A. L., Hsu, Y. & Serpell, J. A. (1999). Evaluation of clomipramine as an adjunct to behavioural therapy in the treatment of separation-related problems in dogs. *Veterinary Record*, 145: 365–9.

Price, E. O. (1984). Behavioral aspects of animal domestication. *Quarterly Review of Biology*, 59: 1–32.

Riedel, J., Schumann, K., Kaminski, J., Call, J. & Tomasello, M. (2008). The early ontogeny of dog-human communication. *Animal Behaviour*, 75: 1003–14.

Roll, A. & Unshelm, J. (1997). Aggressive conflicts among dogs and factors affecting them. *Applied Animal Behaviour Science*, 52: 229–42.

Salman, M. D., New, J. G., Scarlett, J. M., Kass, P. H., Ruch-Gallie, R. & Hetts, S. (1998). Human and animal factors related to the relinquishment of dogs and cats in 12 selected animal shelters in the United States. *Journal of Applied Animal Welfare Science*, 1: 207–26.

Sapolsky, R. M. (2004). Mothering style and methylation. *Nature Neuroscience*, 7: 791–2.

Schmidt, M. V. (2010). Molecular mechanisms of early life stress – lessons from mouse models. *Neuroscience and Biobehavioral Reviews*, 34: 845–52.

Schoon, A. & Berntsen, T. G. (2011). Evaluating the effect of early neurological stimulation on the development and training of mine detection dogs. *Journal of Veterinary Behavior*, 6: 150–7.

Scott, J. P. (1962). Critical periods in behavioral development. *Science*, 138: 949–58.

Scott, J. P. (1963). The process of primary socialization in canine and human infants. *Monographs of the Society for Research in Child Development*, 28: 1–49.

Scott, J. P. & Bielfelt, S. W. (1976). Analysis of the puppy testing program. In *Guide Dogs for the Blind: Their Selection, Development and Training*, eds. C. J. Pfaffenberger, J. P. Scott, J. L. Fuller, B. E. Ginsburg & S. W. Bielfelt. Amsterdam: Elsevier, pp. 39–75.

Scott, J. P. & Fuller, J. L. (1965). *Genetics and the Social Behavior of the Dog*. Chicago, IL: University of Chicago Press.

Scott, J. P. & Marston, M. V. (1950). Critical periods affecting the development of normal and mal-adjustive social behavior of puppies. *Journal of Genetic Psychology*, 77: 25–60.

Scott, J. P., Stewart, J. M. & DeGhett, V. J. (1974). Critical periods in the organization of systems. *Developmental Psychobiology*, 7: 489–513.

Serpell, J. A. (1983). The personality of the dog and its influence on the pet-owner bond. In *New Perspectives on Our Lives with Companion Animals*, eds. A. H. Katcher & A. M. Beck. Philadelphia, PA: University of Pennsylvania Press, pp. 57–71.

Serpell, J. A. (1987). The influence of inheritance and environment on canine behavior: myth and fact. *Journal of small Animal Practice*, 28: 949–56.

Serpell, J. A. (2003). Anthropomorphism and anthropomorphic selection – beyond the "cute response". *Society & Animals*, 11: 83–100.

Serpell, J. A. & Duffy, D. L. (2014). Breeds and their behavior. In *Domestic Dog Cognition and Behavior*, ed. A. Horowitz. Berlin: Springer-Verlag, pp. 31–57.

Serpell, J. A. & Duffy, D. L. (2016). Aspects of juvenile and adolescent environment predict aggression and fear in 12 month-old guide dogs. *Frontiers in Veterinary Science*, 3: 49. doi: 10.3389/fvets.2016.00049

Serpell, J. A. & Jagoe, J. A. (1995). Early experience and the development of behavior. In *The Domestic Dog: Its Evolution, Behaviour and Interactions with People*, ed. J. A. Serpell. Cambridge: Cambridge University Press, pp. 80–102.

Sherman, B. L. & Mills, D. S. (2008). Canine anxieties and phobias: an update of separation anxiety and noise aversions. *Veterinary Clinics Small Animal Practice*, 38: 1081–106.

Shull-Selcer, E. A. & Stagg, W. (1991). Advances in the understanding and treatment of noise phobias. *Veterinary Clinics of North America: Small Animal Practice*, 21: 353–67.

Simmel, E. C. & Baker, E. (1980). The effects of early experiences on later behavior: a critical discussion. In *Early Experiences and Early Behavior: Implications for Social Development*, ed. E. C. Simmell. New York: Academic Press, pp. 3–13.

Slabbert, J. M. & Rasa, O. A. E. (1993). The effect of early separation from the mother on pups in bonding to humans and pup health. *Journal of the South African Veterinary Association*, 64: 4–8.

Smotherman, W. P., Brown, C. P. & Levine, S. (1977). Maternal responsiveness following differential pup treatment and mother-pup interactions. *Hormones and Behavior*, 8: 242–53.

Stanley, W. C. (1970). Feeding behavior and learning in neonatal dogs. In *Second Symposium on Oral Sensation and Perception*, ed. J. F. Bosma. Springfield, IL: Charles Thomas, pp. 242–90.

Stanley, W. C. (1972). Perspectives in behavior organization and development resulting from studies of feeding behavior in infant dogs. In *Third Symposium on Oral Sensation and Perception: The Mouth of the Infant*, ed. J. F. Bosma. Springfield, IL: Charles Thomas, pp. 188–257.

Stur, I. (1987). Genetic aspects of temperament and behavior in dogs. *Journal of Small Animal Practice*, 28: 957–64.

Sweatt, D. J. (2013). The emerging field of neuroepigenetics. *Neuron*, 80: 624–32.

Thorne, F. C. (1944). The inheritance of shyness in dogs. *Journal of Genetic Psychology*, 65: 275–9.

Topál, J., Gácsi, M., Miklósi, A., Virányi, Z., Kubinyi, E. & Csányi, V. (2005). Attachment to humans: A comparative study on hand-reared wolves and differently socialized dog puppies. *Animal Behaviour*, 70: 1367–75.

Tiira, K., Hakosalo, O., Kareinen, L. *et al.* (2012). Environmental effects on compulsive tail-chasing in dogs, *PLoS One*, 7: e41684. http://doi:10.1371/journal.pone.0041684

Trut, L. N., Plyusnina, I.Z. & Oskina, I.N. (2004). An experiment on fox domestication and debatable issues of evolution of the dog. *Russian Journal of Genetics*, 40: 794–807.

Tuber, D. S., Hothersall, D. & Peters, M. F. (1982). Treatment of fears and phobias in dogs. *Veterinary Clinics of North America: Small Animal Practice*, 12: 607–23.

van Hooff, J. A. R. A. M. & Wensing, J. A. B. (1987). Dominance and its behavioral measures in a captive wolf pack. In *Man and Wolf*, ed. H. Frank. Dordrecht, The Netherlands: Dr W. Junk Publishers, pp. 219–51.

Voith, V. L. & Borchelt, P. L. (1982). Diagnosis and treatment of dominance aggression in dogs. *Veterinary Clinics of North America: Small Animal Practice*, 12: 655–63.

Voith, V. L. & Borchelt, P. L. (1985a). Fears and phobias in dogs. *Compendium of Continuing Education for the Practising Veterinarian*, 7: 209–18.

Voith, V. L. & Borchelt, P. L. (1985b). Separation anxiety in dogs. *Compendium on Continuing Education for the Practising Veterinarian*, 7: 42–52.

Weaver, I. C. G., Cervoni, N., Champagne, F. A. *et al.* (2004) Epigenetic programming by maternal behavior. *Nature Neuroscience*, 7: 847–854.

Wells, D. L. & Hepper, P. G. (2006). Prenatal olfactory learning in the domestic dog. *Animal Behaviour*, 72: 681–686.

Weinstock, M. (2008). Long-term behavioural consequences of prenatal stress. *Neuroscience and Biobehavioral Reviews*, 32: 1073–1086.

Whimbey, A. E. & Denenberg, V. H. (1967). Two independent behavioral dimensions in open-field performance. *Journal of Comparative Physiological Psychology*, 63: 500–504.

Wilsson, E. (1984). The social interaction between mother and offspring during weaning in German shepherd dogs:

individual differences between mothers and their effects on offspring. *Applied Animal Behavior Science*, 13: 101–12.

Wolfle, T. L. (1990). Policy, program and people: the three Ps to well-being. In *Canine Research Environment*, eds. J. A. Mench & L. Krulisch. Bethesda, MD: Scientists Center for Animal Welfare, pp. 41–7.

Woolpy, J. H. (1968). The social organisation of wolves. *Natural History*, 77: 46–55.

Woolpy, J. H. & Ginsburg, B. E. (1967). Wolf socialization: a study of temperament in a wild social species. *American Zoologist*, 7: 357–63.

Wright, J. C. (1980). Early development of exploratory behavior and dominance in three litters of German shepherds. In *Early Experiences and Early Behavior: Implications for Social Development*, ed. E. C. Simmel. New York: Academic Press, pp. 181–206.

Wright, J. C. & Nesselrote, M. S. (1987). Classification of behavior problems in dogs: distributions of age, breed, sex and reproductive status. *Applied Animal Behavior Science*, 19: 169–78.

Wynne, C. D. L., Udell, M. A. R. & Lord, K. A. (2008). Ontogeny's impacts on human-dog communication. *Animal Behaviour*, 76: e1–4.

Zimen, E. (1987). Ontogeny of approach and flight behavior towards humans in wolves, poodles and wolf-poodle hybrids. In *Man and Wolf*, ed. H. Frank. Dordrecht, The Netherlands: Dr W. Junk Publishers, pp. 275–92.

7 Breed and gender differences in dog behavior

BENJAMIN L. HART AND LYNETTE A. HART

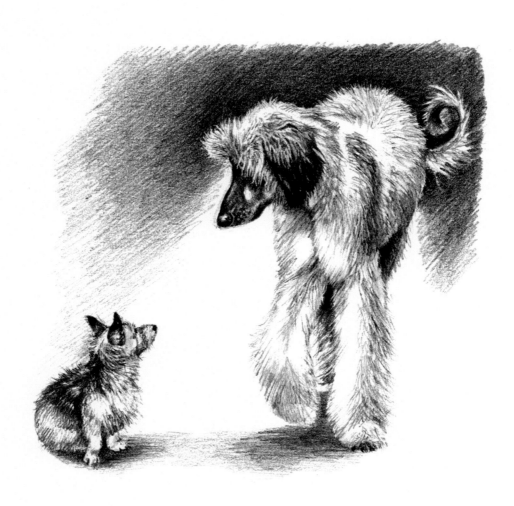

7.1   Introduction

Dogs are absolutely unique among domestic animals in their association with human caregivers. For one thing, their history with us over evolutionary time is the longest of any domestic species. Secondly, they display an almost unbelievable degree of morphological and behavioral diversity – diversity due almost entirely to their association with humans. Over the centuries, as dogs have been bred for various physical attributes, they have also undergone a variety of changes in behavior. Some breeds have been selected for behavioral changes that are useful in hunting, such as pointing at game birds, chasing foxes while vocalizing, or retrieving waterfowl shot by hunters. In other breeds, behavior associated with the performance of complex tasks, such as herding sheep, has been accentuated. These particular behavior functions that have come to characterize the different breeds of dogs are the outcome of the suppression or enhancement of existing "native" canine behavioral characteristics, rather than the emergence of new behavior patterns (Scott & Fuller, 1965; Lord *et al.*, Chapter 4).

This chapter represents a revised, updated and extended version of a previous review (Hart, 1995) of behavioral differences among 56 popular dog breeds (Hart & Hart, 1985; 1988; Hart & Miller, 1985). Here we report some of the main findings using a new data set involving 80 breeds based on breed rankings derived from telephone interviews with 168 small animal veterinarians.

Extensive research on the canine genome has laid the groundwork for investigations of behavioral differences among breeds that may be related to differences in breed-specific genomes. A particularly useful study with regard to understanding behavioral differences and similarities among breeds of dogs is one that used microsatellite DNA markers to study genetic relationships among 85 breeds (Parker *et al.*, 2004). The same technique was subsequently extended and refined (Parker *et al.*, 2007, 2010). These analyses reveal that almost all dog breeds are genetically distinct and that some can be grouped according to genetic similarity. These genetically similar breed groups provided a means to determine whether the observed breed differences in behavior in the present study had at least some genetic basis.

7.2   Background

In the last decade or so, several studies have looked at the reliability of differences in behavior between breeds and factors related to these differences (see also van den Berg, Chapter 5). In a Danish study, breed membership was found to account for differences in inter-dog aggression, along with city of residence and age of owner (Rugbjerg *et al.*, 2003). Using the standardized C-BARQ questionnaire, Serpell & Hsu (2005) investigated levels of "trainability" in 1563 dogs belonging to 11 breeds, and found that show-bred dog breeds tended to score lower than breeds developed for fieldwork. The C-BARQ questionnaire was also used to examine breed differences in the prevalence and severity of aggression towards familiar and unfamiliar humans and dogs in different dog breeds (Duffy *et al.*, 2008). Large and consistent differences were found among the breeds and the authors concluded that the propensity towards aggressive behavior is at least partially rooted in genetics. Studies of breeds registered by the Swedish Kennel Club have documented reliable breed-specific differences in behavior such as sociability, fearfulness, and aggressiveness (Svartberg & Forkman, 2002; Svartberg *et al.*, 2005). As emphasized by one study, breed behavioral development appears to be an ongoing process (Svartberg, 2006). Other studies have looked at certain aspects of what is referred to as personality variables in dogs (Ley *et al.*, 2009). In examining the historical function and genetic relatedness among a sample of breeds, trainability and boldness were two categories of behavior that could be related to the historical function of the breeds (Turcsan *et al.*, 2011).

7.3　Methodology

The methods employed in the present study are based on three assumptions: (1) significant differences exist in many behavioral characteristics among the various breeds of dogs, although the magnitude of differences, and within-breed variability, will differ from trait to trait; (2) some of these behavioral differences are reflected in the perspectives of authorities, particularly small animal veterinarians who have extensive experience with a large number of dog breeds and dog–owner relationships; and (3) the behavioral information about breed differences that exists in the minds of these authorities can be obtained by direct interview with a large number of the authorities with a data collection format that minimizes the opportunity for them to emphasize the breeds in which they may have a personal interest.

The use of a ranking method in this study (ranking a random sample of seven breeds chosen from the master list of 80 breeds), rather than absolute scoring, avoids the situation where different authorities could have different standards about what a score may mean. The extent of agreement among authorities in their cumulative rankings of the various breeds on a trait is an indication of the reliability of breed differences and should be reflected in statistical significance. An absence of breed differences would be indicated by random variability in the cumulative rankings and a lack of statistical significance.

This procedure admittedly measures the perceptions of authorities, not actual breed differences. The methodology does, however, control for consistency among these perspectives. There was no way of checking the validity of the ranking against an independent method of ranking 80 breeds in laboratory tests. The methodology is an up-dated version of the previously developed system that provided behavioral profiles for 56 commonly registered breeds on 13 behavioral characteristics (Hart & Hart, 1985, 1988; Hart & Miller, 1985).

7.3.1　Selection of authorities

In order to achieve maximum uniformity among the individuals serving as authorities for ranking breeds of dogs, small animal veterinarians were chosen as the individuals to be interviewed. Small animal veterinarians have a relatively uniform professional background, they see frequent interactions between owners and their dogs, handle dogs in the hospital wards, and listen to the complaints and boastings about dogs from their clients.

Telephone interviews, rather than mail surveys, were used to reduce the likelihood of response bias. Veterinarians, at least 5 years beyond graduation, were selected from a directory by a modified random selection method, utilizing the total range of names in three regions of the continental US: Eastern, Central, and Western, and with an attempt to interview men and women approximately equally. Following initial telephone contact, a letter explaining the purpose of the interviews was sent, and an interview by a registered veterinary technician or a veterinary student (both women) was arranged. An identical interviewing protocol was followed in each case. The study involved a set of 168 interviews with 72 male and 96 female veterinarians (from about 800 initial telephone contacts). Those being interviewed were not told about the breeds they were presented with until the start of the interview. This approach was expected to yield a balanced data set in which each breed was ranked against other breeds about the same number of times.

7.3.2   Selection of breeds and behavioral characteristics

The project involved 80 of the breeds most frequently registered by the American Kennel Club over a 3-year time span. With rankings from 168 interviews of sets of seven breeds, each breed was potentially ranked against other breeds 14 times.

Based on a review of the 13 behavioral characteristics identified in a previous study (Hart and Hart, 1988), a decision was made to delete the two least reliable traits in terms of their ability to distinguish between breeds – *destructiveness* and *playfulness* – as well as *excitability* which overlapped substantially in ranking with the trait *activity level*. The authorities were therefore asked to rank breeds on the remaining 10 behavioral characteristics. The terminology for the final list of characteristics, considered to be those which could be readily understood by authorities were: *activity level; snapping, especially at children; excessive barking; demand for affection; aggression toward other dogs; aggression towards family members; territorial defense; watchdog barking; trainability;* and *ease of housetraining.*

The behavioral characteristics on which authorities were asked to rank the list of seven breeds were expressed in ways that illustrated the behavior. For example, the characteristic of *activity level* was introduced with the following sentence: "Some dogs may be quite active throughout the day and respond excitedly to stimuli such as a knock on the door, while others are relatively calm in both general activity level and excitability." The authority was then asked to rank the seven breeds presented, from most to least with regard to this characteristic. The order in which questions were presented was systematically varied.

Before ranking breeds on a characteristic, the authorities were first asked to compare neutered male dogs with spayed female dogs as to which was more likely to display the behavior without regard to breed. The question referred only to neutered males and spayed females to make the scoring system uniform because most male and female dogs in the US are neutered or spayed.

7.3.3   Data analysis

The ranking of breeds was recorded on a scale of 1–7 where a ranking of 1 was given to the breed considered to have the highest tendency to display the behavior. If an authority did not know enough about a particular breed to rank it on a particular trait, it was not assigned a rank and all other ranking data were adjusted to utilize the full 7-point scale.

A least squares means procedure was used to derive the ranking of the final 80 breeds on each characteristic (Searle *et al.*, 1980). Analyses of variance (ANOVAs), based on Blom normal scores, were conducted to determine if there were significant breed differences in the rankings for each characteristic by comparing the variability among breeds to the variability within breeds (Blom, 1958). Principal Components Factor Analysis of the breed rankings on the 10 characteristics was also conducted to determine associations between the different behavioral traits.

The formula for expressing the degrees of difference in rankings between male and female dogs was: number of authorities ranking males higher, minus the number of authorities ranking females higher, divided by total number of authorities × 100. Fisher's sign test was performed to designate characteristics for which male dogs and female dogs were ranked as significantly different.

A separate analysis was conducted using the genetic groupings of breeds provided in the published paper by Parker *et al.* (2004) and the supporting online material. There was an overlap of 58 breeds between the genetic study and the present behavior study. Breeds of the three most closely related groupings, the *wolf-like, guarding* and *herding* groups, were examined with regard to placement on each of the 10 behavioral characteristic rankings. The group, referred to as the *wolf-like group*, with a similarity coefficient of 0.99, included the chow chow, shiba inu, Siberian husky, Alaskan malamute, shar-pei and akita. A second group with a coefficient of 0.84, and referred to as *guarding dogs*, included the mastiff, bulldog, boxer, Rottweiler, German shepherd dog and Newfoundland. A third group with a coefficient of 0.61, and referred to as the *herding dogs*, included the collie, Shetland sheepdog, St. Bernard and Irish wolfhound.

It was expected that the *wolf-like* group of breeds with the highest similarity coefficient would show the highest tendency to cluster on at least some behavioral characteristics. Mixed model ANOVAs were used to compare differences in mean clustering on the characteristics (Littell *et al.*, 1996). All statistical tests were 2-tailed, with a significance level of $P < 0.05$.

7.4   Results

7.4.1   Breed rankings and comparisons with genetic structure analysis

Rankings of all 80 breeds based on least squares means were obtained for all characteristics, with a rank of 1 representing the lowest and 80 the highest. For all behavioral characteristics there were statistically significant differences among breeds ($P < 0.0001$) with F-values ranging from 4.2 to 10.6 (Table 7.1).

Table 7.1 Arrangement of behavioral characteristics according to F-values derived from ANOVA models based on Blom normal scores. The higher the F-value, the better the characteristic differentiates among breeds. All F-values reflect statistically significant differences ($P < 0.0001$).

Trait	F value
Activity level	10.6
Snapping at children	9.5
Excessive barking	7.8
Territorial defense	7.7
Aggression to dogs	7.4
Aggression to family members	7.3
Affection demand	6.5
Trainability	5.1
Watchdog barking	4.9
Housetraining ease	4.2

The higher the F-value, the greater the likelihood that the characteristic distinguishes between breeds. Thus, *activity level*, with an F-value of 10.6, distinguishes between breeds the best, and *housetraining ease*, with an F-value of 4.2, distinguishes the least.

Three examples of rankings of selected breeds are presented in Figures 7.1–7.3, for *aggression to other dogs, aggression to human family members* and *demand for affection*. For the breeds represented, the two traits dealing with aggression show similar breed rankings that are much different from rankings on *affection demand*. The *wolf-like* genetic group includes the chow chow, akita, shiba inu, and shar pei.

Four rather divergent breed-specific behavior profiles are illustrated in Figures 7.4–7.7, for the collie and Shetland sheepdog from the genetic *herding* group, and the chow chow and shiba inu from the genetic *wolf-like* group.

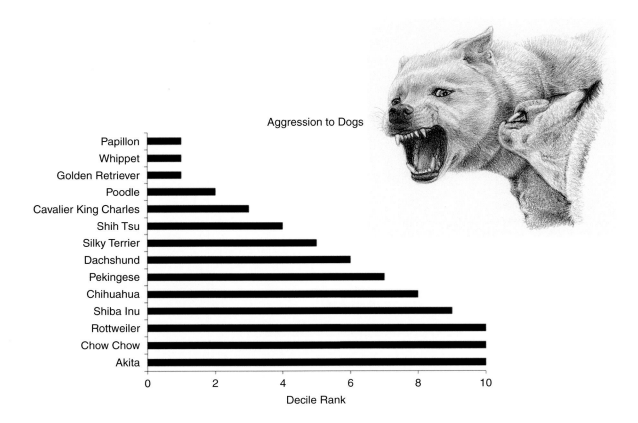

Figure 7.1 Rankings on "aggression to other dogs" among breeds selected from the master list of 80 breeds. For deciles 1 and 10 three breeds are listed to compare a group from the *wolf-like* genetic group – the akita, chow chow and shiba inu – with the group ranking lowest on the trait. (Artwork provided by copyright holders B. L. Hart and L. A. Hart.)

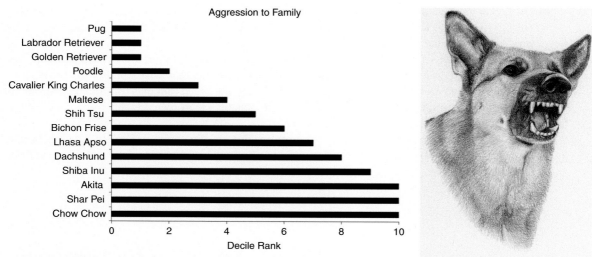

Figure 7.2 Rankings on "aggression to family members" among breeds selected from the master list of 80. For deciles 1 and 10 three breeds are listed to compare a group from the *wolf-like* genetic group – chow chow, shar pei and akita – with the group ranking lowest on the trait. The overlap with Figure 7.1 is very apparent. (Artwork provided by copyright holders B. L. Hart and L. A. Hart.)

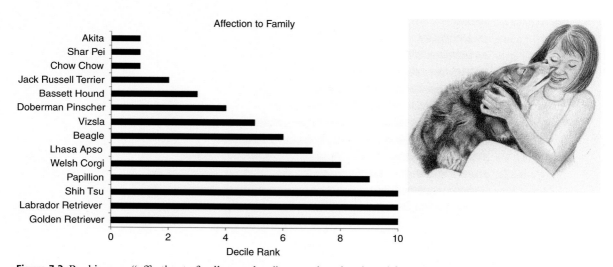

Figure 7.3 Rankings on "affection to family members" among breeds selected from the master list of 80. For deciles 1 and 10 three breeds are listed to compare a group from the *wolf-like* genetic group – akita, shar pei and chow chow – at the lowest decile, with the group of breeds ranking in the highest decile. (Artwork provided by copyright holders B. L. Hart and L. A. Hart.)

While these graphs illustrate visually the differences between the *wolf-like* breeds and the *herding* breeds, this impression is strongly reinforced by the results of statistical analysis. Mixed model ANOVAs revealed significant differences in rankings on five of the behavioral characteristics among breeds belonging to the three genetic groups (*wolf-like, guarding* and *herding*). On the traits of *aggression to family members, aggression towards other dogs, territorial defense* and *snapping*, the *wolf-like* group clustered at the high end of the rankings and significantly differed from the *herding* group which tended to cluster at the lower end of the same characteristics ($P = 0.01$). On *affection demand*, the *wolf-like* breeds ranked significantly lower ($P = 0.01$) than the *guarding* and *herding* breeds. There was no significant clustering of the *wolf-like, guarding* and *herding* breeds on the other five traits.

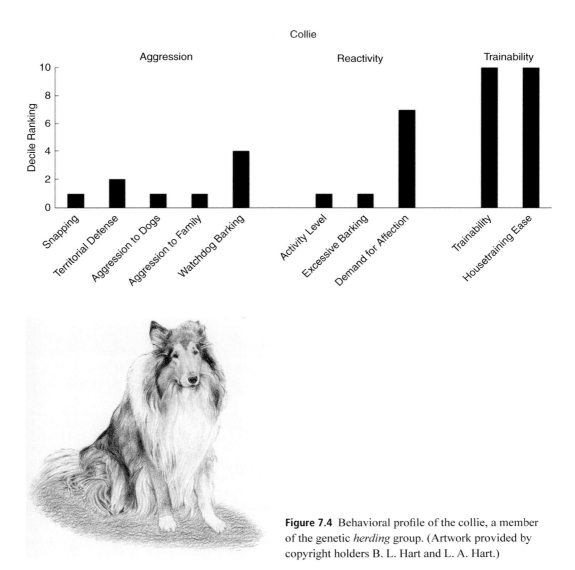

Figure 7.4 Behavioral profile of the collie, a member of the genetic *herding* group. (Artwork provided by copyright holders B. L. Hart and L. A. Hart.)

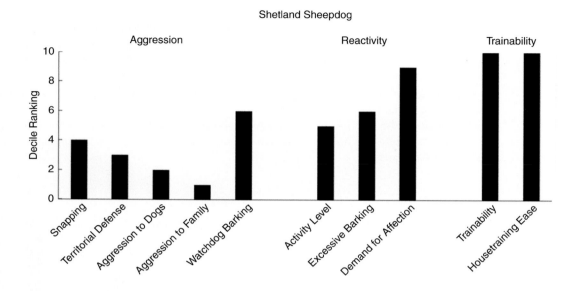

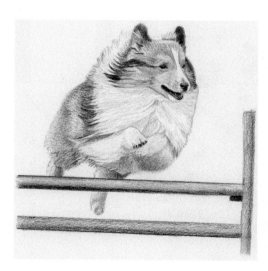

Figure 7.5 Behavioral profile of the Shetland sheepdog, a member of the genetic *herding* group. (Artwork provided by copyright holders B. L. Hart and L. A. Hart.)

7.4.2   Factor analysis

Principal Components Factor Analysis of the breed rankings on the 10 characteristics extracted three factors with eigenvalues greater than 1.0. Major factor loadings of the 10 characteristics were determined for only these three factors, which accounted for 43.6%, 25.2% and 18.7% of the variance, respectively. The characteristics loading most heavily on the first factor (referred to as "aggression") were *aggression to dogs, aggression to family members, territorial defense, snapping* and *watchdog barking*. On the second factor (referred to as "reactivity"), *affection demand, excessive barking* and *activity level* loaded most heavily. On the third factor (referred to as "trainability"), *trainability* and *ease of housetraining* loaded most heavily.

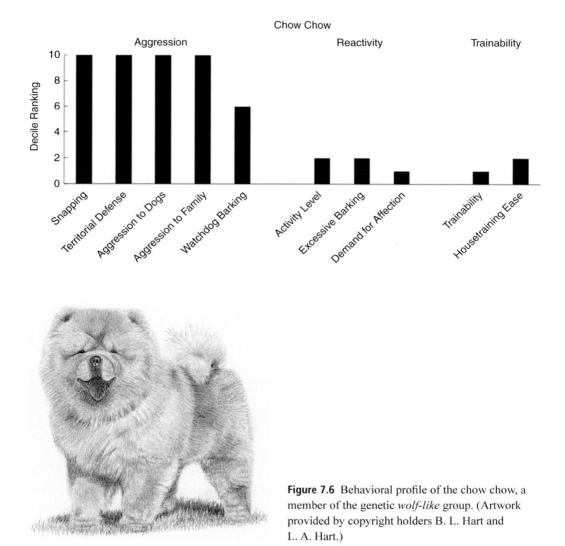

Figure 7.6 Behavioral profile of the chow chow, a member of the genetic *wolf-like* group. (Artwork provided by copyright holders B. L. Hart and L. A. Hart.)

7.4.3 Gender analysis of behavioral characteristics

A statistically significant difference between male and female dogs was found on all characteristics ($P < 0.01$). The mean scores for the various characteristics are portrayed as the magnitude of the degree of consensus shown along an axis extending from –100 to 100, with –100 being a score where all males would be ranked higher than all females, and 100 being a score where all females would be ranked higher than all males (Figure 7.8). The characteristics most strongly associated with males were *aggression to family members, territorial defense* and *aggression to other dogs*. Other characteristics for which males were scored higher were *watchdog barking, activity level, excessive barking* and *snapping*. Characteristics for which female dogs ranked higher were *trainability, ease of housetraining* and *affection demand*.

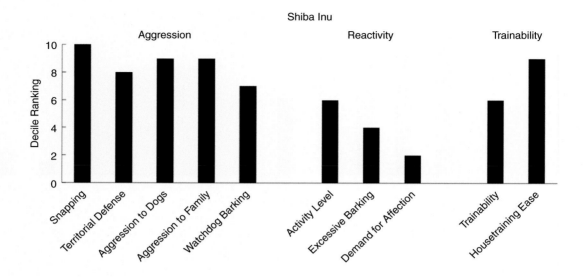

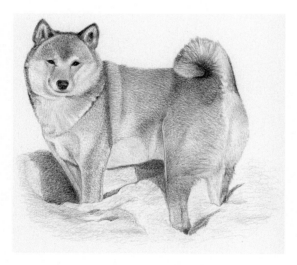

Figure 7.7 Behavioral profile of the shiba inu, a member of the genetic *wolf-like* group. (Artwork provided by copyright holders B. L. Hart and L. A. Hart.)

7.5   Discussion

The statistically significant rankings of 80 breeds on each of 10 characteristics reveal that it is possible to obtain quantitative data that reflect measures of the consensus of authorities about differences in behavior among breeds of dogs. The authorities that contributed to the rankings may have had biased viewpoints, but the study was designed to reduce the degree to which someone being interviewed could make a pitch for a favorite breed, or otherwise have undue influence on the data, i.e. interviewed authorities were selected from a directory, and then presented with a randomly selected group of seven breeds to rank.

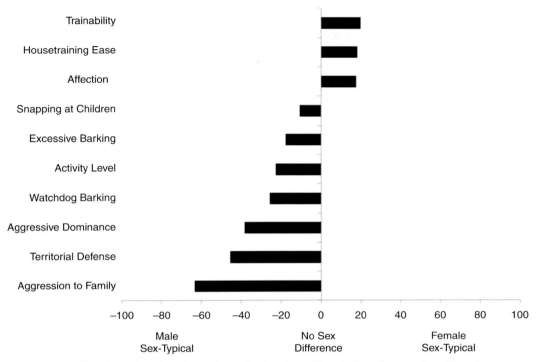

Figure 7.8 Rankings by authorities of gonadectomized male and female dogs, irrespective of breed membership. A score of −100 or 100 would mean that all authorities would have ranked, respectively, males or females always higher on that characteristic. The length of the bar represents the degree of consensus regarding one sex being more likely to show the characteristic under consideration.

Aside from some possible breed-related biases that may have occurred in general, there are some inaccuracies inherent in the data collection system because of the necessarily limited amount of data which could be collected. While a larger sample size would presumably yield more accurate rankings, a larger number of interviews would probably not change the picture in a major way. In fact, given the inevitable difficulty of comparing rankings of one study which involves 80 breeds with one which involves 56 breeds, the results in rankings and Factor Analyses in both the present study and the previous one (Hart, 1995; Hart & Hart, 1988) were similar.

Confidence in the reliability of our system of developing behavioral profiles was reinforced by a comparison with the genetic analyses conducted by Parker *et al.* (2004) on 85 breeds. Breeds that grouped together with relatively high similarity coefficients in genetic structure also tended to cluster on several behavioral characteristics. This is what one would expect if there were a genetic basis for these behavioral traits. The group of breeds referred to as *wolf-like*, and with the highest similarity coefficient, clustered at the low end of *affection demand* and at the high end of *aggression to family members, aggression to dogs, territorial defense* and *snapping*. The *herding* group of breeds clustered on the same characteristics, but at opposite ends, and were significantly different than the wolf-like breeds.

The clustering of genetic groups, such as the *wolf-like* and *herding* breeds, on some characteristics but not others, suggests that historically the related breeds shared some behavioral characteristics, especially in the realm of aggressive behavior and affection. However, selective breeding that was invested in individual breed development apparently resulted in differentiation in other characteristics such as *activity level, watchdog barking* and *trainability*. As mentioned previously, virtually all of the breeds under consideration are genetically distinct, which implies that the breeds within a genetically related group would be expected to differ on a number of behavioral parameters while remaining similar on others. As emphasized by several investigators, the dog offers unparalleled phenotypic diversity among even closely related breeds, with regard to morphology, physiology and behavior. Our experimental approach offers one efficient and relatively low-cost method of acquiring quantitative data on behavioral traits.

The overall results revealed some important conceptual findings with regard to breed-specific analyses. While all characteristics significantly differentiated between breeds at some level, traits such as *activity level* discriminate between breeds better than other traits such as *ease of house training*. It stands to reason there is more impact from early training and environment on those characteristics that discriminate the least well among breeds.

This project did not attempt to obtain information about all registered breeds. This would have diluted the data that provided the rankings because when authorities were not familiar enough with a breed to rank it, the breed was left out of the rankings.

Principal Components Factor Analyses revealed that rankings on some characteristics are related to rankings on others. Three factors accounted for 88% of the variability, a finding in agreement with that obtained in a previous study (Hart, 1995; Hart & Hart, 1988). This analysis implies that the traits associated with a factor tend to occur together. For example, *affection demand* was associated with the reactivity factor and loaded more strongly on this factor than the other characteristics. This finding implies that dogs that are very active, and likely to bark excessively, are also those most predisposed to seek affection. *Ease of housetraining*, while loading positively on trainability, secondarily loaded negatively on reactivity, suggesting that the reduced level of reactivity carries with it a reduced *ease of housetraining*. This is the only characteristic to exhibit significant cross-loading on more than one of the three factors, and in opposite directions. This cross-loading may contribute to housetraining having the lowest F-value and presumably discriminating the least reliably between breeds.

With regard to gender differences, the data extend the understanding of sex differences in behaviors with regard to neutered dogs. The degree of consensus of authorities in ranking one sex more likely to display a behavior than the other sex would appear to represent a reflection of sexual dimorphism in that behavioral characteristic. In the present study the behavioral differences between the sexes (neutered) on all 10 characteristics were derived from the opinions of authorities rather than laboratory observations, but assuming the cumulative rankings of so many authorities reflect real behavioral differences between the sexes, the analysis reveals a continuum in the magnitude of sexually dimorphic traits. For example, while it could be said that both *aggression to family members* and *aggression to dogs* are typically more characteristic of male than female dogs, the difference between the sexes is more pronounced with regard to *aggression to family members* (Figure 7.8). While both of these behavioral characteristics may be altered by castration (Neilson *et al.*, 1997), no evidence is available on the effects of castration on the other, somewhat less male-typical, characteristics. Perhaps it is only the most sexually dimorphic characteristics that are most readily altered by castration.

7.6   Conclusions

In the last decade, several studies using different web-based methodologies have documented differences among dog breeds with regard to types of aggressive behavior and trainability. Using the approach reviewed here, the present study obtained significant differences among 80 popular breeds on 10 different behavioral characteristics, using direct telephone interview rankings from 168 authorities, thereby avoiding response bias and personal standards of scoring. The authorities, small animal veterinarians, have similar educational backgrounds, and see many dogs of all different breeds day-after-day. Significant differences in all characteristics – *activity level; snapping, especially at children; excessive barking; demand for affection; aggression toward other dogs; aggression towards family members; territorial defense; watchdog barking; trainability*, and *ease of housetraining* – were seen among breeds. Significant gender differences were also found with the same behavioral characteristics. Furthermore, the genetic basis for some of these breed-specific behavioral differences was verified by comparison with the results of previous analyses of molecular genetic relationships among most of the dog breeds involved. The results can be of value in helping those who wish to adopt a purebred puppy and wish to make a breed and gender choice that best matches their lifestyle and personality.

Acknowledgements

Financial support for preparation of this chapter was provided by grant (#2009-36-F) from the Center for Companion Animal Health, School of Veterinary Medicine, at the University of California, Davis. The authors are happy to acknowledge artist Emma Mooring for the illustrations.

References

Blom, G. (1958). *Statistical Estimates and Transformed Beta-Variables*. New York: Wiley and Sons, pp. 31–80.

Duffy, D. L., Hsu, Y. & Serpell, J. A. (2008). Breed differences in canine aggression. *Applied Animal Behaviour Science*, 114: 441–60.

Hart, B. L. (1995). Analyzing breed and gender differences in behaviour. In *The Domestic Dog: Its Evolution, Behaviour and Interactions with People*, ed. J. A. Serpell. Cambridge: Cambridge University Press, pp. 65–78.

Hart, B. L. & Hart, L. A. (1985). Selecting pet dogs on the basis of cluster analysis of breed behavior profiles and gender. *Journal of the American Veterinary Medical Association*, 186: 1181–5.

Hart, B. L. & Hart, L. A. (1988). *The Perfect Puppy. How to Choose Your Dog by its Behavior*. New York: W.H. Freeman and Co.

Hart, B. L. & Miller, M. F. (1985). Behavioral profiles of dog breeds. *Journal of the American Veterinary Medical Association*, 186: 175–80.

Ley, J. M., Bennett, P. C. & Grahame, G. J. (2009). A refinement and validation of the Monash Canine Personality Qiestionnaire (MCPQ). *Applied Animal Behaviour Science*, 116: 220–227.

Littell, R. C., Milliken, G. A., Stroup, W. W. & Wolfinge, R. D. (1996). *SAS System for Mixed Models*. Cary, NC: SAS Institute Inc., pp. 87–92.

Neilson, J.C., Eckstein, R.A. & Hart, B. L. (1997). Effects of castration on behavior of male dogs with reference to the role of age and experience. *Journal of the American Veterinary Medical Association*, 211: 180–2.

Parker, H. G., Kim, L. V., Sutter, N. B. *et al.* (2004). Genetic structure of the purebred domestic dog. *Science*, 304: 1161–4.

Parker, H. G., Kukekova, A. V., Akey, D. T. *et al.* (2007). Breed relationships facilitate fine-mapping studies: a 7.8-kb deletion cosegregates with Collie eye anomaly across multiple dog breeds. *Genome Research*, 17: 1562–71.

Parker, H. G., Shearin, A. L. & Ostrander, E. A. (2010). Man's best friend becomes biology's best in show: genome analyses in the domestic dog. *Annual Review of Genetics*, 44: 309–36.

Rugbjerg, H., Proschow, H. F., Ersboll, A. K. & Lund, J. D. (2003). Risk factors associated with interdog aggression and shooting phobias among purebred dogs in Denmark. *Preventive Veterinary Medicine*, 58: 85–100.

Scott, J. P. & Fuller, J. L. (1965). *Genetics and the Social Behavior of the Dog*. Chicago, IL: University of Chicago Press

Searle, S. R., Speed, F. M. & Milliken, G. A. (1980). Population marginal means in the linear model: an alternative to least squares means. *Journal of the American Statistical Association*, 34: 216–21.

Serpell, J. A. & Hsu, Y. (2005). Effects of breed, sex, and neuter status on trainability in dogs. *Anthrozoos*, 18: 196–207.

Svartberg, K., Tapper, I. & Temrin, H. (2005). Consistency of personality traits in dogs. *Animal Behaviour*, 69: 283–91.

Svartberg, K. (2006). Breed-typical behavior in dogs – historical remnants or recent constructs? *Applied Animal Behaviour Science*, 96: 293–313

Svartberg K. & Forkman B. (2002). Personality traits in the domestic dog (*Canis familiaris*). *Applied Animal Behaviour Science*, 79: 133–55.

Turcsan, B., Kubinyi, E. & Miklosi, A. (2011). Trainability and boldness traits differ between dog breed clusters based on conventional breed categories and genetic relatedness. *Applied Animal Behaviour Science*, 132: 61–70.

8 Dog social behavior and communication

JOHN BRADSHAW AND NICOLA ROONEY

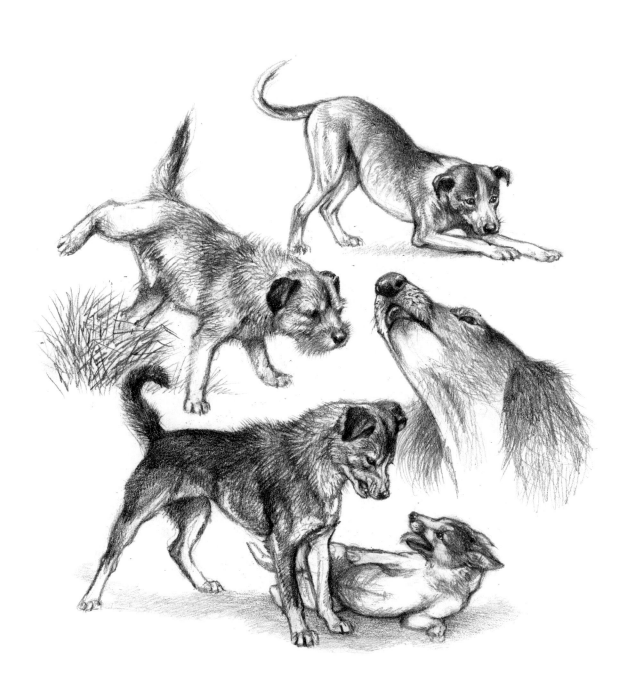

8.1   Introduction

The success of the domestic dog as a species depends upon its ability to interact socially with members of its own species and, crucially, with humankind. Effective interaction depends upon both a repertoire of signals whereby social intentions can be expressed, and also the cognitive ability to interpret the behavior of others. For the dog, both of these abilities must inevitably be derived from those of their ancestral species, the grey wolf, *Canis lupus*, and many traditional accounts of dog behavior have borrowed heavily from studies of wolves (e.g. Fox, 1973). However, over the past decade scientific consensus has shifted dramatically in two areas, both of which call into question the reliability of these comparisons. Firstly, studies of wolf packs in the wild have painted a very different picture of their social organization than had previously emerged from studies of captive wolves. Secondly, the cognitive abilities of the domestic dog have been shown to have been markedly altered by domestication.

Field studies of wild wolf packs have revealed that the natural unit of wolf society is the family (e.g. Mech, 1999), casting doubt on the validity of much previous research using captive packs. Wild packs are usually kin-selected units in which young adults assist their parents for one or two breeding seasons before dispersing. Neighboring packs tend to avoid contact with one another, but when they do meet, unrestrained conflict is likely to occur (Mech & Boitani, 2003). Most of the classic studies of captive wolves (e.g. Rabb *et al*., 1967; Schenkel, 1947; van Hooff & Wensing, 1987; Zimen, 1975) were conducted on artificially assembled groups of unrelated adults. Prevented from dispersing, and presumably perceiving one another as originating from different packs and therefore competitors, most of these wolves were placed in the position of having to fight before they could reproduce. From the outcome of these competitions grew the concept of the wolf "dominance hierarchy," in which one male and one female wolf, the "alphas," suppressed breeding in all the other adults through aggression. By contrast, in most natural packs the non-breeding members, both pre- and post-reproductive, have chosen to remain with the breeding pair rather than disperse.

The term "alpha" is therefore redundant because it simply becomes a synonym for "parent" (Mech, 2008). Aggressive interactions within natural packs are rare and may only ever become intense when sexually mature offspring are on the point of dispersing (Mech & Cluff, 2010). The separate "pecking-order" hierarchies for males and females, that typify captive wolves, are therefore now perceived as artefacts, generated by enforced and unnatural competition between wolves that would, given the opportunity, have set up several well-separated breeding units. The term "dominance" within natural wolf packs simply describes a situation where one male and one female reproduce and lead the pack, and other non-breeding adults accept their leadership without coercion and maintain their affiliations by occasional displays of "submission" (see Section 8.4.3) and appeasement.

In both the scientific and popular dog literature, much has been made of the outward similarity between wolf and dog behavior, but this may be misleading. Often the assumption is made that, if a dog performs a species-typical signal, such as "passive submission" or the "play-bow" (see Section 8.7), its motivation can be most accurately deduced by comparisons with wolf behavior (e.g. Monks of New Skete, 1978). There are, however, at least four reasons why superficially similar dog and wolf behaviors might require different interpretation. One is that much of dog behavior appears to be derived from the repertoire of juvenile, not adult wolves (Kretchmer & Fox, 1975), yet comparisons are usually made with the latter. A second is the radical changes in social cognition, especially in inter-species communication, that appear to have been brought about by domestication (see Range & Viranyi, Chapter 10). A third – probably related to the second – is that interspecific socialization, which characterizes the domestic dog, changes the context within which many signals function. The fourth is the powerful rewarding value of contact with humans, self-evident from the ease with which dogs can be trained using social attention as a reinforcer. The frequency of performance of some signals, and the contexts in which they are performed, may be profoundly altered by the reactions of their human attachment figure.

While some breeds of dog are capable of performing a substantial subset of wolf-type signals, the similarity between their repertoire and that of the wolf needs to be interpreted with caution. No visual signals (postures intended to convey a specific meaning) seem to have evolved *de novo* during domestication in any species, although some may have been lost. Thus the only signals available to the dog are those it has inherited from its canid ancestors. While the signals may remain outwardly similar, the cognitive, emotional and social context within which they are performed has changed radically due to domestication, and therefore both dog-to-dog and dog-to-human communication should logically be examined within that social context, rather than through superficial comparisons with one wild ancestor.

Here we first review the most recent approaches that have been applied to social structure in domestic dogs, breaking with tradition by placing most emphasis on studies of feral and companion dogs rather than on wolves, and looking in depth at the concept of dominance hierarchies. We then examine the main communication channels – sight, sound and smell – relating each to the likely social function of each signal, and paying special attention to play. Finally, we speculate on how these new insights alter our perception of the dog–human relationship.

8.2   Social Structure

The best model for the dog's social capabilities might be most logically sought from feral dogs, which are descended from fully domesticated animals, rather than from wolves. Unfortunately most feral dogs are so disrupted by human interference (e.g. Beck, 1975; Boitani *et al.*, Chapter 17) and disease (Daniels & Bekoff, 1989) that their true social capabilities may only rarely emerge, especially if, like wolves, their preferred pack structure is based on familial alliances built up over several years. However, even in those situations where feral dogs are as undisturbed as wild wolves, they have never been observed to establish wolf-type family packs. Feral dogs, unlike wolves, are not known to assist their parents in the raising of offspring, nor is paternal care the norm.

8.2.1   Dingoes and Indian pariah dogs

Dingoes, the "wild" dogs of Australia, are the descendants of domestic dogs that crossed over from New Guinea or the Indonesian Archipelago several thousand years ago (Clutton-Brock, Chapter 2). Studies of dingoes in captivity (e.g. Corbett, 1988) came to the same conclusions as studies of captive wolves: that packs were "dominated" by a single breeding pair suppressing all other breeding via aggression. However, it is now known that in the wild all the female dingoes in a pack can breed every year (Thomson *et al.*, 1992).

The mating systems of feral dogs have been recorded in detail in West Bengal, India (Pal, 2011; Pal *et al.*, 1999). These free-roaming "pariah" dogs live in groups of 5–10 adults, and their dependent offspring, sharing a territory that they defend against neighboring groups. All adult females come into breeding condition every year, and each is courted by several males, mostly from other groups. Pal (2011) recorded no fewer than six mating strategies among just 14 females: monogamy, polygyny, promiscuity, polyandry, opportunity and "rape." Seasonal monogamy, involving a pair-bond with one male, was the most common, and these males guarded their litters for the first 6–8 weeks of life (Pal, 2005). Both communal denning and paternal care (apart from guarding) were rare. Females usually withdrew from the group before giving birth, and became aggressive towards other group members during at least the first two weeks after parturition. Withdrawal of females from the group, and also male guarding of some but not all litters, appear to be typical for feral dogs (e.g. Macdonald & Carr, Chapter 16; Boitani *et al.*, Chapter 17). The reproductive behavior of these feral groups is quite unlike that of the grey wolf, and much more like that of other species from the dog family, such as the coyote (*C. latrans*), that have less structured social lives (Moehlman, 1989). It is likely that the differences in social organization between feral dogs and wolves are due to genetic differences between them, brought about by the process of domestication.

Exchanges of other types of behavior amongst free-roaming dogs are also strikingly different from those of wolves. Although group membership in free-roaming dogs tends to remain stable outside the breeding season, wolf-like ritualized exchanges – often described as "dominant" and "submissive" (see Section 8.4.3) behavior – are rare in some groups (e.g. Pal *et al.*, 1998), and although they have been observed in others (Bonanni *et al.*, 2010), not all group members appear to perform them (Cafazzo *et al.*, 2010). Dominance hierarchies based on exchange of agonistic or submissive behavior can be calculated, but bear little relation to breeding success (for an exception see Cafazzo *et al.*, 2014), and may be more a reflection of behavioral "style" and age (older dogs tending to be more aggressive) than any underlying social structure (Bradshaw *et al.*, 2009, 2016). Between-group behavior is also strikingly different to that of wolf packs: "submissive behavior," rare in encounters between different wolf packs, is more commonly displayed between members of different free-roaming groups than within those groups (Pal *et al.*, 1998).

8.2.2   Companion dogs

Although it is self-evident that dogs in multi-dog households do not interact randomly, the interpretation of their interactions is not straightforward. Companion dogs exist in multispecies societies in which interactions with humans often take precedence over interactions with other dogs: not only do many dogs benefit more from interacting with humans than with dogs, e.g. experiencing greater amelioration of stress (Tuber *et al.*, 1996), but also their ultimate reproductive success is often determined by human intervention rather than by their ability to select an optimum sexual partner and successfully raise young. From a functional perspective, the reproductive success of ancestral companion dogs will have been determined more by their owner's perception of their behavior (and conformation) than by the way that they interacted with conspecifics. Thus the selection pressures on intraspecific social behavior are qualitatively different from those that apply to feral/free-roaming dogs or any wild canid, including the wolf.

The literature on dog–dog, and especially dog–owner, interactions has also traditionally been couched in terms of a dominance/submission framework (e.g. Bradshaw & Nott, 1995), and attempts continue to be made to characterize relationships based on performance of "dominant" or "submissive" postures (Bauer & Smuts, 2007; Lisberg & Snowdon, 2009; van der Borg *et al.*, 2015). While putative social structures can be mathematically extracted from such data, it is unclear whether these have any meaning for the dogs involved. For example, it used to be asserted that the outcomes of games played between dog and owner are an important determinant of the "dominance" relationship between them, with the apparent winner of the game gaining "status" (O'Farrell, 1992; Rogerson, 1992). However, we were unable to find any evidence to support this hypothesis in a series of observational and experimental studies of dog–owner games (Rooney & Bradshaw 2002, 2003; summarized in Bradshaw et al., 2015).

8.2.3   The concepts of dominance and hierarchy

"Dominance" is both a word in everyday use, with connotations of importance, power and influence, and also a technical term in animal behavior. Dog owners and dog trainers with no formal education in ethology may therefore inadvertently use it in ways that are not supported by canine science (McGreevy et al., 2012). For example, certain individual dogs or breeds may be referred to as more "dominant" than others, even though in ethology "dominance" is used to characterise relationships, not personalities (Bradshaw et al., 2009, 2016; see Schilder et al., 2014 for a conflicting view).

Among free-roaming and feral dogs, rankings (or hierarchies) based upon exchange of aggressive behavior are generally rather indeterminate (Bradshaw et al., 2009; Cafazzo et al., 2010) except among males competing over receptive females (Cafazzo et al., 2010). Directional exchanges of submissive and affiliative behavior (see Section 8.4.3) generally provide more reliable hierarchies (Bradshaw et al., 2009; Cafazzo et al., 2010), of which asymmetries in low-posture (as expressed in both active and passive submission – see Section 8.4.3), may be the most consistent (van der Borg et al., 2015). Rankings derived for such groups might thus be described more logically as *deference* hierarchies, since they reflect the flow of "submissive" behavior "up" the hierarchy rather than aggressive behavior "down" it. Moreover, group cohesion appears to be expressed more in so-called "affiliative submissive" behavior performed spontaneously in greeting ceremonies than in submissive behavior performed in response to aggression (Bonanni et al., 2010). This suggests that it is primarily affiliative behavior that forms the social "glue" that holds such groups together, counteracting the potentially disruptive, even dangerous, effects of competition over resources that inevitably occurs between individual dogs. Furthermore, affiliative submission is strongly age-stratified, flowing from the youngest individuals to the oldest (Bonanni et al., 2010; Cafazzo et al., 2010), indicating that it is probably derived from infantile food-begging behavior.

While hierarchies in free-roaming dogs may predict access to food (Cafazzo et al., 2010), they generally do not predict frequency of mating (Pal et al., 1999; see Cafazzo et al., 2014 for an exception) and no clear connection has been made with lifetime reproductive success. Thus the selective pressures that have given rise to such apparent hierarchies remain unclear, at least in the narrow context of intra-specific interactions. Free-roaming populations of dogs are rarely self-sustaining, relying on immigration from dogs with stronger associations with humans, such as abandoned pets (Daniels & Bekoff, 1989; Boitani et al., Chapter 17). Therefore the social behavior of free-roaming groups may reflect strategies, such as "affiliative submission" (Bonanni et al., 2010), that have contributed to breeding success for successive generations of owned dogs, but are selectively neutral in the feral state.

8.2.4   Cognitive aspects of hierarchy

Hierarchy is a property that is extracted by human observers from encounters between animals; there is no requirement for the animals themselves to be aware of their relationships. It has proved possible to construct simple robots that establish very convincing and stable dominance hierarchies, based on straightforward stimulus-and-response rules and limited recall of previous encounters (Funato et al., 2011; Vaughan et al., 2000). Clearly such robots cannot be "aware" of the "relationships" that they appear to have established with their neighbors. The mere existence of a hierarchy cannot be used as evidence that the actors within it possess their own cognitive representation of that hierarchy.

Dogs are clearly more complex entities than robots: for example, they are capable of recognising other dogs, even after considerable periods of separation (e.g. Hepper, 1994). However, it is possible to explain dominance hierarchies among non-primate mammals in terms of simple pairwise relationships (Appleby, 1993), without invoking any capacity on the animals' part to appreciate the existence of the hierarchy. Recently, it has been demonstrated that dogs alter their behavior according to their own observations of third-party interactions (Kundey *et al.*, 2010; Marshall-Pescini *et al.*, 2011; Rooney & Bradshaw, 2006). However, dogs appear cognitively limited in the extent to which they can extract this information (e.g. Kaminski *et al.*, 2012), and so far, cognitive science has failed to demonstrate more than rudimentary "theory of mind" in dogs (Horowitz, 2011; Range & Viranyi, Chapter 10). Many, perhaps all, of their supposedly "insightful" actions can be explained more parsimoniously by associative learning (e.g. Elgier *et al.*, 2012), coupled with highly selective attention (Horowitz, 2009); similar conclusions have been drawn from studies of arguably the most socially sophisticated of the Carnivora, the spotted hyena (Holekamp & Engh, 2002). It is therefore doubtful whether dogs understand the relationships that they have with the dogs around them; it is more likely that they are simply responding to combinations of stimuli that have gained meaning through previous encounters.

In short, there is little evidence to support the notion that "status" is a concept that has any meaning for dogs. Thus it seems highly improbable that status could be a motivation for dog behavior, or a quality that dogs try to optimize in an analogous way to physiological goals such as metabolic homeostasis or the minimization of stress. Despite this, until recently, a hypothetical "status drive" was widely used as an intervening variable in characterizing unwanted aggression towards both dogs and people (e.g. Landsberg *et al.*, 2003), and some dog training techniques still rely heavily on this concept (see AVSAB, 2008).

Although it is self-evident that dogs do behave "assertively" when competing for valued resources, such behavior can be accounted for more parsimoniously using simple learning rules. In contrast to the unitary construct of the wolf pack, no single framework has yet emerged to describe the social structure of owned dogs as a replacement for the simplistic "multi-species pack" concept. This is perhaps not surprising, given the diversity of such social groups, both in terms of their size and the variety of types of dog involved, and also the complexity and variability of the behavior of the human participants.

8.2.5   Replacements for the "dominance" framework

The Resource Holding Potential (RHP) model (Parker, 1974) has been proposed by several authors as an alternative framework for explaining relationships between dogs (Lindsay, 2005; Shepherd, 2002; Wickens, 1993). It has the advantage that it predicts that the outcome of disputes depends on the subjective value of the resource to each of the individuals, allowing for "dominance" relationships to be reversed depending on context. It therefore explains why an otherwise "submissive" member of a group may be permitted access to a resource that it values highly, because it does not pay the usually more "'dominant'" member to escalate the dispute. However, unlike most other species, companion dogs often appear to pay scant attention to relative size when encountering one another, despite the large weight differences between the largest and smallest individuals; for example, size was not a predictor of the outcome of encounters between dogs being exercised by their owners (Bradshaw & Lea, 1993). Many dogs also do not appear to place much importance on the apparent fighting ability of their opponent, allowing differences in motivation (how much the dog values the resource), perceived motivation (what the behavior of the other dog signifies about the likelihood that it will escalate), and the previous experiences of both dogs, to all play a much greater role in determining the outcome of the encounter than is typical for other animals.

Patterns of interactions between dogs, and between dogs and their owners, appear to fit better into a framework in which prior experience and context are the major determinants of subsequent encounters (Bradshaw *et al.*, 2009). For example, a dog that has been physically punished in a context where it has been unable to make an association between the punishment and any cue other than the person carrying out the punishment, may feel anxious when that person approaches again. The behavioral strategy that it adopts will depend on its prior experience; it may show any one of appeasement, avoidance or aggression, or some combination of these. Any strategy that is successful will be reinforcing, and over subsequent encounters the dog will become more confident in showing this behavior in that specific context. Thus an aggressive display that was originally performed with a fearful posture and was thus clearly defensive, may, if repeatedly successful in reducing the dog's anxiety, become the dog's strategy of choice, metamorphosing into a display commonly if misleadingly labeled "dominance aggression" (Bradshaw *et al.*, 2009). Agonistic behavior between dogs, and especially between dogs and their owners, may thus be more parsimoniously explained by associative learning than by the concept that dogs are constantly striving to achieve "status" within a mixed-species social group.

Conceptually, it may be more useful to place domestic dogs in the context within which they have evolved – human society. Given the emerging consensus that domestic dogs have evolved a unique sensitivity to human gaze and gesture (Range & Viranyi, Chapter 10), and the extreme rapidity with which abandoned dogs appear to form attachments to individual people (Blackwell *et al.*, 2010; Mendl *et al.*, 2010), indicating great motivation for human contact, dog–human relationships generally (with individual exceptions) take precedence in any mixed-species group over those between the dogs themselves. It may therefore be appropriate to place the primary focus on affiliative relationships between dogs and their owners rather than "dominance" when considering inter-specific relationships, and also as an important factor in relationships between companion dogs. It is evident, however, that domestication has not altered dogs' communicative repertoires to anything like the same extent as it has their cognitive abilities.

8.3   Canine communication – general considerations

Communication is not an entirely straightforward concept, especially when dogs are exchanging information with humans. Here we will use a simple definition of communication, " … a stylised signal or display by one individual modifying the response of another" (Barnard, 2004), but we will also discuss the passive transmission of information such as individual identity, gender, reproductive status, etc., even though this is not communication in the strictest sense.

In social species, signals can be used either to manipulate the behavior of recipients, for example by raising hackles or baring teeth to increase apparent size or ferocity, or to convey "honest" information about the sender's intentions (Krebs & Dawkins, 1984). Unfortunately, most studies of communication in dogs pre-date these insights and thus have not emphasised this distinction sufficiently. The relative extent to which dogs use visual, olfactory and auditory signals, both when signaling and when assimilating information from other dogs and people, is unknown. However, probably due to the perceptual bias of humans, visual communication is relatively well studied in dogs, although interpretations are often marred by misunderstandings of, and over-reliance upon, analogies with wolf communication. Comparisons of the relative importance of the various sensory modalities are rare, but do tend to support the importance of olfaction. Discrimination learning may be achieved quicker using olfactory (Williams & Johnson, 2002) than using auditory (Kowalska *et al.*, 2001) and visual (Miklósi, 2014) cues, and trained explosives dogs have been shown to use mainly olfaction over vision, even in good light (Gazit & Terkel, 2003).

8.4   Visual communication

8.4.1   Vision

Dogs are visual generalists, able to operate in a range of ambient light levels (Pretterer *et al.*, 2004), although their eyes show several adaptations to dim light, including a predominance of rods in the central region of the retina, the presence of rhodopsin pigment with a peak sensitivity to light of wavelengths 506–510 nm, a large cornea and a superiorly located *tapetum lucidum*, which reflects back light that has already passed through the retina, thereby optimizing low-light vision, but with some consequent trade-off in acuity in bright light.

Dogs' visual acuity is thought to equate to 20/75, so a dog would be able to distinguish the same detail at 20 feet that the average person could at 75 feet. However, their ability to distinguish stationary objects may be considerably less (Miller & Murphy, 1995); like humans, dogs are more sensitive to moving than to stationary objects (Walls, 1963). Unsurprisingly, movement is integral to many attention-gaining visual signals, such as tail wagging. Dogs generally have a limited range of accommodation, only 2–3 dioptres, and are only capable of focusing on objects more than 50 cm from their eyes, whilst closer objects appear blurred (Miller & Murphy, 1995). Therefore, vision at close range is often augmented by the use of smell or taste.

In mixed breed dogs the average field of view is 240 degrees (Sherman & Wilson, 1975). However, large interbreed differences exist, due to the wide variation in skull shape (Murphy & Pollock, 1993). Height differences also affect the visual perspectives of different breeds, and potentially impact upon their ability to communicate (Miller & Murphy, 1995). In addition, a large number of heritable ocular diseases exist in dogs, many of which show predispositions in particular breeds (Summers *et al.*, 2010), and can limit their visual capabilities.

Dogs have dichromatic color vision; they cannot distinguish between green and grey, or between yellow and orange, and red likely appears as black. There is little evidence for any role of color in visual communication. Overall, dogs' visual abilities probably place more emphasis on movement than on color or texture, but the consequences of this for their communicative abilities remain under-investigated.

8.4.2   Intraspecific visual communication

Many of the wolf's visual signaling structures have been retained in the less modified breeds of dog. The overall body shape and height can be altered from an upright pose, exaggerating the animal's size and indicating confidence and an impression of high RHP, to the low body position characteristic of a juvenile wolf approaching a parent, or a fearful dog crouching in front of an angry owner. Facial expressions can convey varying amounts of tension, by moving the lips from a horizontally retracted "appeasement" grin to a loose play face, or a threatening expression with lips vertically retracted and teeth bared (Fox, 1970).

Relative eye contact is an important signal. Whilst a full-faced challenging stare can serve to intimidate (Simpson, 1997) and, if reciprocated, lead to escalation of a conflict, an anxious dog or one wanting to appease will usually avoid direct eye contact, and thereby diffuse conflict. Dog breeds with mobile ears can move them between upright confident positions to a relaxed positioning or can pull their ears back flat against their skull defensively (Fox, 1970). The coat is also important and hair can be moved during piloerection, most noticeably to raise the hackles, thereby emphasising body size, or threatening an opponent (Fox, 1970).

The tail is an effective signaling structure, extending the dog's silhouette against its environment (Endler, 1992), often further aided by a contrast of color of the tail tip (e.g. Ortolani, 1999). Both tail height and movement can be varied. High positions have historically been described as indicating dominance, and are usually assumed by apparently confident animals, whilst tails held low or tucked between the legs signal a fearful or anxious state. Tail movements are used in a variety of contexts related to differing moods (Fox & Bekoff, 1975). Loose free tail-wagging indicates affiliative intentions, low wagging may serve to draw attention to the tucked tail or deference, whilst high wagging can indicate confidence, or if stiff, can be symptomatic of anxiety. The importance of the tail has been highlighted by studies using a robotic dog when large dogs were more likely to approach a long/wagging tail rather than a long/still tail (Leaver & Reimchen, 2008).

Finally, wolves and dogs can use specific actions or gestures that are often interpreted as indicating emotional states. Some examples include paw-lifting and lip licking – described as appeasement or displacement activities (Beerda et al., 1999; Schilder & van der Borg, 2004), or as signs of fear and anxiety (Loftus et al. 2012) – and the raised leg that is a component of urine marking, which is said to be indicative of confidence.

The different signaling structures are best suited to communication over different distances. When dogs initially come into sight of one another, overt signals, body size and height are likely the first signals visible, although tails, especially if moving, may also be important and raised hackles will soon be apparent. On the basis of these signals a "receiver" dog can decide whether to retreat, to ignore and show no change in behavior, or to approach and potentially interact with the signaling dog, and if so what manner of approach to adopt. Such choices are limited if dogs are on a leash, when the chance of interaction occurring is significantly reduced (Westgarth et al., 2010), partly as a result of physical restraint, but also because the capacity for signals to be displayed and viewed is reduced. Preliminary studies suggest that when on-leash, dogs tend to show lower tail, ear and body positions, and are more likely to be approached tentatively, than when off-leash (Rooney, unpublished data).

Researchers vary in opinion as to how important relative size is to interactions between dogs (see Bradshaw & Nott, 1995), and undoubtedly some very small dogs appear to exhibit disproportionate confidence when interacting with conspecifics many times their weight. Since size is an honest (non-deceptive) signal this highlights how much value dogs must place on other, potentially deceptive, signals. However, large dogs were significantly more likely than smaller ones to approach a medium-sized robotic dog (Leaver & Reimchen, 2008). As with encounters between real dogs (Bradshaw & Lea, 1993) some approaches were continuous, but many included tentative pauses or were aborted as the dog got closer and more subtle signaling was noticed. Fewer dogs approached when the robot's tail was short, presumably due to the recipient's inability to interpret the model's intention or mood. It is also likely that dogs behave differently dependent upon the breed (Rooney, in press), and even the color of the dog they encounter, likely a result of generalizing from past experiences.

At closer range, individual recognition and memory of past interactions, as well as olfactory and tactile information, may affect subsequent behavior, and signals from ears and facial expressions will also affect the course of the interaction. At each stage, participants modify their behavior according to the signals given by their partner, hence signals in general serve to maximise the chances of a positive amicable encounter ensuing and minimise the risk of conflict or injury.

8.4.3   Affiliative and "submissive" postures

Most previous accounts of dog behavior have described two types of "submissive" posture. In one, "passive submission," the dog rolls over on its back and exposes its inguinal region (Figure 8.1). In the other, "active submission," one dog approaches another from the side, with its tail wagging, and may attempt to lick or paw the other's muzzle (Figure 8.2); if the dog perceives the recipient as a potential threat it may approach using a crouched posture with tail held low, or even not complete its approach, stopping some distance away. These terms originated in an early ethogram, based initially on observations of captive wolves (Schenkel, 1947) and subsequently other canids, including domestic dogs (Schenkel, 1967, see Figure 8.1).

It seems likely that both postures are ritualized versions of behavior that originally evolved in the context of care-soliciting by infant canids. "Active submission" resembles the behavior used by pups to induce their mother to regurgitate food (Schenkel, 1967), and passive submission may originate in the posture they adopt when their mother grooms their perineal region in order to stimulate the elimination of urine and faeces.

As defined by Schenkel (1967), "active submission" encompasses a range of greeting displays that are morphologically linked, but appear to be modified by the performing animal's specific goal. Sometimes the performing wolf may adopt a normal carriage and appears to be entirely relaxed apart from some flattening of the ears (Figure 8.2a), but more usually the display is performed with a partially crouched posture (Figure 8.2b) and/or tension around the muzzle and eyes, suggesting an attempt at appeasement. These displays occur in several contexts in wolf

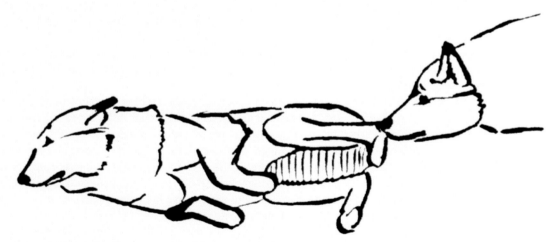

Figure 8.1 Passive submission. (From Schenkel, R. Submission: Its Features and Function in the Wolf and Dog, *Amer. Zool.* (1967) 7 (2): 319–329 © Oxford University Press, reprinted with permission.)

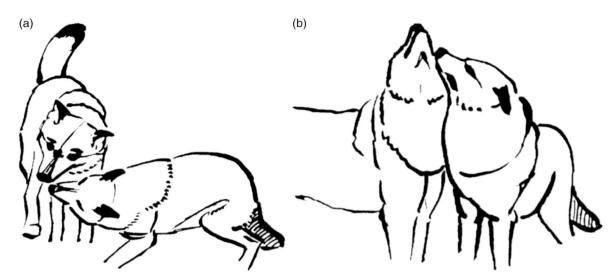

Figure 8.2 Active submission. (From Schenkel, R. Submission: Its Features and Function in the Wolf and Dog, *Amer. Zool.* (1967) 7 (2): 319–329 © Oxford University Press, reprinted with permission.)

behavior, including the "group ceremony," and except in captive wolves are rarely performed in response to actual threat. Mech (1999) states that in wolves, "active submission appears to be primarily a food-begging gesture or a food-gathering motivator." Any wolf (or dog) performing these postures is actually placing itself in a good position to attack the recipient's throat, so it is difficult to imagine how it could have evolved as a way of de-escalating an agonistic encounter, which is the conventional definition of a submissive behavior. Indeed Schenkel himself (1967, p. 325) characterized this posture as "begging for love," and it appears likely that it is primarily performed to enhance cohesion within an established group, rather than to deflect aggression. It is unclear whether this posture is effective in de-escalating conflicts between wolves (Harrington & Asa, 2003), or between dogs. Thus in both the wolf and dog it appears to be used primarily to reinforce affectionate bonds, rather than to deflect overt aggression. We therefore propose that it is more accurately termed the *affiliative display*, in order to avoid the connotation that it is routinely motivated by deference or is a standard response to physical threat. Rather, it is an attempt by the performer to enhance or restore a social bond to its target, and is often performed from a posture that is also indicative of appeasement.

By contrast, when performing "passive submission" (i.e. lying on its back; Schenkel, 1967) a dog (or wolf) appears to be inviting a potentially lethal attack, thereby conveying the strong impression that it is unwilling to escalate a conflict. In both artificial and natural wolf packs alike, this behavior has been observed as a response to agonistic behavior, for example that performed by a parent towards same-sex mature offspring, where the parent appears to be persuading the offspring to disperse (Mech & Cluff, 2010). Under these circumstances the posture does appear to inhibit the attack, and by that token is genuinely submissive. Domestic dogs, however, often adopt this posture when there is no immediate threat but rather when they appear anxious, possibly because they have learned that it induces rewarding (anxiety-relieving) attention from their owners. In dogs, therefore, it may only be submissive in limited circumstances, and hence it might be more neutrally described morphologically rather than functionally, as the "belly-up display."

8.4.4   Breed differences in signaling

Artificial selection has resulted in a wide variety of morphologies in different breeds of dog. Many breeds are anatomically modified in ways that not only compromise their physical health (Asher *et al*., 2009; Hubrecht *et al*., Chapter 14; Rooney & Sargan, 2010), but reduce their capacity to signal (Beaver, 1981, 1982; Blackshaw, 1985). For example, the stiff legs of the French bulldog prevent it from signaling by subtle adjustments of height, commonly used by dogs of many other breeds (Netto *et al*., 1992). Breeds with flat faces (brachycephalic) are less able to utilise facial expressions; dogs with very short, tightly curled or surgically docked tails, or with immobile drooping or permanently erect ears are less able to signal their intentions. Breeds with very short coats or permanently erect fur are unable to raise their hackles; and for breeds with very long or dense fur, nearly all body language communication is obscured. Short legs and long bodies can limit a dog's ability to play-bow to invite playful interactions with other dogs (Figure 8.3: Rooney, 2009). By assessing a dog's ability to use each signaling structure, researchers have compared the breeds for relative modification on signaling capacity (Kerswell *et al*., 2009a; Rooney, 2011).

Extreme anatomical breed traits affect a dog's ability to interact with other dogs and engage in normal social interactions (Goodwin *et al*., 1997; McGreevy & Nicholas, 1999; Rooney, 2011); the most modified breeds perform the fewest visual signals, all of which appear early during lupine ontogeny (Goodwin *et al*., 1997). Puppies do not appear to compensate for a reduced repertoire by more frequent use of those visual signals they can produce (Kerswell *et al*., 2009a). It has been hypothesized that ambiguity of signaling in the most modified breeds will result in less amicable interactions with other dogs, due to their inability to diffuse negative interactions and/or to elicit positive ones (Goodwin *et al*., 1997; Rooney, 2011). Recent observations made at socialization classes suggest that, once in close proximity, encounters between puppies vary according to the snout length of the dyad (for example, puppies with shorter snouts sniffed others more and elicited more pouncing), coat length (Kerswell *et al*., 2010), and the extent to which their eyes are covered by fur (puppies with less visible eyes were bitten more), but at longer range, body shape and tail length may be more important. The full picture of the relative importance of each signaling structure, in both inter- and intra-group encounters, remains to be fully determined (Rooney, 2011).

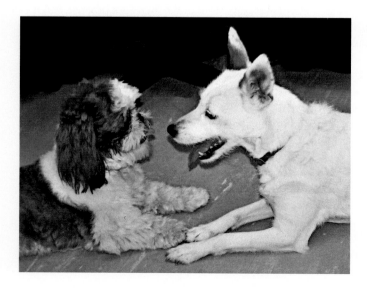

Figure 8.3 Breed differences in visual signaling capacities. (© N. J. Rooney.)

8.4.5   Dog–human visual signaling

Dog are very sensitive to human visual signals: they can follow a variety of pointing gestures (Range & Viranyi, Chapter 10), and have been shown to attend more to hand signals than to words during training (Soproni *et al.*, 2001). They can distinguish between pictures showing the heads of unfamiliar people (Racca *et al.*, 2010), between the faces of familiar people (Racca *et al.*, 2011), and can match visual images and voices (Adachi *et al.*, 2007; Gergely *et al.*, 2012). Dogs can learn to distinguish smiling from non-smiling faces, and once trained using images of their owners, can generalize to images of strangers of the same but not the opposite gender (Nagasawa *et al.*, 2011). When dogs communicate with humans, they utilize the same repertoire of signals used for intraspecific communication, but the context is distinct and hence some meanings may have changed. For example, some of the signals and actions traditionally described as intraspecific "submission," including paw-lifting, nuzzling, lip-licking, gaze aversion and low tail and ear positions, are used inter-specifically to gain attention from, or to appease, a human when a dog feels anxious (Loftus *et al.*, 2012).

Visual signals are the primary means by which humans interpret dogs' intentions and emotional states. Yet people's abilities to do so varies greatly (Tami & Gallagher, 2009) and is generally poor, even amongst those living and working with dogs (e.g. Kerswell *et al.* 2009b; Mariti *et al.*, 2012). Pet dogs rarely bite without showing subtle signals, yet 50% of owners describe their dogs as having given no "warning" before biting someone (O'Sullivan *et al.*, 2008). After watching standardized video footage, owners recall vocal signals of aggression (growling, barking) more readily than they do visual signals (Correia *et al.*, 2007). Behavioral signs are often mislabeled or misinterpreted (Tami & Gallagher, 2009), and owners show limited ability to identify stress behaviors even in their own dog (Mariti *et al.*, 2012). One study suggests that the dog's posture affects brain activity in dog experts but not in non-experts, implying that the former are more sensitive to potential signaling capacity (Kujala *et al.*, 2012). Overall it appears that dogs may be innately more skilled in interpreting visual information emanating from humans (Range & Viranyi, Chapter 10) than vice versa.

8.5   Auditory communication

8.5.1   Dog hearing and sound production

The canine hearing system has evolved primarily to optimize predation, to localize sounds produced by likely prey species of small rodents. The pinna is very mobile in many breeds, with more than 20 separate muscles providing 180° of movement, helping to scan the environment, capture, and direct sound further into the ear. Dogs can distinguish arrival times in the left and right ears of as little as 55 microseconds apart (Kalmykova, 1981), which facilitates accurate pinpointing of sound direction. Dogs' peak sensitivity is in the range 4–8 kHz; they have a similar low-frequency limit to that of humans (67 Hz compared to 31 Hz; Heffner, 1998), but considerably higher upper limits (41–47 kHz, compared to 15–20 kHz in humans; Heffner, 1983). In spite of the area of tympanic membrane varying with body size, upper hearing limits differ little between breeds (Heffner, 1983). Overall, dogs' hearing is more sensitive than that of humans, especially at high frequencies and in the human "ultrasonic" range (Miklósi, 2014; Prescott *et al.*, 2004). Dogs differentially learn to attend to different aspects of complex sounds. So, for example, when presented with two sounds that differ in both location and quality, they predominantly used the location of the sounds as a cue when learning a spatial task, yet the quality of the sound when learning a go/no-go task (Heffner, 1978).

As in most mammals, dogs generate a variety of sounds in the vocal folds of the larynx. For example, barking is staccato but variable in form, while whining is produced by the movement of the tongue within the vocal cavity alternately blocking and opening air passages. Yelping is a high-amplitude piercing variant of whining; growls are non-cyclical and vary in length dependent upon the situation (Cohen & Fox, 1976). Agonistic tooth-snapping, not vocal but mechanical, has low volume and hence is reserved for close encounters (Cohen & Fox, 1976).

Whilst sounds can be used to enhance or draw attention to visual and olfactory displays (for example, vocalizing while giving a visual play signal – see Section 8.7), they are also used for communication in their own right (Cohen & Fox, 1976). Cohen and Fox (1976) identified a total of 12 different vocal sounds in the Canidae, together with the contexts in which they occur. Of these, 10 are produced by dogs, all of which (with the possible exception of panting) occur also in wolves.

8.5.2   Effects of domestication

Dogs are more vocal than wolves, relying less on long distance howling and more on close range barking (Feddersen-Petersen, 2000). Wolves can bark but do so rarely (Schassburger, 1987). In contrast, most dogs bark frequently, in numerous contexts, and sometimes to excess (Juarbe-Diaz, 1997). There have been various theories posed regarding this difference. Barking has been suggested to be a paedomorphic trait, but a lack of difference in its developmental rate between the two species suggests this is unlikely (Pongracz et al., 2010). Dogs are generally no longer under selection pressure to be quiet predators whereas feral dogs, which may still be, rarely bark (Pongracz et al., 2010), and only in limited contexts (MacDonald & Carr, 1995). It is therefore likely that learning contributes to how much an individual dog barks. Human-directed vocalizations, including barking, increase when selection favours tameness (Belyaev, 1979), and hence a propensity to bark may be an incidental by-product of domestication (Coppinger & Feinstein, 1991). However, humans are also likely to have deliberately selected individual dogs showing "watchdog" behavior involving an increased propensity and/or reduced latency to bark.

Acoustic features of dog vocalizations vary predictably with context. Play growls differ acoustically from food guarding growls (Farago et al., 2010a). Barks are reliably context-specific (Molnár et al., 2008), ranging from harsh, low-frequency, unmodulated vocalizations, commonly directed at strangers, to more tonal, higher pitch, modulated barks commonly given in isolation and play situations (Yin & McCowan, 2004). Individual dogs can also be identified from their bark spectrograms irrespective of the context of the bark (Yin & McCowan, 2004). Such differences in structure indicate the potential for barks to convey information about both their target and the identity of the vocalizing dog.

8.5.3   Dog–dog vocal communication

Indian pariah dogs appear to prevent individuals from outside the social group approaching via vocalizations, mostly initiated by males, but both sexes take part in group vocalizations (Pal et al., 1999). Feral dogs in Italy were noted to vocalize primarily ahead of group scavenging trips and during aggressive encounters with neighboring groups (Macdonald & Carr, Chapter 16).

Unsurprisingly, dogs can be trained to respond differentially to dog and other noises (Heffner, 1975), but their discriminatory abilities extend beyond this without training. For example, they can distinguish between playbacks of conspecifics in different contexts (e.g. when left alone or when a stranger enters (Maros *et al.*, 2008), and between different individuals barking in the same context (Molnár *et al.*, 2009). They also respond differently to digitally reversed vocalizations, indicating that temporal features are important (Siniscalchi *et al.*, 2012).

Perception of growls is also context-specific; those recorded during food-guarding have been shown to deter another dog from taking a seemingly unattended bone more effectively than growls recorded in a stranger's presence (Faragó *et al.*, 2010a). Growls also convey information about the caller's body size: dogs tend to look sooner and for longer at a picture matching the size of the caller, as compared to one 30% larger or smaller (Faragó *et al.*, 2010b), although they perceive play growling dogs to be bigger then their actual size (Bálint *et al.*, 2013), and they show similar responses when the growls are re-synthesized (Taylor *et al.*, 2011). If the sender dog is larger than the receiving dog, the receiver tends to avoid further agonistic signaling, whilst dogs of the same size or larger are more likely to challenge the opponent (Taylor *et al.*, 2010a). This suggests that the perceptual and cognitive mechanisms at the basis of size assessment in dogs have a multisensory nature, and it is at least possible that dogs have some degree of mental representation of the caller from hearing it vocalize (Taylor *et al.*, 2010a).

8.5.4   Dog–human vocal communication

Dogs' vocalizations also convey information to human companions. At the most basic level, dogs use vocalizations to attract attention and solicit care from humans. This is evident from the very high levels of vocalizations in some kennel environments (Scheifele *et al.*, 2012), and during separation from owners or carers (Sherman & Mills, 2008) often resulting in nuisance barking (Steiss *et al.*, 2007). Whilst such vocalization may initially be motivated by a desire to decrease the distance between dog and human, levels may be increased further due to inadvertent reinforcement by carers or owners (similar to that which occurs with repetitive behaviors; Denham *et al.*, 2014) and by social contagion causing barking to spread to other dogs (e.g. Adams & Johnson, 1994).

Humans can also derive important contextual information from listening to dogs' vocalizations. When hearing barks, people use the fundamental frequency and formant dispersion to estimate aggressiveness (Taylor *et al.*, 2010b), while growls are primarily categorised from their temporal features. People generally interpret growls from large dogs as being more aggressive than those from smaller dogs, and struggle to identify the context in which the growl occurred (Taylor *et al.*, 2009). But when listening to barks, people are able to categorise context and motivational states, above chance levels (though far from perfectly), regardless of whether they have owned dogs (Pongrácz *et al.*, 2005), and from a very young age (Pongrácz *et al.*, 2011). However, people generally categorize low-frequency, low-tonality, rapid-pulsing barks as more aggressive, whilst high-pitched and slow-pulsing barks are thought to be happier (Pongrácz *et al.*, 2005). People follow the same rules when classifying artificially assembled bark sequences (Pongrácz *et al.*, 2006), adopting previously learnt rules which mimic those used in human communication.

8.5.5   Human–dog vocal communication

Humans communicate with dogs primarily with words. Whether the dogs comprehend that these words possess semantic meaning, or simply learn each word as an arbitrary sound cue (phoneme), has been debated (e.g. Griebel & Oller, 2012; Kaminski *et al.*, 2004; Pilley & Reid, 2011). Studies have demonstrated that two border collies (Kaminski *et al.*, 2004; Pilley & Reid 2011) and a

Yorkshire terrier (Griebel & Oller, 2012) could retain sound cues ("names") for 120, 1022 and 117 objects respectively, but it is unclear whether dogs comprehend such words as elements of a vocabulary in the same way that human infants do (Bloom, 2004; Range & Viranyi, Chapter 10).

Nonverbal acoustic signals, such as whistles, are widely used in dog training: sounds used to stimulate dogs tend to be short, rapidly repeated notes, often rising in frequency, whereas inhibiting signals tend to be prolonged, descending single notes (McConnell & Bayliss, 1985). Four short notes have been shown to be more effective at eliciting a "come" response in sheepdogs and increasing motor activity levels than one longer continuous note, and young dogs are more easily trained to return to their trainer by rising sounds as compared to long descending ones (McConnell, 1990).

The effectiveness of human communication, and hence the dog's responsiveness, is affected by non-semantic features of the vocalization (or command). For example, taped commands are less effective than those spoken by a person, and vocal commands are less likely to be obeyed when the person turns their back (Fukuzawa *et al.*, 2005). Also, working dog ability is hampered when aspects of the handler's voice are altered (Coutellier, 2006). Thus auditory communication from man to dog is, in practice, almost always modified by non-verbal elements.

8.6   Olfactory communication

8.6.1   Canine olfaction

Dogs are renowned for their acute sense of smell, and it would be surprising if they did not use this sense extensively when communicating with one another, both at close range, when individual odors can be discerned, and over substantial distances, as when oestrous females attract males. However, relatively little research attention has been directed towards chemical signaling in domestic dogs, perhaps due to our own lack of sensitivity to such odors, which results in communication from dog to owner having to rely almost entirely upon visual and auditory signals. Despite the expanding reliance on dogs' olfactory abilities, especially in the detection of contraband, it is remarkable how little is known about the details of the dog's olfactory capacity (see Walker *et al.*, 2006), especially the respective roles of the olfactory apparatus *per se* and the vomeronasal organ (Adams & Wiekamp, 1984).

8.6.2   Olfactory recognition

The great sensitivity and resolution of their olfactory systems provides dogs with the ability to distinguish between individual dogs and humans on the basis of their odor alone. Dogs are able to identify other dogs based on the odor of their urine (Brown & Johnston, 1983) and distinguish kin from non-kin even following two years' separation (Hepper, 1994). Dogs can be trained to identify individual people based on their scent (Settle *et al.*, 1994), even identical twins living together (Pinc *et al.*, 2011), and some react spontaneously to major metabolic changes (e.g. changes in blood glucose levels) in their owners (e.g. Chen *et al.*, 2000; Rooney *et al.*, 2013). The extent to which dogs in everyday life identify humans on the basis of scent as compared to facial features, body shape, posture and gait is yet to be determined.

While individual recognition does not fall within the strict definition of communication (because an odor that is specific to an individual is not considered to be a signal as such), dogs appear to

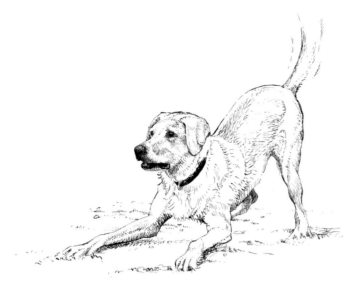

Figure 8.4 Play bow. (© Alan Peters, reprinted with permission.)

place a high priority on obtaining olfactory information from each other. Approximately 8 out of 10 encounters between adult dogs meeting off-leash in public spaces culminate in the two dogs at least attempting to sniff one another (Bradshaw & Lea, 1993, Rezác *et al.*, 2011). The areas sniffed most intensely are the sides of the face and neck (Figure 8.4), and around the inguinal area. Exocrine glands in these areas include those in the ear pinnae and at the corners of the mouth, the preputial gland in males, the vagina in females, and the anal sacs. The sequence of behavior within such interactions suggests that for many dogs, the goal is to obtain as much olfactory information about the other without allowing itself to be sniffed, explaining the protracted mutual circling that may precede such encounters (Bradshaw & Lea, 1993). Individual odors may therefore emanate from several different areas of the body and different types of gland, both apocrine and eccrine, and are therefore likely to vary depending on which part of the body is sniffed. Presumably the sniffing dog memorises some kind of combination of odors.

Such odors are likely to change over time, since many of their volatile components will be produced not by the dog itself, but by micro-organisms on the skin or within the glands themselves (Archie & Theis, 2011). For example, the anal sacs are essentially fermentation vessels, supplied by the anal glands, in which a cocktail of micro-organisms produce particularly pungent odors that presumably make up a significant proportion of each dog's characteristic smell. The odor profiles of these sacs vary considerably between individuals and remain stable over periods of at least several weeks (Natynczuk *et al.*, 1989), although it is unclear how this level of control is achieved. Nevertheless, each dog's odor must change gradually over time, so in order to maintain an accurate association between the visual and olfactory characteristics of a particular individual, dogs must need to sniff one another regularly.

8.6.3   Olfactory communication

Discrete scent signals, sometimes referred to as "pheromones," have not been extensively studied in domestic dogs. The maternal pheromone that attracts and calms puppies is produced by sebaceous glands near to the teats (Pageat & Gaultier, 2003; see Reisner, Chapter 11; Zawistowski & Reid,

Chapter 12 for applications in behavior modification), but most other signals are carried in urine. Oestrus bitches produce a scent that is universally attractive to males, so is presumably species-specific, although its active volatiles have not been identified (Schultz *et al.*, 1985). Both female and male dogs scent-mark with urine, the latter usually raising one hind leg before urinating and frequently directing the urine on to prominent objects (Sprague & Anisko, 1973). Ground-scratching may be used to produce an additional visual indicator of the urine deposit, although this behavior is more common in males and spayed females than in entire females (Wirant & McGuire, 2004). Because their activities are controlled largely by humans, urine-marking by pet dogs is difficult to interpret. Among free-roaming dogs, males may urine-mark as a component of territorial behavior, while females mark most frequently around their den sites. Over-marking by males on top of female urine marks is a component of courtship (Pal, 2003). The raised-leg display, with or without associated deposition of urine, has been interpreted as an indicator of readiness to escalate a conflict (Cafazzo *et al.*, 2012). The possible use of faeces and anal sac secretions in scent-marking does not appear to have been studied in detail in domestic dogs, although they are thought to function in territorial demarcation in the grey wolf (e.g. Zub *et al.*, 2003).

Dogs' great interest in sniffing urine-marks presumably stems from a motivation to gain information about other dogs within their home range. In addition to information about the sex and reproductive status of the producer of the urine-mark (Lisberg & Snowdon 2009), dogs are also likely to be comparing the odor of scent-marks with the odor of dogs that they have sniffed during encounters – a form of scent-matching (Gosling, 1982) – thereby assessing the home ranges of those dogs.

8.7   Play signals

Play is an important aspect of the social behavior of dogs. Playing is not only intrinsically pleasurable and self-rewarding (Burghardt, 2005), it also has multiple potential benefits, both delayed and immediate, including inducing positive welfare (Held & Spinka, 2011), reducing social tension (Arelis, 2006), and its presence can be indicative of positive wellbeing (Boissy *et al.*, 2007), and a successful dog–human relationship (Rooney & Bradshaw, 2003). Dogs engage in locomotor-rotational (running and circular body movements), object (manipulation of inanimate objects) and social (two or more individuals interacting with one another) play, unusually with both conspecifics and with humans, although their play with each is structurally, and likely motivationally, distinct (Rooney *et al.*, 2000). Compared to undomesticated animals, dogs show particularly high levels of play, since although play peaks in puppyhood at 8–9 weeks of age (Pal, 2010), it continues into adulthood at relatively high levels. This may be due to specific selection for playfulness or a result of neotenization. However, captive adult wolves also play (Cordoni, 2009), suggesting that this "luxury" activity has immediate benefits to canids in general.

Play is typically composed of action patterns used in other contexts such as predation, fighting and mating (Bekoff & Allen, 1998). When performed in the non-play context, these have obvious, often immediate, consequences for the actors. During play, however, function is less apparent. A bite delivered during a dog-fight, for example, may have significant fitness consequences for the actor (and recipient), whilst an inhibited bite delivered during play does not. It is therefore crucial that both players are aware whether an action is performed playfully or not. The context is maintained via play signals – unambiguous actions used primarily in the context of play (Bekoff, 1976) – performed at the beginning to solicit play, and throughout subsequent play bouts (Bekoff,

1974, 1975, 1995). In addition, they function in metacommunication – defining the context of other signals, and thereby the significance of the acts which follow (Bateson, 1955).

Play signals involve a range of sensory modalities. Two commonly documented visual signals used by dogs and some other mammals are the play face (Darwin, 1898 in Fagen, 1981; Bekoff, 1974), characterized by "the mouth being held open with unretracted lips slightly exposing unclenched teeth" (Fedigan, 1972, p. 349), and the play bow (Figure 8.4), involving the dog "crouching on its forelegs and elevating its hind-end, from which position it is able to perform a wide range of other movements" (Bekoff, 1974, p. 324). Other common canid signals include face pawing (extending a forelimb towards a playmate's face), exaggerated approaches made with a loose bouncy gait at a speed greater than walking (Bekoff, 1975); staring followed by head turns (Biben, 1982; Fox et al., 1976), and leaping. The ability to exhibit these signals is affected by morphology and hence some very modified breeds may find it difficult to signal their playful intentions (Rooney, 2011; see also Figure 8.3). Our own observations suggest that the likelihood of dogs reacting to a dog playfully on a walk vary depending on its relative ability to signal play intention unambiguously (Rooney, 2011). Other studies suggest that the degree of facial modification or neotenization may be the defining feature increasing playful responses in close-range interactions (Kerswell et al., 2010). Dogs are sensitive to the attentional state of their play partner: they use attention-gaining behaviors when a playmate is facing away, and play signals only when they are facing (Horowitz, 2009).

Not all play signals are visual. Dogs exhibit play-panting (Aldis, 1975), growling and barking (Feddersen-Petersen, 1986, 1991), which differ acoustically from their agonistic counterparts (Farago et al., 2010a; Yin and McCowan, 2004). It has also been suggested that self-handicapping (Bauer & Smuts, 2007; Ward et al., 2008) and simple contagion (Bekoff, 2001) may also serve to instigate play.

Dogs communicate play to humans using many of the same signals, but they also make use of learned behaviors; for example, toy presentations, physical contact, and specific vocalizations (Rooney, 1999). Play solicitation signals such as the "play bow" are among the most well recognized types of dog behavior (Tami & Gallagher, 2009), whereas play itself is often confused, and play growls, though acoustically distinct from those used in other contexts, are often misinterpreted as aggressive (Taylor et al., 2009).

Intraspecific play signaling in humans shows some similarities to that of dogs' (Aldis, 1975), specifically when using vocalizations and a "play face" (Blurton-Jones, 1967). However, there are also substantial differences, The signaling area is generally reduced to the face, and human play signals usually take the form of laughter and smiling (Blurton-Jones, 1967; Fry, 1990; van Hooff, 1972). Full motor invitations are rare (Loizos, 1966). This raises the question as to how humans communicate their play intentions to dogs. Humans commonly initiate and maintain play with dogs using a repertoire of over 30 actions (Rooney et al., 2001), although these actions vary considerably in their effectiveness. They include postures, vocalizations, and physical contact with the dog, which would be avoided during intraspecific play due to its potential riskiness. However, individualized signaling repertoires which are unique to particular dog–owner relationships may be an example of ontogenetic ritualization (the process of mutual anticipation by which particular social behaviors come to function as intentional communicative signals: Halina et al., 2013; Tomasello et al., 1994), in which there is joint adjustment in signaling through learning by both sender and receiver.

During dog–human play, the human play partner can vary the play signals delivered systematically, and the dog's behavior can be compared in signaled and unsignaled situations. (In contrast, for intraspecific play, function can only be inferred indirectly, usually from temporal contingency (Bekoff, 1974, 1975), i.e. actions that occur simultaneously or very close together in time.) We have been able to test whether putative human–dog play signals really fulfil a play-soliciting role. We examined the effect of two composite play signals, on the behavior of 20 Labrador retrievers. Both "bow" and "lunge" performed by a human caused increases in play, and the efficiency of both these postural signals was enhanced when they were accompanied by play vocalizations (Rooney *et al.*, 2001). Dogs that had observed structured dog–human interactions were quicker to approach a dog that had previously won the game, but only when the interaction was clearly playful. When no play signals were present, their speed of approach to the players was reduced (Rooney & Bradshaw, 2006). The presence of play signals is therefore likely to affect the meaning of the dog–human interactions that follow, not only for the participants, but also for any spectators.

As with other interactions, some authors have asserted that dominance hierarchies are formed during intra- as well as inter-specific play (O'Farrell, 1992; Rogerson, 1992). Indeed asymmetries in attacks and pursuits and self-handicapping do reflect asymmetries in posturing (often described as dominance relationships) in dog dyads playing in parks (Bauer & Smuts, 2007), and observations suggest that third-party dogs are more likely to join in attacking a losing as compared to a winning dog (Ward *et al.*, 2009), which may appear to support status-enhancement. However, the cause and effect of these observations should be interpreted with caution. Asymmetries, both during dog–dog and dog–human play (e.g. Rooney & Bradshaw, 2003), may reflect existing relationships, and even when dogs do not know one another, they may join in playing with winners simply because this is more rewarding than joining losers. Hence the expression of so-called competitive ability, as assessed either during well-signaled play (Pal, 2008), or in other contexts, may be better interpreted in terms of each dog's previous experiences rather than being motivated by the desire to enhance social status.

8.8   Conclusions

The relevance of wolf social biology to furthering our comprehension of the behavior of domestic dogs has recently been cast into doubt, partly because wolves and dogs are now known to be significantly different in their cognitive abilities, and partly because studies of free-roaming dogs have revealed a preferred social structure that is pack-based but otherwise quite unlike that of the wolf. The apparent certainties of the wolf-pack model, which was still universally adopted as recently as two decades ago, have not yet been replaced by any new consensus.

To explain dog behavior functionally ("what is it for?") requires an understanding of the adaptive pressures that have shaped dogs since their divergence from the wolf. It is likely that these are essentially anthropogenic, and that each dog's lifetime reproductive success is influenced more by interactions with people than by interactions with other dogs. If so, it follows that any social structure adopted by free-roaming dogs may not be fully adapted to feral life.

The suggestion made by Boitani & Ciucci (1995) that free-roaming dog behavior is an epiphenomenon of artificial selection may help to explain why adaptive models, such as Resource Holding Potential, fit dog behavior much less well than they do that of wild living animals. In particular, most dogs show less regard for the size of their opponent, or its apparent strength, than other animals usually do. Human interventions in fights between dogs, and favouritism for the (literal) underdog, may have partially released dogs from the evolutionary pressure to de-escalate a fight that cannot, or does not need to be, won, which is a key assumption of the RHP model. Instead, early domestic dog evolution would have been shaped primarily by the need to develop behavioral strategies that were effective at gaining human attention and approval.

In the absence of an unambiguous functional framework, many canine scientists, especially those involved in the treatment of behavioral disorders, have turned to proximate explanations for both normal and abnormal canine behavior. Using this approach, dogs are conceived as little different to any other mammal, their minute-to-minute behavior being driven by changes in emotional state (underpinned by changes in hormones and neurochemistry) and individual reactions to external stimuli, which are moderated by past experiences (Casey *et al.*, 2013).

The term "dominance aggression," derived from the captive wolf-pack model, is still widely used and supported (e.g. Pérez-Guisado & Muñoz-Serrano, 2009; Weiss, 2009), although generally not by behavior specialists (e.g. McGreevy *et al.*, 2012; Sherman *et al.*, 2009; Reisner, Chapter 11; Zawistowski & Reid, Chapter 12). In its place, approaches based on the cumulative experience of each animal are becoming widely adopted. These emphasize the roles of experiential and emotional (rather than motivational) factors as internal contributors to aggression (Serpell *et al.*, Chapter 6). There is a growing consensus that the concept of dog–human relationships being based on continually enforcing dominance status, for example during training, is not only ill-founded, but also potentially detrimental to both owner safety and dog welfare (Herron *et al.*, 2009; Reisner, Chapter 11).

Effective communication between dog and owner is clearly crucial to the establishment of a successful relationship, but this has received relatively little research attention. Miscommunication between dog and owner is often based upon sensory differences between the two species. Humans and dogs alike produce and respond to visual and auditory signals, but when communicating with dogs, humans emphasize verbal signals, while dogs attend mainly to human gaze, and hand signals. Dogs also use olfaction extensively, both for signaling and when assimilating information from other dogs and people. Intentional olfactory communication between dog and human is virtually impossible, due to the extreme mismatch in their olfactory sensory abilities. Our inability to even imagine much of the olfactory world that dogs inhabit also manifests itself in a powerful anthropocentric bias in our research into communication. For example, the current interest in canine cognition has focused almost entirely on visual communication, the primary means whereby we communicate with dogs. Likewise, far more research attention has been paid to dog–dog visual signals than to their olfactory communication and information-gathering, despite the obvious fact that the dogs themselves often prioritise sniffing over looking, and are now known to learn more efficiently during olfactory than visual discrimination tasks.

Even when there is no sensory barrier, when humans interpret dog signaling they are most attentive to and better able to recognise auditory cues, frequently missing or misinterpreting postural signs of fear, and hence potential signs of impending anxiety and consequent aggression. People can, however, be taught how to better recognise and interpret dog behavior (e.g. Mariti *et al.*, 2012, Loftus *et al.*, 2012), and hence be trained to communicate more effectively with their dogs. Such training has the potential both to ameliorate the risk of behavior problems emerging, and also to improve the welfare of our canine companions.

Acknowledgements

We would like to thank Emily Blackwell, Rachel Casey and Kendal Shepherd for valuable discussions, and Corinna Clark for critical review of the manuscript. We acknowledge the support of the Biotechnology and Biological Sciences Research Council, the Waltham Centre for Pet Nutrition and the RSPCA for our research described here.

References

Adachi, I., Kuwahata, H. & Fujita, K. (2007). Dogs recall their owner's face upon hearing the owner's voice. *Animal Cognition* 10: 17–21.

Adams, D. R. & Wiekamp, M. D. (1984). The canine vomeronasal organ. *Journal of Anatomy*, 138: 771–87.

Adams, G. J. & Johnson, K. G. (1994). Sleep, work and the effects of shift work in drug detector dogs, *Canis familiaris*. *Applied Animal Behaviour Science*, 41: 115–26.

Aldis, O. (1975). *Play Fighting*. New York: Academic Press.

American Veterinary Society of Animal Behavior (AVSAB) (2008). Position statement on the use of dominance theory in behavior modification of animals. [Online]. Available: http://avsabonline.org/uploads/position_statements/dominance_statement.pdf

Appleby, M. C. (1993). How animals perceive a hierarchy – reactions to Freeman *et al*. *Animal Behavior*, 46: 1232–33.

Archie, E. A. & Theis, K. R. (2011). Animal behavior meets microbial ecology. *Animal Behaviour*, 82: 425–36.

Arelis, C. L. (2006). *Stress and the power of play*. MSc Thesis. Alberta, Canada: University of Lethbridge. [Online]. Available: https://www.uleth.ca/dspace/handle/10133/342

Asher, L., Diesel, G., Summers, J. F., McGreevy, P. D. & Collins, L. M. (2009). Inherited defects in pedigree dogs. Part 1: Disorders related to breed standards. *Veterinary Journal*, 182: 402–11.

Bálint A, Faragó T., Dókaa, A., Miklósi, A. & Pongrácz, P. (2013). Beware, I am big and non-dangerous!" – Playfully growling dogs are perceived larger than their actual size by their canine audience *Applied Animal Behaviour Science*, 148, 128–37.

Barnard, C. J. (2004). *Animal Behaviour: Mechanism, Development, Function and Evolution*. Harlow, UK: Prentice Hall.

Bateson, G. (1955). A theory of play and fantasy. *Psychiatric Research Reports*, 2, 39–51.

Bauer, E. B. & Smuts, B. B. (2007). Cooperation and competition during dyadic play in domestic dogs, *Canis familiaris*. *Animal Behaviour*, 73, 489–99.

Beaver, B. (1981). Friendly communication by the dog. *Veterinary Medicine & Small Animal Clinician*, 76: 647–9.

Beaver, B. V. (1982). Distance-increasing postures of dogs. *Veterinary Medicine & Small Animal Clinician*, 77: 1023–4.

Beck, A. M. (1975). The ecology of "feral" and free-roving dogs in Baltimore. In *The Wild Canids*, ed. M. W. Fox. New York: Van Nostrand Reinhold, pp. 380–90.

Beerda, B., Schilder, M. B. H., van Hooff, J. A. R. A. M., de Vries, H. W. & Mol, J. A. (1999). Chronic stress in dog subjected to social and spatial restriction. I: Behavioral responses. *Physiology & Behavior*, 66: 233–42.

Bekoff, M. (1974). Social play and play-soliciting by infant canids. *American Zoologist*, 14: 323–40.

Bekoff, M. (1975). The communication of play intention: are play signals functional? *Semiotica* 15: 231–40.

Bekoff, M. (1976). Animal play; problems and perspectives. In *Perspectives in Ethology, vol. 2*, eds. P. P. G. Bateson & P. H. Klopfer. New York: Plenum Press, pp. 165–88.

Bekoff, M. (1995). Play signals as punctuation: the structure of social play in canids. *Behavior*, 132: 419–29.

Bekoff, M. (2001). The evolution of animal play, emotions, and social morality: on science, theology, spirituality, personhood, and love. *Zygon*, 36: 615–55.

Bekoff, M. & Allen, C. (1998). Intentional communication and social play: how and why animals negotiate and agree to play. In *Animal Play: Evolutionary, Comparative and Ecological Perspectives*, eds. M. Bekoff & J. A. Byers. Cambridge: Cambridge University Press, pp. 97–114.

Belyaev, D. K. (1979). Destabilising selection as a factor in domestication. *Journal of Heredity*, 70: 301–8.

Biben, M. (1982). Object play and social treatment of prey in bush dogs and crab-eating foxes. *Behaviour*, 79: 201–11.

Blackshaw, J. K. (1985). Human and animal inter-relationships, Review Series 3. Normal behavior patterns of dogs. *Australian Veterinary Practitioner*, 15: 110–12.

Blackwell, E.-J., Bodnariu, A., Tyson, J., Bradshaw, J. W. S. & Casey, R. A. (2010). Rapid shaping of behavior associated with high urinary cortisol in domestic dogs. *Applied Animal Behaviour Science*, 124: 113–20.

Bloom, P. (2004). Can a dog learn a word? *Science*, 304: 1605–6.

Blurton Jones, N. G. (1967). An ethological study of some aspects of social behavior in children in nursery school. In *Primate Ethology*, ed. D. Morris. London: Morrison and Gibb, pp. 347–68.

Boissy, A., Manteuffel, G., Jensen, M. B. *et al*. (2007). Assessment of positive emotions in animals to improve their welfare. *Physiology & Behavior*, 92: 375–97.

Boitani, L. & Ciucci, P. (1995). Comparative social ecology of feral dogs and wolves. *Ethology Ecology & Evolution* 7: 49–72.

Bonanni, R., Cafazzo, S., Valsecchi, P. & Natoli, E. (2010). Effect of affiliative and agonistic relationships on leadership behavior in free-ranging dogs. *Animal Behaviour*, 79: 981–91.

Bradshaw, J. W. S. & Lea, A. M. (1993). Dyadic interactions between domestic dogs during exercise. *Anthrozoös*, 5: 245–53.

Bradshaw, J. W. S. & Nott, H. M. R. (1995). Social and communication behaviour of companion dogs. In *The Domestic Dog: its Evolution, Behaviour and Interactions with People*, ed. J. A. Serpell. Cambridge: Cambridge University Press, pp. 115–30.

Bradshaw, J. W. S., Blackwell, E. J. & Casey, R. A. (2009). Dominance in domestic dogs – useful construct or bad habit? *Journal of Veterinary Behavior*, 4: 135–44.

Bradshaw, J. W. S., Pullen, A. J. & Rooney N. J. (2015). Why do adult dogs "play"? *Behavioural Processes*, 110: 82–7.

Bradshaw, J. W. S., Blackwell, E. J. & Casey, R. A. (2016). Dominance in domestic dogs – a response to Schilder et al. (2014). *Journal of Veterinary Behavior*, 11: 102–8.

Brown, D. S. & Johnston, R. E. (1983). Individual discrimination on the basis of urine in dogs and wolves. In *Chemical Signals in Vertebrates 3*, eds. D. Müller-Schwarze & R. M. Silverstein. New York: Plenum, pp. 343–436.

Burghardt, G. M. (2005). *The Genesis of Animal Play: Testing the Limits*. Cambridge, MA: MIT Press.

Cafazzo, S., Natoli, E. & Valsecchi, P. (2012). Scent-marking behavior in a pack of free-ranging domestic dogs. *Ethology*, 118: 955–66.

Cafazzo, S., Valsecchi, P., Bonanni, R. & Natoli, E. (2010). Dominance in relation to age, sex, and competitive contexts in a group of free-ranging domestic dogs. *Behavioural Ecology*, 21: 443–55.

Cafazzo, S., Valsecchi, P., Bonanni, R. & Natoli, E. (2014). Social variables affecting mate preferences, copulation and reproductive outcome in a pack of free-ranging dogs. *PLoS ONE* 9(6): e98594. http://doi:10.1371/journal.pone.0098594

Casey, R. A., Loftus, B. A., Bolster, C., Richards, G. J. & Blackwell, E.-J. (2013). Inter-dog aggression in a UK owner survey: prevalence, co-occurrence in different contexts and risk factors. *Veterinary Record*, 172: 127.

Chen, M., Daly, M., Natt, S., Candy, Williams, G. (2000). Non-invasive detection of hypoglycaemia using a novel, fully biocompatible and patient friendly alarm system. *British Medical Journal*, 321: 1565–6.

Cohen, J. A. & Fox, M. W. (1976). Vocalization in wild canids and possible effects of domestication. *Behavioural Processes*, 1: 77–92.

Coppinger, R. & Feinstein, M. (1991). Hark-hark, the dogs do bark and bark. *Smithsonian*, 21: 119–29.

Corbett, L. K. (1988). Social dynamics of a captive dingo pack: population regulation by dominant female infanticide. *Ethology*: 78, 177–98.

Cordoni, G. (2009). Social play in captive wolves (*Canis lupus*): not only an immature affair. *Behaviour*, 146: 1363–85.

Correia, C., Ruiz De La Torre, J. L., Manteca, X. & Fatjo, J. (2007). Accuracy of dog owners to describe and interpret the canine body language during aggressive episodes. In *Proceedings of the Sixth International Veterinary Behaviour Meeting*, eds. G. Landsberg, S. Matteillio & D. S. Mills. Riccione, Italy: Tipografia Camuna, p. 33.

Coutellier, L. (2006). Are dogs able to recognize their handler's voice? A preliminary study. *Anthrozoos*, 19: 278–84.

Daniels, T. J. & Bekoff, M. (1989). Population and social biology of free-ranging dogs, *Canis familiaris. Journal of Mammalogy*, 70: 754–62.

Denham, H. D. C., Bradshaw, J. W. S. & Rooney, N.J. (2014). Repetitive behaviour in kennelled domestic dog: stereotypical or not? *Physiology & Behavior*. http://dx.doi.org/10.1016/j.physbeh.2014.01.007

Elgier, A. M., Jakovcevic, A., Mustaca, A. E. & Bentosela, M. (2012). Pointing following in dogs: are simple or complex cognitive mechanisms involved? *Animal Cognition*, 15: 1111–19.

Endler, J. A. (1992). Signal, signal conditions, and the direction of evolution. *American Naturalist*, 139: S125–53.

Fagen, R. M. (1981). *Animal Play Behavior*. New York: Oxford University Press.

Faragó, T., Pongrácz, P., Range, F., Viranyi, Z. & Miklósi, Á. (2010a). "The bone is mine": affective and referential aspects of dog growls. *Animal Behaviour*, 79: 917–25.

Faragó, T., Pongrácz, P., Miklósi, Á., Huber, L., Virányi, Z. & Range, F. (2010b). Dogs' expectation about signalers' body size by virtue of their growls. *PLoS ONE*, 5: e15175. http://doi:10.1371/journal.pone.0015175

Feddersen-Petersen, D. (1986). Observations on social play in some species of Canidae. *Zoologischer Anzeiger*, 217: 130–44.

Feddersen-Petersen, D. (1991). The ontogeny of social play and agonistic behavior in selected canid species. *Bonner Zoologische Beiträge*, 42: 97–114.

Feddersen-Petersen, D. U. (2000). Vocalization of European wolves (*Canis lupus lupus* L.) and various dog breeds (*Canis lupus familiaris*). *Archiv für Tierzucht*, 43: 387–97.

Fedigan, L. (1972). Social and solitary play in a colony of vervet monkeys (*Cercopithecus aethiops*). *Primates*, 13: 347–64.

Fox, M. (1970). A comparative study of the development of facial expressions in canids; wolf, coyote and foxes. *Behavior*, 36: 49–73.

Fox, M. W. (1973). *Behavior of Wolves, Dogs and Related Canids*. London: Jonathan Cape.

Fox, M. W. & Bekoff, M. (1975). The behavior of dogs. In *The Behavior of Domestic Animals*, 3rd edition, ed. E. S. E. Hafez. London: Baillière Tindall, pp. 370–409.

Fox, M. W., Halperin, S., Wise, A. & Kohn, E. (1976). Species and hybrid differences in frequencies of play and agonistic actions in canids. *Zeitschrift fier Tierpsychologie*, 40: 194–209.

Fry, D. P. (1990). Play aggression among Zapotec children: implications for the practice hypothesis. *Aggressive Behavior*, 16: 321–40.

Fukuzawa, M., Mills, D. S. & Cooper, J. J. (2005). More than just a word: non-semantic command variables affect obedience in the domestic dog (*Canis familiaris*). *Applied Animal Behaviour Science*, 91: 129–41.

Funato, T., Nara, M., Kurabayashi, D., Ashikaga, M. & Aonuma, H. (2011). A model for group-size-dependent behavior decisions in insects using an oscillator network. *Journal of Experimental Biology*, 214: 2426–34.

Gazit, I. & Terkel, J. (2003). Domination of olfaction over vision in explosives detection by dogs. *Applied Animal Behaviour Science*, 82: 65–73.

Gergely, A., Hernádi, A., Petró, E., Miklósi, B., Kanizsár, O., Miklósi, A. & Topál, J. (2012). Matching pictures with the appropriate sound: results from an eye-tracking study of dogs and 14-month-old infants. In *Proceedings of 3rd Canine Science Forum*, 25–27 July 2012. Barcelona, Spain, p. 82.

Goodwin, D., Bradshaw, J. W. S. & Wickens, S. M. (1997). Paedomorphosis affects agonistic visual signals of domestic dogs. *Animal Behaviour*, 53: 297–304.

Gosling, L. M. (1982). A reassessment of the function of scent marking in territories. *Zeitschrift für Tierpsychologie*, 2: 89–118.

Griebel, U. & Oller, D. K. (2012). Vocabulary learning in a Yorkshire terrier: slow mapping of spoken words. *PLoS ONE*, 7: e30182.

Halina, M., Rossano, F. & Tomasello, M. (2013). The ontogenic ritualization of bonobo gestures. *Animal Cognition*, 16: 653–66.

Harrington, F. H. & Asa, C. S. (2003). Wolf communication. In *Wolves: Behavior, Ecology, and Conservation*, eds. L. D. Mech & L. Boitani. Chicago, IL: University of Chicago Press, pp. 66–103.

Heffner, H. E. (1975). Perception of biologically meaningful sounds by dogs. *Journal of the Acoustic Society of America*, 58: S124.

Heffner, H. (1978). Effect of auditory cortex ablation on localization and discrimination of brief sounds. *Journal of Neurophysiology*, 41: 963–76.

Heffner, H. E. (1983). Hearing in large and small dogs: absolute thresholds and size of the tympanic membrane. *Behavioral Neuroscience*, 97: 310–18.

Heffner, H. E. (1998). Auditory awareness in animals. *Applied Animal Behaviour Science*, 57: 259–68.

Held, S. & Spinka, M. (2011). Animal play and animal welfare. *Animal Behaviour*, 81: 891–9.

Hepper, P. G. (1994). Long-term retention of kinship recognition established during infancy in the domestic dog. *Behavioural Processes*, 33: 3–14.

Herron, M. E., Shofer, F. S. & Reisner, I. R. (2009). Survey of the use and outcome of confrontational and non-confrontational training methods in client-owned dogs showing undesired behaviors. *Applied Animal Behaviour Science*, 117: 47–54.

Holekamp, K. E. & Engh, A. L. (2002). Field studies of social cognition in spotted hyenas. In *The Cognitive Animal: Empirical and Theoretical Perspectives on Animal Cognition*, eds. M. Bekoff, C. Allen & G. M. Burghardt. Cambridge, MA: MIT Press, pp. 371–8.

Horowitz, A. (2009). Attention to attention in domestic dog (*Canis familiaris*) dyadic play. *Animal Cognition*, 12: 107–18.

Horowitz, A. (2011). Theory of mind in dogs? Examining method and concept. *Learning & Behavior*, 39: 314–17.

Juarbe-Diaz, S. V. (1997). Social dynamics and behavior problems in multiple-dog households. *The Veterinary Clinics of North America Small Animal Practice*, 27: 497–514.

Kalmykova, I. V. (1981). Localization of dichotically presented sounds in dogs. *Neuroscience and Behavioral Physiology*, 11: 268–72.

Kaminski, J., Call, J. & Fischer, J. (2004). Word learning in a domestic dog: evidence for "fast mapping". *Science*, 304: 1682–3.

Kaminski, J., Schulz, L. & Tomasello, M. (2012). How dogs know when communication is intended for them. *Developmental Science*, 15: 222–32.

Kerswell, K. J., Bennett, P., Butler, K. L. & Hemsworth, P. H. (2009a). The relationship of adult morphology and early social signaling of the domestic dog (*Canis familiaris*). *Behavioural Processes*, 81: 376–82.

Kerswell, K. J., Bennett, P., Butler, K. L. & Hemsworth, P. H. (2009b). Self-reported comprehension ratings of dog behavior by puppy owners. *Anthrozoös*, 22: 183–93.

Kerswell, K. J., Butler, K. L., Bennett, P. & Hemsworth, P. (2010). The relationships between morphological features and social signaling behaviors in juvenile dogs: The effect of early experience with dogs of different morphotypes. *Behavioural Processes*, 85: 1–7.

Kowalska, D. M., Kusmierek, P., Kosmal, A. & Mishkin, M. (2001). Neither perirhinal/entorhinal nor hippocampal lesions impair short-term auditory recognition memory in dogs. *Neuroscience*, 104: 965–78.

Krebs, J. R. & Dawkins, R. (1984). Animal signals: mind-reading and manipulation. In *Behavioral Ecology: An Evolutionary Approach*, 2nd edition, eds. J. R. Krebs & N. B. Davies. Sunderland, MA: Sinauer, pp. 380–402.

Kretchmer, K. R. & Fox, M. W. (1975). Effects of domestication on animal behavior. *Veterinary Record*, 96: 102–8.

Kujala, M. V., Kujala, J., Carlson, S. & Hari, R. (2012). Dog experts' brains distinguish socially relevant body postures similarly in dogs and humans. *PLoS ONE*, 7: e39145. http://doi:10.1371/journal.pone.0039145

Kundey, S. M. A., De Los Reyes, A., Royer, E. et al. (2010). Reputation-like inference in domestic dogs (*Canis familiaris*). *Animal Cognition*, 14: 291–302.

Landsberg, G., Hunthausen, W. & Ackerman, L. (2003). *Handbook of Behavior Problems in the Dog and Cat*. Philadelphia, PA: W. B. Saunders, pp. 385–426.

Leaver, S. D. A. & Reimchen, T. E. (2008). Behavioral responses of *Canis familiaris* to different tail lengths of a remotely-controlled life-sized dog replica. *Behaviour*, 145: 377–90.

Lindsay, S. R. (2005). *Handbook of Applied Dog Behavior and Training, Volume 3, Procedures and Protocols*. Ames, IA: Iowa State University Press, pp. 532–4.

Lisberg, A. E. & Snowdon, C. T. (2009). The effects of sex, gonadectomy and status on investigation patterns of unfamiliar conspecific urine in domestic dogs. *Canis familiaris. Animal Behaviour*, 77: 1147–54.

Loftus, B., Rooney, N. J. & Casey R. A. (2012). Recognising fear and anxiety in dogs. [Online]. Available: www.bris.ac.uk/vetscience/services/behaviour-clinic/dogbehaviouralsigns

Loizos, C. (1966). Play in mammals. In *Play, Exploration and Territory in Mammals*, ed. P. A. Jewell. London: Academic Press, pp. 1–9.

Macdonald, D. W. & Carr, G. (1995). Variation in dog society: between resource dispersion and social flux. In *The Domestic Dog: Its Evolution, Behaviour and Interactions with People*, ed. J. Serpell. Cambridge: Cambridge University Press, pp. 199–216.

Mariti, C., Gazzano, A., Moore, J. L., Baragli, P., Chelli, L. & Sighieri, C. (2012). Perception of dogs' stress by their owners. *Journal of Veterinary Behavior*, 7: 213–9.

Maros, K., Pongrácz, P., Bárdos, Gy., Molnár, Cs., Faragó, T. & Miklósi, Á. (2008). Dogs can discriminate barks from different situations. *Applied Animal Behaviour Science*, 114: 159–67.

Marshall-Pescini, S., Passalacqua, C., Ferrario, A., Valsecchi, P. & Prato-Previde, E. (2011). Social eavesdropping in the domestic dog. *Animal Behaviour*, 81: 1177–83.

McConnell, P. B. (1990). Acoustic structure and receiver response in domestic dogs, *Canis familiaris. Animal Behaviour*, 39: 897–904.

McConnell, P. B. & Baylis, J. R. (1985). Interspecific communication in cooperative herding: Acoustic and visual signals from shepherds and herding dogs. *Zeitschrift für Tierpsychologie*, 67: 302–28.

McGreevy, P. D. & Nicholas, F. W. (1999). Some practical solutions to welfare problems in dog breeding. *Animal Welfare*, 8: 329–41.

McGreevy, P. D., Starling, M., Branson, N. J., Cobb, M. L. & Calnon, D. (2012). An overview of the dog–human dyad and ethograms within it. *Journal of Veterinary Behavior*, 7: 103–17.

Mech, L. D. (1999). Alpha status, dominance, and division of labor in wolf packs. *Canadian Journal of Zoology*, 77: 1196–203.

Mech, L. D. (2008). Whatever happened to the term alpha wolf? *International Wolf*, 18: 4–8.

Mech, L. D. & Boitani, L. (2003). Wolf social ecology. In *Wolves: Behavior, Ecology, and Conservation*, eds. L. D. Mech & L. Boitani. Chicago, IL: University of Chicago Press, pp. 1–34.

Mech, L. D. & Cluff, H. D. (2010). Prolonged intensive dominance behavior between Gray Wolves, *Canis lupus. Canadian Field-Naturalist*, 124: 215–8.

Mendl, M., Brooks, J., Basse, C., Burman, O., Paul, E., Blackwell, E. & Casey, R. (2010). Dogs showing separation-related behavior exhibit a "pessimistic" cognitive bias. *Current Biology*, 20: R939–40.

Miklósi, Á. (2014). *Dog Behaviour, Evolution and Cognition*, 2nd edition. Oxford: Oxford University Press.

Miller, P. E. & Murphy, C. J. (1995). Vision in dogs. *Journal of the American Veterinary Medical Association*, 207: 1623–34.

Moehlman, P. D. (1989). Intraspecific variation in canid social systems. In *Carnivore Behavior, Ecology and Evolution*, Vol. 1, ed. J. L. Gittleman. Ithaca, NY: Cornell University Press, pp. 143–63.

Molnár, C. S., Kaplan, F., Roy, P., Pachet, F., Pongrácz, P., Dóka, A. & Miklósi, Á. (2008). Classification of dog barks: a machine learning approach. *Animal Cognition*, 11: 389–400.

Molnár, C. S., Kaplan, F., Faragó, T., Dóka, A. & Miklósi, Á. (2009). Dogs discriminate between barks: the effect of context and identity of the caller. *Behavioural Processes*, 82: 198–201.

Monks of New Skete (1978). *How To Be Your Dog's Best Friend: A Training Manual For Dog Owners*. Boston, MA: Little, Brown & Co., pp. 11–12.

Murphy, C. J. & Pollock, R. V. S. (1993). The eye. In *Miller's Anatomy of the Dog*, 3rd edition, ed. H. Evans. Philadelphia, PA: Saunders, pp. 1009–58.

Nagasawa, M., Murai, K., Mogi, K. & Kikusui, T. (2011). Dogs can discriminate human smiling faces from blank expressions. *Animal Cognition*, 14: 525–33.

Natynczuk, S., Bradshaw, J. W. S. & Macdonald, D. W. (1989). Chemical constituents of the anal sacs of domestic dogs. *Biochemical Systematics & Ecology*, 17: 83–7.

Netto, W. J., van der Borg, J. A. M. & Slegers, J. F. (1992). The establishment of dominance relationships in a dog pack and his relevance for the man-dog relationship. *Tijdschrift voor Diergeneeskunde*, 117(Suppl.): 51S–52S.

O'Farrell, V. (1992). *Manual of Canine Behaviour*, 2nd edition. Cheltenham, UK: British Small Animal Veterinary Association.

O'Sullivan, E. N., Jones, B. R., O'Sullivan, K. & Hanlon, A. J. (2008). The management and behavioral history of 100 dogs reported for biting a person. *Applied Animal Behavior Science*, 114: 149–58.

Ortolani, A. (1999). Spots, stripes, tail tips and dark eyes: predicting the function of carnivore color patterns using the comparative method. *Biological Journal of the Linnean Society*, 67: 433–76.

Pageat, P. & Gaultier, E. (2003). Current research in canine and feline pheromones. *Small Animal Practice*, 33: 187–211.

Pal, S. K. (2003). Urine marking by free-ranging dogs (*Canis familiaris*) in relation to sex, season, place and posture. *Applied Animal Behaviour Science*, 80: 45–59.

Pal, S. K. (2005). Parental care in free-ranging dogs, *Canis familiaris. Applied Animal Behaviour Science*, 90: 31–47.

Pal, S. K. (2008). Maturation and development of social behaviour during early ontogeny in free-ranging dog puppies in West Bengal, India. *Applied Animal Behaviour Science*, 111: 95–107.

Pal, S. K. (2010). Play behavior during early ontogeny in free-ranging dogs (*Canis familiaris*). *Applied Animal Behaviour Science*, 126: 140–53.

Pal, S. K. (2011). Mating system of free-ranging dogs (*Canis familiaris*). *International Journal of Zoology*. http://doi:10.1155/2011/314216

Pal, S. K., Ghosh, B. & Roy, S. (1998). Agonistic behavior of free-ranging dogs (*Canis familiaris*) in relation to season, sex and age. *Applied Animal Behaviour Science*, 59: 331–48.

Pal, S. K., Ghosh, B. & Roy, S. (1999). Inter- and intra-sexual behavior of free-ranging dogs (*Canis familiaris*). *Applied Animal Behaviour Science*, 62: 267–78.

Parker, G. A. (1974). Assessment strategy and the evolution of fighting behavior. *Journal of Theoretical Biology*, 47: 223–43.

Pérez-Guisado, J. & Muñoz-Serrano, A. (2009). Factors linked to dominance aggression in dogs. *Journal of Animal and Veterinary Advances*, 8: 336–42.

Pilley J. W. & Reid, A. K. (2011). Border collie comprehends object names as verbal referents. *Behavioural Processes*, 86: 184–95.

Pinc, L., Bartoš, L., Reslová, A. & Kotrba, R. (2011). Dogs discriminate identical twins. *PLoS ONE*, 6: e20704.

Pongrácz, P., Molnár, C. S., Miklósi, Á. & Csányi, V. (2005). Human listeners are able to classify dog (*Canis familiaris*) barks recorded in different situations. *Journal of Comparative Psychology*, 119: 136–44.

Pongrácz, P., Molnár, C. S. & Miklósi, Á. (2006). Acoustic parameters of dog barks carry emotional information for humans. *Applied Animal Behaviour Science*, 100: 228–40.

Pongrácz, P., Molnár, C. S. & Miklósi, Á. (2010). Barking in family dogs: An ethological approach. *Veterinary Journal*, 183: 141–7.

Pongrácz, P., Molnár, C., Doka, A. & Miklósi, Á. (2011). Do children understand man's best friend? Classification of dog barks by pre-adolescents and adults. *Applied Animal Behaviour Science*, 135: 95–102.

Prescott, M. J., Morton, D. B., Anderson, D. *et al.* (2004). Refining dog husbandry and care. 8th Report of the BVA/AWF/FRAME/RSPCA/UFAW Joint Working Group on refinement. *Laboratory Animals*, 38(Suppl 1): S1–S94.

Pretterer, G., Bubna-Littitz, H., Windischbauer, G., Gabler, C. & Griebel, U. (2004). Brightness discrimination in the dog. *Journal of Vision*, 4: 241–9.

Rabb, G. B., Woolpy, J. H. & Ginsberg, B. E. (1967). Social relationships in a group of captive wolves. *American Zoologist*, 7: 305–11.

Racca, A., Amadei, E., Ligout, S., Guo, K., Meints, K. & Mills, D. (2010). Discrimination of human and dog faces and inversion responses in domestic dogs (*Canis familiaris*). *Animal Cognition*, 13: 525–33.

Racca, A., Range, F., Virányi, Z. & Huber, L. (2011). Discrimination of familiar human faces in domestic dogs. *Journal of Veterinary Behaviour*, 8: e46.

Řezáč, P., Viziová, P., Dobešová, M., Havliček, Z. & Pospíšilová, D. (2011). Factors affecting dog–dog interactions on walks with their owners. *Applied Animal Behaviour Science*, 134: 170–6.

Rogerson, J. (1992). *Training Your Dog*. London: Popular Dogs Publishing.

Rooney, N. J. (1999). Play behavior of the domestic dog (*Canis familiaris*) and its effects on the dog–human relationship. Unpublished Ph.D. thesis, University of Southampton.

Rooney, N. J. (2009). The welfare of pedigree dogs: Cause for concern. *Journal of Veterinary Behavior*, 4: 180–6.

Rooney, N. J. (in press). Deleterious effects on behavior associated with pedigree dog breeding in the UK. *European Journal of Companion Animal Practice*.

Rooney, N. J. & Bradshaw, J. W. S. (2002). An experimental study of the effects of play upon the dog-human relationship. *Applied Animal Behaviour Science*, 75: 161–76.

Rooney, N. J. & Bradshaw, J. W. S. (2003). Links between play and dominance and attachment dimensions of dog-human relationships. *Journal of Applied Animal Welfare Science*, 6: 67–94.

Rooney, N. J. & Bradshaw, J. W. S. (2006). Social cognition in the domestic dog: behavior of spectators toward participants in interspecific games. *Animal Behaviour*, 72: 343–52.

Rooney, N. J. & Sargan, D. R. (2010). Welfare concerns associated with pedigree dog breeding in the UK. *Animal Welfare*, 19: 133–40.

Rooney, N. J., Bradshaw, J. W. S. & Robinson, I. H. (2000). A comparison of dog–dog and dog–human play behavior. *Applied Animal Behaviour Science*, 66: 235–48.

Rooney, N. J., Bradshaw, J. W. S. & Robinson, I. H. (2001) Do dogs respond to play signals given by humans? *Animal Behaviour*, 61: 715–22.

Rooney, N. J., Morant, S. & Guest, C. (2013) Investigation into the value of trained glycaemia alert dogs to clients with Type I diabetes. *PLoS ONE*, 8: e69921.

Schassburger, R. M. (1987). Wolf vocalizations: An integrated model of structure, motivation and ontogeny. In *Man and Wolf: Advances, Issues, and Problems in Captive Wolf Research*, ed. H. Frank. Dordrecht, The Netherlands: Dr W. Junk Publishers, pp. 313–47.

Scheifele, P., Martin, D., Clark, J. G. R., Kemper, D. & Wells, J. (2012.) Effect of kennel noise on hearing in dogs. *American Journal of Veterinary Research*, 73: 482–9.

Schenkel, R. (1947). Ausdrucks-Studien an Wölfen: Gefangenschafts-Beobachtungen. *Behavior*, 1, 81–129.

Schenkel, R. (1967). Submission: its features and function in the wolf and dog. *American Zoologist*, 7: 319–29.

Schilder, M. B. H. & van der Borg, J. A. M. (2004). Training dogs with help of the shock collar: short and long term behavioral effects. *Applied Animal Behaviour Science*, 85: 319–34.

Schilder, M. B. H., Vinke, C. M. & van der Borg, J. A. M. (2014). Dominance in domestic dogs revisited: useful habit and useful construct? *Journal of Veterinary Behavior: Clinical Applications and Research*, 9: 184–191.

Schultz, T. H., Kruse, S. M. & Flath, R. A. (1985). Some volatile constituents of female dog urine. *Journal of Chemical Ecology*, 11: 169–75.

Settle, R. H., Sommerville, B. A., McCormick, J. & Broom, D. M. (1994). Human scent matching using specially trained dogs. *Animal Behavior*, 48: 1443–8.

Shepherd, K. (2002). Development of behavior, social behavior and communication in dogs. In *BSAVA Manual of Canine and Feline Behavioral Medicine*, eds. D. F. Horwitz, D. S. Mills & S. Heath. Quedgeley, UK: BSAVA, pp. 8–20.

Sherman, B. L. & Mills, D. S. (2008). Canine anxieties and phobias: an update on separation anxiety and noise aversions. *Veterinary Clinics of North America, Small Animal Practice*, 38: 1081–106.

Sherman, B. L., Meyer, E. K. & Hetts, S. (2009). More on canine dominance aggression. *Journal of the American Veterinary Medical Association*, 234: 1254–5.

Sherman, S. M. & Wilson, J. R. (1975). Behavioral and morphological evidence for binocular competition in post-natal development of dogs visual system. *Journal of Comparative Neourology*, 161: 183–95.

Simpson, B. S. (1997). Canine communication. *Veterinary Clinics of North America: Small Animal Practice*, 27: 445–464.

Siniscalchi, M., Lusito, R., Sasso, R. & Quaranta, A. (2012). Are temporal features crucial acoustic cues in dog vocal recognition? *Animal Cognition*, 15: 815–821.

Soproni, K., Miklosi, A., Topal, J. & Csanyi, V. (2001). Comprehension of human communicative signs in pet dogs (*Canis familiaris*). *Journal of Comparative Psychology*, 115: 122–6.

Sprague, R. H. & Anisko, J. J. (1973). Elimination patterns in the laboratory beagle. *Behaviour*, 47: 257–67.

Steiss, J. E., Schaffer, C., Ahmad, H. A. & Voith, V. L. (2007). Evaluation of plasma cortisol levels and behavior in dogs wearing bark control collars. *Applied Animal Behaviour Science*, 106: 96–106.

Summers, J. F., Diesel, G., Asher, L., McGreevy, P. D. & Collins, L. M. (2010). Inherited defects in pedigree dogs. Part 2: Disorders that are not related to breed standards. *Veterinary Journal*, 183: 39–45.

Tami, G. & Gallagher, A. (2009). Description of the behavior of domestic dog (*Canis familiaris*) by experienced and inexperienced people. *Applied Animal Behaviour Science*, 120: 159–69.

Taylor, A. M., Reby, D. & McComb, K. (2009). Context-related variation in the vocal growling behavior of the domestic dog (*Canis familiaris*). *Ethology*, 115: 905–15.

Taylor, A. M., Reby, D. & McComb, K. (2010a). Size communication in domestic dog, *Canis familiaris*, growls. *Animal Behaviour*, 79: 205–10.

Taylor, A. M., Reby, D. & McComb, K. (2010b). Why do large dogs sound more aggressive to human listeners: acoustic bases of motivational misattributions. *Ethology*, 116: 1155–62.

Taylor, A. M., Reby, D. & McComb, K. (2011). Cross modal perception of body size in domestic dogs (*Canis familiaris*). *PLoS ONE*, 6: e17069.

Thomson, P. C., Rose, K. & Kok, N. E. (1992). The behavioral ecology of dingoes in North-western Australia. V. Population dynamics and variation in the social system. *Wildlife Research*, 19: 565–84.

Tomasello, M., Call, J., Nagell, K., Olguin, R. & Carpenter, M. (1994). The learning and use of gestural signals by young chimpanzees: a trans-generational study. *Primates*, 35: 137–54.

Tuber, D. S., Hennessy, M. B., Sanders, S. & Miller, J. A. (1996). Behavioral and glucocorticoid responses of adult domestic dogs (*Canis familiaris*) to companionship and social separation. *Journal of Comparative Psychology*, 110: 103–8.

van der Borg, J. A. M., Schilder, M. B. H., Vinke, C. M. & de Vries, H. (2015). Dominance in domestic dogs: a quantitative analysis of its behavioural measures. *PLoS ONE*, 10: e0133978. http://doi:10.1371/journal.pone.0133978

van Hooff, J. A. R. A. M. (1972). A comparative approach to the phylogeny of laughter and smiling. In *Non-Verbal Communication*, ed. R. A. Hinde. Cambridge: Cambridge University Press, pp. 209–41.

van Hooff, J. A. R. A. M. & Wensing, J. A. B. (1987). Dominance and its behavioral measures in a captive wolf pack. In *Man and Wolf: Advances, Issues, and Problems in Captive Wolf Research*, ed. H. Frank. Dordrecht, the Netherlands: Dr W. Junk, pp. 219–52.

Vaughan, R. T., Stoy, K., Sukhatme, G. S. & Mataric, M. J. (2000). Go ahead, make my day: Robot conflict resolution by aggressive competition. In *From Animals to Animats 6*, eds. J. A. Meyer, A. Berthoz, D. Floreano, H. Roitblat & S. W. Wilson. Cambridge, MA: MIT Press, pp. 491–500.

Walker, D. B., Walker, J. K., Cavnar, P. J. *et al.* (2006). Naturalistic quantification of canine olfactory sensitivity. *Applied Animal Behaviour Science*, 97: 241–254.

Walls, G. L. (1963). *The Vertebrate Eye and its Adaptive Radiation*. New York: Hafner Publishing Co.

Ward, C., Bauer, E. B. & Smuts, B. B. (2008). Partner preferences and asymmetries in social play among domestic dog, *Canis lupus familiaris*, littermates. *Animal Behavior*, 76: 1187–99.

Ward C., Trisko, R. & Smuts, B. B. (2009). Third-party interventions in dyadic play between littermates of domestic dogs, *Canis lupus familiaris*. *Animal Behaviour*, 78: 1153–60.

Weiss, T. (2009). Thoughts on canine dominance aggression. *Journal of the American Veterinary Medical Association*, 234: 731.

Westgarth, C., Christley, R. M., Pinchbeck, G. L., Gaskell, R. M., Dawson, S. & Bradshaw, J. W. S. (2010). Dog behavior on walks and the effect of use of the leash. *Applied Animal Behaviour Science*, 125: 38–46.

Wickens, S. M. (1993). Social relationships in the domestic dog (*Canis familiaris*): the effect of learning and breed on behaviour within status relationships. Unpublished Ph.D., University of Southampton, UK.

Williams, M. & Johnston, J. M. (2002). Training and maintaining the performance of dogs (*Canis familiaris*) on an increasing number of odor discriminations in a controlled setting. *Applied Animal Behaviour Science*, 78: 55–65.

Wirant, S. C. & McGuire, B. (2004). Urinary behavior of female domestic dogs (*Canis familiaris*): influence of reproductive status, location and age. *Applied Animal Behavior Science*, 85: 335–48.

Yin, S. & McCowan, B. (2004). Barking in domestic dogs: context specificity and individual identification. *Animal Behavior*, 68: 343–55.

Zimen, E. (1975). Social dynamics of the wolf pack. In *The Wild Canids: Their Systematics, Behavioral Ecology and Evolution*, ed. M. W. Fox. New York: Van Nostrand Reinhold, pp. 336–62.

Zub, K., Theuerkauf, J., Jedrzejewski, W., Jedrzejewska, B., Schmidt, K. & Kowalczyk, R. (2003). Wolf pack territory marking in the Bialowieza primeval forest (Poland). *Behavior*, 140: 635–48.

9

Ethology, ecology and epidemiology of canine aggression

RANDALL LOCKWOOD

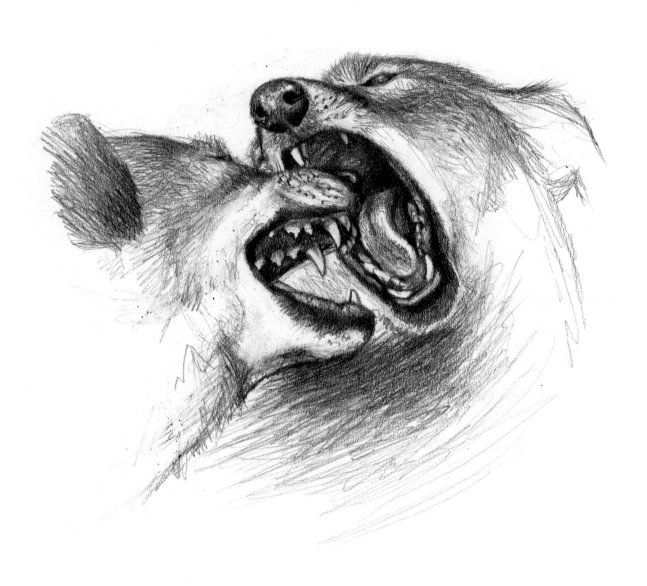

9.1   Introduction

In *Man Meets Dog* (1953), Konrad Lorenz praised the wonders of domestication that, in a few thousand years, had transformed the wolf into the docile Alsatian dog that his children could playfully and fearlessly torment. Lorenz admitted in his later years that much of what he had written about dogs was simply incorrect. His assumption that domestication had largely purged the wolf of the behavior that made it potentially dangerous to man was one of his more serious errors.

For many years the phrase "dog bites man" was a cliché for an event that is the antithesis of news, largely because it is such a common occurrence. In the last two decades, however, media around the world have given enormous attention to dog attacks and dog aggression in general. This has created the popular impression that such attacks have become more numerous or severe. Much of this attention has focused on specific breeds assumed to have a greater propensity for aggression, and the various legal and legislative attempts to protect the public from "vicious dogs." In addition, increased law enforcement attention to dogfighting and several high-profile prosecutions, including that of National Football League quarterback, Michael Vick, have led to widespread discussion of the breeding, raising, training and potential rehabilitation of dogs used in organized dogfighting (Gorant, 2010; Huss, 2008; Lockwood, 2011) and have renewed the debate over the genetic, environmental and sociological contributions to canine aggression.

The issue of aggression problems in dogs has also attracted growing attention as a welfare concern. Salman *et al.* (1998, 2000) surveyed 12 animal shelters in the US and noted that 40% of relinquishing owners cited behavioral problems as one of the reasons for surrendering a dog. When behavior was the only reported reason for relinquishment, aggression was the most frequently cited problem (40% of dogs). In addition, surveys of owner's complaints about canine behavior indicate that the most common problem reported is aggression (Beaver, 1993, 1994) and such problems produce a significant risk for euthanasia (Fatjo *et al.*, 2007; Galac & Knol, 1997; Hart & Hart, 1997; Reisner *et al*, 1994). Thus identifying animals at risk for such problems, and identifying potentially effective solutions, has been a major effort for animal behaviorists working within rescue and shelter settings.

From an epidemiological perspective, dog bites continue to be a significant problem. Several factors have led to increased recognition of the problem. First, a growing body of epidemiological reports have clearly described the extent of the dog bite problem in the US and other countries (Avis, 1999; AVMA Task Force, 2001; Beck, 1981; Beck *et al.*, 1975; Berzon, 1978; Gershman *et al.*, 1994; Guy *et al.*, 2001a, 2001b, 2001c; Holmquist & Elixhauser, 2010; Langley, 2009; Mead, 2006; Overall & Love, 2001; Patronek & Slavinski, 2009; Pinckney & Kennedy, 1982; Podberscek & Blackshaw, 1993; Reisner *et al.*, 2011; Roll & Unselm, 1997; Sacks *et al.*, 1989, 1996; Weiss *et al.*, 1998). Second, there has been widespread reporting of some of the more shocking fatal dog attacks in the media (Jones, 2003) and many serious bite cases have been brought before the civil and criminal courts. Third, insurance industry reports as to the prevalence of bite claims have raised the issue of the costs of dog bites (Insurance Information Institute, 2012). In the United States, settlements in excess of $1 million have not been uncommon. Dog bites reportedly accounted for more than one third of homeowners insurance liability claims paid in 2011, totaling $479 million.

This chapter will first review the natural history of canid aggression, and some of the factors involved in dog bite incidents. This will include attempts to identify breed-specific differences in the incidence of different forms of aggressive behavior and to clarify possible underlying genetic and physiological influences. I will also review recent efforts to associate problems of dog aggression with patterns of dog owner behavior. Finally, possible solutions to problems associated with canine aggression will be considered.

9.2   Forms of canine aggression

Aggression is one component of a range of agonistic behaviors that serve to regulate individuals' ability to compete for various resources (food, shelter, territory, mates, social status). Agonistic behaviors may include attacks, threats, displays, retreats, placating aggressors, and conciliation (Scott & Frederickson, 1951). Various authors provide a wide range of definitions of canine aggression and the forms it can take. Aggression was identified as a key component in most of the earliest efforts to describe dog behavior or personality (Goddard & Beilharz, 1983; Lorenz, 1953; Pavlov, 1941; Royce, 1955; Scott & Fuller 1965). More recently, some definitions have been based on the function or implied motive of the behavior, including predatory, maternal, protective, territorial, dominance or play aggression, or the context in which it occurs such as pain-elicited or fear-elicited aggression (Landsberg et al., 1997; Lindsay, 2000; Overall, 1997). Studies focusing on dog welfare and risk assessments have looked most closely at the specific *target* of aggressive behaviors, distinguishing between aggression to familiar and unfamiliar dogs and familiar and unfamiliar people (Borchelt, 1983; Goodloe & Borchelt, 1998; Hsu and Serpell, 2003) and examining specific responses to various standardized test situations (Dowling-Guyer et al., 2011; Jones & Gosling, 2005; Netto & Planta, 1997; Svartberg, 2005). This chapter will focus on those aspects of canine aggression most relevant to animal welfare and human safety, including dog-to-human (stranger or familiar) and dog-to-dog aggression.

9.3   Domestication and canine aggression

The domestication of the dog from the wolf is well-accepted, although debate continues regarding the specific subspecies involved and the sites and/or timing of the process, since multiple origins are possible (Druzhkova et al. 2013; Vila et al., 1997; vonHoldt et al., 2010; see also Clutton-Brock, Chapter 2; vonHoldt & Driscoll, Chapter 3)

Canids in general and wolves in particular show a high degree of diversity on a variety of behavioral measures (aggression, boldness/timidity, playfulness, sociability) as well as physical measures (size, coat-color) even within litters or among closely related animals (Fox, 1969, 1971; Lockwood, 1976, 1979; Mech, 1970). This inherent phenotypic variability contributed to the wolf's ability to occupy the largest range of habitats, from deserts to tundra, of any large non-human land mammal. This diversity likely reflected rich genotypic variability that provided much of the raw material needed to produce the many forms of the domestic dog (Shearin & Ostrander, 2010).

It is likely that the process of domestication of the dog involved both selecting segments of the wolf genome associated with desirable traits for different purposes (and discarding others), as well as taking advantage of existing canine mechanisms for enhancing genetic diversity to produce or amplify some of the more recent changes associated with specific breeds. Gray et al. (2009) modeled the demographic history of wild canid populations and domestic dog breeds and suggested that domestication resulted in a 5% loss of nucleotide diversity, while breed formation caused a 35%

loss, which would suggest that some of the genetic programming present in the wolf was "edited out" in the production of physically and behaviorally diverse dog breeds.

Shearin & Ostrander (2010) suggest several major mechanisms for producing high levels of phenotypic variation in dogs starting with the raw material of the wolf genome. The first is variability in simple sequence repeats (SSRs). They identify five genes with large repeat expansions or contractions in members of the Canidae and suggest that this is one source of potentially large phenotypic variation in the domestic dog not requiring major changes in the genome. A second mechanism is carnivore-specific short-interspersed nuclear elements (SINEs), which have been related to some morphological traits such as merle coat color and behavioral abnormalities including narcolepsy. Finally, they list a variety of other mechanisms for producing variations common to other species including chromosomal fission and gene duplication.

As discussed below, the significance of such findings to issues of canine aggression are currently uncertain since the genetic mechanisms underlying dog aggression, in any of its many forms, are not well-established. However, if we assume that there are likely genetic mechanisms that influence certain aspects of aggression such as threshold, latency, persistence, target and bite inhibition, it is reasonable to suggest that a wide range of aggression-related behaviors could be influenced by a relatively small number of interacting genes (see also van den Berg, Chapter 5).

The classic work on tameness in silver foxes (*Vulpes vulpes*) (Belyaev, 1969) is often suggested as a model of behavior genetic processes that might have occurred during the domestication of the wolf (Spady & Ostrander, 2008; Trut, 1999; Lord *et al*., Chapter 4). This work is relevant to issues of the origins of canine aggression since a major alteration seen over 30 to 35 generations of selective breeding of ranched foxes was a decrease in fear and aggression toward humans and a rise in dog-like behaviors such as tail-wagging and licking. In addition, these behavioral changes were accompanied by morphological changes including altered coat colors, floppy ears, shortened tails, curly tails and other dog-like characteristics. Lindberg *et al*. (2005) found only small differences between three brain regions in tamed vs. unselected lines of foxes, suggesting that the behavioral and physiological changes caused by selection for tameness might be associated with only limited changes in gene expression in the fox brain. However, even if only a small number of genes are involved in tameness/aggression, the interactions with other components of the genome may be complex. Kukekova *et al*. (2011) mapped two VVU12 loci associated with tame behavior across various fox hybrids and concluded that the suite of traits that provide variations in the tame form of foxes are quite complex. Similarly, Jazin (2007) notes that multiple regions of the genome may be involved in the expression of a single gene and many complex interactions could produce quantitative changes associated with behavioral traits.

In the course of domestication of the wolf into the dog, it is certain that much of the selective pressure put on the dog's ancestors involved the regulation of various components of inter- and intra-specific aggression to suit a variety of human needs. Scott & Fuller (1965) commented that agonistic behavior in dogs has been subjected to great modifications in different breeds and noted that, "compared with wolves, they are highly specialized in their choice and patterns of agonistic behavior" (p. 78). Most social canids show surprisingly low levels of serious intraspecific aggression and lethal intraspecific encounters are relatively rare except in captive populations or wild populations whose territories have been reduced to the extent that territorial disputes between different groups become more common (Lockwood, 1976; Mech, 1970). Despite the strong restraint on the use of aggression – i.e. "bite inhibition" that Lorenz correctly recognized to be at the core of wolf social structure – agonistic behavior can occur in many contexts including expressions of dominance, territorial defense, food competition, protection of young or other pack members, pain-elicited aggression and fear-elicited aggression. Domestic dog aggression can occur in any of these contexts, and may also involve components of interspecific predatory behavior.

It is important to recognize that artificial selection, which has resulted in the production of various breeds of dogs, frequently produces exaggerated physical or behavioral characteristics that would be maladaptive in free-living wild canids. For example, racing breeds such as greyhounds and whippets can outrun most wolves, yet the changes mankind has produced in these animals would render them relatively helpless and vulnerable in the world of the wild wolf.

Many of the problems we associate with canine aggression, including increased inter- or intra-specific aggression, originate from the fact that a major human objective in the production of many dog breeds has been the creation of animals that are *more* likely to show aggression than their wolf ancestors. It is likely that one of the earliest uses of tamed or domesticated wolves was to alert humans to the presence of human or animal intruders and to repel or attack such threats. This is a more likely scenario for the initial keeping of tamed wolves than other potential advantages such as using such animals to aid in tracking and killing prey. Throughout recorded history a major purpose of the dog has been to provide protection through interspecific aggression (e.g. most guard and attack breeds), to alert to or repel human and other animal intruders, or for use as offensive weapons in warfare (Varner & Varner, 1983). In addition, in some breeds, there have been centuries of selection for participation in so-called "blood sports" including gladiatorial combat against humans and the heightened intraspecific aggression of a variety of other fighting breeds used around the world (Fleig, 1996; Semencic, 1991). As Overall and Love (2001, p. 1929) note, "some dogs' behavioral problems are simply different manifestations of traits that have been selected for by humans." They further note that when breeds become popular, selection against less favorable traits is relaxed and, behaviors seen as "tough" or "sharp" may be selected for.

9.4   Factors contributing to canine aggression

Although canine agonistic behavior can take many forms, the greatest concern from the standpoint of human health and safety and animal welfare is dog-to-human aggression and, to a slightly lesser degree, dog-to-dog aggression. Thus most analyses of dog aggression have focused on those factors associated with greater risk for aggression.

Dog bite incidents are ultimately the outcome of many interrelated factors including the type of dog(s) involved, the behavior of the owner, the behavior of the victim, and so on. Prior to the mid-1950s, a primary concern about dog bite was the fear of rabies. Thus approaches to animal control and bite prevention tended to follow a "disease" model of dog bite – identifying the "vector" (e.g. type of dog involved) and containing or eliminating it. As greater understanding of the complexity of the human–canine relationship developed, the focus changed to a "societal" model, recognizing dog bite as a problem that required a community response to a complex issue (AVMA Task Force, 2001).

In reviewing problems of canine aggression, Overall & Love (2001) noted that there is a need for more detailed description of the biological features of the dogs involved in aggressive incidents and identification of the risks caused by canine and human behavior. The major factors affecting canine aggression and its impact include:

1. Biological variables associated with the dog – sex, spay/neuter status, health, diet and nutritional status, breed, lineage within a breed (e.g. field vs. show).
2. Development/socialization of the dog to people, other animals, and environments.
3. Housing/supervision/restraint.
4. Training and other interactions with people, including abuse.
5. Victim behavior and demographics.

9.4.1   Biological factors

Sex and spay/neuter status

Many studies using various measures of aggression have indicated higher levels of aggressive behavior in male dogs in general (Beaver, 1993, 1994; Hart & Hart, 1997; Line & Voith, 1986; Roll & Unshelm, 1997). Serious dog bite seems to be a phenomenon primarily associated with male dogs. In the Beck *et al.* (1975) survey, 70% of the biting animals were male. Moore *et al.* (1977) were able to collect more detailed information on biting animals, recording information on breed, sex and reproductive status. Overall, 87% of all biting animals in that survey were males and 60% were unneutered males. Of the remaining 13% of bites attributed to females, half were by unspayed females. Podberscek & Blackshaw (1993) also reported a preponderance of bites attributed to male dogs in studies from Australia. Gershman *et al.* (1994) looked at risk factors revealed by comparing biting dogs with non-biting matched controls. Being a male increased the likelihood of a bite by an odds-ratio of 6.2.

Some of this difference is often attributed to elevated levels of testosterone in male dogs. One of the most common controlled substances found in association with illegal dogfighting activity is testosterone proprionate, allegedly for its ability to enhance muscle mass and fighting performance (Lockwood, 2011). However, evidence from behavioral studies looking at canine aggression as a function of spay/neuter status is inconsistent. Neilson *et al.* (1997) studied 57 male dogs over 2 years of age at time of castration for aggression-related problems. An improvement of at least 50% in various aggressive behaviors was seen in only 30%, with the lowest improvement seen for aggression to strange dogs. There was no significant effect on aggression toward unfamiliar people. Greater improvement was seen in roaming, mounting and marking. Farhoody (2010) compared aggression scores of male dogs neutered at different ages with intact dogs. There was a significantly *higher* aggression score in neutered dogs as compared to intact dogs regardless of the age at which the dogs were neutered. When aggression scores in female dogs spayed at different ages were compared with intact female dogs, there was significant increase in aggression score of dogs spayed at 12 months or earlier as compared to intact dogs. This is consistent with similar findings for spayed females reported by Wright & Nesselrote (1987) and Guy *et al.* (2001a).

In a large-scale survey of over 3800 dog owners regarding their pet's human directed aggression, Casey *et al.* (2014) found that female neutered dogs were 2.3 times less likely to show family directed aggression than neutered males and 1.8 times less likely to show aggression to strangers entering the house than neutered males.

It is likely that spay/neuter status is confounded with other measures of dog-owner responsibility, at least in US populations where resistance to neutering male dogs is high in areas where there is also resistance to licensing and other indicators of lower levels of responsible pet ownership.

Size

Harris *et al.* (1974) report that larger dogs (regardless of breed) are implicated in more attacks on humans, which is consistent with other epidemiological studies. While size is related to the *risks* associated with dog aggression, it is not necessarily related to the *incidence* of such behavior. Duffy *et al.* (2008) reviewed owner reports using the Canine Behavioral Assessment Research Questionnaire (C-BARQ) and noted that all the breeds that stood out as being rated relatively high for aggression to household members were in the small to medium-size range. This relationship between small body size and aggressive behavior problems has recently been confirmed in a larger study of the relationship between morphology and behavior in dogs (McGreevy *et al.*, 2013). The authors note that the biological basis for this association remains to be determined and suggest that the high correlation of small size with undesirable behaviors may reflect that small dogs may be more likely to be retained as companions despite behaviors that would be unwelcome in larger dogs.

Health and physiology

Overall health can impact the expression of aggressive behavior in a variety of ways. Poor general condition, such as is often encountered with dogs rescued from serious neglect (e.g. puppy mill or hoarding situations) or abuse may result in a short-term general depression of *all* behaviors. Some animals may demonstrate an increase in aggression to people or other dogs in the days or weeks after rescue as they become better able to express their behavioral repertoire. Abuse or neglect may also produce chronic painful conditions that result in greater risk of pain-elicited aggression.

Pain may also be a significant factor in aggression in non-abused animals. Camps *et al.* (2012) report on 12 clinical cases of pain-related aggression. The most common cause of pain was hip dysplasia (66.7%), but no relationship was found between the cause of pain and the characteristics of the aggressive behavior. Dogs that had not been aggressive before the onset of the pain-eliciting condition were more impulsive, showed aggression as a result of manipulation more frequently and adopted a defensive body posture more frequently than dogs that had been aggressive before the onset of pain.

Fighting breeds are often described as being "stoic" and appearing to have a higher tolerance of pain, or at least an inhibition of behaviors indicating a response to painful stimuli such as a toe pinch. This may be mediated by peculiarities in neurotransmitters or opiate receptor sites. A single anecdotal report of unusual responsiveness to morphine and naloxone in a pit bull suggests that there may be physiological differences in the breed (Brown *et al.*, 1987), although no definitive studies have been reported in the literature.

Fox & Andrews (1973) identified some individual differences in corticosteroid levels associated with dominance aggression in wolves. Hennessy *et al.* (2001) found that cortisol levels were negatively correlated with behavior problems at 6 months and suggested that measures of behavior and endocrine activity obtained in shelters might prove useful for screening dogs for adoption, or targeting dogs for behavioral intervention.

Other clinical conditions, including certain endocrine, neurological and neurochemical issues, may contribute to reactivity and aggressiveness (Reinhard, 1978; Reisner, 1991). Other physiological findings related to aggression have been somewhat inconsistent across different clinical populations. It is likely that there are complex interactions between internal physiological states and the possible expression of genes potentially involved in aggressive behavior. Studies of possible behavioral genes, such as those involved in serotonergic, catecholaminergic, and glutamatergic pathways, have failed to find significant differences in populations with different profiles of aggressive behavior (Masuda *et al.*, 2004; van den Berg *et al.*, 2003, 2005; van den Berg, Chapter 5). Våge *et al.* (2010) studied the expression of nine genes in different brain parts of 11 dogs euthanized for aggressive behavior and nine non-aggressive dogs. An initial PCR-based cDNA subtraction method, with the amygdala of an aggressive dog as the primary target, indicated that these genes were expressed differentially in the two populations.

Diet

The possible involvement of serotonin levels and other elements of the hypothalamic–pituitary–adrenal (HPA) axis in aggressive behaviors suggests that dietary variations related to biochemical precursors of elements of this system could have an effect on some forms of aggression. Although there are many anecdotal accounts of the influence of different dietary regimens on behavior, there have been few controlled studies. Dodman *et al.* (1996) fed diets containing a low (17%), medium

(25%), or high (32%) protein content to 12 dogs with dominance aggression, 12 dogs with hyper-activity, 12 dogs with territorial aggression, and 14 control dogs without behavioral problems. Territorial aggression was significantly reduced when dogs were fed the low- or medium-protein diet, compared with territorial aggression when fed the high-protein diet, but they concluded that a reduction in dietary protein content is not generally useful in the treatment of behavior problems in dogs, but may be appropriate in dogs with territorial aggression that is a result of fear. DeNapoli *et al*. (2000) looked at the effect of dietary protein content and tryptophan supplements on small samples (11 dogs each) of animals with dominance aggression, territorial aggression and hyperactivity. For dogs showing dominance aggression, owners' behavioral scores of aggression were highest in dogs fed unsupplemented high-protein rations. Tryptophan-supplemented low-protein diets were associated with significantly lower aggression scores than low-protein diets without tryptophan supplements (see also Zawistowski & Reid, Chapter 12).

Breed and lineage

The most controversial issue surrounding the understanding and prediction of aggressive behavior in dogs has been the role of breed, largely because breed designations have been at the core of legislation and litigation regarding dog aggression (Lockwood, 1988; Patronek *et al*., 2010). An understanding of the connections between breeds and various forms of canine aggression is important for several reasons. First, an understanding of significant and consistent behavioral differences in genetically different populations may provide better potential understanding of different forms of aggression and other potentially problematic behaviors. Such an understanding requires the identification of reproducible behavioral phenotypes and clearly defined genotypes. Second, improved understanding of genetic and other factors underlying undesirable or dangerous canine behaviors may result in improved breeding and selection. Third, much of the public's selection of companion animals is based on assumptions of likely behavior based on perception of breed stereotypes rather than the assessment of behavior in specific individuals. If such expectations are invalid or inconsistent, it is important to communicate this to potential owners. Finally, a better understanding of the limitations of breed stereotypes is essential for informing public policy.

Information on canine aggression and the breed-related factors that may influence it comes from several sources:

1. Breeding and cross-breeding studies.
2. Epidemiological studies of dog bites.
3. Analysis of caseloads from animal behaviorists and/or veterinarians and physiological and neurological studies of dogs with different aggression profiles.
4. Surveys of dog-owners or dog experts (trainers, veterinarians, behaviorists).
5. Behavioral assessments and standardized testing (e.g. by breed clubs or animal shelters).

Each of these approaches has potential drawbacks, particularly when attempting to evaluate breed differences in risks and/or when making recommendations for animal care and control policies.

Breeding and cross-breeding studies: Clearly many canine behaviors that are considered characteristic of particular breeds are influenced by genetic factors that increase the likelihood of expression of such behaviors (see van den Berg *et al*, 2003; van den Berg, Chapter 5). Pointers point, setters set, retrievers retrieve, herding dogs herd, guarding dogs guard and fighting dogs fight. However, none of these patterns of behavior is without some environmental influence and none is found at the same level in all animals sharing very similar genetic histories. Even among bloodlines of champion fighting dogs maintained for illegal dogfighting, it is common that many of the offspring of accomplished fighters will show little or no inclination toward dog–dog aggression, leading to high incidence of culling within even these highly inbred lines (Lockwood, 2011). As Parker & Ostrander (2005, p. 512) point out, despite major advances in canine genetics in the last decade, "We still don't know … why herding dogs herd and pointing dogs point."

The classic approach to sorting out genetic contributions to breed-related behaviors has been to systematically study the development of a range of behaviors in a group of dogs from diverse breeds, as well as their hybrids. This was the costly and time-consuming approach used in the pioneering work of Scott and Fuller (1965) and their students. They selected wire-haired fox terriers as one of the breeds to focus on in their studies in part because of their recognition that terrier breeds had been selected for, "a tendency to attack prey and keep on attacking regardless of any injury suffered" (p. 77). Ironically, this academic description parallels the definition of "gameness" in fighting dogs provided in an underground dogfighting publication:

A game dog has no fear of "Man" nor "Beast", "Life" or "death". Although he has no fear of "Death", he will fight for "Life", be it his or his master's … Gameness is a quality inherent in some but not in others. It's a quality that when found must be cherished and cared for. (Mize, 2010, p. 22)

The other breeds studied by Scott and Fuller – basenji, beagle, cocker spaniel and sheltie – did not share this history and were selected for other presumed genetic predispositions (e.g. herding, sociability and barklessness). They reported a (presumably) genetically based decrease in the latency to show intraspecific aggression in terriers, but did not witness any serious attacks.

Epidemiology of aggression by breed of dog: One of the most debated issues involving the assessment of canine aggression is the use of dog bite epidemiology to develop breed-specific profiles of the association between breed and incidence of dog-to-human aggression (Lockwood, 1995; Patronek et al., 2010). From an epidemiological perspective, it is difficult to draw scientifically sound conclusions about the relative dangers posed by different breeds. Accurate breed-specific bite rates are hard to obtain. Such statistics require good information for both the numerator (number of all bites attributed to each specific *reliably identified* breed) and the denominator (number of animals of that breed in the population). None of these conditions is met in most bite epidemiological studies. Most bites go unreported, with estimates of the percentage of bites captured by existing reporting systems ranging from 10% in Kansas City, MO, to 36% in Pittsburgh, PA (Chang et al., 1997), and 44–83% in different Atlanta communities (Tan et al., 2004). Bites requiring medical attention are more likely to be reported, which can lead to an over-representation of larger breeds in bite statistics.

The source of breed identification of biting dogs is rarely specified in bite reports. Breeds are often unverified and Voith et al. (2009, 2013) have demonstrated that even people who work with dogs on a daily basis in an expert capacity show little inter-observer reliability in breed identification, and cannot reliably identify breed mixtures. As a result, dogs whose appearance may lead to identification as a particular breed may in fact have little or no genetic relationship to that breed.

Overall and Love (2001) provide a meta-analysis of 11 US dog bite epidemiological studies from 1970 to 1996 and did not find a clear trend for breeds coming to the top of the list. The only breed appearing in the top group on most lists was the German shepherd.

Dog-related human fatalities are usually investigated and publicized in much greater detail than the estimated four million non-fatal dog bites occurring each year. In part for this reason, such incidents have had a disproportionate influence on public policy if the objective of such policies is to reduce the overall incidence of human injury attributed to dogs (Bradley, 2006; Cunningham, 2005; Hattaway, 1997). Only 20–30 such instances occur annually in the US, comprising less than 0.01% of all dog bites and involving less than 0.004% of the US dog population. Such instances are usually not simply a conventional dog bite that ends in a human death. Fatal dog attacks represent a "perfect storm" combining many factors associated with bite risk (i.e. the wrong dog, in the wrong hands, with improper rearing and supervision, and a vulnerable and unprotected victim) (Gladwell, 2006). Therefore breed-specific policies based on this exceedingly rare and aberrant occurrence should not be used as the basis for public policy (AVMA Task Force, 2001; Sacks *et al.*, 1996, 2000)

Because such data are so frequently misused to justify breed-specific legislation and other restrictions, following the publication of Sacks *et al.* (2000) the American Veterinary Medical Association (AVMA) issued a "To Whom it May Concern" letter noting:

In contrast to what has been reported in the news media, the data contained within this report **CANNOT be used to infer any breed-specific risk** for dog bite fatalities (e.g., neither pit bull-type dogs nor Rottweilers can be said to be more "dangerous" than any other breed based on the contents of this report). To obtain such risk information it would be necessary to know the numbers of each breed currently residing in the United States. Such information is not available. (AVMA, 2000)

Patronek *et al.* (2013) conducted a more detailed analysis of 256 dog bite related fatalities (DBRFs) occurring between 2000 and 2009 using additional data that had not been available in previous studies (including Sacks *et al.*, 1996, 2000). Unlike previous studies, they limited valid determination of breed to those cases with documented pedigree, parentage information or DNA analysis as well as assessment of breed attribution by a Certified Applied Animal Behaviorist. They compared breed identifications reported by the media with those made by law enforcement or animal control. Media reports were often discordant, differing from law enforcement or animal control records in 34.9% of cases. DNA or pedigree data were available for only 19 dogs and seven of these were discordant with media reports (36.8%). There were 45 cases (17.6%) in which there was consistent concordance of breed by pedigree, parentage, DNA or vet, animal control and media. These cases included 20 recognized breeds and two known mix breeds. The authors conclude that these data support the recommendations of the AVMA Task Force on Canine Aggression and Human-Canine Interaction (AVMA Task Force, 2001) and the CDC, who have consistently stressed the multifactorial nature of dog bites and the need for multiple approaches to address this complexity rather than a focus on breed.

Clinical case loads: Duffy *et al.* (2008) note that reviews of clinical case loads related to aggression provide little insight into breed-related correlates of different problems since clients having issues with larger or more powerful dogs are more likely to seek help. In addition, clients are more likely to present cases involving owner or family-directed aggression than cases involving dog–dog or dog–stranger aggression.

Survey methods: Two different survey methods have been used to attempt to associate dog breeds with specific behavior profiles, including the incidence of different forms of aggression. The first approach has been to survey presumed experts in canine behavior (veterinarians, trainers, obedience judges) for their ranking of various behavior and personality traits of many breeds (Hart & Hart, 1985, 1997, Chapter 7). Usually this has been used in an attempt to advise potential dog owners of breed-related tendencies to allow for more informed selection of pets. As noted by Duffy *et al.* (2008), such rankings are usually not based on any objective criteria or breed-specific experience and may simply reflect common breed stereotypes. In addition, surveys of similar experts in other countries (UK and Japan) using almost identical methods to those of Hart and Hart showed concordance rates of only 50–60% (Bradshaw & Goodwin, 1998; Takeuchi & Mori, 2006).

A more promising approach is the collection of very detailed behavioral information from questionnaires completed by large samples of owners. Duffy *et al.* (2008) report aggression-related data based on use of the Canine Behavioral Assessment Research Questionnaire (CBARQ) with owners of 30 breeds, as well as a sample of breed club members. They report that some breeds appeared to be aggressive in several contexts (e.g. Dachshunds, Chihuahuas and Jack Russell terriers) while others were more specific. Akitas, Siberian huskies, and pit bull terriers were more often reported to show aggression directed toward unfamiliar dogs, suggesting that independent mechanisms may mediate the expression of different forms of aggression.

Although their findings were consistent with earlier breed profiles (e.g. Hart & Hart, 1985), they emphasize that the high within-breed variation in C-BARQ scores suggests that it is "inappropriate to make predictions about a given dog's propensity for aggressive behavior based solely on its breed" (p. 451). They further note the C-BARQ scores for stranger-directed aggression found among pit bull terriers were about average and were inconsistent with their reputation as a "dangerous breed." About 7% of pit bull owners indicated that their dogs had bitten or attempted to bite an unfamiliar person in the recent past, somewhat higher than the overall average (4.7%). However, 22% reported bites were directed at other dogs. This pattern is consistent with the view that certain lineages within this breed, like other terriers, have been selectively bred for aggression toward other animals rather than humans (Lockwood, 1995; Lockwood & Rindy, 1987).

Some of the within-breed variability in behavior measures, including aggression scores, can be the result of different recent selective histories in different lineages that appear physically the same. Svartberg's (2005) study of 31 different breeds found that, in general, breeding for show was associated with lower levels of aggression, curiosity and playfulness, and with higher levels of fearfulness, while selection for use in field trials was correlated with higher levels of playfulness and aggression. Duffy et al. (2008) comment that within Springer spaniels, aggression is more common in dogs from show breeding lines than from working gun dog lines.

The conclusion from these diverse approaches to looking at the influence of breed on canine aggression is that breeds *do* differ in how they regulate different patterns of aggression (i.e. to familiar and unfamiliar people and familiar and unfamiliar animals), *but* breed alone, even when reliably determined, provides limited power for predicting the aggressive behavior of an individual dog in a particular context. For these reasons, much of the current focus on canine aggression has shifted to looking at other factors related to aggression, and examining the utility of different assessment tools and techniques to evaluate individual animals.

9.4.2   Environmental factors

Socialization

Dog behaviorists have long recognized that the moderation of agonistic behavior and the development of bite inhibition in social contexts (e.g. interactions with other dogs or people) requires an opportunity to interact with potential social partners (human and/or animal) during sensitive periods (Scott & Fuller, 1965; Serpell et al., Chapter 6). Dogs deprived of sufficient social contact with other dogs, people, or both can be at risk for responding to future interactions with fear, aggression or both.

Patronek et al. (2013) looked at the opportunities for socialization in dogs involved in fatal attacks on people. They note that 76.2% of these dogs were kept as "resident dogs" rather than "family dogs," i.e. they were "isolated from regular, positive human interactions" (p. 1728), including 37.9% of resident dogs that were kept chained and 34.9% isolated in a fenced area or pen. They identify the lack of opportunity for socialization as one of several significant preventable risk factors for serious or fatal attacks.

McMillan et al. (2011) looked at the mental health of dogs formerly kept as breeding stock in commercial breeding establishments (CBE's, i.e. "puppy mills") by having adopters of these dogs complete the C-BARQ. Although such dogs are kept in proximity to other dogs, they have limited opportunity for interaction and little human contact. Compared to matched controls the CBE dogs had higher rates of fear and house-soiling but significantly lower rates of aggression to strangers and other dogs. Similar studies of animals rescued from abusive situations have also been conducted (McMillan *et al*., 2015, 2016).

Communication

Another important part of socialization is the development of the ability to accurately communicate and interpret the mood and intention of others (human and non-human) and regulate one's behavior accordingly. Under natural conditions, the aggression of wild canids is held in check by a detailed set of postural and facial signals that clearly indicate mood and intent (Fox, 1971; Schenkel, 1967). In addition, aggressive encounters are normally ended rapidly when one individual emits the appropriate "cut-off" behavior, such as infantile vocalizations (whining, yelping) and submissive displays. Goodwin *et al*. (1997; see also Bradshaw & Rooney, Chapter 8) suggest that domestication has reduced the complexity of signaling in some breeds, with more "wolf-like" breeds having at least nine threat signals compared with two in Norfolk terriers. In addition, dogs from fighting lineages may have been under selective pressure to suppress or eliminate accurate communication of aggressive motivation or intent because, according to accounts from dog fighters, it is to a fighting dog's advantage for its attack to be unexpected (Lockwood, 2011). Many accounts of dog attacks on people note that the incident occurred "without warning." This may be due to human inexperience in appropriately reading subtle warning signals preceding an attack, or may reflect true suppression of signaling of threat in some fighting and guarding lineages. Kujala *et al*. (2012) offer evidence from functional magnetic resonance imaging that experience with dogs leads dog experts to distinguish socially relevant body postures in dogs and humans using similar pathways.

9.4.3   Housing and restraint

The manner in which dogs are housed or restrained can also affect the likelihood of an attack. Sacks *et al*. (1989) reported that 28% of the animals in the fatal attacks they studied were chained at the time of the attack. In their case-controlled comparison of biting and non-biting dogs, Gershman *et al*. (1994) indicated that chaining raised the odds ratio of a dog being involved in a bite by a factor of 2.8. As noted above, Patronek *et al*. (2013) also identified chaining as a significant risk factor associated with fatal dog attack.

The question remains whether dogs are chained or tethered because they are aggressive or whether they become aggressive because chaining or tethering reflects inadequate opportunity for socialization or abusive treatment. Because chaining is seen as a significant risk factor associated with dog aggression, 22 US states and many communities have placed various restrictions on the nature and duration of chaining or tethering (AVMA, 2013a).

Studies of the effect of size of housing on aggression have been relatively uninformative, in part because they have involved laboratory Beagles that had a history of selection for low dog–dog aggression and tolerance of confined housing. Hughes & Campbell (1989) found no differences in aggression or play in Beagles housed in 12 m × 1 m pens *vs*. 1 m × 2 m pens. Yeon *et al*. (2001) looked at the behavior of 30 Alaskan sled dogs kept on 3.5 m tethers vs. 5.9 m^2 pens and found no significant differences but noted that these dogs had been housed on tethers for most of their lives and concluded that tethering may be intuitively less acceptable but its impact on a dog's behaviors can depend on the breed and experience of the dog.

9.4.4   Training

The last decade has seen applied animal behaviorists, veterinary behaviorists and other certified trainers shift away from coercive and even violent training methods that were in vogue with previous generations of trainers and which still remain popular with some trainers (Herron *et al.*, 2009; Reisner, Chapter 11; Zawistowski & Reid, Chapter 12). Such tactics can exacerbate rather than correct undesired behaviors (Bradshaw & Rooney, Chapter 8).

Hiby *et al.* (2004) found significantly fewer behavior problems in dogs that had been trained using rewards only, as compared with dogs that had been trained using some form of punishment only, or a combination of both. O'Sullivan *et al.* (2008) conducted telephone interviews of volunteer owners of 21 dogs having no history of perceived aggressive behavior prior to the reported bite incident and 79 that had a record of aggression. Owners reprimanding the dog by physical and verbal means were a significant predictor of aggressive behavior, as was owner tolerance of significant degrees of aggressive behavior, inadequate or ineffective obedience training and biting of adult household members. Herron *et al.* (2009) surveyed responses of 140 dog owners regarding the outcomes of a variety of interventions with dogs showing undesirable behaviors. The most common confrontational methods used by dog owners included hitting or kicking the dog (43%), growling at dog (41%) and alpha roll (e.g. forcing the dog onto its back) (31%). Such responses elicited an aggressive response from at least 25% of dogs, with alpha roll having the greatest likelihood of resulting in an aggressive response in dogs with aggression to familiar people.

9.4.5   Victim behavior

Under the principles of Common Law that shaped many dangerous dog laws there is the assumption that dogs are harmless unless they have previously demonstrated a vicious propensity. This often leads to the related assumption that victims of dog attack have provoked or otherwise precipitated the attack. Some bite reports equate "provocation" with any victim behavior that might be expected to increase the likelihood of aggression from a dog (e.g. running or screaming), but in legal terms "provocation" applies primarily to inappropriate actions (teasing, tormenting, inflicting pain, trespass, attempting to commit a crime) that might initiate an attack.

Studies that have documented the context in which an attack has occurred generally show that bite victims are rarely engaging in activity that could legally be considered provocation. In the bites surveyed by Beck *et al.* (1975), the victims had no interaction with the dog, or were walking or sitting in 75% of the cases. In 9.6% of the cases, the victim was playing with the dog and in only 6.5% of the cases could the victim's behavior be classified as provocation. Reisner *et al.* (2011) examined the circumstances of dog bites by interviewing 203 children ≤17 years (or parent proxies for children ≤6 years) presenting with dog bite injuries to a children's hospital. Most children (72%) knew the biting dog, and most bites to younger children occurred during positive interactions, initiated by the child, with familiar dogs, indoors. Most of the older children bitten had been active (e.g. outdoors), were unfamiliar with the dog, and had not interacted with it.

Because bites to children commonly involve avoidable interactions, most bite prevention outreach has focused on alerting children to warning signs and avoidance of such risk through appropriate caution and defensive behaviors if threatened (Chapman *et al.*, 2000; Jalongo, 2008; Love & Overall, 2001; Spiegel, 2000; Wilson *et al.* 2003).

9.4.6   Other human behaviors

Although much of the past discussion of canine aggression and its origins focused on issues of breed and biology, the growing recognition that dog bites are also a sociological concern has led to increased attention to the human behaviors associated with the ownership of dogs that are at risk for aggression.

Sudden increases in breed popularity can result in relaxed selection and increased ownership of potentially difficult breeds by inexperienced owners. The sudden rise of Rottweilers in pediatric bite surveys between 1990 and 1995 (Kaye *et al.*, 2009) may be associated the rapid increase in AKC registration of the breed during that period (Herzog, 2006), partly in response to growing restrictions on pit bull type dogs.

Several studies have attempted to address the patterns of ownership associated with dogs considered vicious or potentially dangerous. A report from the UK (Hughes *et al.*, 2011) addressed concerns over irresponsible ownership of "status dogs" (also termed "weapon dogs," "bling dogs" or "combat dogs") by young men, particularly in blighted urban areas. Schuler *et al.* (2008) looked at risk factors associated with bite incidents in Portland, Oregon and noted that biting dogs were more likely than non-biting dogs to be kept in neighborhoods with incomes below the county median. Dog bite has been associated with other social problems, including child abuse and other forms of family violence. DeViney *et al.* (1983) noted that the incidence of injuries from a family pet in homes with a documented history of child maltreatment and animal cruelty was six times the rate of injury seen in families without such history. Jonker & Jonker-Bakker (1991) reported that 48 of 62 children interviewed as victims of sexual abuse (77%) had been attacked by their abuser's dog. Vaisman-Tzachor (2001) expands on this with three additional case histories of this type.

Several studies have attempted to look at the potential association between ownership of "vicious" dogs and anti-social behaviors. The underlying idea is that the ownership of animals that are selected for, or are at risk of exhibiting, aggression may be characteristic of general deviance on the part of the dog owner. Barnes *et al.* (2006) looked at 166 Ohio owners of "vicious" dogs compared with 189 owners of "low-risk" dogs. They indicated that vicious dog owners had up to 10 times more criminal convictions than other dog owners. Specifically, vicious dog owners were 6.8 times more likely to be convicted of an aggressive crime, 2.8 times more likely to have carried out a crime involving children, 2.4 times more likely to have perpetrated domestic violence, and 5.4 times more likely to have an alcohol conviction when compared to low-risk dog owners. A major flaw of this study was that "vicious" dog was not defined based on any report of aggressive behavior on the part of the dog, but only on the basis of the selected breed, making use of Ohio's dangerous dog law that defined pit bulls as automatically fitting this category – a law that was rescinded in 2012. "Vicious" was also interpreted to mean any akitas, chow chows, Dobermans, Rottweilers, or wolf-mixes. In fact, only 1% of the owners in the study had actually been cited for incidents involving dog aggression.

Ragatz *et al.* (2009) followed a similar methodology examining dog owners in four categories: vicious dog vs. large dog vs. small dog vs. control. As with Barnes *et al.* (2006) the identification of someone as the owner of a "vicious dog" was not based on any history of the animals' behavior, but solely on the basis of the dog allegedly belonging to a supposedly "vicious" breed drawing from the same list as Barnes *et al.* (2006). They reported that owners of vicious dogs were significantly more likely to admit to violent criminal behavior, compared to large dog owners, small dog owners, and controls. The vicious dog owner sample also engaged in more types (i.e. violent, property, drug, and status) of criminal behavior compared to all other participant groups.

Personality traits were examined and owners of vicious dogs were reported to score significantly higher than controls on impulsive sensation-seeking and primary psychopathy (e.g. carelessness, selfishness, and manipulative tendencies) than small dog owners. It is important to note that this sample is composed of only *college student* dog owners. No information was gathered about the certainty of their dog's breed identification or whether the dog had ever been involved in "vicious" behavior.

Schenk *et al.* (2012) reported additional data using the same sample and flawed methodology. "Vicious" dog owners reported significantly higher criminal thinking, entitlement, sentimentality, and superoptimism tendencies. Vicious dog owners were arrested, engaged in physical fights, and used marijuana significantly more than other dog owners.

While these studies may provide insights into the human personality characteristics influencing the *selection* of animals that may be at risk, they tell us little about the actual human behaviors that may directly contribute to the production of canine aggression. However, they add some credence to the perception of dog bites as a public health problem with a substantial *human* behavior component.

Patronek *et al.* (2013) applied a much more rigorous analysis of fatal dog attacks to identify preventable human actions that were associated with such attacks. They identified six factors that were associated with fatalities:

1. No able bodied person was present to control the dog.
2. The victim was compromised in ability to interact appropriately either because of age (very young or old) or impairment.
3. The dog was a "resident dog," i.e. not kept as a socialized household pet.
4. Reproductively intact dog.
5. Prior history of mismanagement (dog reported "at large").
6. Prior history of abuse or neglect of the dog.

They note that four or more of the above factors were present in 80.5% of the fatal attacks that were reviewed.

One of the most effective approaches to addressing dangerous dog issues has been to specifically respond to the human behavior associated with irresponsible keeping of dogs that have been involved in bite incidents. In 1986 Multnomah County, Oregon, passed stringent laws responding to bite incidents that held owners increasingly accountable for future problems. In the five years prior to the implementation of the program, 25% of those dogs that had caused injury to people or other animals through attacking or biting repeated that same behavior within one year. After the implementation of the program, that rate of repeat incidence has been reduced to 7% (Oswald, 1991).

9.5   Assessing individual animals

A lesson that clearly emerges from the analysis of the biology and behavior of canine aggression is that dogs are individuals and that, although there are broad trends in behavior associated with breeds, these are of limited value for assessing how a given individual may behave in different situations. Thus there has been increasing interest in determining best practices for assessing risks for the most problematic behaviors related to dog aggression, as well as developing protocols for addressing these potential risks.

The primary reasons for assessing aggressive behavior in dogs are to aid in the selection of suitable companion animals, improve lasting shelter adoptions and identify animals that may be predisposed to aggression in order to limit liability and welfare concerns. These goals are somewhat different from more established dog behavior assessment methods that have focused on evaluating working dogs for potential job performance (Jones & Gosling, 2005).

Aggression assessments are not temperament tests, they are intended to be a snapshot of behavior to determine the likelihood of aggression in some circumstances (e.g. to children, unfamiliar adults, unfamiliar dogs, etc.) and identify resources that may be needed to address the issue (Reid, 2013; Weiss & Mohan-Gibbons, 2013; Zawistowski & Reid, Chapter 12). It is recognized that there is no gold standard for such assessments, although several, including the ASPCA's SAFER test, are in widespread use (ASPCA 2011a, 2011b). Marston & Bennett (2003) and Christensen *et al.* (2007) point out how shelter assessments may fail to screen for aggression since shelter animals may suffer from hidden disease, sleep deprivation, noise pollution, social stress and other factors that may inhibit some dogs from exhibiting aggressive tendencies, or the test situation may fail to adequately simulate potential triggers.

Several studies aimed at validating aggression tests using pet dog populations report general validity with respect to owner accounts, but in more than 20% of cases dogs passed aggression tests despite having a history of biting (Kroll *et al.*, 2004; Netto & Planta, 1997). Stephen & Ledger (2007) assessed whether relinquishing owners' reports of their dogs behavior predicted behavior problems post adoption. Although many behavior problems were not correlated between old and new homes, aggression to unfamiliar dogs, unfamiliar people and the veterinarian were significantly correlated, suggesting that such information can be useful (see also Duffy *et al.*, 2014).

Canine behavioral assessment continues to evolve, particularly the evaluation of risk for various forms of aggression. Additional work is needed to review the best ages, situations and protocols for reliable and valid assessments, as well as the long-term accuracy of such assessments and factors that may limit the predictive value of such efforts.

9.6   Canine aggression and public policy

Problems associated with canine aggression are the result of complex interactions of genetic, physiological, developmental, environmental and social factors. For many years the most expedient political solution has been to apply the "disease" model and attempt to eliminate the "vector" by banning or otherwise restricting particular breeds, usually those most associated with the extremely rare phenomenon of fatal attacks on humans. This approach has been resoundingly and universally opposed by professionals in veterinary medicine, animal behavior, animal care and control, and animal protection as an approach that is ineffective, costly, epidemiologically unsound, and unfair to responsible owners of affected breeds (AVMA Task Force, 2001; Patronek *et al.*, 2010).

Several studies have reviewed the effectiveness of such policies. In the UK, the Dangerous Dog Act of 1991 did not seem to reduce the number of dog bites to humans caused by restricted breeds over the following two years (Klassen *et al.*, 1996). Longer-term analysis showed bites to have increased 25% since passage of the act (Collier 2006). Martinez *et al.* (2011) report that breeds listed as dangerous in Spain did not display aggressiveness more often than those not listed. Schalke *et al.* (2008) and Ott *et al.* (2008) looked at the results of temperament tests in Germany of 415 dogs receiving compulsory standardized tests and found no significant differences between Golden Retrievers and restricted breeds, resulting in the withdrawal of breed-specific legislation in Lower Saxony. Patronek *et al.* (2010) report additional recent instances of breed-specific regulations being removed in the Netherlands and Italy.

Raghavan *et al.* (2013) looked at a variety of urban and rural jurisdictions in Manitoba, Canada where pit bull bans were identified, and examined differences in dog bite injury hospitalization rates with and without breed-specific legislation (BSL). No actual measures of the degree of implementation or enforcement of BSL were used (e.g. numbers of citations, animals seized, etc.), only whether a community had such legislation on the books and when it was enacted.

Although the authors suggest that, "BSL may have resulted in a reduction of DBIH [dog bite injury hospitalizations] in Winnipeg," the most directly applicable comparison data do not support that conclusion. The only urban population studied other than Winnipeg was Brandon, the second largest city in Manitoba. Brandon has had non-breed-specific dangerous dog legislation since 1994. All the other data analyzed came from rural settings with no documentation of the actual degree of implementation of BSL. No significant differences were observed in the dog bite injury hospitalization rates in Winnipeg relative to Brandon after the implementation of BSL in Winnipeg, with an average overall incidence of 2.84 DBIH per 100 000 person-years in Winnipeg compared to 2.50 in Brandon. The results for victims aged 0 to 20 years followed the same pattern, with an incidence of 5.26 DBIH per 100 000 person years and a rate of 5.99 in Winnipeg pre-BSL and 5.02 post-BSL ($P = 0.247$, NS).

The current legislative landscape remains a patchwork. As of this writing, 13 states in the US currently specifically prohibit the passage of breed-specific laws, while such laws have been upheld in 10 states, although one of these, Ohio, rescinded the breed-specific provisions in 2012 (AVMA, 2013b). Many communities continue to consider such restrictions as a simple "quick-fix" for perceived problems that are deeply rooted in the social, economic and political problems of irresponsible animal ownership and inadequate public health and animal care and control resources.

Problems of irresponsible ownership are not unique to any breed, nor will they be in the future. Effective animal control legislation must emphasize responsible and humane ownership of genetically sound animals, as well as the responsible supervision of children and animals when they interact. Additional recommendations include:

1. Strengthening and enforcing laws against animal cruelty in general and dog fighting in particular.
2. Eliminating the mass-production of poorly bred, unhealthy and unsocialized animals in large-scale "puppy mills."
3. Introducing and enforcing strong animal control laws that place the burden of responsibility for an animal's actions on its owner and providing communities with sufficient resources to enforce these laws.
4. Encouraging programs that educate the public about responsible dog ownership and the problems of dog bite.
5. Refining and evaluating tools for the assessment of dogs in shelters with particular attention to identifying animals at risk of aggression and evaluating the best protocols for addressing such risks through behavioral and/or medical intervention.

9.7   Conclusions

Aggression in general, and aggression to humans, is one of the most complex behaviors in the canine repertoire. It likely has complex genetic, epigenetic, environmental, experiential and even human cultural influences. However, recent research has helped identify those factors that contribute to the risk of adverse consequences of this behavior for dogs and people.

It is possible to protect the health and safety of the public and at the same time preserve the rights of responsible dog owners. By placing greater emphasis on responsible and humane animal care, we can go a long way toward solving these problems and preserving the special human–dog relationship that has developed over thousands of years.

References

American Society for the Prevention of Cruelty to Animals (ASPCA) (2011a). ASPCA SAFER. [Online]. Available: www.aspcapro.org/aspca-safer.php [accessed June 2, 2013].

American Society for the Prevention of Cruelty to Animals (ASPCA) (2011b). *Meet Your Match*. [Online]. Available: www.aspcapro.org/aspcas-meet-your-match.php [accessed June 2, 2013].

American Veterinary Medical Association (AVMA) (2000). *To Whom It May Concern*. [Online]. Available: www.avma.org/Advocacy/StateAndLocal/Documents/javma_000915_fatalattacks.pdf [accessed June 2, 2013].

American Veterinary Medical Association (AVMA) (2013a). *Animal Tethering Prohibitions*. [Online]. Available: https://www.avma.org/Advocacy/StateAndLocal/Pages/sr-animal-tethering-prohibitions.aspx [accessed June 2, 2013].

American Veterinary Medical Association (AVMA) (2013b). *Breed Ordinances*. [Online]. Available: https://www.avma.org/Advocacy/StateAndLocal/Pages/sr-breed-ordinances.aspx [accessed June 2, 2013].

American Veterinary Medical Association Task Force on Canine Aggression and Human-Canine Interactions (AVMA Task Force) (2001). A community approach to dog bite prevention. *Journal of the American Veterinary Medical Association*, 218: 1732–49.

Avis, S. P. (1999) Dog pack attack: hunting humans. *American Journal of Forensic Medicine and Pathology*, 20: 243–6.

Barnes, J. E., Boat, B. E., Putnam, F. W., Dates, H. F. & Mahlman, A. R. (2006). Ownership of high risk ("vicious") dogs as a marker for deviant behaviors: implications for risk assessment. *Journal of Interpersonal Violence*, 21: 1616–34.

Beaver, B. V. (1993). Profiles of dogs presented for aggression. *Journal of the American Animal Hospital Association*, 31: 595–8.

Beaver, B. V. (1994). Owner complaints about canine behaviour. *Journal of the American Veterinary Medical Association*, 204: 1953–5.

Beck, A. M. (1981). The epidemiology of animal bite. *The Compendium on Continuing Education for the Practicing Veterinarian*, 3: 254–8.

Beck, A. M., Loring, H. & Lockwood, R. (1975). The ecology of dog bite. *Public Health Reports*, 90: 262–7.

Berzon, D. R. (1978). The animal bite epidemic in Baltimore, Maryland: review and update. *American Journal of Public Health*, 68: 593–5.

Belyaev, D. K. (1969). Domestication of animals. *Science* 5: 47–52.

Borchelt, P. (1983). Aggressive-behavior of dogs kept as companion animals – classification and influence of sex, reproductive status and breed. *Applied Animal Ethology*, 10: 45–61.

Bradley, J. (2006). *Dog Bites: Problems and Solutions*. Baltimore, MD: Animals and Society Institute.

Bradshaw, J. W. S. & Goodwin, D. (1998). Determination of behavioural traits of pure-bred dogs using factor analysis and cluster analysis; a comparison of studies in the USA and UK. *Research in Veterinary Science*, 66: 73–76.

Brown, S. A., Crowell-Davis, S., Malcom, T. & Edwards, P. (1987). Naloxone-responsive compulsive tail chasing in a dog. *Journal of the American Veterinary Medical Association*, 183: 654–7.

Camps, T., Amat M., Mariotti, V. M., Le Brech, S. & Manteca, X. (2012). Pain-related aggression in dogs: 12 clinical cases. *Journal of Veterinary Behavior: Clinical Applications and Research*, 7: 99–102.

Casey, R. A., Loftus, B., Bolster, C., Richards, G. J. & Blackwell, E. J. (2014). Human directed aggression in domestic dogs (*Canis familiaris*): Occurrence in different contexts and risk factors. *Applied Animal Behaviour Science*, 152: 52–63.

Chang, Y. F., McMahon, J. E., Hennon D. L. *et al.* (1997) Dog bite incidence in the city of Pittsburgh: a capture-recapture approach. *American Journal of Public Health*, 87: 1703–5.

Chapman S., Cornwall, J., Righetti, J. & Sung, L. (2000). Preventing dog bites: randomized controlled trial of an educational intervention. *British Medical Journal*, 320: 1512–13.

Christensen, E., Scarlett, J., Campagna, M. & Houpt, K. A. (2007). Aggressive behavior in adopted dogs that passed a temperament test. *Applied Animal Behaviour Science*, 106: 85–95.

Collier, S. (2006). Breed-specific legislation and the pit bull terrier: are the laws justified? *Journal of Veterinary Behavior*, 1: 17–22.

Cunningham, L. (2005). The case against dog breed discrimination by homeowners' insurance companies. *Connecticut Insurance Law Journal*, 11: 61–129.

DeNapoli J. S., Dodman, N. H., Shuster, L., Rand, W. M. & Gross, K.L. (2000). Effect of dietary protein content and tryptophan supplementation on dominance aggression, territorial aggression, and hyperactivity in dogs. *Journal* of the *American Veterinary Medical Association*, 217: 504–8.

DeViney, L., Dickert, J. & Lockwood, R. (1983). The care of pets within child abusing families. *International Journal for the Study of Animal Problems*, 4: 321–36.

Dodman N. H., Moon R. & Zelin, M. (1996). Influence of owner personality type on expression and treatment outcome of dominance aggression in dogs. *Journal of the American Veterinary Medical Association*, 209: 1107–9.

Dowling-Guyer, S., Marder, A. & D'Arpino, S. (2011). Behavioral traits detected in shelter dogs by a behavior evaluation. *Applied Animal Behaviour Science*, 130: 107–14.

Druzhkova A. S., Thalmann, O., Trifonov, V. A., Vorobieva, N.V. *et al.* (2013). Ancient DNA analysis affirms the canid from Altai as a primitive dog. *PLoS One*, 8: e57754.

Duffy D. L., Hsu, Y. & Serpell, J. A. (2008). Breed differences in canine aggression. *Applied Animal Behaviour Science*, 114: 441–60.

Duffy, D. L., Kruger, K. A. & Serpell, J. A. (2014). Evaluation of a behavioral assessment tool for dogs relinquished to shelters. *Preventive Veterinary Medicine*, 117: 601–9.

Fatjo, J., Amat, M., Mariotti, V. M. *et al.* (2007). Analysis of 1040 cases of canine aggression in a referral practice in Spain. *Journal of Veterinary Behavior: Clinical Applications and Research*, 2: 158–65.

Farhoody, P. (2010). *Behavioral and Physical Effects of Spaying and Neutering Domestic Dogs (Canis familiaris)*. Masters thesis, Hunter College, New York.

Fleig, D. (1996). *Fighting Dog Breeds*. (Translated by W. Charlton). Neptune City, NJ: T.F.H. Publications.

Fox, M. W. (1969). The anatomy of aggression and its ritualization in Canidae: a developmental and comparative study. *Behaviour*, 35: 242–58.

Fox, M. W. (1971). *The Behaviour of Wolves, Dogs and Related Canids*. New York: Harper and Row.

Fox, M. W. & Andrews, R. (1973). Physiological and biochemical correlates of individual differences in behavior of wolf cubs. *Behaviour*, 46: 129–40.

Galac, S. & Knol, B. W. (1997). Fear-motivated aggression in dogs: patient characteristics, diagnosis and therapy. *Animal Welfare*, 6: 9–15.

Gershman, K., Sacks, J. & Wright, J. (1994). Which dogs bite – a case-control study of risk-factors. *Pediatrics* 93: 913–17.

Gladwell, M. (2006). Troublemakers: what pit bulls can teach us about profiling. *New Yorker*, February 6. [Online]. Available: www.gladwell.com/pdf/pitbull.pdf [accessed June 2, 2013].

Goddard, M. E. & Beilharz, R. G. (1983). Genetics of traits which determine the suitability of dogs as guide-dogs for the blind. *Applied Animal Ethology*, 9: 299–315.

Goodloe, L. P. & Borchelt, P. L. (1998). Companion dog temperament traits. *Journal of Applied Animal Welfare Science*, 1: 303–38.

Gorant, J. (2010). *The Lost Dogs: Michael Vick's Dogs and Their Tale of Rescue and Redemption*. New York: Gotham Books.

Goodwin, D., Bradshaw, J. W. S. & Wickens, S. M. (1997). Paedomorphosis affects visual signals of domestic dogs. *Animal Behaviour*, 53: 297–304.

Gray, M. M., Granka, J. M., Bustamante, C. D., Sutter, N. B., Boyko, A. R., Zhu, L., Ostrander, E. A. & Wayne, R. K. (2009). Linkage disequilibrium and demographic history of wild and domestic canids. *Genetics*, 181: 1493–1505. http://doi:10.1534/genetics.108.098830

Guy, N. C., Luescher, U. A., Dohoo, S. E. *et al.* (2001a). A case series of biting dogs: characteristics of the dogs, their behaviour, and their victims. *Applied Animal Behaviour Science*, 74: 43–57.

Guy, N. C., Luescher, U. A., Dohoo, S. E. *et al.* (2001b). Risk factor for dog bites to owner in a general veterinary caseload. *Applied Animal Behaviour Science*, 74: 29–42.

Guy, N. C., Luescher, U. A., Dohoo, S. E. *et al.* (2001c). Demographic and aggressive characteristics of dogs in a general veterinary caseload. *Applied Animal Behaviour Science*, 74: 15–28.

Harris, D., Imperato, P. & Oken, B. (1974). Dog bites – an unrecognized epidemic. *Bulletin of the New York Academy of Medicine*, 50: 81–100.

Hart, B. L. & Hart, L. A. (1985). Selecting pet dogs on the basis of cluster-analysis of breed behavior profiles and gender. *Journal of the American Veterinary Medical Association*, 186: 1181–1185.

Hart, B. L. & Hart, L. A. (1997). Selecting, raising, and caring for dogs to avoid problem aggression. *Journal of the American Veterinary Medical Association*, 210: 1129–34.

Hattaway, D. (1997). Dogs and insurance. *Journal of the American Veterinary Medical Association*, 210: 1143–4.

Hennessy, M. B., Voith, V. L., Mazzei, S. J. *et al.* (2001). Behavior and cortisol levels of dogs in a public animal shelter, and an exploration of the ability of these measures to predict problem behavior after adoption. *Applied Animal Behaviour Science*, 73: 217–33.

Herron, M. E., Shofer, F. S. & Reisner, I. R. (2009). Survey of the use and outcome of confrontational and non-confrontational training methods in client-owner dogs showing undesired behaviors. *Applied Animal Behaviour Science*, 117: 47–54.

Herzog, H. (2006). Forty-two thousand and one Dalmatians: fads, social contagion, and dog breed popularity. *Society and Animals*, 4: 383–98.

Hiby, E. F., Rooney, N. J. & Bradshaw, J. W. S. (2004). Dog training methods: their use, effectiveness and interaction with behavior and welfare. *Animal Welfare*, 13: 63–9.

Holmquist, L. & Elixhauser, A. (2010). Emergency department visits and inpatient stays involved dog bites, 2008. *Healthcare Cost and Utilization Project, Statistic Brief #11*. Rockville (MD): Agency for Health Care Policy and Research.

Hsu, Y. & Serpell, J. A. (2003). Development and validation of a questionnaire for measuring behavior and temperament traits in pet dogs. *Journal of the American Veterinary Medical Association*, 223: 1293–300.

Hughes, G., Maher, J. & Lawson, C. (2011). Status dogs, young people and criminalisation: towards a preventative strategy. RSPCA/Cardiff University Working Paper 139. [Online]. Available: www.cardiff.ac.uk/socsi/research/publications/workingpapers/paper-139.html [accessed December 4, 2013].

Hughes, H. C. & Campbell, S. A. (1989). Effect of primary enclosure size and human contact. In *Canine Research Environment*, eds. J. Mench and L. Krulich. Bethesda, MD: Scientists Center for Animal Welfare, pp. 66–73.

Huss, R. (2008). Lessons learned: acting as guardian/special master in the Bad Newz Kennel case. *Animal Law*, 15: 69–90.

Insurance Information Institute (2012). Prevent dog bites – and a lawsuit; average cost of dog bite claims is on the rise. Press Release May 17, 2012. [Online]. Available: www.iii.org/press_releases [accessed May 3, 2013].

Jalongo M. R. (2008). Beyond a pets theme: teaching young children to interact safely with dogs. *Early Childhood Education*, 36: 39–45.

Jazin, E. (2007). Behaviour genetics in canids. In *The Behavioural Biology of Dogs*, ed. P. Jensen. Cambridge, MA: CABI, pp. 76–90.

Jones, A. (2003) *Red Zone: The Behind the Scenes Story of the San Francisco Dog Mauling*. New York: William Morrow.

Jones, A. C. & Gosling, S. D. (2005). Temperament and personality in dogs (*Canis familiaris*): A review and evaluation of past research. *Applied Animal Behaviour Science*, 95: 1–53.

Jonker F. & Jonker-Bakker, P. (1991). Experiences with ritualistic child sexual abuse: a case study from the Netherlands. *Child Abuse and Neglect*, 15: 191–6.

Kaye A. E., Belz J. M. & Kirschner R. E. (2009). Pediatric dog bite injuries: a 5-year review of the experience at the children's hospital of Philadelphia. *Plastic and Reconstructive Surgery*, 124: 551–558.

Klassen, B., Buckley, J. R. & Esmail, A. (1996). Does the dangerous dog act protect against animal attacks: a prospective study of mammalian bites in the accident and emergency department. *Injury – International Journal of the Care for the Injured*, 27: 89–91.

Kroll, T. L., Houpt, K. A. & Erb, H. N. (2004). The use of novel stimuli as indicators of aggressive behavior in dogs. *Journal of the American Animal Hospital Association*, 40: 13–19.

Kujala M. V., Kujala J., Carlson S. & Hari, R. (2012). Dog experts' brains distinguish socially relevant body postures similarly in dogs and humans. *PLoS One*, 7: e39145.

Kukekova, A. V., Trut, L. N., Chase, K. et al. (2011). Mapping loci for fox domestication: deconstruction/reconstruction of a behavioral phenotype. *Behavior Genetics*, 41: 593–606.

Landsberg, G., Hunthausen, W. & Ackerman, L. (1997). *Handbook of Behaviour Problems of the Dog and Cat*. Oxford: Butterworth Heinemann.

Langley. R. L. (2009). Human fatalities resulting from dog attacks in the United States, 1979–2005. *Wilderness & Environmental Medicine*, 20: 19–25.

Lindberg, J., Bjornerfeldt, S., Saetre, P. et al. (2005). Selection for tameness has changed brain gene expression in silver foxes. *Current Biology*, 15: R915–16.

Lindsay, S. R. (2000). *Handbook of Applied Dog Behavior and Training, Vol. 1*. Iowa City, IA: Iowa State Press.

Line, S. & Voith, V.L. (1986). Dominance aggression of dogs towards people: behavior profile and response to treatment. *Applied Animal Behaviour Science*, 16: 77–83.

Lockwood, R. (1976). *An ethological analysis of social structure and affiliation in captive wolves (Canis lupus)*. Unpublished Ph.D. dissertation, Washington University, St. Louis, Missouri.

Lockwood, R. (1979). Dominance in wolves: useful construct or bad habit? In *The Ecology and Behavior of Wolves*, ed. E. Klinghammer. New York: Garland STM Press, pp. 225–44.

Lockwood, R. & Rindy, K. (1987). Are pit bull terriers different? An analysis of the pit bull terrier controversy. *Anthrozoös*, 1: 2–8.

Lockwood, R. (1988). Humane concerns about dangerous dog laws. *University of Dayton Law Review*, 13: 267–77.

Lockwood, R. (1995). The ethology and epidemiology of canine aggression. In *The Domestic Dog: Its Evolution, Behaviour and Interactions with People*, ed. J. A. Serpell. Cambridge: Cambridge University Press, pp. 131–8.

Lockwood, R. (2011). *Dogfighting Toolkit for Law Enforcement: Addressing Dogfighting in Your Community*. Washington, DC: Community Oriented Policing Services, US Department of Justice.

Lorenz, K. Z. (1953). *Man Meets Dog*. Harmondsworth: Penguin Books.

Love, M. & Overall K. L. (2001), How anticipating relationships between dogs and children can help prevent disasters. *Journal of the American Veterinary Medical Association*, 219: 446–53.

Martinez, A. G., Pernas, G. S., Casalta, J. D., Rey, M. L. S. & Palomino, L. F. D. (2011). Risk factors associated with behavioral problems in dogs. *Journal of Veterinary Behavior*, 6: 225–31.

Marston, L. C. & Bennett, P. C. (2003). Reforging the bond-towards successful canine adoption. *Applied Animal Behaviour Science*, 95: 103–22.

Masuda, K., Hashizume, C., Kikusui, T., Takeuchi, Y. & Mori, Y. (2004). Breed differences in genotype and allele frequency of catechol o-methyltransferase gene polymorphic regions in dogs. *Journal of Veterinary Medical Science*, 66: 183–7.

McGreevy, P. D., Georgevsky, D., Carrasco, J. et al. (2013). Dog behavior covaries with height, bodyweight and skull shape. *PloS One* 8: e80259.

McMillan, F. A., Duffy, D. L. & Serpell, J. A. (2011). Mental health of dogs formerly used as "breeding stock" in commercial breeding establishments. *Applied Animal Behaviour Science*, 135: 86–94.

McMillan, F. D., Duffy, D. L., Zawistowski, Stephen L. & Serpell, J. A. (2015). Behavioral and psychological characteristics of canine victims of abuse. *Journal of Applied Animal Welfare Science*, 18: 92–111.

McMillan, F. D., Vanderstichel, R., Stryhn, H., Yu, J. & Serpell, J. A. (2016). Differences in behavioral characteristics between dogs removed from hoarding situations and a convenience sample of pet dogs. *Applied Animal Behaviour Science*, 178: 69–79.

Mead, P. C. (2006). Police and domestic dog bite injuries: what are the differences? What are the implications about police dog use? *Injury Extra*, 37: 395–401.

Mech, L. D. (1970). *The Wolf*. New York: Natural History Press.

Mize, M. D. (2010). Definition of "gameness." *Sporting Dog Journal*, September, p. 22.

More, R. M., Zehmer, R. B., Moultbrop, J. I. & Parker, R. L. (1977). Surveillance of animal bites cases in the United States: 1971–1972. *Archives of Environmental Health*, 32: 267–70.

Neilson, J. C., Eckstein, R. A. & Hart, B. L. (1997). Effects of castration on male dogs with reference to the role of age and experience. *Journal of the American Veterinary Medical Association*, 211: 180–2.

Netto, W. J. and Planta, D. J. U. (1997). Behavioural testing for aggression in the domestic dog. *Applied Animal Behaviour Science*, 52: 243–63.

O'Sullivan E. N., Jones, B. R., O'Sullivan, K. & Hanlon, A. J. (2008). The management and behavioural history of 100 dogs reported for biting a person. *Applied Animal Behaviour Science*, 114: 149–58.

Oswald, M. (1991). Report on the Potentially Dangerous Dog Program: Multnomah County, Oregon. *Anthrozoös*, 4: 247–54.

Ott, S. A., Schalke, E., von Gaertner, A. M. & Hackbarth, H. (2008). Is there a difference? Comparison of golden retrievers and dogs affected by breed-specific legislation regarding aggressive behavior. *Journal of Veterinary Behavior: Clinical Applications and Research*, 3: 134–40.

Overall, K. L. (1997). *Clinical Behavioral Medicine for Small Animals*. St. Louis, MO: Mosby.

Overall, K. L. & Love, M. (2001). Dog bites to humans – demography, epidemiology, injury, and risk. *Journal of the American Veterinary Medical Association*, 218: 1923–34.

Parker, H. G. & Ostrander, E. A. (2005). Canine genomics and genetics: Running with the pack. *PLoS Genetics*, 1: e58.

Patronek, G. J. & Slavinski, S. A. (2009). Animal bites. *Journal of the American Veterinary Medical Association*, 234: 336–45.

Patronek, G. J., Slater, M. & Marder, A. (2010). Use of a number-needed-to-ban calculation to illustrate limitations of breed-specific legislation in decreasing the risk of dog bite-related injury *Journal of the American Veterinary Medical Association*, 237, 788–92.

Patronek, G. J., Sacks, J. J., Delise, K. M., Cleary, D. V. & Marder, A. R. (2013). Co-occurrence of potentially preventable factors in 256 dog bite-related fatalities in the United States (2000–2009). *Journal of the American Veterinary Medical Association*, 243: 1726–36.

Pavlov, I. P. (1941). *Lectures on Conditioned Reflexes, vol. 2. Conditioned Reflexes and Psychiatry*. (Translated by W. Horsley Gantt). New York: International Publishers.

Pinckney, L. E. & Kennedy, L. A. (1982). Traumatic deaths from dog attacks in the United States. *Pediatrics*, 39: 193–6.

Podberscek, A. L. & Blackshaw, J. K. (1993). A survey of dog bites in Brisbane, Australia. *Australian Veterinary Practitioner*, 23: 178–83.

Ragatz, L., Fremouw, W., Thomas, T. & McCoy, K. (2009). Vicious dogs: the antisocial behaviors and psychological characteristics of owners. *Journal of Forensic Science*, 54: 699–703.

Raghavan, M., Martens, P. J., Chateau, D. & Burchill, C. (2013). Effectiveness of breed-specific legislation in decreasing the incidence of dog-bite injury and hospitalizations in people in the Canadian province of Manitoba. *Injury Prevention*, 19: 177–83.

Reid, P. (2013). Animal behavior forensics: evaluation of dangerous dogs and cruelty victims. In *Shelter Medicine for Veterinarians and Staff*, 2nd edition, eds. L. Miller and S. Zawistowski. Ames, IA: John Wiley & Sons, pp. 559–67.

Reinhard, D. W. (1978). Aggressive behavior associated with hypothyroidism. *Canine Practice*, 5: 69–70

Reisner, I. R. (1991). The pathophysiologic basis of behavior problems. *Veterinary Clinics of North America*, 1: 207–24.

Reisner, I. R., Erb, H. N. & Houpt, K. A. (1994). Risk factors for behaviour-related euthanasia among dominant-aggressive dogs: 110 cases (1989–1992). *Journal of the American Veterinary Medical Association*, 205: 855–63.

Reisner I. R., Nance, M. L, Zeller, J. S. *et al.* (2011). Behavioural characteristics associated with dog bites to children presenting to an urban trauma centre. *Injury Prevention*, 17: 348–53.

Roll, A. & Unshelm, J. (1997). Aggressive conflicts amongst dogs and factors affecting them. *Applied Animal Behaviour Science*, 52: 229–42.

Royce, J. R. (1955). A factorial study of emotionality in the dog. *Psychological Monographs: General and Applied*, 69: 1–27.

Sacks, J. J., Sattin, R. W. & Bonzo, S. E. (1989). Dog bite-related fatalities from 1979 through 1988. *Journal of the American Medical Association*, 262: 1489–92.

Sacks, J. J., Lockwood, R., Hornreich, J. & Sattin, R. W. (1996). Fatal dog attacks, 1989–1994. *Pediatrics*, 97: 891–5.

Sacks, J. J., Sinclair, L., Gilchrist, J., Golab, G. & and Lockwood, R. (2000). Breeds of dogs involved in fatal human attacks in the United States between 1979 and 1998. *Journal of the American Veterinary Medical Association*, 217: 836–40.

Salman, M. D., New Jr., J. G., Scarlett, J. M. *et al.* (1998). Human and animal factors related to relinquishment of dogs and cats in 12 selected animal shelters in the United States. *Journal of Applied Animal Welfare Science*, 1: 207–26.

Salman, M. D., Hutchison, J., Ruch-Gallie, R. *et al.* (2000). Behavioral reasons for relinquishment of dogs and cats to 12 shelters. *Journal of Applied Animal Welfare Science*, 3: 93–106.

Schalke E., Ott, S. A., Gaertner, A. M., Mittmann, A. & Hackbarth, H. (2008). Is breed specific legislation justified: Study of the results of the temperament test of Lower Saxony. *Journal of Veterinary Behavior*, 3: 97–103.

Schenk, A. M., Ragatz, L. L. & Fremouw, W. J. (2012). Vicious dogs part 2: criminal thinking, callousness, and personality styles of their owners. *Journal of Forensic Science*, 57: 152–9.

Schenkel, R. (1967). Submission: its features and function in the wolf and dog. *American Zoologist*, 7: 319–29.

Schuler, C. M., DeBess, E. E., Lapidus, J. A. & Hedberg, K. (2008). Canine and human factors related to dog bite injuries. *Journal of the American Veterinary Medical Association*, 232: 542–6.

Scott, J. P. & Frederickson, E. (1951). The causes of fighting in mice and rats. *Physiological Zoology*, 26: 273–309.

Scott, J. P. & Fuller, J. L. (1965). *Genetics and Social Behavior of the Dog*. Chicago, IL: University of Chicago Press.

Semencic, C. (1991). *Pit Bulls and Tenacious Guard Dogs*. Neptune City, NJ: T.F.H. Publications.

Shearin A. L. & Ostrander E. A. (2010) Canine morphology: Hunting for genes and tracking mutations. *PLoS Biol*, 8: e1000310.

Spady T. C. & Ostrander, E. A. (2008). Canine behavioral genetics: Pointing out the phenotypes and herding up the genes. *The American Journal of Human Genetics*, 82: 10–18.

Spiegel, I. B. (2000). A pilot study to evaluate an elementary school-based dog bite prevention program. *Anthrozoös*, 13: 164–73.

Stephen, J. & Ledger, R. (2007). Relinquishing dog owners' ability to predict behavioural problems in shelter dogs post adoption. *Applied Animal Behaviour Science*, 107: 88–99

Svartberg, K. (2005). A comparison of behavior in test and in everyday life: evidence of three consistent boldness-related personality traits in dogs. *Applied Animal Behaviour Science*, 91: 103–28.

Takeuchi, Y. & Mori, Y. (2006). A comparison of the behavioral profiles of purebred dogs in Japan to profiles of those in the United States and the United Kingdom. *Journal of Veterinary Medical Science*, 68: 789–96.

Tan, R. L., Powell, K. E., Lindemer, K. M. *et al.* (2004). Sensitivities of three county health department surveillance systems for child-related dog bites: 261 cases (2000). *Journal of the American Veterinary Medical Association*, 225: 1680–3.

Trut, L. N. (1999). Early canid domestication: The farm-fox experiment. *American Scientist*, 87, 160–9.

Våge, J., Bønsdorf, T. B., Arnet, E., Tverdal, A. & Lingaas, F. (2010). Differential gene expression in brain tissues of aggressive and non-aggressive dogs. *BMC Veterinary Research 2*, 6: 34. [Online]. Available: www.biomedcentral.com/1746–6148/6/34 [accessed April 15, 2013].

van den Berg, L., Schilder, M. B. H. & Knol, B. W. (2003). Behavior genetics of canine aggression: behavioral phenotyping of golden retrievers by means of an aggression test. *Behaviour Genetics*, 33: 469–83.

van den Berg, L., Kwant, L., Hestand, M. S., van Oost, B. A. & Leegwater, P. A. (2005). Structure and variation of three canine genes involved in serotonin binding and transport: the serotonin receptor 1a gene (htr1a), serotonin receptor 2a gene (htr2a), and serotonin transporter gene (slc6a4). *Journal of Heredity*, 96: 786–96.

Vaisman-Tzachor, R. (2001). Could family dog bites raise suspicion of child abuse? *The Forensic Examiner*, September/October, pp. 18–25.

Varner, J. G. & Varner, J. J. (1983). *Dogs of the Conquest*. Norman, OK: University of Oklahoma Press.

Vila, C., Savolainen, P., Maldonado, J. E. *et al.* (1997). Multiple and ancient origins of the domestic dog. *Science*, 276: 1687–9.

Voith, V. L., Ingram, E. & Mitsouras, K. (2009). Comparison of adoption agency breed identification and DNA breed identification of dogs. *Journal of Applied Animal Welfare Science*, 12: 253–62.

Voith, V. L., Trevejo, R. & Dowling-Guyer, S. *et al.* (2013). Comparison of visual and DNA breed identification of dogs and inter-observer reliability. *American Journal of Sociological Research*, 3: 17–29

vonHoldt, B. M., Pollinger, J. P., Lohmueller, K. E. *et al.* (2010). Genome-wide SNP and haplotype analyses reveal a rich history underlying dog domestication. *Nature*, 464: 898–902.

Weiss, H. B., Friedman, D. I. & Jeffrey, H. (1998). Incidence of dog bite injuries treated in emergency departments. *Journal of the American Medical Association*, 279: 51–3.

Weiss, E. & Mohan-Gibbons, H. (2013). Behavior evaluation, adoption and follow-up. In *Shelter Medicine for Veterinarians and Staff*, 2nd edition., eds. L. Miller and S. Zawistowski. Ames, IA: John Wiley & Sons, pp. 531–9.

Wilson F., Dwyer F. & Bennett P. C. (2003). Prevention of dog bites: evaluation of a brief educational intervention program for preschool children. *Journal of Community Psychology*, 31: 75–86.

Wright, J. C. & Nesselrote, M. (1987). Classification of behavior problems in dogs – distributions of age, breed, sex and reproductive status. *Applied Animal Behaviour Science*, 19: 169–78.

Yeon, S. C., Golden, G., Sung, W. *et al.* (2001). A comparison of tethering and pen confinement of dogs. *Journal of Applied Animal Welfare Science*, 4: 257–70.

10 Social cognition and emotions underlying dog behavior

FRIEDERIKE RANGE AND ZSÓFIA VIRÁNYI

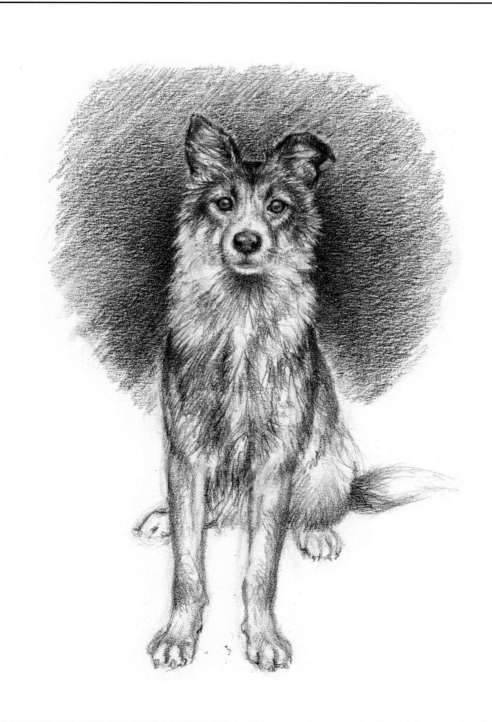

10.1   Introduction

Since domestication began more than 10 000 years ago (Pang *et al.*, 2009; see also Clutton-Brock, Chapter 2; vonHoldt & Driscoll, Chapter 3), dogs have been living in a human-dominated niche in which they are likely to enjoy advantages if they are able to communicate and cooperate success-fully with people (Miklósi *et al.*, 2004; Bradshaw & Rooney, Chapter 8). As such, dogs are thought to have evolved cognitive-emotional traits analogous to the social skills that differentiate humans from other primates (Hare *et al.*, 2005; Topál *et al.*, 2009a). Accordingly, investigating the cognition of domestic dogs provides a potentially exciting opportunity to reveal which cognitive traits have functional relevance in the present social life of humans (Virányi *et al.*, 2008a).

Recent intensive research focusing on dogs' social interactions and communication with humans has revealed that dogs perform more like humans in some communicative and cooperative tasks than any other animal species (Lakatos *et al.*, 2009; Soproni *et al.*, 2001). In some of these tasks, dogs outperform other species that are more closely related to humans, such as chimpanzees (*Pan troglodytes*) (Brauer *et al.*, 2006; Hare *et al.*, 2002; but see Mulcahy & Hedge, 2012). These intrigu-ing dog–human similarities are often assumed to originate from the dog's adaptation to the human environment, and are partly due to their life-long experiences with humans and the influence that this exerts on their cognitive development (Udell *et al.*, 2010, Miklósi & Tópal, 2011). Dogs typically grow up in human families and develop attachments and dependent relationships analogous to those between children and their parents (Topál *et al.*, 1998). This developmental environment can foster a variety of mechanisms ranging from classical conditioning (Bentosela *et al.*, 2008) to more complex modifications of cognitive and emotional processes, such as the ontogenetic process of "encultura-tion" that has been proposed to result in enhanced cognitive abilities in non-human primates raised by humans (Hare *et al.*, 2005). Consequently, many argue that dog behavior and cognition have been modified in ways that help dogs to be socially integrated into human groups.

For both theoretical and practical reasons, it is important to ask to what extent aspects of dog behavior and cognition have either been genetically modified during the course of domestication or altered by individual experiences and training. The domestic dog offers a special opportunity to hypothesize about the evolutionary changes that contributed to the cognitive abilities of both dogs and humans. Since it is generally assumed that wolves, the closest wild-living relatives of dogs (Savolainen *et al.*, 2002; Scott & Fuller, 1965), still strongly resemble the common ancestor of dogs and wolves, we can investigate how domestication changed the behavior and cognition of dogs in comparison to that of wolves. For this purpose, however, we need to raise dogs and wolves in identical conditions in order to provide them with similar learning opportunities and developmental influences (Frank & Frank, 1982a; Kubinyi *et al.*, 2007; Range & Virányi, 2015). And we need to compare differently reared populations of both dogs and wolves to uncover the relative impor-tance of the genetic predispositions and learning processes that enable dogs to live in human groups (Miklósi & Topál, 2011; Udell *et al.*, 2012).

10.2   Social cognition and emotions: Tools to live in human groups

Because of the unique evolutionary and individual histories of dogs, the scientific study of their cognition and behavior is mainly focused on searching for skills that may be analogous to human characteristics (see Topál *et al.*, 2009a for a review). Dogs have been selected, and learn individually, to live in human groups, to accept humans as social partners, and to cooperate and communicate with humans. Comparing the cognitive abilities of dogs, wolves, and humans can therefore teach us indirectly about the evolution and development of human cognition. This research also has considerable practical relevance by contributing to the development of socialization and training techniques that can facilitate the cooperation and coexistence of humans and the many millions of dogs living in the human environment. Thus, there are good practical and theoretical reasons why the domestic dog has been studied from an anthropocentric perspective in recent decades. Here we review the available literature using a structure based on the current categorization of human cognitive skills. In humans, some of these skills are relatively simple while others are thought to involve more advanced cognitive processes, and accordingly are developed at earlier or later ages.

10.3   The focus of dogs' attention: Whom do they observe?

In social species, one of the most crucial sources of information is the behavior and interactions of other individuals. Paying attention to companions and monitoring their behavior enables individuals to make better decisions when engaging in cooperative or competitive social interactions, or when responding to changes in their environment. Paying attention to others is obviously needed for communication as well as for learning from others. For domestic dogs, the behavior of human social partners is probably just as important as the behavior of conspecifics. However, the human world is also exceedingly complex with an enormous amount of information available and new situations occurring every day. Dogs therefore need to be highly selective about what they pay attention to. Moreover, when we interact and work with our dogs, we also want them to be primarily attentive to us and not to another dog, cat, or person who happens to be in the vicinity. Confirming this, it has been shown that dogs pay more attention to a person than to a remotely moved object, even at earlier ages when they tend to be most interested in such objects (Wallis et al., 2014).

In other animals, especially primates, visual attention between group members is related systematically to hierarchical ranks (McNelis et al., 1998). Moore et al. (1991) suggested that looking at others provides a direct measure of social interest, and dominant animals have repeatedly been found to receive the most visual attention within a group compared to other group members (e.g. Chance & Jolly, 1970). Other studies have found an influence of familiarity and relatedness on the pattern of transmission of socially acquired behaviors, indicating higher attentiveness towards familiar individuals – e.g. chickens, Gallus g. domesticus (Nicol & Pope, 1994), chimpanzees (Menzel, 1974, 1997), and Japanese macaques, Macaca fuscata (Nishida, 1987).

Only a few studies to date have focused on social attention in dogs (see Virányi et al., 2008a for a review). One study, investigating the selectivity of attention towards various partners – human and dog – used a "two-hole" procedure (Range et al., 2009a). The dogs were separated from a conspecific or a human model by an opaque screen with two holes that allowed visual access to the activities of the models on the other side. Results showed that overall the dogs paid more attention to the human demonstrator than to the dog demonstrator. Dogs looked for a longer duration in the case of a human demonstrator but not more often, which means that a human could hold the attention of the dogs longer than a conspecific could. The finding that the dogs' attentiveness is not necessarily affected by the identity of the human demonstrator was further supported by a detour task in which dogs learnt with the same efficiency from their owner and from a stranger how to detour around a V-shaped fence to gain access to a reward (Pongrácz *et al.*, 2001, 2004). However, a later study, using a different paradigm in which the owner and a stranger walk simultaneously through a room (thereby forcing the dogs to be selective about who to attend to), found that the dogs showed clear preferential attention towards their owners (Mongillo *et al.*, 2010). This study was the first to demonstrate that the nature of the dog–human relationship influences dogs' attention towards human companions.

Another study investigated whether this preference towards the owner was driven by the familiarity between owner and dog or by the quality of the relationship (Horn *et al.*, 2013). In this experiment, dogs watched the owner, another familiar person living with the dog in the same household, and an unfamiliar experimenter, one at a time visit three boxes that they either merely looked at, touched, or manipulated. Interestingly, the dogs attended significantly more to the familiar humans from their household than to an unfamiliar experimenter when both familiar humans shared responsibility for the care of the dog (e.g. both went for walks, did training with the dog, and fed the dog regularly). However, if only the owner spent active time with the dog, the dogs paid the same amount of attention to the familiar person as to the completely unfamiliar experimenter. A part of this effect may be that training exercises seem to increase the amount of time dogs are ready to spend focusing on their human partner at least in situations that the dogs may perceive as training or working (Wallis *et al.*, 2015).

Overall, these findings confirm that pet dogs pay special attention to humans and especially to their owners with whom they usually have a more interactive relationship. Given the strong attachment between owners and dogs (Tópal *et al.*, 2005), this is not very surprising. Still, it is an intriguing question whether this close and selective attention is an expression of emotional dependency or a form of information seeking. Initial evidence for the latter comes from a study in which dogs were tested for their ability to use emotional information about a novel (scary) object or person provided by the owner – so-called social referencing. It was found that over 80% of the dogs looked back at their owner after looking at the object, suggesting that they were seeking information from their owner rather than seeking emotional support (Duranton *et al.*, 2016; Merola *et al.*, 2012a). This conclusion was supported by the fact that it was primarily the less confident dogs that looked back at their owners, and they did so rather than approaching them, a result that would not have been expected if they were seeking emotional reassurance. Even more convincingly, a further study showed that social referencing occurs equally regardless of whether a stranger or a familiar person conveys the emotional message about the object (Merola *et al.*, 2012b).

10.4   Social learning

Learning from others what kind of food to eat, where to find it, how to behave with conspecifics, and where to hide in case of a predator attack, is thought to be less costly, both in regard to the energy that needs to be invested as well as the risk of making mistakes (e.g. eating poisonous food), than if each individual has to gather the necessary information independently. Accordingly, it has been shown in many species that individuals can benefit from observing others. However, while many species can learn from others about a specific location or where to manipulate an object to obtain food (local and stimulus enhancement; Spence, 1997), learning new behaviors by copying the movements of a demonstrator (imitation; Heyes, 1993; Thorndike, 1898; Thorpe, 1956) is probably rare in the animal kingdom. Here we review the various mechanisms of social learning in dogs.

10.4.1   Learning about places and objects via observation

Almost every dog owner has observed his/her dog investigating a spot on the ground that another dog has inspected shortly beforehand. Heberlein & Turner (2009) used a similar scenario to show that having snout contact with a demonstrator dog immediately after observing it finding food in a location invisible to the observer increased the latter's motivation to search for food in this location. This suggests that while the dogs used the visual information provided by the demonstrator, further cues (e.g. smell of food on the other's muzzle) were necessary to provide the right context to use it. One situation in which dogs typically perform quite poorly is if they have to make a detour in order to reach an attractive goal. Pongrácz *et al.* (2001) used this problem to investigate how demonstrations of a human or dog influence if and what adult dogs learn from a demonstration. In their paradigm, a reward (food or toy) was placed at the inside apex of a V-shaped fence and the dogs had to detour around the fence in order to reach the reward (Figure 10.1). Dogs benefited from both human and dog demonstrations, but without the demonstrations they usually tried to reach the reward by

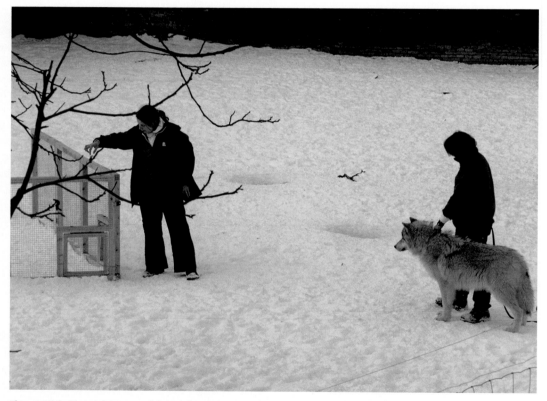

Figure 10.1 General set-up of the V-shape fence studies. The food is dropped in the corner of the V so that the animal can see it (in the present picture a wolf). Afterwards the demonstrator either returns directly to the starting position behind the waiting subject or first demonstrates how to detour the fence to get to the food. Once the demonstrator has reached her position behind the subject, the subject is released and the time it takes to detour the fence to get to the reward is measured. Without a demonstration, dogs usually paw or dig at the place closest to the food reward. (© Lisa Wallis, reprinted with permission.)

digging at the spot closest to it (Pongrácz *et al.*, 2001). Other studies have used a box with a reward (food or toy) hidden inside that could be opened by manipulating a lever. In general, dogs also performed better in these tasks after observing a human (Kubinyi *et al.*, 2003; Range *et al.*, 2009b) or dog (Range *et al.*, 2009b) demonstration.

How much dogs can profit from a human or dog demonstrator in the detour task depends on the communicative cues used by the human (see below) as well as on the demonstrator dog's social status (as assessed by their owners) relative to the observer dog: socially subordinate dogs learn better from an unfamiliar dog demonstrator than dominant ones do, while socially dominant dogs learn better from humans (Pongrácz *et al.*, 2008, 2012). Although this and other studies show that dogs pay attention to the details of a demonstration (e.g., to whether or not the model hides food at a certain location; Range & Virány, 2013), the demonstration need not involve a social component. Mersmann *et al.* (2011) showed that dogs were just as successful at solving a detour problem when a partial "demonstration" was provided by an object (a box on wheels) that was pulled around the end of the fence by means of a concealed rope.

10.4.2   Imitation

Whether or not dogs can imitate is an on-going debate. One recent study showed that wolves are better imitators than pack-living dogs (Range & Virányi, 2014), and there are contradictory results also on pet dogs. Tennie and colleagues (2009) examined whether dogs that observed another dog that had been trained to "sit" or "lie down" in response to an unfamiliar command would imitate the same action when placed in the same situation and exposed to the same command. No evidence for imitation was found in a group of 180 dogs, regardless of whether or not they had been previously trained on the action (sit or lie down). In contrast, two other studies found some evidence that, under certain circumstances, dogs are able to imitate. The first study showed that dogs imitated the direction a screen was pushed more often if another dog pushed it than in a control situation when the screen was moved remotely while the demonstrator dog observed passively (Miller *et al.*, 2009). Interestingly, if a human was used as a demonstrator, the dogs still matched the direction the screen was pushed but they also did so if the human was present but the screen moved independently. The latter observation suggests that the dogs were emulating (i.e. learning how the environment works) rather than imitating.

Another study using a dog demonstrator also reported positive findings for imitative abilities in dogs. In this case, two groups of dogs were required to pull down a wooden rod to open a food container to gain a reward after observing another dog perform this action with her paw. The first group saw the demonstrator do this while carrying a ball in her mouth and the second group saw her do the same thing without a ball (Range *et al.*, 2007) (Figure 10.2). In a previous trial, a control group of dogs (who saw no demonstration) showed that they preferred to use their mouths to pull down the wooden rod, but in the experiment only the dogs in the second group copied the demonstrated paw action to obtain food from the apparatus. In other words, the observers only copied the demonstrated action when the demonstrator had the opportunity to use the preferred action (because her mouth was free) but used the paw instead to solve the problem. When the demonstrator was seemingly obliged to perform the less preferred action by the constraint of carrying a ball in her mouth, the observers used the preferred action (their mouths) to solve the problem (although see Kaminski *et al.*, 2011a, for an alternative interpretation, and Huber *et al.*, 2011, for a commentary on that paper). Selective imitation of this type has been observed in human infants, and it has been argued that it is important for the transmission of cultural knowledge where learners have to identify what relevant information to retain from observing others' behavior (Gergely *et al.*, 2002).

(a)

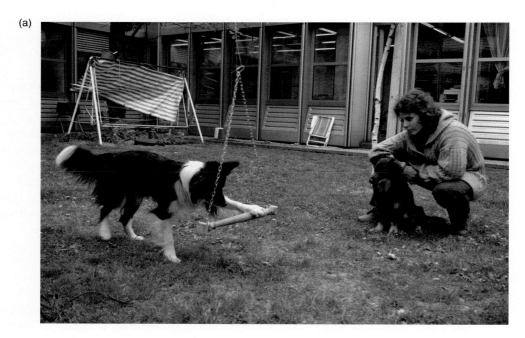

(b)

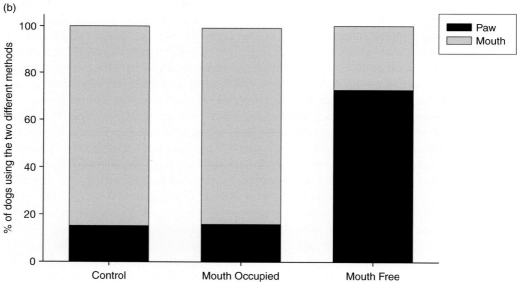

Figure 10.2 The procedure for a social learning experiment in which the "model" dog demonstrates the action (pushing the rod down with the paw), while the observer watches. After several demonstrations, the observer is allowed to try to manipulate the apparatus (a). The graph (b) depicts the proportion of dogs using their paw or only their mouth to manipulate the apparatus in the control group (left bar) and after watching the paw action used by the demonstrator dog under the two experimental conditions (middle bar, model had mouth occupied; right bar, model had mouth free), recorded in the first trial. Black, paw action was imitated; light grey, only mouth action was used. (© Friederike Range; Range *et al.*, 2007.) (A black and white version of this figure will appear in some formats. For the color version, please refer to the plate section.)

Further support for the claim that dogs are capable of imitation comes from two other studies using a "Do-As-I-Do" paradigm to investigate how well dogs are able to match the actions of a human demonstrator. In this paradigm, the dog is first taught to repeat a set of human-demonstrated actions on command ("Do it!") (Figure 10.3). In the testing phase, the dog is then confronted with untrained novel actions that it is asked to repeat. Two dogs, a male Belgian Tervueren "Philip" (Topál *et al.*, 2006) and a female Weimaraner "Joy" (Huber *et al.*, 2009), learned the task, but showed the same limitations with regard to the degree of matching of novel actions. As with apes (Call, 2001), the dogs were not particularly sensitive to the details of the actions, but mostly achieved a functional fit. They also showed superior performance with object manipulations (e.g. putting a ball into a basket) in comparison to body-oriented movements (e.g. lifting a paw). Their actions seemed to be goal-directed and object-bound. For example, if a demonstrator pretended to jump over a hurdle, Joy did not repeat this "senseless" action, but went to the actual hurdle to jump over it. Finally, shortcuts revealed that the dogs were often driven by efficiency (Range *et al.*, 2007).

10.4.3   Teaching dogs: Evoking attention and facilitating social learning?

Earlier we suggested that social learning may depend strongly on how much the observer uses the opportunity of watching a model during a demonstration. In humans, we usually make sure that the observer is actually paying attention to us when we demonstrate something new by establishing eye contact and actively calling the attention (so-called ostensive-communicative cues) of the observer to our actions. This is an important aspect of teaching (Caro & Hauser, 1992). In animals, the "models" typically do not address the observers – only a few studies report active "teaching" behavior on the part of an animal demonstrator (Boesch, 1991; Thornton & Mcauliffe, 2006). Importantly, however, although animal demonstrators do not typically call the attention of their observers, this does not exclude them from being influenced by a human demonstrator's ostensive-communicative cues addressing them and calling their attention.

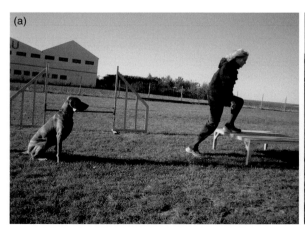 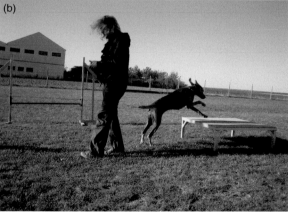

Figure 10.3 The "Do-As-I-Do" paradigm: The owner demonstrates an action (a), and then the owner tells the dog to "do-it." Here, the dog copies the correct action by jumping on the table (b), even though other possibilities were present e.g. jumping over the hurdle. (© Friederike Range.) (A black and white version of this figure will appear in some formats. For the color version, please refer to the plate section.)

Compared to other animals, domestic dogs seem to be especially sensitive to human attention-calling cues (Kis *et al.*, 2012; Topál *et al.*, 2009b). For example, in a test situation in which they had to choose one of two containers, dogs relied more on human direction than on their own first-hand knowledge of where a reward could be found (Szetei *et al.*, 2003). Dogs also chose one treat instead of eight, if a human called their attention to the single treat, even if previously they had displayed a preference for the larger number of treats (Marshall-Pescini *et al.*, 2011a).

Similar sensitivity of dogs to human ostensive communicative cues has also been shown in social learning situations. Kupán *et al.* (2011) let dogs observe either a communicative or a non-communicative demonstration in which a human retrieved a tennis ball from an opaque container by manipulating another distant and obviously empty (transparent) one. Invisible to the dogs, the two containers were connected by means of a string so that the demonstrator could lift the opaque container by moving the empty transparent one horizontally. Dogs that observed a communicative demonstration were more successful than dogs observing a non-communicative demonstration in retrieving the tennis ball when they had to make their own choice. Similarly, in the V-fence studies mentioned above, observing a human walk around the fence only enhances the dogs' detouring performance if the human is talking to the do∂g during the demonstration (Pongrácz *et al.*, 2004). Interestingly, although communicative cues were required if a human demonstrated the detour, this was not necessary if another dog demonstrated the detour, suggesting that dogs actually have different expectations of a human than of a conspecific demonstrator in regards to communication.

In another study, the influence of (1) human ostensive cues and (2) the type of demonstrator (human vs. dog), as well as the interaction between these two factors, was investigated systematically (Range *et al.*, 2009b). Despite slight differences in attention to the different demonstrators, the presence of human or dog demonstrators exerted equal influence on the test performance of the dogs. However, in this experiment the ostensive-communicative cues during the demonstrations were given by somebody other than the demonstrator, and this appeared to distract the test dogs from closely watching the demonstration. This distraction increased the dogs' level of excitement as noted by increased pulling on the leash, and thereby may have reduced their performance. This suggests that precise timing and synchronization of attention-getting ostensive signals are necessary to avoid this distraction effect.

It is clear that dogs can learn from observing humans as well as conspecifics, but it seems that the former process is more dependent on ostensive communication than learning from other dogs. While dogs seem to be capable of imitation, this is clearly not their most typical way of learning from others. Moreover, it is important to pay attention to several factors to facilitate social learning in dogs, such as giving communicative cues in a way that is not too distracting or over-motivating, and choosing a demonstrator with the appropriate social status relative to the observer dogs. Care must also be exercised to avoid dogs selectively learning something other than what is intended. Nevertheless, simple forms of social learning (e.g. local enhancement) probably constitute strong mechanisms to learn about the social and physical environment, and should be integral to the training and education of dogs. One of the first studies on social learning in working dogs showed that watching their mothers locating and retrieving sachets of narcotics improved the pups' ability to perform the same task three months later in comparison to a control group lacking this experience (Slabbert *et al.*, 1997). More recently, the "Do as I do!" paradigm has been proposed and utilized broadly to train dogs (Fugazza & Miklósi, 2014). Using social learning in addition to indvidual learning based techniques (operant and classical conditioning) could significantly reduce the time to train dogs in particular tasks.

10.5   Referential communication

The previous examples illustrate clearly that a dog's approach towards an object can be strongly influenced by the way humans manipulate the object while communicating with the dog. However, this kind of referential communication is still very different in comparison to how humans typically communicate: we can talk about persons and objects that are not even present in the given situation and still our partner will know to whom or what we are referring. Humans use not only words but also other symbols (e.g. sign language, traffic signs) to recall different referents (objects, persons, situations, etc.) in others' minds. In contrast, dogs do not communicate using symbolic language. They do, however, produce context-specific barks (Yin & McCowan, 2004) that humans can correctly classify as aggressive, fearful, distressed, playful, or happy even if they have little experience with dogs (Pongrácz et al., 2005, 2006). Thus, dog barks are functionally informative, and can call our attention to something we might not notice otherwise, for example during hunting or guarding.

10.5.1   Comprehension of referential communication: humans informing dogs

The inability of dogs to speak our language does not mean that they are incapable of understanding our words, or of connecting objects and persons to their names. Indeed, a handful of studies have demonstrated that dogs can learn the names of several hundreds of objects such as toys. If asked, they can fetch the right object based on its individual name even if it is located in another room and the owner or experimenter cannot give any visual cues to help the dogs choose (Griebel & Oller, 2012; Kaminski et al., 2004; Pilley & Reid, 2011). While these dogs can also retrieve the correct object if shown a small replica of the toy, photos of the toy are not sufficient to trigger retrieval (Kaminski et al., 2009a). Interestingly, these dogs do not just have a prodigious memory for hundreds of words but they seem to learn the words by reasoning by exclusion (which is defined as the selection of the correct alternative by logically excluding other potential alternatives; Call, 2006). If sent into a room containing lots of familiar toys, they can map a newly heard word to the *one* new toy in the room and retain that information – a process referred to as fast mapping. The same process supports rapid word learning in human toddlers.

Although learning by exclusion seems to be within the capacities of many dogs (Aust et al., 2008), knowing the names of hundreds of objects seems to remain the privilege of a few exceptionally motivated and extensively trained individuals. This is not so surprising given that, in everyday situations, dogs tend to rely on non-semantic aspects of verbal commands, such as the tone of voice, body posture and proximity of humans (i.e. Fukuzawa et al., 2005). It has been proposed, however, that certain directional behaviors, e.g. pointing and gazing at an object, can be the evolutionary (or, in prelinguistic infants, developmental) precursor of linguistic referential signals (Senju & Csibra, 2008). For example, looking at an object can help the receiver to identify what the signaler is referring to. It is likely that using such non-verbal forms of referential communication is more typical of the majority of dogs than being able to identify numerous objects based on their names.

A wide range of animal species (primates, corvids, goats, wolves, and tortoises) has been shown to follow the direction of others' gaze (Fitch et al., 2010; see Range & Virányi, 2011 for a review). This suggests that this behavior is based on a socially facilitated orientation response (i.e. a predisposition to look where others are looking) (Povinelli & Eddy, 1996) that requires no more than an intrinsic tendency to co-orient with others, combined with associative learning (Tomasello et al., 1999;

Triesch *et al.*, 2006). In spite of this, for a long time the only study that had been published on dogs following others' gaze into distant space without having a well-defined object to look at, reported negative results (Agnetta *et al.*, 2000). More recently, however, it has been found that pack-living dogs follow the gaze of their conspecific pack mates as well as wolves (Werhahn *et al.*, 2016), and pet dogs also follow human gaze if it has clearly been addressed to them (Met *et al.*, 2014; Wallis *et al.*, 2015). The latter study also showed that, paradoxically, training dogs for eye-contact with humans actually hinders gaze following, which is one factor contributing to the astonishing difference between dogs and other animals in regard to this simple form of gaze following.

In contrast, dogs perform well when following human-given directional cues in another situation; e.g. if a human is indicating which of two containers is baited with food (Gácsi *et al.*, 2009a; Riedel *et al.*, 2008; Soproni *et al.*, 2002) (Figure 10.4). This task is very simple. Two containers are placed on the floor at a distance of roughly 1.5 meters from the subject. An experimenter is standing in the middle, but slightly behind the containers. Only one of the containers is baited out of sight of the subject. To give the subject a clue to where the food is located, the experimenter either looks or points at the baited container after calling the dog's attention. After the cue is given, the dog is released to

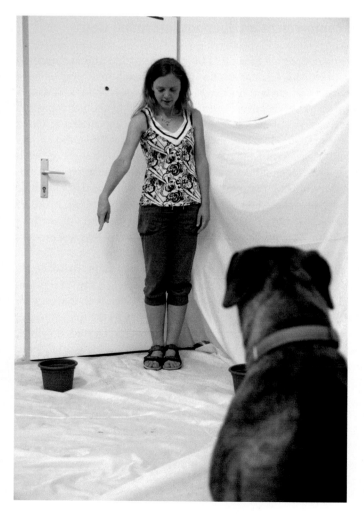

Figure 10.4 In the momentary distal pointing task, the dog is sitting about 2–3 meters in front of two bowls, one of which is baited. The experimenter is pointing towards the bowl that is baited after establishing eye contact with the subject. (© L. Wallis, reprinted with permission.)

make a choice and is only rewarded if it follows the cue. Among all animals, dogs are considered to be the masters of this task (though see Udell *et al.*, 2012) leading to an immense interest in this area of dog cognition (see Miklósi & Soproni, 2006 for a review). Hand cues can vary greatly in terms of the distance between the pointing hand and the indicated container, as well as of the number of pointing gestures and the length of each point. The most relevant cue for our current topic is *momentary distal pointing*. Here the pointing hand is at least 50 cm from the baited container, the action is performed for only a short duration and is no longer present when the subject is making its choice. Hence, it has been suggested that following momentary distal pointing may inform us whether subjects can comprehend referential communication (Anderson *et al.*, 1996; Povinelli *et al.*, 1997).

Since this early interpretation, however, various alternative mechanisms have been proposed including: (1) the local enhancement effect of the pointing hand that is closer to the baited than to the non-baited container; (2) a hand–food association the subjects formed during prior feeding sessions; or (3) because the dogs perceive the point as a command to move in the indicated direction (see also a similar interpretation of the effects of human ostensive-communicative cues in Social learning, Section 10.4) without actually expecting to find a referent in the pointed location (Kaminski, 2008). Kaminski and her colleagues conducted a series of studies in order to dissect the mechanisms underlying the success of dogs in following human pointing cues, but obtained contradictory results that do not allow for a firm conclusion (Grassmann *et al.*, 2012; Kaminski *et al.*, 2012; Pettersson *et al.*, 2011; Scheider *et al.*, 2011) and also later studies confirm that dogs likely interpret pointing as an imperative that sends them to a certain location (Tauzin *et al.*, 2015). As such, although dogs apparently respond to pointing as to a communicative gesture, it is relatively safe to conclude that current tests of whether dogs can follow human pointing do not necessarily inform us about comprehension of referential communication in dogs.

In contrast to pointing, following others' gaze to identify a third object in the environment would be free of some of these alternative explanations (e.g. local enhancement), and indeed, one study has demonstrated that dogs may understand the referential nature of human gaze. Soproni *et al.* (2001) found that dogs chose one of two containers, if an experimenter looked at it, but that they chose randomly if she turned her face to the side but upward, looking above the container. They argued that both gaze cues had a similar discriminative component (right or left side) but only the first one had a referential component. It may be worthwhile to note that these gazing probe trials were interspersed in a longer series of pointing trials, potentially facilitating the dogs' success by learning. A few additional studies confirmed the conclusion that dogs can follow human gaze to locate hidden food, but all of them tested dogs repeatedly, and not only with gaze but also with various simpler cues (Agnetta *et al.*, 2000; Miklósi *et al.*, 1998). More recently, Kaminski *et al.* (2012) used methods that are more similar to the ones in pointing studies and found that dogs do not reliably follow human gaze without the experimental training that characterized the former studies. Even more puzzling, in another study dogs not only did not follow a human gaze cue but they even avoided it and rather approached the second container than the one the experimenter had looked at (Oliva *et al.*, 2015). This latter finding suggests that dogs may interpret directional human gaze differently to pointing.

10.5.2 Communicating referentially: Dogs informing humans

Studies have shown that dogs can inform their owners which of three out-of-reach hiding places is baited with food (Gaunet, 2010; Lakatos *et al.*, 2012; Miklósi *et al.*, 2000). They indicate the baited location by alternating their gaze between the hiding place and the owner, moving back and forth between these two locations, and by soliciting the owner's attention by barking while looking at the baited container. However, it has been debated whether this is true communication or rather the result of learned associations between these behaviors and the desired outcome. Looking back and forth between the food and the owner could simply reflect that there are two interesting things present in the room that catch their attention, or that they expect that the owner will do something with the food and check repeatedly to appraise the situation (Horn *et al.*, 2012). These explanations, however, cannot account for the finding that dogs indicate the location of a hidden toy more often if the owner was absent when the toy was hidden compared with trials when the owner was present during the hiding process (Virányi *et al.*, 2006). These results seem to confirm that the dogs intend to inform the owner about the location of the desired object. However, Kaminski *et al.* (2011b) showed that dogs only inform humans about the location of objects they want, not objects interesting only for the humans. Whether this is due to a lack of cooperative/helping motivation or reflects limited cognitive skills in recognizing what information humans need to solve a problem, is unclear.

In sum, it is surprising how little scientific knowledge we have about the forms and mechanisms of referential communication between dogs and humans, despite the fact that dog–human pairs regularly engage in joint behaviors that involve objects: dogs lead us to the kitchen to ask for food, or bring their bowl to ask for water, and people ask their dogs to bring their shoes or to open the door. In the first case it is hard to know if the dogs intend to communicate with us or if we simply reinforced some behaviors that originally were not intended for us. In the latter case, it is unclear whether the dogs understand that "Close the door!" refers to the door or if it codes only the action of closing the door that includes its object as well. Dogs and humans regularly gain information about objects, persons and events from others' behavior, and this capacity merits more intensive research.

10.6   Dogs read humans' behavior. Can they also read our minds?

One of the most exciting questions in relation to dog cognition is whether dogs can also reason about our mental states. In short, do dogs have a "theory of mind"? When they try to predict or influence our behavior do they attribute mental states to us: what we pay attention to, what we intend to do, what we do and do not know about, and what kind of false beliefs we may have if we are misinformed about reality? When we talk about "reading human minds," we do not mean any kind of telepathic skill. As with humans, it is possible for dogs to use the behavioral signs of others (being absent, looking into the wrong direction, having the eyes closed, etc.) as well as certain contextual cues (e.g. presence of a barrier blocking one's view) to infer whether someone had the chance to see something and, thus, to know about it (Whiten, 1996).

10.6.1   Inferring knowledge states and beliefs

The finding that dogs will indicate the location of a hidden toy more intensively to their owners if the owner was absent than if she was present during the hiding (Virányi *et al.*, 2006) is exactly the kind of behavior one would expect if dogs tailored their indicating behavior according to the knowledge or ignorance of their owners. Being rigorous regarding the underlying cognitive mechanisms, however, one must consider whether these results can be explained by other, less sophisticated mechanisms. For instance, it is possible that dogs use simple behavioral heuristics that get reinforced during repeated interactions with humans. For example, the above, apparently insightful, performance of the dogs could be explained if the dogs communicate with their owners following this rule: "if your owner was not there when something important happened communicate about this more intensively." In this case the dogs need to adjust their signaling behavior directly to the previous presence or absence of their owners without having to think about their knowledge state. Kaminski *et al.* (2011b) proposed an even lower level explanation suggesting that dogs might have been simply more excited after their owner was absent. Therefore, in the "ignorant owner" condition, being left alone with the experimenter during the toy hiding process and then more aroused upon the owner's return to the room might have led to more indicating behaviors. In other words, these findings can be explained without attributing *Theory of Mind* to dogs.

Similar arguments can be made based on Maginnity & Grace (2014) and Ashton, Cooper and West's unpublished experiments (reported in Cooper *et al.*, 2003). In these studies, after being trained to locate food in three or four hiding places, the dogs were prevented from seeing the hiding during the test trials. However, they could observe if two experimenters did or did not have visual access to the hiding process: one experimenter was watching the hiding while the other one could not do so (e.g., had left the room or had her eyes covered). Each experimenter then indicated a hiding place and the subjects were allowed to choose between their different suggestions. Most dogs chose the location indicated by the human who could see the hiding process in the first trial, but there was no preference for the knowledgeable partner in the subsequent five trials. Interestingly, when the partners were dogs (pre-trained to choose a fixed location) that had been waiting either in a covered or an uncovered box during the hiding, the subjects always followed one of the dog-partners but failed to discriminate between them.

Finally, Kaminski *et al.* (2009b) found clear negative results with a different test paradigm. In this case, a group of 53 pet dogs were first pre-trained to bring a toy to a seated experimenter on command. Once reliably trained, two identical toys were placed behind two opaque screens in view of the test dog but where the experimenter could not see them. The experimenter, however, was in the room and able to witness one of the toys being concealed behind the screen but out of the room when the other toy was concealed. The rationale being that, if the dogs recognized which concealed toy the experimenter knew about, they would bring this one to her rather than the other when asked to do so. The dogs, however, appeared to choose the toys at random without taking into account the knowledge of the experimenter. Accordingly, to date, there is still no convincing evidence that dogs can think about others' mental states, or impute knowledge, ignorance or false beliefs to humans.

10.6.2 Taking others' attentional states and perspectives into account

Dogs seem to adjust very well to what we pay attention to and seem to know what humans can or cannot see. This is understandable if we consider that in these cases our behavior and the momentary arrangement of all participants and objects of the actual situation provide observable cues to which the dogs can adjust their behavior. For instance, the above test paradigm using two toys hidden behind two screens can be modified so that the dogs do not need to remember what happened in the past. If one screen is transparent and the other one is opaque, only one toy, the one behind the transparent screen, is visible to the experimenter. In this case, the dogs fetch the toy that is visible from the experimenter's perspective despite the fact that they themselves can see both toys from their position (Kaminski *et al.*, 2009b). Moreover, the dogs can use not only the transparency of screens but also their size and the presence of a window to judge what humans can see from a position different from theirs (Bräuer *et al.*, 2004). This has been demonstrated in a competitive situation where a piece of food was placed on the floor and the dogs were prohibited from taking it. The dogs were very skilled in knowing when a screen was positioned so that the human could not see whether or not they took the food and thus could choose when to ignore the prohibition. Similarly, they knew that they had a better chance of stealing the food, and of doing so unnoticed, in situations where the owners had their backs turned towards them, their eyes closed or their faces covered by a book, than when they were looking at them (Call *et al.*, 2003; Schwab & Huber, 2006) and when the food could be removed silently from its container in contrast to a more noisy container (Kundey *et al.*, 2010). Dogs adjust to the visual orientation of humans not only when trying to avoid some punishment but also when they want to communicate with humans. When begging from a pair of humans, dogs prefer to approach the person who is looking at them with her eyes uncovered in contrast to the one who turns away or has her eyes blindfolded (Gácsi *et al.*, 2004). The owner's orientation also helps them to decide whether a given command was intended for them (Virányi *et al.*, 2004). In a triadic situation, it has been shown that dogs quickly obeyed the "Down!" command, if the owner was looking at them, but did not obey if the owner turned to an experimenter when the command was given. Most importantly, if the owner kept the same position as in the experimental trial (turning her side to the dog) but the experimenter moved out from the focus of the owner's orientation, and thus, the owner seemed to "talk to the wall," the dogs did obey the command after it was repeated three times. It is an important finding because it shows that dogs do not automatically respond to some cues given by the owner but take other components of the situation into account and adjust their behavior accordingly.

10.6.3　Attributing intentions

Since dogs are quite skilled at reading the behavioral cues of humans, the question arises whether they can go a step further and recognize some of our intentions. For example, if we step on a dog's foot accidentally rather than intentionally, it seems intuitively likely that aspects of our behavior indicate to the dog that the act was unintended. Interestingly, however, there are contradictory findings regarding whether dogs can differentiate between intentional and accidental actions (Kundey *et al.*, 2011; Riedel *et al.*, 2006). Dogs respond more to similar hand gestures and gaze cues if the experimenter expresses her communicative intentions by establishing eye-contact with the dog and calling its name than in the absence of such cues (Kaminski *et al.*, 2012). They are also able to discriminate between a "cooperative" human experimenter who consistently points at a container baited with food and a "deceptive" one who points consistently at an empty container (Petter *et al.*, 2009). However, these dogs make the same discriminations when the cooperative and deceptive humans are replaced by inanimate black and white boxes, which suggests that the intentions of the humans are probably irrelevant. The cognitive mechanisms underlying dogs' preferences for partners who behave generously in a begging situation *versus* those who are possessive remain open to question (Kundey *et al.*, 2011; Marshall-Pescini *et al.*, 2011b). It is clear that dogs take others' behaviors into account when these indicate cooperative intentions, but currently little is known about the cognitive and emotional processes underlying such preferences.

Based on these results, we can conclude that currently we have no evidence showing that dogs are capable of attributing mental states to humans. To be fair, it is important to note that some would form a similar conclusion about other animals as well, including great apes (Heyes, 1998; Povinelli & Vonk, 2003). Also, humans do not always think about the mental states of others but sometimes form their decisions based on simple cues involved in the situation (Gagliardi *et al.*, 1995). Nevertheless, dogs should at least get credit for showing highly flexible responses to human behavioral cues that often quite closely resemble the kinds of behaviors we would expect from partners who take our mental states into account.

10.7   The interplay between cognition and emotions

As humans, if we see a child falling down, we offer a helping hand and some sympathetic words to ease the pain. While we have the capacity to understand that the child is experiencing pain and also that by helping the child we might gain a positive reputation among bystanders, this (usually) does not cross our mind in the specific situation. Instead, feelings of empathy are thought to trigger such behaviors spontaneously in humans, as well as provoking feelings of guilt if we simply passed by without helping. Can dogs also feel guilty, or be empathetic, or even have a sense of fairness? A recent study showed that at least 74% of dog owners ascribe guilty feelings to their dogs, and 81% think that their dogs are jealous, e.g. when attention is unequally given to themselves and another person or dog (Morris *et al.*, 2008). Both of these emotions are generally thought to be non-basic emotions.

10.7.1   Empathy

Empathy, the ability to understand and vicariously experience the emotional and motivational states of others, is thought to be an important prerequisite for social interactions and especially cooperation (De Waal & Suchak, 2010; Preston & De Waal., 2002). At present there is little direct evidence that dogs are empathetic, although they may be susceptible to emotional contagion (Joly-Mascheroni *et al.*, 2008), which is considered to be a rudimentary form of empathy. In their study, these authors found that 21 of 29 pet dogs yawned after seeing and hearing a human yawn while they did not yawn after seeing silent mouth openings. These results led to speculation that the tendency of dogs to mimic human yawns is driven by an underlying desire to affiliate with humans, and thus, might have facilitated early human-canine interactions (Yoon & Tennie, 2010). However, two studies that further investigated contagious yawning in dogs, found (1) that when dogs were shown silent videotaped yawns, the vast majority did not show contagious yawning (Harr *et al.*, 2009), and (2) that dogs did not yawn more in response to a familiar, closely bonded partner than to an unfamiliar one, nor did pet dogs in a stable emotional relationship respond more than shelter dogs (Madsen & Persson, 2013; O'Hara & Reeve, 2011). These results cast doubt on contagious yawning in dogs and furthermore suggest that, if it does exist, it is probably not based on an empathetic response, but might be better explained by reactions to specific stimuli (O'Hara & Reeve, 2011). Another recent study, however, showed that the mere sound of a human yawn was sufficient to elicit yawning in dogs. Moreover, unexpectedly, the authors found that dogs yawned more at familiar than unfamiliar yawns, suggesting that dogs may be able to show empathy-based, contagious yawning after all (Silva *et al.*, 2012).

Further positive evidence for empathy-like behavior in dogs comes from a study using an experimental protocol first used with human infants. Here dogs were confronted with different humans crying (test) or talking (control 1) or humming (control 2). The dogs oriented (showing submissive rather than playful behavior) toward their owner or a stranger more often in the test than in the control situations. While these dogs' response patterns were behaviorally consistent with expressions of empathic concern, one cannot, however, rule out the possibility that they had learned this behavior from being previously rewarded for approaching distressed human companions in the past (Custance & Mayer, 2012).

One study shows that pet dogs can respond with empathy-like behavior also to conspecifics (Quervel-Chaumette *et al.*, 2016). Dogs that had lived at least for a year together with another dog were separated from their fellow dog. In the experimental room the subject dog, together with its owner, stayed on one side of a visual barrier while its partner dog was lead to the other side of the barrier and, without the subject knowing it, outside the room. After this, whines of the partner or an unfamiliar dog recorded previously during separation from the owner or a computer-generated control sound were played back. After the playback, the partner dog re-entered the room and the subject's behaviour was recorded. During this reunion phase the dogs demonstrated more comfort-offering behaviors toward their familiar partners after they had heard whines of their partner dogs than after control stimuli or after being exposed to unfamiliar whines. Furthermore, familiar whines tended to evoke higher cortisol levels than stranger whines, indicating that the distress-calls of a fellow dog evoke a stress-reaction in dogs.

Familiarity plays a role also in the pro-social behaviour of dogs. Pro-social behaviours, or other-regarding preferences, are defined as voluntary actions that benefit others. For example, pet dogs display a readiness to donate food to another dog if it is familiar to them whereas they do so less often to benefit a stranger dog (Quervel-Chaumette *et al.*, 2015).

10.7.2   Guilt

Almost every dog owner has experienced occasions when some food has disappeared from a low table while answering the door. The prime suspect in that situation is the dog, who often instantly droops the ears and looks guilty when we turn towards it with anger and disapproval. But does the dog actually feel guilty, or does it simply react to a learned situation? Perhaps the dog is expressing anticipation of punishment, or it may have learned that looking "guilty" will help to placate its owner. Two recent studies have explored whether dogs really react to such situations based on a sense of guilt or are simply responding to the behavior of the owner. Horowitz (2009a) modeled a situation similar to the one described above in which the owner left the dog in a familiar room with a treat that the dog was instructed not to eat. The researcher then manipulated two aspects of the experiment: (1) whether or not the treat disappeared (either because it was removed immediately after the owner left the room or it was fed to the dog), and (2) the beliefs of the owner regarding the obedience of the dog (the owner was either informed that the dog ate the food or not and, accordingly, was asked to either scold the dog upon his/her return or to greet it in a friendly manner). The results revealed that the dogs did not show more "guilty" behaviors when they had actually eaten the treat as opposed to when they hadn't, and that their responses were dependent on whether or not the owner scolded them. Interestingly, however, those dogs that were scolded unfairly (because they did not eat the treat) showed more "guilty" behaviors than the dogs that had actually been disobedient.

Another study used a slightly different paradigm to avoid the problem of scolding the dog, and the fact that the dogs were not really disobedient since they were offered the food by an experimenter (Hecht *et al.*, 2012). In this case, after the social rule was established that the dogs were not allowed to eat a food reward left on a table, the dogs were left alone with the food. When the owners returned shortly afterwards, they were required to stand still while their dog greeted them and then asked to judge whether or not the dog was guilty of having eaten the food (they could not see if the dog had really eaten the food). The results confirmed the previous findings in that the guilty dogs did not react any differently than dogs who were not guilty of a misdeed. Altogether, the results of these studies call for further investigations of whether or not dogs really feel guilty or if they are mainly reacting to their owners' perceptions of their guilt.

10.7.3 Fairness

Whether dogs have a sense of fairness has been examined in several contexts in recent decades. The earliest studies focused on social play behavior, which is considered to be a balance between cooperation and competition (Bekoff, 2001; Cordoni, 2009; Palagi, 2006). During play sessions, conflicts about "winning" occur regularly, requiring individuals to cooperate in order to keep play interactions attractive for all participants, and to prevent play from escalating into real aggression (Bauer & Smuts, 2007; Bekoff, 2001). For example, dogs may engage in role reversals and self-handicapping during play, especially when the partners are not evenly matched – e.g. they differ in age, sex or size (Bauer *et al.*, 2007; Bekoff, 2001; Horowitz, 2009b). During role reversal, play roles switch and a dominant animal acts subordinate while the subordinate acts dominant (Bekoff, 1995), while during self-handicapping an individual performs a behavioral pattern that might compromise itself (Bekoff, 2001); for example, if a dominant individual inhibits the intensity of its bites towards a subdominant individual during play. Although self-handicapping and role-reversals do not seem necessary for play to occur, they help to maintain a play session (Bauer & Smuts, 2007). Interestingly, this is not only true if dogs play with dogs, but dogs are also more motivated during play sessions with humans, if they are allowed to win (Rooney & Bradshaw, 2002). Based on these observations, it has been proposed that a sense of fairness is crucial to negotiate playful interactions in dogs and other canids (Bekoff, 1995). This is supported by anecdotal observations of dogs, young coyotes and wolves that, if the rules of social play are not respected, the other animals involved react to the lack of fairness by ending the encounter or avoiding play with rule-breakers (Bekoff, 2004). Although it seems to be in line with the fact that these canids also cooperate during the rearing of young, territorial defense, and probably hunting (Mech, 1970; Mech & Boitani, 2003), the first systematic study on captive wolves did not confirm this expectation (Essler *et al.*, 2016).

It has been argued that for such cooperation to evolve it is crucial that the individual animal is sensitive to others' efforts and pay-offs in comparison to its own costs and gains. It has been investigated whether domestic dogs show a response to the inequity of rewards received for the same action in pairs of familiar dogs (Brucks *et al.*, 2016; Range *et al.*, 2009c). In these experiments, dogs' willingness to obey a simple command (e.g. giving the paw) was tested when either (a) the focal dog and its partner both received the same low-value reward (a piece of dry bread – condition 1: baseline), (b) the focal dog received no reward while the partner received the low-value reward (condition 2), or (c) when the partner was absent from the experiment and the focal dog received no reward for giving the paw (control condition 3) (Figure 10.5 and Table 10.1). The dogs refused to cooperate with the experimenter and showed increased stress levels when unrewarded in the presence of a rewarded

Table 10.1 Summary of experimental conditions and focal dog responses to the inequity aversion experiment.

Test Conditions	Focal Task	Focal Reward	Partner Task	Partner Reward	Response of Focal
Equity (condition 1)	+	Low	+	Low	–
Reward inequity (condition 2)	+	–	+	Low	Refusal
No reward control (condition 3)	+	–	No partner		–

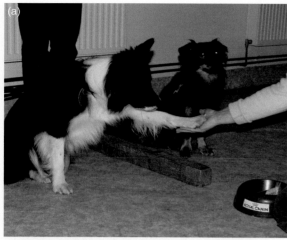
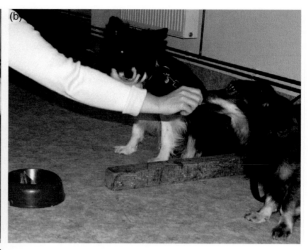
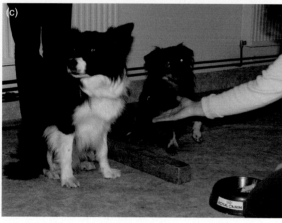

Figure 10.5 The pictures present the set-up of the experiment in condition 2: (a) first the focal dog is asked for the paw but is not rewarded, then (b) the partner is asked for the paw and is rewarded. (c) Finally, the focal dog is asked once again to give the paw. (© Friederike Range.)

partner compared to the baseline and asocial control situations. When, after the test, the subject and its partner had the chance to share some food, they co-fed for a shorter time if only the partner had been rewarded for giving the paw or if the partner had received better quality food than the subject in comparison to the equal rewarding condition. This suggested that the presence of a rewarded partner mattered (i.e. the dogs reacted to the unequal reward distribution). In a follow-up study, we analyzed whether individual characteristics, motivation and personality, determined the response of each subject to unequal reward distributions, or whether the subjects' responses depended on the specific relationship they had with their partner (Range *et al.*, 2012). We found that the dogs' motivation – as measured in a separate test of their persistence in trying to solve an unsolvable problem – influenced their persistence in giving the paw without being rewarded for it when tested alone (condition 3), but not in the reward inequity condition (condition 2). This supports the view that the aversion of dogs toward inequity relies on their partner's action and is independent of other non-social aspects of the situation. Furthermore, we found that dog pairs with a close relationship (i.e. sleeping regularly in body contact) were more inequity averse than dogs in a less affiliative relationship (the opposite of what has been found in primates). Overall, these two findings suggest that inequity aversion in dogs is conditional on their and their partner's rewards. However, the difference between the dogs' behavior and that of human and non-human primates may point towards a difference in the underlying mechanisms: e.g. whether dogs actually see the situation as unfair or whether they simply react to some sort of behavioral cue from the partner.

In another study that investigated dogs' reactions to an unequal reward situation, a subject dog and a control dog were able to approach two trainers in turn, each of whom asked the dogs to sit (Horowitz, 2012). While one of the trainers always rewarded the test and control dog equally, the other trainer either over-rewarded or under-rewarded the control dog. After the test dogs had gathered experience with the two trainers, they could choose whom to approach. Subjects showed a preference for the over-rewarding compared to the fair trainer, but did not differentiate between the under-rewarding and the fair trainer. Accordingly, dogs selected the "unfair" trainer if this meant that he had also the overall larger quantity of food and thus potentially offered the greater opportunity for future rewards.

In general, these studies on empathy, guilt and fairness in dogs demonstrate that we are far from understanding whether our best friend shares similar emotions with us, even if sometimes the behavior looks very much as we would react if confronted with a similar situation.

10.7.4   Recognizing human emotions

There is a growing body of evidence that dogs are responsive to humans' emotional expressions. Pet dogs can differentiate between happy, neutral, sad, disgusted and angry expressions on human (and conspecific) faces, and, moreover, show some understanding of their relevance. In one study, dogs were trained to discriminate between faces of the same person with either a happy or angry emotional expression presented on a touch screen monitor. Although during the training the dogs saw only either the lower or upper halves of these faces, in the test they readily categorized pictures that showed the other half of the faces as expressing happy or angry emotions (Müller *et al.*, 2015). A second study (Albuquerque *et al.*, 2016) demonstrated that dogs not only have a knowledge of the complex visual expressions of emotions on human and conspecific faces but they combine these with vocalizations specific to happy/playful *versus* angry/aggressive emotions. Although rather sophisticated techniques, such as eye-tracking and functional MRI, have been applied in this field of research (Barber *et al.*, 2016; Cuaya *et al.*, 2016), a lot of work is still needed to determine to what extent this performance reflects skills homologous to face-processing in other species (modified by the extensive experiences of dogs with humans) and to what extent it relies on evolutionary adaptations to living with humans.

10.8   Triple origin of behavioral similarities between dogs and humans

It is a challenging task collecting data that are sufficiently detailed and sophisticated to allow firm conclusions to be drawn about the cognitive mechanisms underlying dogs' behavior. However, it should be emphasized that investigating the origins of these abilities (ontogenetic as well as evolutionary) as well as their underlying mechanisms will yield complementary explanations of dog behavior (Tinbergen, 1963). Determining the cognitive mechanisms requires a different analysis than reproducing the learning processes a dog went through when acquiring a certain behavior. Thus, while the previous sections of this chapter were concerned with the underlying mechanisms, we will now focus on the developmental and evolutionary origins of dog behavior.

10.8.1   Development, learning and training

Most of the studies reviewed in this chapter focused on pets for the simple reason that most of the findings suitable for cognitive analysis are based on studies of this group of dogs. However, we will only gain an exhaustive understanding of the cognitive abilities of dogs if we also investigate other populations, such as shelter or feral/free-roaming dogs (Coppinger & Coppinger, 2001). These kinds of dogs may not tolerate the proximity of humans (feral dogs), or may be so keen on contact with humans that this motivation overshadows everything else (shelter dogs). Examining these animals in rigorous cognitive experiments can therefore be extremely challenging, and it is clear that developmental and learning processes have a strong influence on their behavioral performance. For instance, the experiences of dogs with humans' everyday behavior or training experiences can affect how they communicate and interact with us. Tópal et al. (1997) showed that dogs kept habitually in backyards tend to solve problems more independently than dogs kept in apartments; the latter needing more encouragement from their owners to be similarly successful. At the same time, dogs that have been extensively trained either with a clicker, or as search and rescue or agility dogs, are not only more pro-active problem-solvers than dogs with no or just basic obedience training, but also communicate differently with humans (Marshall-Pescini et al., 2008; Osthaus et al., 2003, 2005; Range et al., 2009b). Even the different training methods seem to produce different behavioral outcomes. For instance, agility training increases dogs' tendencies to look at humans, search and rescue training increases their level of barking, while guide dogs for the blind tend to lick their mouths more noisily when trying to get humans' attention (Gaunet, 2008; Marshall-Pescini et al., 2010). Even shorter-term effects have been demonstrated, with dogs flexibly learning within a given experiment, or adjusting their human-directed gazing according to whether their owner was previously encouraging them or not (Horn et al., 2012; Wallis et al., 2015; Wynne et al., 2008). In light of this flexibility, Elgier et al. (2009) have suggested that based on their experiences dogs can quickly adapt to any given situation and learn to respond to those cues associated with subsequent rewards.

10.8.2   Evolutionary adaption to the human environment: Domestication

Observing how adaptively dogs can adjust their behavior at an individual level, the question arises whether similar processes might have taken place during the evolution of the species. Breed differences, as well as associations between behavior and morphological traits (e.g. length of the skull, ranging from pugs to Afghan hounds) or genetic polymorphisms, indicate that there is a genetic influence on human-directed behavior in dogs, such as attentiveness, following human pointing, and trainability (Gácsi et al., 2009b; Jakovcevic et al., 2010; Kubinyi et al., 2012; Serpell & Hsu, 2005; Wobber et al., 2009). As outlined earlier, it has been proposed that the domestic dog and the human species went through convergent evolution, suggesting that dog–human similarities rest on evolutionary changes that happened during the course of domestication (Hare & Tomasello, 2005; Topál et al., 2009b). To confirm this hypothesis, comparisons between dogs and wolves with identical learning opportunities are needed. With comparisons of pet dogs and zoo-kept wolves (Agnetta et al., 2000; Hare et al., 2002), we cannot be sure to what extent the observed differences are caused by genetic differences or by the different experiences of the animals (Virányi et al., 2008b). We are well aware, of course, that even providing the same environment and similar exposure to social stimuli does not necessarily mean that dogs and wolves extract the same information and go through the same learning processes. They may easily perceive different behaviors of the partner and different components of the social situation as relevant, and thus, gain differential knowledge. If their environment is comparable, however, then the resulting behavioral differences will ultimately be based on their different genetic make-up and can be traced back to evolutionary differences across species.

Currently, few comparisons of cognitive abilities exist that were conducted on wolves and dogs raised and kept in an identical way (Frank & Frank, 1982a; Miklósi *et al.*, 2003). Surprisingly, some of these studies show that the differences between dogs and wolves may be smaller than originally thought. For instance, until recently it was assumed that only dogs could follow human momentary distal pointing, and that even human-raised wolves could not do this (Hare *et al.*, 2002). However, in 2009, Gácsi and her colleagues showed that, as adults, wolves can follow the pointing cue (Gácsi *et al.*, 2009c; see also Udell *et al.*, 2012). Whether the behavioral difference stems from emotional, attentional or cognitive characteristics of dogs that develop faster compared to wolves is still unclear. After an initial proposal that dogs were selected for human-like, complex social cognition (Hare *et al.*, 2002), Miklósi *et al.* (2003) suggested that young dogs are predisposed to pay more attention to humans than young wolves and thus have a better chance of noticing their pointing gestures. Similarly, the discovery that farm foxes selected for tameness will also follow certain forms of human pointing (Trut *et al.*, 1999), led Hare *et al.* (2005) to propose that selection for reduced fear and aggression towards humans – in the experimental foxes and possibly also in dogs – might be enough to enable the use of species-specific cognitive abilities when interacting with humans. This hypothesis implies that the social cognitive abilities of dogs and wolves are rather similar but that domestication prepared the dogs to interact not only with conspecifics but also human social partners (see also Gácsi *et al.*, 2009c).

10.8.3   Wolf origins of dog–human interactions

Interestingly, the behavior of young dogs and wolves does not differ in every human-related situation. At an early age, human-raised wolves can follow human gaze into distant space and around a barrier (Range & Virányi, 2011), and can learn from a human demonstration in a local enhancement task (Range & Virányi, 2013). Thus, despite being naturally fearful and avoidant of people, hand-raised wolves can learn to accept humans as partners at least to the extent that they pay sufficient attention to them and coordinate their behavior with them. Since the ability to follow conspecific and human gaze, or learn socially from them, appears at similar ages during development, it is unlikely that being hand-raised influences the development of these abilities *per se*, but rather that it enables wolves to use their species-specific cognitive abilities also with humans. Gaze following and social learning are both likely to have adaptive value in family packs of wolves. Wolves are cooperative breeders in which non-breeding pack members help the dominant pair to raise their young (Mech, 1970; Mech *et al.*, 2003). Moreover, wolves rely on close action coordination with pack members when defending their territories and hunting large game (Mech, 1970; Mech *et al.*, 2003). Consequently, the overall higher dependency on cooperative interactions with conspecifics predicts that wolves will pay close attention to others and coordinate their actions with them. We propose that due to their social organization, several cognitive and emotional characteristics (e.g., high tolerance) that make dogs special may also be present in wolves (Range & Virányi, 2015; Range *et al.*, 2015). In other words, instead of placing too much emphasis on the domestication history of dogs, it is important to investigate to what extent and in what form the evolutionary precursors of dogs' social behavior exist in wolves.

10.9   Conclusions

The emotional and cognitive characteristics that help dogs to become an integral part of human groups originate from at least three different sources. First, it is likely that wolves were already equipped with social skills that are either analogous or homologous with human abilities. Second, dogs may have evolved additional adaptations to the human environment during the course of domestication. Finally, individual learning and training processes can further enhance the success of dogs in building relationships and co-working with humans. In order to gain a full understanding of how these evolutionary and ontogenetic processes contribute to dog behavior and its underlying cognitive-emotional mechanisms, a complex study of wolf and dog populations living in different conditions and socialized and trained differently by humans and conspecifics is necessary.

References

Agnetta, B., Hare, B. & Tomasello, M. (2000). Cues to food location that domestic dogs (*Canis familiaris*) of different ages do and do not use. *Animal Cognition*, 3: 107.

Albuquerque, N., Guo, K., Wilkinson, A., Savalli, C., Otta, E. & Mills, D. (2016). Dogs recognize dog and human emotions. *Biology Letters*, 12: 20150883

Anderson, J., Montant, M. & Schmitt, D. (1996). Rhesus monkeys fail to use gaze direction as an experimenter-given cue in an object choice task. *Behavioral Processes*, 37: 47–55.

Aust, U., Range, F., Steurer, M. & Huber, L. (2008). Inferential reasoning by exclusion: a comparative study of pigeons, dogs, and humans. *Animal Cognition*. http://doi10.1007/s10071-008-0149-0

Barber A. L. A., Randi, D., Müller, C. A. & Huber, L. (2016). The processing of human emotional faces by pet and lab dogs: Evidence for lateralization and experience effects. *PLoS ONE*, 11: e0152393

Bauer, E. B. & Smuts, B. B. (2007). Cooperation and competition during dyadic play in domestic dogs, *Canis familiaris. Animal Behavior*, 73: 489–99.

Bekoff, M. (1995). Play signals as punctuation – the structure of social play in canids. *Behavior*, 132: 419–29.

Bekoff, M. (2001). Social play behavior – cooperation, fairness, trust, and the evolution of morality. *Journal of Consciousness Studies*, 8: 81–90.

Bekoff, M. (2004). Wild justice, cooperation and fair play: Minding manners, being nice, and feeling good. In *The Origins and Nature of Sociality*, eds. Sussman, R. & Chapman, A. Chicago, IL: Aldine.

Bentosela, M., Barrera, G., Jakovcevic, A., Elgier, A. M. & Mustaca, A. E. (2008). Effect of reinforcement, reinforcer omission and extinction on a communicative response in domestic dogs (*Canis familiaris*). *Behavioral Processes*, 78: 464–9.

Boesch, C. (1991). Teaching among wild chimpanzees. *Animal Behavior*, 41: 530–2.

Bräuer, J., Call, J. & Tomasello, M. (2004). Visual perspective taking in dogs (*Canis familiaris*) in the presence of barriers. *Applied Animal Behavior Science*, 88: 299–317.

Brauer, J., Kaminski, J., Riedel, J., Call, J. & Tomasello, M. (2006). Making inferences about the location of hidden food: social dog, causal ape. *Journal of Comparative Psychology*, 120: 38–47.

Brucks, D., Essler, J. L., Marshall-Pescini, S. & Range, F. (2016). Inequity aversion negatively affects tolerance and contact-seeking behaviours towards partner and experimenter. *PLoS ONE*, 11(4): e0153799. doi: 10.1371/journal.pone.0153799.

Call, J. (2001). Chimpanzee social cognition. *Trends in Cognitive Science*, 5: 388–93.

Call, J. (2006) Inferences by exclusion in the great apes: the effect of age and species. *Animal Cognition*, 9: 393–403.

Call, J., Bräuer, J., Kaminski, J. & Tomasello, M. (2003). Domestic dogs (*Canis familiaris*) are sensitive to the attentional state of humans. *Journal of Comparative Psychology*, 117: 257–63.

Caro, T. M. & Hauser, M. D. (1992). Is there teaching in nonhuman animals? *Quarterly Review of Biology*, 67: 151–74.

Chance, M. R. A. & Jolly, C. (1970). *Social Groups of Monkeys, Apes and Men*. London, Jonathan Cape.

Cooper, J. J., Ashton, C., Bishop, S., West, R., Mills, D. S. & Young, R. J. (2003). Clever hounds: social cognition in the domestic dog (*Canis familiaris*). *Applied Animal Behavior Science*, 81: 229–44.

Coppinger, R. & Coppinger, L. (2001). *Dogs: A New Understanding of Canine Origin, Behavior and Evolution*. Chicago, IL: The University of Chicago Press.

Cordoni, G. (2009). Social play in captive wolves (*Canis lupus*): not only an immature affair. *Behavior*, 146: 1363–85.

Cuaya, L. V., Hernández-Pérez, R. & Concha, L. (2016). Our faces in the dog's brain: functional imaging reveals temporal cortex activation during perception of human faces. *PloS ONE*, 11: e0149431

Custance, D. & Mayer, J. (2012). Empathic-like responding by domestic dogs (*Canis familiaris*) to distress in humans: an exploratory study. *Animal Cognition*, 15: 851–9.

De Waal, F. B. M. & Suchak, M. (2010). Prosocial primates: selfish and unselfish motivations. *Philosophical Transactions of the Royal Society B*, 365: 2711–22.

Duranton, C., Bedossa, T. & Gaunet, F. (2016). When facing an unfamiliar person, pet dogs present social referencing based on their owners' direction of movement alone. *Animal Behaviour*, 113: 147–56.

Elgier, A. M., Jakowevic, A., Barrera, G., Mustaca, A. E. & Bentosela, M. (2009). Communication between domestic dogs (*Canis familiaris*) and humans: dogs are good learners. *Behavioral Processes*, 81: 402–8.

Essler, J. L., Cafazzo, S., Marshall-Pescini, S., Virányi, Z., Kotrschal, K., & Range, F. (2016). Play behavior in wolves: using the '50: 50' rule to test for egalitarian play styles. *PloS ONE*, 11: e0154150

Fitch, W. T., Huber, L. & Bugnyar, T. (2010). Social cognition and the evolution of language: constructing cognitive phylogenies. *Neuron*, 65: 795–814.

Frank, H. & Frank, M. G. (1982a). On the effects of domestication on canine social-development and behavior. *Applied Animal Ethology*, 8: 507–25.

Frank, H. & Frank, M. G. (1982b). Comparison of problem-solving performance in 6-week-old wolves and dogs. *Animal Behavior*, 30: 95–8.

Fugazza, C. & Miklósi, Á. (2014). Should old dog trainers learn new tricks? The efficiency of the Do as I Do method and shaping/clicker training method to train dogs. *Applied Animal Behaviour Science*, 153: 53–61.

Fukuzawa, M., Mills, D. S. & Cooper, J. J. (2005). More than just a word: non-semantic command variables affect obedience in the domestic dog *(Canis familiaris)*. *Applied Animal Behavior Science*, 91: 129–41.

Gácsi, M., Győri, B., Virányi, Z. et al. (2009c). Explaining dog wolf differences in utilizing human pointing gestures: selection for synergistic shifts in the development of some social skills. *PLoS ONE*, 4: e6584.

Gácsi, M., Kara, E., Belényi, B., Tópal, J. & Miklósi, A. (2009a). The effect of development and individual differences in pointing comprehension of dogs. *Animal Cognition*, 12: 471–9.

Gácsi, M., Mcgreevy, P., Kara, E. & Adam, M. (2009b). Effects of selection for cooperation and attention in dogs. *Behavioral and Brain Functions*, 5.

Gácsi, M., Miklósi, A., Varga, O., Tópal, J. & Csányi, V. (2004). Are readers of our face readers of our minds? Dogs (*Canis familiaris*) show situation-dependent recognition of human's attention. *Animal Cognition*, 7: 144–53.

Gagliardi, J. L., Kirkpatricksteger, K. K., Thomas, J., Allen, G. J. & Blumberg, M. S. (1995). Seeing and knowing – knowledge attribution versus stimulus-control in adult humans (*Homo sapiens*). *Journal of Comparative Psychology*, 109: 107–14.

Gaunet, F. (2008). How do guide dogs of blind owners and pet dogs of sighted owners (*Canis familiaris*) ask their owners for food? *Animal Cognition*, 11: 475–83.

Gaunet, F. (2010). How do guide dogs and pet dogs (*Canis familiaris*) ask their owners for their toy and for playing? *Animal Cognition*, 13: 311–23.

Gergely, G., Bekkering, H. & Kiraly, I. (2002). Rational imitation in preverbal infants. *Nature*, 415: 755.

Grassmann, S., Kaminski, J. & Tomasello, M. (2012). How two word-trained dogs integrate pointing and naming. *Animal Cognition*, 15: 657–65.

Griebel, U. & Oller, D. K. (2012). Vocabulary learning in a Yorkshire Terrier: slow mapping of spoken words. *PLoS ONE*, 7: e30182

Hare, B., Brown, M., Williamson, C. & Tomasello, M. (2002). The domestication of social cognition in dogs. *Science*, 298: 1634–6.

Hare, B., Plyusnina, I., Ignacio, N. et al. (2005). Social cognitive evolution in captive foxes is a correlated by-product of experimental domestication. *Current Biology*, 15: 226–30.

Hare, B. & Tomasello, M. (2005). Human-like social skills in dogs? *Trends in Cognitive Sciences*, 9: 439–44.

Harr, A. L., Gilbert, V. R. & Phillips, K. A. (2009). Do dogs (*Canis familiaris*) show contagious yawning? *Animal Cognition*, 12: 833–7.

Hecht, J., Miklósi, Á. & Gácsia, M. (2012). Behavioral assessment and owner perceptions of behaviors associated with guilt in dogs. *Applied Animal Behavior Science*, 139: 134–42.

Herberlein, M. & Turner, D. (2009). Dogs, *Canis familiaris*, find hidden food by observing and interacting with a conspecific. *Animal Behavior*, 78: 385–91

Heyes, C. M. (1993). Imitation, culture and cognition. *Animal Behavior*, 46: 999–1010.

Heyes, C. M. (1998). Theory of mind in nonhuman primates. *Behavioral and Brain Sciences*, 21: 101–48.

Horn, L., Range, F. & Huber, L. (2013). Dogs' attention towards humans depends on their relationship, not only on social familiarity. *Animal Cognition*, 16: 435–43.

Horn, L., Viranyi, Z., Miklósi, A., Huber, L. & Range, F. (2012). Domestic dogs (*Canis familiaris*) flexibly adjust their human-directed behavior to the actions of their human partners in a problem situation. *Animal Cognition*, 15: 57–71.

Horowitz, A. (2009a). Disambiguating the "guilty look": salient prompts to a familiar dog behavior. *Behavioral Processes*, 81: 447–52.

Horowitz, A. (2009b). Attention to attention in domestic dog (*Canis familiaris*) dyadic play. *Animal Cognition*, 12: 107–18.

Horowitz, A. (2012). Fair is fine, but more is better: limits to inequity aversion in the domestic dog. *Social Justice Research*, 25: 195–212.

Huber, L., Range, F., Voelkl, B., Szucsich, A., Viranyi, Z. & Miklósi, A. (2009). The evolution of imitation: what do the capacities of non-human animals tell us about the mechanisms of imitation? *Philosophical Transactions of the Royal Society B – Biological Sciences*, 364: 2299–309.

Huber, L., Range, F. & Virányi, Z. (2011). Dogs imitate selectively, not necessarily rationally: reply to Kaminski et al. *Animal Behavior*, 83: e1–3.

Jakovcevic, A., Elgier, A. M., Mustaca, A. E. & Bentosela, M. (2010). Breed differences in dogs' (*Canis familiaris*) gaze to the human face. *Behavioral Processes*, 84: 602–7.

Joly-Mascheroni, R. M., Senju, A. & Shepherd, A. J. (2008). Dogs catch human yawns. *Biology Letters*, 4: 446–8.

Kaminski, J. (2008). Dogs (*Canis familiaris*) are adapted to receive human communication. In *Neurobiology of "Umwelt": How Living Beings Perceive the World, Research and Perspectives in Neurosciences*, eds. A. Berthoz & Y. Christen. Heidelberg: Springer, pp. 103–7.

Kaminski, J., Bräuer, J., Call, J. & Tomasello, M. (2009b). Domestic dogs are sensitive to a human's perspective. *Behaviour*, 146: 979–98.

Kaminski, J., Call, J. & Fischer, J. (2004). Word learning in a domestic dog: evidence for "fast mapping." *Science*, 304: 1682–3.

Kaminski, J., Neumann, M., Brauer, J., Call, J. & Tomasello, M. (2011b). Dogs, *Canis familiaris*, communicate with humans to request but not to inform. *Animal Behavior*, 82: 651–8.

Kaminski, J., Nitzschner, M., Wobber, V. *et al.* (2011a). Do dogs distinguish rational from irrational acts? *Animal Behaviour*, 81: 195–203.

Kaminski, J., Schulz, L. & Tomasello, M. (2012). How dogs know when communication is intended for them. *Developmental Science*, 15: 222–32.

Kaminski, J., Tempelmann, S., Call, J. & Tomasello, M. (2009a). Domestic dogs comprehend human communication with iconic signs. *Developmental Science*, 12: 831–7.

Kis, A., Topál, J., Gácsi, M. *et al.* (2012). Does the A-not-B error in adult pet dogs indicate sensitivity to human communication? *Animal Cognition*, 15: 737–43

Kubinyi, E., Topál, J., Miklósi, Á. & Csányi, V. (2003). The effect of human demonstrator on the acquisition of a manipulative task. *Journal of Comparative Psychology*, 117: 156–65.

Kubinyi, E., Vas, J., Hejjas, K. *et al.* (2012). Polymorphism in the Tyrosine Hydroxylase (TH) gene is associated with activity-impulsivity in German shepherd dogs. *PLoS ONE*, 7: e30271

Kubinyi, E., Virányi, Z. & Miklósi, A. (2007). Comparative social cognition: from wolf and dog to humans. *Comparative Cognition & Behavior Reviews*, 2: 26–46.

Kundey, S. M. A., De Los Reyes, A., Royer, E. *et al.* (2011). Reputation-like inference in domestic dogs (*Canis familiaris*). *Animal Cognition*, 14: 291–302.

Kundey, S. M. A., De Los Reyes, A., Taglang, C. *et al.* (2010). Domesticated dogs (*Canis familiaris*) react to what others can and cannot hear. *Applied Animal Behavior Science*, 126: 45–50.

Kupán, K., Adam, M., Gyoergy, G. & Jozsef, T. (2011). Why do dogs (*Canis familiaris*) select the empty container in an observational learning task? *Animal Cognition*, 14: 259–68.

Lakatos, G., Gácsi, M., Tópal, J. & Miklósi, A. (2012). Comprehension and utilisation of pointing gestures and gazing in dog-human communication in relatively complex situations. *Animal Cognition*, 15: 201–13.

Lakatos, G., Soproni, K., Doka, A. & Miklósi, A. (2009). A comparative approach to dogs' (*Canis familiaris*)

and human infants' comprehension of various forms of pointing gestures. *Animal Cognition*, 12: 621–31.

Madsen, E. A. & Persson, T. (2013). Contagious yawning in domestic dog puppies (*Canis lupus familiaris*): the effect of ontogeny and emotional closeness on low-level imitation in dogs. *Animal Cognition*, 16: 233–40.

Maginnity, M. E. & Grace, R. C. (2014). Visual perspective taking by dogs (*Canis familiaris*) in a Guesser–Knower task: Evidence for a canine theory of mind? *Animal Cognition*, 17: 1375–92.

Marshall-Pescini, S., Passalacqua, C., Ferrario, A., Valsecchi, P. & Prato-Previde, E. (2011b). Social eavesdropping in the domestic dog. *Animal Behavior*, 81: 1177–83.

Marshall-Pescini, S., Passalacqua, C., Valsecchi, P. & Prato-Previde, E. (2010). Comment on "Differential sensitivity to human communication in dogs, wolves, and Human infants". *Science*, 329: 142.

Marshall-Pescini, S., Prato-Previde, E. & Valsecchi, P. (2011a). Are dogs (*Canis familiaris*) misled more by their owners than by strangers in a food choice task? *Animal Cognition*, 14: 137–42.

Marshall-Pescini, S., Valsecchi, P., Petak, I., Accorsi, P. A. & Previde, E. P. (2008). Does training make you smarter? The effects of training on dogs' performance (*Canis familiaris*) in a problem solving task. *Behavioral Processes*, 78: 449–54.

McNelis, N. L. & Boatright-Horowitz, S. L. (1998). Social monitoring in a primate social group: the relation between visual attention and hierarchical ranks. *Animal Cognition*, 1: 65–70.

Mech, D. (1970). *The Wolf: The Ecology and Behavior of an Endangered Species*. Garden City, NY: Natural History Press.

Mech, L. D. & Boitani, L. (2003). Wolf social ecology. In *Wolves: Behavior, Ecology, and Conservation*, eds. L. D. Mech & L. Boitani. Chicago, IL: University of Chicago Press, p. 448.

Menzel, E. W. (1974). A group of young chimpanzees in a one acre-field. In *Behavior of Nonhuman Primates*. eds. A. M. Schrier & F. Stollnitz. New York: Academic Press, p. 509.

Menzel, E. W. (1997). Leadership and communication in young chimpanzees. In *Precultural Primate Behavior*, ed. E.W. Menzel. Basel: Karger, p. 258.

Merola, I., Prato-Previde, E. & Marshall-Pescini, S. (2012a). Social referencing in dog-owner dyads? *Animal Cognition*, 15: 175–85.

Merola I., Prato-Previde, E. & Marshall-Pescini, S. (2012b). Dogs' social referencing towards owners and strangers. *PLoS ONE*, 7: e47653. http://doi:10.1371/journal.pone.0047653

Mersmann, D., Tomasello, M., Call, J., Kaminski, J. & Taborsky, M. (2011). Simple mechanisms can explain social learning in domestic dogs (*Canis familiaris*). *Ethology*, 117: 675–90.

Met, A., Miklósi, Á., & Lakatos, G. (2014). Gaze-following behind barriers in domestic dogs. *Animal Cognition*, 17: 1401–5.

Miklósi, A., Kubinyi, E., Tópal, J., Gácsi, M., Viranyi, Z. & Csanyi, V. (2003). A simple reason for a big difference:

wolves do not look back at humans, but dogs do. *Current Biology*, 13: 763–6.

Miklósi, A., Polgardi, R., Topál, J. & Csányi, V. (2000). Intentional behavior in dog–human communication: an experimental analysis of "showing" behavior in the dog. *Animal Cognition*, 3: 159.

Miklósi, A., Polgardi, R., Tópal, J. & Csanyi, V. (1998). Use of experimenter-given cues in dogs. *Animal Cognition*, 1: 113.

Miklósi, A. & Soproni, K. (2006). A comparative analysis of animals' understanding of the human pointing gesture. *Animal Cognition*, 9: 81–93.

Miklósi, A. & Tópal, J. (2011). On the hunt for the gene of perspective taking: pitfalls in methodology. *Learning & Behavior*, 39: 310–13.

Miklósi, A., Tópal, J. & Csanyi, V. (2004). Comparative social cognition: what can dogs teach us? *Animal Behavior*, 67: 995–1004.

Miller, H. C., Rayburn-Reeves, R. & Zentall, T. R. (2009). Imitation and emulation by dogs using a bidirectional control procedure. *Behavioral Processes*, 80: 109–14.

Mongillo, P., Bono, G., Regolin, L. & Marinelli, L. (2010). Selective attention to humans in companion dogs, *Canis familiaris. Animal Behavior*, 80: 1057–63.

Moore, K., Cleland, J. & McGrew, W. C. (1991). Visual encounters between families of cotton-top tamarins (*Saguinus oedipus*). *Primates*, 32: 23–33.

Morris, P. H., Doe, C. & Godsell, E. (2008). Secondary emotions in non-primate species? Behavioral reports and subjective claims by animal owners. *Cognition & Emotion*, 22: 3–20.

Mulcahy, N. J. & Hedge, V. (2012). Are great apes tested with an abject object-choice task? *Animal Behavior*, 83: 313–21.

Müller, C. A., Schmitt, K., Barber, A. L. & Huber, L. (2015). Dogs can discriminate emotional expressions of human faces. *Current Biology*, 25: 601–5.

Nicol, C. J. & Pope, S. J. (1994). Social learning in small flocks of laying hens. *Animal Behavior*, 47: 1289–96.

Nishida, T. (1987). Local traditions and cultural transmission. In *Primate Societies*, eds. B. B. Smuts, D. Cheney, R. Seyfarth, R. Wrangham & T. Struhsaker. Chicago, IL: University of Chicago Press, p. 578.

O'Hara, S. & Reeve, A. (2011). A test of the yawning contagion and emotional connectedness hypothesis in dogs, *Canis familiaris. Animal Behavior*, 81: 335–40.

Oliva, J. L., Rault, J. L., Appleton, B. & Lill, A. (2015). Oxytocin enhances the appropriate use of human social cues by the domestic dog (*Canis familiaris*) in an object choice task. *Animal Cognition*, 18: 767–75.

Osthaus, B., Lea, S. E. G. & Slater, A. M. (2003). Training influences problem-solving abilities in dogs (*Canis lupus familiaris*). *Proceedings of the Annual BSAS Conference*, p. 103.

Osthaus, B., Lea, S. E. G. & Slater, A. M. (2005). Dogs (*Canis lupus familiaris*) fail to show understanding of means-end connections in a string-pulling task. *Animal Cognition*, 8: 37–47.

Palagi, E. (2006). Social play in bonobos (*Pan paniscus*) and chimpanzees (*Pan troglodytes*): Implications for natural social systems and interindividual relationships. *American Journal of Physical Anthropology*, 129: 418–26.

Pang, J.-F., Kluetsch, C., Zou, X.-J. *et al.* (2009). MtDNA data indicate a single origin for dogs south of Yangtze River, less than 16,300 years ago, from numerous wolves. *Molecular Biology and Evolution*, 26: 2849–64.

Petter, M., Musolino, E., Roberts, W. A. & Cole, M. (2009). Can dogs (*Canis familiaris*) detect human deception? *Behavioral Processes*, 82: 109–18.

Pettersson, H., Kaminski, J., Herrmann, E. & Tomasello, M. (2011). Understanding of human communicative motives in domestic dogs. *Applied Animal Behavior Science*, 133: 235–45.

Pilley, J. W. & Reid, A. K. (2011). Border collie comprehends object names as verbal referents. *Behavioral Processes*, 86: 184–95.

Pongrácz, P., Banhegyi, P. & Miklósi, A. (2012). When rank counts – dominant dogs learn better from a human demonstrator in a two-action test. *Behavior*, 149: 111–32.

Pongrácz, P., Miklósi, A., Kubinyi, E., Gurobi, K., Tópal, J. & Csanyi, V. (2001). Social learning in dogs: the effect of a human demonstrator on the performance of dogs in a detour task. *Animal Behavior*, 62: 1109–17.

Pongrácz, P., Miklósi, A., Timar-Geng, K. & Csanyi, V. (2004). Verbal attention-getting as a key factor in social learning between dog (*Canis familiaris*) and human. *Journal of Comparative Psychology*, 118: 375–83.

Pongrácz, P., Molnar, C. & Miklósi, A. (2006). Acoustic parameters of dog barks carry emotional information for humans. *Applied Animal Behavior Science*, 100: 228–40.

Pongrácz, P., Molnar, C., Miklósi, A. & Csanyi, V. (2005). Human listeners are able to classify dog (*Canis familiaris*) barks recorded in different situations. *Journal of Comparative Psychology*, 119: 136–44.

Pongrácz, P., Vida, V., Bánhegyi, P. & Miklósi, Á. (2008). How does dominance rank status affect individual and social learning performance in the dog (*Canis familiaris*)? *Animal Cognition*, 11: 75–82.

Povinelli, D. J., Reaux, J. E., Bierschwale, D. T., Allain, A. D. & Simon, B. B. (1997). Exploitation of pointing as a referential gesture in young children, but not adolescent chimpanzees. *Cognitive Development*, 12: 327–65.

Povinelli, D. J. & Vonk, J. (2003). Chimpanzee minds: suspiciously human? *Trends in Cognitive Science*, 7: 157–60.

Povinelli, D. J. & Eddy, T. J. (1996) Factors influencing young chimpanzees (*Pan troglodytes*) recognition of attention. *Journal of Comparative Psychology*, 110: 336–45.

Preston, S. D. & De Waal, F. B. M. (2002). Empathy: its ultimate and proximate bases. *Behavioral and Brain Sciences*, 25: 1–72.

Quervel-Chaumette, M., Dale, R., Marshall-Pescini, S. & Range, F. (2015). Familiarity affects other-regarding preferences in pet dogs. *Scientific Reports*, 5: 18102.

Quervel-Chaumette, M., Faerber, V., Faragó, T., Marshall-Pescini, S. & Range, F. (2016). Investigating empathy-like responding to conspecifics' distress in pet dogs. *PloS ONE*, 11: e0152920

Range, F., Heucke, S. L., Gruber, C., Konz, A., Huber, L. & Virányi, Z. (2009b). The effect of ostensive cues on dogs' performance in a manipulative social learning task. *Applied Animal Behavior Science*, 120: 170–8.

Range, F., Horn, L., Bugnyar, T., Gajdon, G. K. & Huber, L. (2009a). Social attention in keas, dogs, and human children. *Animal Cognition*, 12: 181–92.

Range, F., Horn, L., Virányi, Z. & Huber, L. (2009c). The absence of reward induces inequity aversion in dogs. *Proceedings of the National Academy of Sciences of the United States of America*, 106: 340–5.

Range, F., Leitner, K. & Virányi, Z. (2012). The influence of the relationship and motivation on inequity aversion in dogs. *Social Justice Research*, 25: 170–94.

Range. F., Ritter, C. & Virányi, Z. (2015). Testing the myth: tolerant dogs and aggressive wolves. *Proceedings of the Royal Society B*, 282: 20150220

Range, F. & Virányi, Z. (2011). Development of gaze following abilities in wolves (*Canis lupus*). *PLoS ONE*: e16888. http://doi:10.1371/journal.pone.0016888

Range, F. & Virányi, Z. (2013). Social learning from humans or conspecifics: differences and similarities between wolves and dogs. *Frontiers in Psychology*. 4: 868. http://doi:10.3389/fpsyg.2013.00868

Range, F. & Virányi, Z. (2014). Wolves are better imitators of conspecifics than dogs. *PLoS ONE*, 9: e86559.

Range, F. & Virányi, Z. (2015). Tracking the evolutionary origins of dog-human cooperation: the "Canine Cooperation Hypothesis." *Frontiers in Psychology*, 5: 1582.

Range, F., Virányi, Z. & Huber, L. (2007). Selective imitation in domestic dogs. *Current Biology*, 17: 868–872.

Riedel, J., Buttelmann, D., Call, J. & Tomasello, M. (2006). Domestic dogs (*Canis familiaris*) use a physical marker to locate hidden food. *Animal Cognition*, 9: 27–35.

Riedel, J., Schumann, K., Kaminski, J., Call, J. & Tomasello, M. (2008). The early ontogeny of human-dog communication. *Animal Behavior*, 75: 1003–14.

Rooney, N. J. & Bradshaw, J. W. (2002). An experimental study of the effects of play upon the dog-human relationship. *Applied Animal Behavior Science*, 75: 161–76.

Savolainen, P., Zhang, Y. P., Luo, J., Lundeberg, J. & Leitner, T. (2002). Genetic evidence for an East Asian origin of domestic dogs. *Science*, 298: 1610–13.

Scheider, L., Grassmann, S., Kaminski, J. & Tomasello, M. (2011). Domestic dogs use contextual information and tone of voice when following a human pointing gesture. *PLoS ONE*: e21676. http://doi:10.1371/journal.pone.0021676

Schwab, C. & Huber, L. (2006). Obey or not obey? Dogs (*Canis familiaris*) behave differently in response to attentional states of their owners. *Journal of Comparative Psychology* 120: 169–75.

Scott, J. P. & Fuller, J. L. (1965). *Genetics and the Social Behavior of the Dog*. Chicago, IL: University of Chicago Press.

Senju, A. & Csibra, G. (2008). Gaze following in human infants depends on communicative signals. *Current Biology*, 18: 668–71.

Serpell, J. & Hsu, Y. (2005). Effects of breed, sex, and neuter status on trainability in dogs. *Anthrozoos*, 18: 196–207.

Silva, K., Bessa, J. & de Sousa, L. (2012). Auditory contagious yawning in domestic dogs (*Canis familiaris*): first evidence for social modulation. *Animal Cognition*, 15: 721–4.

Slabbert, J. M. & Rasa, O. A. E. (1997). Observational learning of an acquired maternal behavior pattern by working dog pups: an alternative training method? *Applied Animal Behavior Science*, 53: 309–16.

Soproni, K., Miklósi, A., Tópal, J. & Csanyi, V. (2001). Comprehension of human communicative signs in pet dogs (*Canis familiaris*). *Journal of Comparative Psychology*, 115: 122–126.

Soproni, K., Miklósi, A., Tópal, J. & Csanyi, V. (2002). Dogs' (*Canis familiaris*) responsiveness to human pointing gestures. *Journal of Comparative Psychology*, 116: 27–34.

Spence, K. W. (1997). Experimental studies of learning and higher mental processes in infra-human primates. *Psychological Bulletin*, 34: 806–850.

Szetei, V., Miklósi, A., Tópal, J. & Csanyi, V. (2003). When dogs seem to lose their nose: an investigation on the use of visual and olfactory cues in communicative context between dog and owner. *Applied Animal Behavior Science*, 83: 141–52.

Tauzin, T., Csík, A., Kis, A. & Topál, J. (2015). What or where? The meaning of referential human pointing for dogs (*Canis familiaris*). *Journal of Comparative Psychology*, 129: 334.

Tennie, C., Glabsch, E., Tempelmann, S., Bräuer, J., Kaminski, J. & Call, J. (2009). Dogs, *Canis familiaris*, fail to copy intransitive actions in third-party contextual imitation tasks. *Animal Behavior*, 77: 1491–9.

Thorndike, E. L. (1898). Animal intelligence: an experimental study of the associative process in animals. *Psychological Review Monograph*, 2: 8.

Thorpe, W. H. (1956). *Learning and Instinct in Animals*. London: Methuen.

Thornton, A. & Mcauliffe, K. (2006). Teaching in wild meerkats. *Science*, 313: 227–9.

Tinbergen, N. (1963). On aims and methods of ethology. *Zeitschrift fur Tierpsychologie*, 20: 410–33.

Tomasello, M., Hare, B. & Agnetta, B. (1999) Chimpanzees, *Pan troglodytes*, follow gaze direction geometrically. *Animal Behaviour*, 58: 769–77.

Tópal, J., Byrne, R. W., Miklósi, A. & Csányi, V. (2006). Reproducing human actions and action sequences: "Do as I Do!" in a dog. *Animal Cognition*, 9: 355–367.

Tòpal, J., Gácsi, M., Miklósi, Á., Virányi, Z., Kubinyi, E. & Csányi, V. (2005). Attachment to humans: a comparative study on hand-reared wolves and differently socialized dog puppies. *Animal Behaviour*, 70: 1367–75.

Topál, J., Gergely, G., Erdohegyi, Á., Csibra, G. & Miklósi, Á. (2009b). Differential sensitivity to human communication in dogs, wolves, and human infants. *Science*, 325: 1269–72.

Tópal, J., Miklósi, Á. & Csányi, V. (1997). Dog-human relationship affects problem solving behavior in the dog. *Anthrozoös*, 10: 214–24.

Tópal, J., Miklósi, Á., Csányi, V. & Doka, A. (1998). Attachment behavior in dogs (*Canis familiaris*): a new application of Ainsworth's (1969) Strange Situation Test. *Journal of Comparative Psychology*, 112: 219–29.

Tópal, J., Miklósi, A., Gácsi, M. *et al.* (2009a). The dog as a model for understanding human social behavior. *Advances in the Study of Behaviour*, 39: 71–116.

Triesch, J., Teuscher, C., Teak, G. & Carlson, E. (2006) Gaze following: why (not) learning it? *Developmental Science*, 9: 125–47.

Trut, L. N. (1999). Early canid domestication: the farm-fox experiment: foxes bred for tamability in a 40-year experiment exhibit remarkable transformations that suggest an interplay between behavioral genetics and development. *American Scientist*, 87: 160–9.

Udell, M. A. R., Dorey, N. R. & Wynne, C. D. L. (2010). What did domestication do to dogs? A new account of dogs' sensitivity to human actions. *Biological Reviews*, 85: 327–45.

Udell, M. A. R., Spencer, J. M., Dorey, N. R. & Wynne, C. D. L. (2012). Human-socialized wolves follow diverse human gestures ... and they may not be alone. *International Journal of Comparative Psychology*, 25: 97–117.

Virányi, Z., Gácsi, M., Kubinyi, E. *et al.* (2008b). Comprehension of human pointing gestures in young human-reared wolves and dogs. *Animal Cognition*, 11: 373–87.

Virányi, Z., Range, F. & Huber, L. (2008a). Attentiveness toward others and social learning in domestic dogs. In *Learning from Animals?* eds. L. N.-H. Röska-Hardy & E. M. Neumann-Held. London: Psychology Press, p. 280.

Viranyi, Z., Tópal, J., Gácsi, M., Miklósi, A. & Csanyi, V. (2004). Dogs respond appropriately to cues of humans' attentional focus. *Behavioral Processes*, 66: 161–72.

Viranyi, Z., Tópal, J., Miklósi, A. & Csanyi, V. (2006). A nonverbal test of knowledge attribution: a comparative study on dogs and children. *Animal Cognition*, 9: 13–26.

Wallis, L. J., Range, F., Müller, C. A., Serisier, S., Huber, L. & Virányi, Z. (2014) Lifespan development of attentiveness in domestic dogs: drawing parallels with humans. *Frontiers in Psychology*, 5: 71.

Wallis, L. J., Range, F., Müller, C. A., Serisier, S., Huber, L. & Virányi, Z. (2015) Training for eye contact modulates gaze following in dogs. *Animal Behaviour*, 106: 27–35.

Werhahn, G., Virányi, Z., Barrera, G., Sommese, A., & Range, F. (2016). Wolves (*Canis lupus*) and dogs (*Canis familiaris*) differ in following human gaze into distant space but respond similar to their packmates' gaze. *Journal of Comparative Psychology*: http://dx.doi.org/10.1037/com0000036.

Whiten, A. (1996). When does smart behavior-reading become mind-reading? In *Theories of Theories of Mind*, eds. P. Carruthers & P. K. Smith. Cambridge: Cambridge University Press, p. 390.

Wobber, V., Hare, B., Koler-Matznick, J., Wrangham, R. & Tomasello, M. (2009). Breed differences in domestic dogs' (*Canis familiaris*) comprehension of human communicative signals. *Interaction Studies*, 10: 206–24.

Wynne, C. D. L., Udell, M. A. R. & Lord, K. A. (2008). Ontogeny's impact on human–dog communication. *Animal Behaviour*, 76: e1–4.

Yin, S. & McCowan, B. (2004). Barking in domestic dogs: context specificity and individual identification. *Animal Behaviour*, 68: 343–55.

Yoon, J. M. D. & Tennie, C. (2010). Contagious yawning: a reflection of empathy, mimicry, or contagion? *Animal Behaviour*, 79: e1–3

11 The learning dog: A discussion of training methods

ILANA REISNER

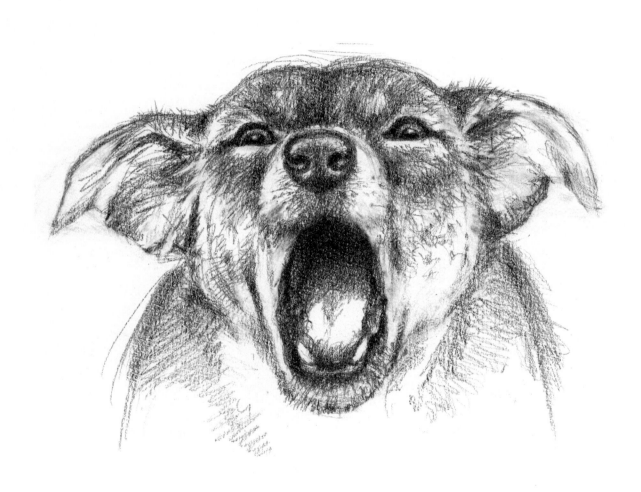

11.1   Introduction

There are currently over 78 million pet dogs in the United States, living in 39% of all US households (American Pet Products Association, 2012), and an undetermined but very large population globally, with highest numbers documented in Brazil, China, Mexico, Japan, Russia and in the European Union (Batson, 2008). Most dogs are kept as companion animals by owners whose training experience and abilities range from naïve to highly skilled. In contrast to guide dogs for the blind, hunting dogs, military, police or other working dogs, pet dogs typically do not have one particular "job" for which a specific, targeted training plan is required. However, through interaction with the physical and social environment, learning is nonetheless important throughout the life of the dog. For example, convincing a young puppy that the yard is the preferred spot for elimination requires learning, as does the middle-aged dog's acceptance of a new baby, or of walking on a leash without pulling. Social learning is continuous and important throughout the life cycle. Whether through planned, deliberate training sessions or more passive associations, the behavior of dogs is largely related to their experiences (see also Serpell *et al.*, Chapter 6). Training should therefore be viewed as a lifelong habit whether or not the dog participates in basic obedience classes.

Canine behavior problems are common (Vacalopoulos & Anderson, 1993) and are the most frequently cited reason for euthanasia, rehoming, or relinquishment of dogs to shelters (Salman *et al.*, 2000). Even owners who forego formal obedience training find it necessary to manage common dog behaviors such as jumping up or excessive barking; after all, any behavior – including aggression at times – that results in a positive outcome for the dog is likely to be repeated. Behavior problems are thus often a consequence of unintentional learning (reinforcement). Furthermore, because many behavior problems in dogs are based in fear or anxiety, the specific method used to modify behavior can also influence its outcome.

Many dog owners seeking help with managing their pets' behavior do so through friends and neighbors, books, the internet, and television. Unfortunately, the choice of local dog training clubs or individual trainers is often a matter of geographic serendipity, and astonishingly little may be known about the experience, competence and even the ethics of local trainers. Techniques that are used are often wildly variable and have become a polarizing topic among professionals and the dog-owning public between those who favor aversive, intimidation-based training and those who advocate for reward-based, gentler methods. Harsh training methods work by inducing fear (Koehler, 1984), which can quickly escalate to active avoidance (escape), learned helplessness (Overmier & Seligman, 1967) or aggression.

11.2   A brief history

The appearance of dog training in print publications began in the nineteenth century, with instructions for sporting or gun dog training, touching on both the positive and the punitive. It is interesting to note that positive reinforcement training appeared in print as early as 1848: "Caresses and substantial rewards are far greater incentives to exertion than any fears of punishment" (Hutchinson, 1848, p. 23). In a 1909 publication, *Breaking and Training Dogs: Being Concise Directions for the Proper Education of Dogs Both for the Field and as Companions*, the author states:

With regard to the subject of rewards, cheese will play a prominent part in the education of our puppy. As the first principles of the said education will be based on the system of as many rewards and as few punishments as possible …. If you decide on using cheese as a medium …. [it] places you in a position to reward your charge at a moment's notice; and be careful not to keep him waiting for his *bonne bouche*. (Pathfinder & Dalziel, 1909, p. 14)

In contrast to gun dog training, military or police dog training appeared to invite a more regimented and even severe approach. The 1910 publication, *Training Dogs: A Manual*, by Colonel Konrad Most, for example, considered by many to be a major landmark in the development of modern dog training, was based upon the training of military or police dogs (Most, 2000). Most was a German police dog trainer who served as director of the Berlin State Breeding and Training Establishment for police dogs and head of the Canine Research Department of the Army from 1919–1937. Most (2000) put forward the concept that unacceptable canine behavior must result in unpleasant consequences. In contrast to the primarily hunting-dog-focused trainers before him, Most emphasized the use of intimidation-based methods. He justified the use of harsh training methods with dogs by stating that successful management, " … can be achieved only by exercising compulsion whenever the dog does not spontaneously do what is required of him" (Most, 2000, p. 24), and that:

[The switch] … should be employed until the animal submits and his will to resist … is replaced by fear. So long as the dog does not submit, but continues to resist, a flexible switch should be used, if necessary, on the head and jaws, but not on the top of the nose. It may also be used on the neck, ears, legs and tail, but not on the sexual parts or on the lower regions of the belly and chest. Apart from such exceptional cases *heavy* cuts should only be applied to the powerful muscles on the fore- and hindquarters and on the back. (Most, 2000, p. 36)

Training Dogs: A Manual quickly formed the foundation upon which generations of dog trainers justified "compulsion" or heavy-handed training methods even for companion dogs, focusing attention on forceful control of the dog's behavior as a struggle for authority, in order to achieve "the permanent and unconditional surrender of the dog" (Most, 2000, p. 37).

During the 1930s and 1940s, pet dog training methods underwent significant changes. Josef Weber (*The Dog in Training*, 1939) and Hans Tosutti (*Companion Dog Training*, 1948), both students of Konrad Most, had emigrated to the United States to launch dog training schools and thereby extend Most's influence internationally. At about the same time, B. F. Skinner published his first book, *The Behavior of Organisms* (1938), elaborating on operant conditioning (instrumental or "trial-and-error" learning) and the significance of its behavioral consequences. Also in the 1930s, a standard poodle breeder and dog fancier, Helene Whitehouse Walker, helped to establish obedience trialing through the American Kennel Club, which published its first official "Regulations and Standard for Obedience Test Field Trials" in April, 1936 (American Kennel Club). Together with Blanche Saunders, who had studied with Josef Weber, Walker traveled throughout the United States educating the public about companion dog training. Among Saunders' students and followers were many of the well-known trainers of the 1950s and 1960s, including Winifred Strickland, whose popular book *Expert Obedience Training for Dogs* (1966) advocated a mix of techniques, such as the use of choke collars and kneeing the dog in the chest for jumping up, but also using food as positive reinforcement – with the ultimate objective of weaning the dog from food (Strickland, 1966).

The use of clickers (markers) as secondary or conditioned reinforcers was developed in the 1940s by Marian Kruse (later Marian Kruse Breland) and Keller Breland, both formerly graduate students studying under B. F. Skinner. Together, the Brelands formed Animal Behavior Enterprises (ABE) with the goal of using positive-reinforcement based operant conditioning techniques for animal training. Through their work they successfully trained a variety of animal species, from marine mammals to land mammals (including dogs) and birds, creating commercial animal exhibits and shows. After the death of Keller Breland in 1965, Marian married Bob Bailey, formerly the first Director of Training in the United States Navy, and together they continued the work of ABE. Although the Brelands were the first to implement clickers as secondary reinforcers, clicker-training was not widely used in dogs until the 1990s when Karen Pryor, a behavioral biologist who had worked with marine mammals and other species, popularized its use in operant conditioning (Pryor, 1999). The clicker (or other salient stimulus, for example a whistle in the case of marine mammals, or a flashlight for deaf dogs) is first paired with food or another unconditioned stimulus (US) until it becomes a conditioned stimulus (CS). It is then used as an event marker to reinforce the target behavior. As Pryor has stated, clicker training differs from traditional dog training in several important ways. For example, training sessions can and should be relatively brief, and include a sufficient amount of variety, so that the animal is more motivated and interested. Clicker training allows the dog to offer behaviors which are then shaped. Most important, in clicker training there is no need or purpose for positive punishment or negative reinforcement (Pryor, 1999).

11.3   Is dominance relevant?

Much of dog training from the mid-twentieth century to the present has relied upon – and continues to evoke – the concept of canine dominance over human owners (so-called "dominance theory") (Bradshaw et al., 2009; Bradshaw & Rooney, Chapter 8). The notion that dogs, by default, will attempt to achieve social dominance over the owner/handler is an extension of Konrad Most's premise that human–dog relationships inevitably involve a struggle for authority, making it necessary to use compulsion training, " … to obtain the permanent and unconditional surrender of the dog. The intimidated state that accompanies it soon disappears, simply because peace again reigns as soon as the man is victorious" (Most, 2000, p. 37). In addition to its basis in Konrad Most's experiences with military and police working dogs, the theory of canine dominance was bolstered by observations of captive wolves whose behavior was assumed to correspond to the social behavior of their wild relatives (Mech, 1981; Schenkel, 1947). While wolf ethologists such as L. David Mech (1981) and others have observed both wild and captive groups of wolves, conclusions about pack social behavior were in part based on captive wolves forced to live with unrelated wolves in close quarters, whereas, " … in natural wolf packs, the alpha male or female are merely the breeding animals, the parents of the pack, and dominance contests with other wolves are rare, if they exist at all" (Mech, 1999). Although it has been argued that free-roaming dogs are socially solitary at times (Berman & Dunbar, 1983; Daniels, 1983), dominance-related group dynamics are indeed a recognized phenomenon among them (Cafazzo et al., 2010). The point is not whether social dominance is an ethological reality in wolves or dogs – it is – but rather whether the dominance hierarchy is a relevant drive for canine aggression to people, and whether dominance-based "firm handed" training is therefore appropriate (Bekoff, 2012). Unfortunately, the relevance of dominance-related behavior in the human–dog relationship has been broadly misunderstood, leading to coercive dog training practices in some cases (Millan, 2013).

The misinterpretation of "dominance theory" as a basis for human–dog interactions thus led to its being accepted, absorbed and widely practiced among dog trainers and behaviorists justifying the need for discipline and often harsh methods in training and handling dogs. In their popular dog training book, the Monks of New Skete advocated the use of physical discipline in response to human- and dog-directed aggression, house-soiling, stealing, and persistent destructiveness, for example with the "shakedown": "Grasp both sides of the dog's neck fur … and raise the dog's front slightly. Make eye contact and give a quick shake as you scold" (Monks of New Skete, 2002, p. 72).

Although the Monks of New Skete previously prescribed the "alpha wolf rollover" as a form of discipline, a revised edition of their popular book states that it is no longer recommended because it might lead to owner-directed aggression, "particularly with a dominant dog" (Monks of New Skete, 2002, p. 76). (The contention that some individual dogs are dominant by temperament has been challenged (Luescher & Reisner, 2009).) It is interesting to note that both the Monks and Konrad Most worked primarily with German shepherd dogs, thus perhaps sharing a dog-handling philosophy with roots in the training of military dogs.

In the field of veterinary behavioral medicine, dominance-related aggression was the clinical diagnosis for dogs displaying aggression toward owners in contexts such as being disturbed while resting, guarding resources, being hugged, kissed, bent over, or otherwise a target of human affection, or in response to (positive) punishment (Reisner et al., 1994; Voith & Borchelt, 1982). At one time, it was recognized as the most common problem for which dogs were referred to behavior specialists (Landsberg, 1991). Treatment of dominance-related aggression centered on reclaiming dominance over the dog by firmly lowering its social status within the human family, although there was some early recognition that more benign management of aggression was preferred (Mugford, 1995). Among those who subscribed to the "dominance theory," who tended to predominate in the United States, owner-directed aggression was often countered with more dominance (aggression) from the owner/handler. Unfortunately, this tendency to escalate conflict reinforced, and in turn was reinforced by, the popular notion that dog training and behavior management *required* physical or emotional (psychological) force. The "alpha roll," based on the misconception that the alpha wolf will "roll" a subordinate wolf onto its back, has resulted in failed interventions and even owner injury (Herron et al., 2009).

In spite of the argument that interspecies (dog to human) dominance-related aggression makes little sense ethologically, and attempts to challenge it can result in injury to owners, the dominance-embracing culture continues to make claims about its training methods (Littlefield, 2014) rallying the financial support of dog owners who continue to believe those claims. In the parlance of dominance, the family dog is a member of the "pack" and, since misinformation about canine social behavior includes the struggle for control, the owner must assert him- or herself to maintain "leader" or "alpha" status.

The subject of dog training has thus developed into one with emotionally polarized points of view. The controversy might be viewed as analogous to the debate over corporal punishment of children. Spanking is discouraged by the American Academy of Pediatrics because of its often negative consequences, and because of the evidence that positive punishment is no more effective than non-punitive, positive reinforcement approaches to changing undesirable behavior (American Academy of Pediatrics, 1998). Yet, in spite of evidence that spanking is associated with long-term negative consequences (Mackenzie et al., 2013), corporal punishment of children continues to be supported by some parents and special interest groups (Gershoff et al., 1999; Ingram, 2006). Perhaps a common denominator in both cases (dogs and children) is ultimate powerlessness when confronted by those in control.

11.4   The science of training

Learning can be defined as the acquisition of new knowledge or behavior through experience or study. To the average pet owner, dog training often stops after formal obedience or house training. The new puppy, for example, is taken to an obedience group class, learns to "sit," "stay" and "come" in response to the handler's commands, and is then considered to be set for life with no further training needed. Appropriately, however, such a limited view of training is being supplanted by the more progressive notion that dogs (like people) learn and therefore continue to be "trained" throughout their lives and in all kinds of ordinary contexts. Both classical conditioning ("I heard a thunderclap in this room last night, therefore I fear this room") and operant conditioning ("I found a delicious sandwich on the counter, therefore I will check the counter again") are continuous.

Any stimulus change that *increases* the probability of occurrence of the behavior preceding it is a *reinforcement* of the behavior. Conversely, a stimulus change that *decreases* the probability of occurrence of the preceding behavior is a *punishment*. The "four quadrants" of operant conditioning, which shape behavior based on its consquences, are best understood by considering whether the stimulus is added to (*positive*) or removed from (*negative*) the situation. Applying this principle, positive reinforcement would be adding something pleasant, while negative reinforcement would be removing something unpleasant. Positive punishment would be the addition of something unpleasant, while negative punishment would be the removal of something pleasant (Clayton, 2013; Mace, 2010). Examples help to illustrate these concepts:

- **Positive reinforcement**: Food, toys, praise, petting,[1] opportunity to do desirable things such as go through doorways.
- **Positive punishment**: Leash correction (jerking leash), hitting, shock, pointing, yelling, "alpha-roll," "dominance down," poking, rolling up newspaper (when the newspaper has previously been associated with hitting), scolding.
- **Negative reinforcement**: Loosening a tightened lead on choke collar, discontinuation of shock, discontinuation of ear pinch and other aversive stimuli.
- **Negative punishment**: Turning one's back on the dog, leaving dog abruptly, removing toy, withholding food.

At its simplest, the difference between the two polarized camps of dog training is that one routinely includes the use of positive punishment and negative reinforcement while the other does not. Although the positive punishment group also uses positive reinforcement at times, it is primarily the use of positive punishment that distinguishes one from the other. Positive punishment and negative reinforcement may work together as "aversive" methods, as do positive reinforcement and negative punishment as "positive" methods (Blackwell *et al.*, 2012). It is interesting to note that dog owners and even some dog professionals continue to confuse these concepts, for example mistaking negative reinforcement for positive punishment.

11.5   Stopping undesirable behavior

Canine behavior problems are common, and whether a given behavior is actually undesirable is often a matter of perception. For example, jumping up on people's laps might be tolerated or even desirable at home when only the family is present, but discouraged when strangers are visiting.

For many pet owners who have taken their puppy or new adult dog through a group obedience class, subsequent training efforts are rekindled only when a behavior problem develops. The focus then is on stopping or changing an undesirable behavior, which leads the owners to seek outside help. Clearly, positive punishment can be effective in stopping or reducing the frequency of undesirable

[1] Whether a behavioral consequence functions as reinforcement, punishment or neither is determined by the recipient. For some dogs, praise may be ineffective, and reaching to pet the dog may be aversive (Overall & Love, 2001).

behaviors quickly (although, in some cases, the inhibition is only temporary); hence the popularity of dog training "celebrities" in books and on television.

Positive punishment is not recommended because, in order for it to be effective, it must be sufficiently aversive, and aversive interactions (e.g. hitting, poking, or rolling a dog onto his back) cause pain and fear that can, in turn, result in defensive aggression towards the punisher (Herron *et al.*, 2009). Equally important, they interfere with trust, and teach the dog that human–dog interactions are unpredictable and unsafe. Considering that problem behavior is often associated with anxiety, the behavior itself may be aggravated by positive punishment. Rather than learning an alternative behavior, a physically punished and aroused dog tends to focus only on his own pain and self-defense – true as well for children who are physically punished (Gershoff, 2002).

How, then, should the average or inexperienced dog owner go about stopping an undesirable behavior? Let's consider the previously mentioned problem of jumping up on people, which can be viewed in two ways. First, it is frequently "tried" by young or new dogs, is unintentionally reinforced by petting and attention, and therefore quickly becomes an operantly conditioned behavior. Second, and perhaps just as important, seeking attention by jumping up on people is a common characteristic of nervous or anxious dogs. If the "jumpee" is unhappy with this behavior and wants to change it, there are several options, discussed below.

11.5.1 Punishment

The following conditions must be met in order for punishment to be effective:

- It must be a consistent consequence of the behavior, i.e. it has to occur every time the behavior is performed.
- It must occur during or immediately following the behavior.
- It must be strong or intense enough to immediately interrupt the behavior.

Positive punishment is not recommended in clinical behavior modification because it may cause fear or pain, and most animals presenting to behaviorists already exhibit some degree of fear or anxiety. However, with these cautions and when the above criteria are met, punishment may still be useful if the dog isn't frightened or hurt (see also Zawistowski & Reid, Chapter 12). For example, a motion-detector spray[2] is aversive, intended to immediately and consistently trigger an air/water spray each time (for example) a dog puts his paws up on the kitchen counter. Several points on the use of punishment should be made here:

- If an aversive stimulus is to be applied in training, it should not be associated with the owner (who might then become the conditioned stimulus by association, causing fear reactions in the dog).
- Strongly motivated behavior may not respond to punishment, especially if the behavior is also intermittently reinforced. The solution is not to increase the severity of the aversive stimulus, but instead to offer alternative, appropriate behavior choices that can be positively reinforced.
- Even a relatively "mild" aversive stimulus such as a motion-detector spray can be too intense for sensitive dogs and lead to the development of anxiety and fear problems.
- There are some behaviors – particularly fearfulness, aggression and submissive behaviors – which should never be managed with positive punishment of any kind because they are likely to worsen the problem behavior and create severe conflict for the dog.

[2] StayAway Motion-Activated Pet Deterrent (Contech Enterprises, Inc., Victoria, BC, Canada).

In the case of the jumping dog, commonly encountered advice is to put a knee into the dog as he jumps, to snap the leash, to squeeze the front paws that are up on the owner, and/or to push the dog backwards (Curtis, 2002; Kilcommons & Wilson, 1999; Monks of New Skete, 2011). All of these are examples of positive punishment. Dogs often continue to jump in spite of these efforts, presumably because (a) as aversive as they sound, they might not be aversive "enough"; (b) the behavior might be intermittently reinforced by friends and family members who pet and interact with the dog as he jumps, thereby making the punishment ineffective; and (c) the motivation for jumping up, which can include anxiety and displacement behavior, might be strong enough to override the punishment.

11.5.2   Extinction

An intermittently reinforced behavior will persist over time, but if all reinforcement is stopped the behavior will eventually be lost, or *extinguished*. The animal learns that the specific behavior does not "pay" (i.e. is not reinforced), and the frequency or intensity of the behavior will fade to the baseline level before reinforcement (Griggs, 2012). For example, the owners of jumping dogs can attempt to extinguish the behavior by folding their arms and looking off into the distance, without talking to, petting, or even "scolding" the dog (because even unpleasant attention can serve as positive reinforcement). The offered behavior – in this case, jumping – often will worsen or intensify in an *extinction burst* before it fades. Generally speaking, extinction can be difficult to apply in the average dog's home because visitors and unmotivated family members may continue to reinforce the behavior inadvertently. Another important disadvantage of extinction as a training method is that it takes more time to produce the desired effect than many owners will tolerate.

11.5.3   Response substitution

The aim of response substitution is to replace undesirable or inappropriate behavior with acceptable behavior. Response substitution is often used together with desensitization, exposing the dog to the stimulus in gradually increasing intensities. Our jumping dog could be asked, for example, to "sit" or to "bring a toy" instead of jumping up. Response substitution is the preferred choice for most pet homes. By teaching the dog to perform an alternate behavior, the owner provides an opportunity to reward (positively reinforce) the dog, and to avoid unpleasant, scary or confusing interactions. Equally important, by being given the opportunity to do the "right" and familiar thing, the dog is also given some control over the environment, which may decrease anxiety (Chorpita & Barlow, 1998).

11.6   Training methods and behavior problems

Behavior problems in pet dogs range from minor annoyances to severe anxieties and aggression. Aggression to people is considered by many to be the most severe behavior problem, but even problems considered objectively to be minor, such as excessive barking, can be serious to owners (Blackwell *et al.*, 2008) and result in relinquishment (Salman *et al.*, 2000). Obedience or other training has been associated with a decrease in behavior problems by some investigators (Bennett & Rohlf, 2007; Clark & Boyer, 1993; Jagoe & Serpell, 1996) but not by others (Voith *et al.*, 1992). Training without positive punishment has been linked to fewer behavior problems in dogs (Blackwell *et al.*, 2008).

Temperamental fearfulness or anxiety is common among dogs and, as evidenced by its association with specific breeds, perhaps an unintentionally selected trait over centuries of breeding (Svartberg, 2005). Whether the result of genes, epigenetic influences, or environmental factors (learning), anxiety is often identified as a longstanding problem in behavior patients, and may generalize to several contexts. For example, anxious puppies and juvenile dogs that back away from the well-meaning strangers who try to greet them will commonly develop fear-related aggression to unfamiliar people as they mature unless this is recognized early and appropriate positive reinforcement and classical training put in place. Anxious dogs are more likely to display territorial aggression in the home, yard and family car, and are susceptible to environmental fears and phobias, and separation and confinement distress (Overall & Dunham, 2001). The owners of such dogs might be naïve about dog training options and, at the prospect of a trainer's "guarantee" or promises of a "cure" (neither of which is a reasonable claim), will agree to training with a harsh hand, which can simply exacerbate any problems. The frustration of living with a problematic dog seems to create a kind of vulnerability to suggestion – hence, perhaps, the popularity of trainers who offer a "quick fix" through punishment. More than a quarter of surveyed dog owners reported that intimidation-based training techniques such as hitting, growling, grabbing and shaking the jowls or scruff, or punitively rolling the dog on its back resulted in aggression by the dog (Herron *et al.*, 2009). Clearly, force-based training can increase the risk that dogs will bite their owners, and may in turn lead to relinquishment or euthanasia because the problem seems intractable or dangerous. Indeed, the most common reason for aggression is self-defense, making it understandable that positive punishment can aggravate further aggression. Moreover, owners using reward-based training reported that their dogs were more obedient, overall, than dogs whose owners used predominantly punishment, whereas those using mainly punishment reported more inappropriate attention-seeking, fear- and aggression-related problems in their pets (Hiby *et al.*, 2004).

For the average family seeking training for a newly acquired puppy or adult dog, the choices can be confusing, with a mind-boggling range of advice and training methods on offer. Breeders, pet stores, rescue organizations and veterinarians may refer owners to local trainers and behavior consultants, or to books and internet resources containing contradictory recommendations. A popular dog trainer in the 1960s and 1970s, Arthur Joseph Haggerty (Captain Haggerty), asserted that trainers who, "sit down with the owners, hypothesize, talk philosophy and whisper in the dog's ear kissy face nice-nice and click a clicker," were almost always ineffectual (Fox, 2006). Some of the methods touted are undeniably harsh, yet are accepted and practiced by many owners. The puzzling popularity of force-based training might be explained by several points:

- Behavior problems in pet dogs are common.
- Behavior problems in pet dogs are frustrating and difficult to resolve.
- People will agree to use forceful methods if such methods "fix" the problem quickly and effectively – however briefly.
- People will agree to use forceful methods if such methods are promoted by someone considered to be knowledgeable and well respected.

Given the relentless stream of "expertise" in the media, social networking sites and other sources, consumers are best advised to ask questions and gather information before they make a commitment. Rational guidelines for choosing a trainer or consultant are available and can help dog owners make the right decision for themselves and for their dogs (American Veterinary Society of Animal Behavior, 2012). Dog owners might ask whether the dog professional:

- has earned credentials from a reputable source;
- uses positive reinforcement including food, toys, tug ropes and clickers;
- attends continuing education conferences, seminars or workshops;

- can provide references from previous clients, if requested;
- welcomes observers (with no dog) at group classes.

Red flags should be raised and the trainer avoided if he or she:

- attributes dog behavior or misbehavior to "dominance" towards people, the need for the owner to establish himself/herself as "alpha," and the view that the family is therefore a "pack";
- uses punishment-based equipment such as choke or check chains, prong, pinch or shock collars;
- promotes poking, jabbing, saying "shhht," biting or growling at the dog, "alpha rolls" or "dominance downs";
- uses positive punishment – including shock or leash corrections, "kneeing," scolding, throwing items to startle, water spraying, hitting or scruffing;
- offers a guarantee for solving the behavior problem;
- refuses to use food for food-motivated dogs (especially because the dog should simply want to "please" the handler).

Central to the ethical practice of canine education and training is the principle to "do no harm." In the last 20–30 years there has been strident advocacy of humane training methods, with emphasis on the use of positive reinforcement. While positive reinforcement is certainly not a novel concept in dog training, in some cases it is recommended exclusively, with complete avoidance of positive punishment and negative reinforcement (Stillwell, 2012).

The use of rewards or positive reinforcement is incorporated into many types of training methods. It may not always be effective (for example, when it is limited to praise alone, regardless of the individual dog's preferences), but the intention to reward is widespread. The emphasis in "positive training" is that positive reinforcement and negative punishment – both of which are non-aversive – are the *predominant* methods used, with little or no positive punishment or negative reinforcement. Positive trainers contend that these methods are more effective as well as more humane; dog owners have reported greater success in training using positive rather than coercive methods (Blackwell *et al.*, 2012). In positive-reinforcement training, the dog is given the opportunity to make decisions and is granted increased control over its environment, which has been associated with improved welfare (Laule *et al.*, 2003). Rather than having its undesirable behavior "corrected," there is simply no reinforcement if the dog does not cooperate and does not perform the cued task. While dogs trained with positive reinforcement are motivated by food, play or social reinforcements, those trained with aversive methods perform the target behavior in order to avoid an aversive stimulus (e.g. a leash correction or shock). In addition, use of aversive stimuli can unintentionally create a learned association between the stimulus (such as shock) and the setting or even the trainer (Schilder & van der Borg, 2004).

At the other end of the behavior modification spectrum are trainers who contend that assertiveness is necessary while food is not. For example, one successful training franchise asserts that its methods are:

based on dogs' natural communication methods and instincts, which do not involve treats. Treats are a form of bribery, and while they might cause dogs to be distracted from their naughty behavior, they do not command respect. Our techniques result in the dog respecting the owner and doing it with simple communication methods that are always available, unlike treats. (Bark Busters Home Dog Training, 2012)

Food, however, is one of the most effective forms of positive reinforcement in the operant conditioning of dogs and was promoted in the training of working spaniels as long ago as the seventeenth century:

when he does something to deserve it, that he may thereby know, that food is a thing that cometh not by chance, or by a liberal hand, but only for a reward for well-doing; and this will make him not only willing to learn, but apt to remember what he is taught without blows, ... (Fairfax, 1760, p. 111)

The effectiveness of a given reinforcer depends on the recipient, in this case the dog. Although some unquestionably enjoy verbal or physical praise and happy talk from the owner/handler, such stimuli may not be compelling reinforcers of behavior for others. Knowledgeable trainers will understand that the reinforcement must fit the individual dog. Also important, when a behavioral response is learned and on cue, reinforcement not only *can* but *should* result from the behavior intermittently rather than continuously, so that food will not always be necessary (Skinner, 1958). The exception would be use of food in classically counterconditioning emotional responses to stimuli. For example, a dog frightened of (or reactive to) children on bicycles can be managed by: (1) keeping the dog on a secure collar or harness and lead; (2) maintaining a safe distance from children, and a distance at which the dog's attention can be redirected; and (3) using a learned cue such as "watch me" to redirect attention and reinforce as rapidly as needed to maintain the dog's attention; or (4) using counterconditioning with food to decrease the dog's fear and reactivity. Without food, toys or other individually tailored positive reinforcers or counterconditioning tools, it cannot be expected that the dog's fearful behavior will be lessened.

Contrary to the beliefs of most pet owners and even some dog trainers, counterconditioning is not equivalent to positive reinforcement when the behavior – such as fear – is an involuntary physiological response to a stimulus. Thus, feeding a frightened dog during a thunderstorm is likely to *decrease*, not reinforce (or thereby increase), its fear. (Desensitization is also useful in cases of fear, but should not be relied upon (alone) when the dog is aggressive. For example, dogs afraid of children can be trained *at a distance* to associate children with food or toys, without putting either party into an unsafe situation.)

An often-misused technique in dog training is *flooding* – that is, forced exposure to the frightening stimulus without the possibility of escape – to manage fear-related aggression and other problems associated with fear in pet dogs. Flooding has been promoted to the general public by Cesar Millan (Derr, 2006). While flooding may be an effective technique for the treatment of mild fears, dogs with more intense reactions to frightening stimuli can be harmed by it, with the additional result that fear and aggression may be increased. Generally speaking, desensitization (gradual and measured exposure to the frightening stimulus) and counterconditioning (pairing something "good" with low-intensity exposure to the stimulus) are preferred.

11.7   What about punishment?

Although reward-based training is used commonly by dog owners, the use of punishment is also extensive. In most cases, surveyed owners used a mix of both methods with 84% using punishment to some degree (Hiby *et al.*, 2004). Whether a given stimulus is "aversive" enough to punish effectively, again, depends upon the individual dog's sensitivity, temperament and experience. This variability should be kept in mind especially with stimuli considered to be "mild" by the humans delivering them.

Positive punishment can adversely affect the behavior of the punished dog by measurably increasing stress and fearfulness. While stress may not impact learning in all cases, it can cause acute or long-term impairment of previously learned behaviors (Shors, 2006); even relatively benign corrections can thus interfere with learning (Beerda *et al.*, 1997; Blackwell & Casey, 2006; Rooney & Cowan, 2011; Schalke *et al.*, 2007; Schilder & van der Borg, 2004). Harsh training methods have been linked to lowered posture, lip-licking, paw-lifting and other appeasement signals consistent with fear or efforts to escape (Beerda *et al.*, 1997). Aggression and other problem behaviors may be increased rather than inhibited, especially in subsequent reactions to people or to other dogs (Arhant *et al.*, 2010; Haverbeke *et al.*, 2008; Hiby *et al.*, 2004). Furthermore, while there is a positive correlation between reward-based training and the degree of obedience reported in pet dogs (Hiby *et al.*, 2004), there is a *negative* correlation between the use of aversive stimuli and the performance of military working dogs (Haverbeke *et al.*, 2008). Because positive punishment alone was not effective in training specific tasks, researchers concluded that there is no evidence of its value in training and that use of " … punishment-based methods, as compared to reward-based methods, does not result in a more obedient dog" (Hiby *et al.*, 2004, p. 67). Beyond simple obedience, dogs trained predominantly with punishment were less interactive when an unfamiliar person tried to solicit play, while those trained with high levels of positive reinforcement showed higher learning scores when trained to perform a new task (Rooney & Cowan, 2011). For impressionable audiences, the term "whispering" (Rarey, 1859) is now associated with the use of physical and psychological force for managing dog behavior (Derr, 2006). As ubiquitous and popular as these methods now are, they are not recommended by veterinary behaviorists (Herron *et al.*, 2009; Kirn, 2009; Luescher, 2014) because of the potential danger for both dog and handler, and because of welfare implications for the dog. The cultural trend towards a one-size-fits-all, cookie-cutter approach to dog training perhaps makes for interesting prime-time television, but it is ultimately misguided (Derr, 2006).

Positive punishment is commonly used to subdue aggression, in spite of the likelihood that much aggression is caused by fear. Trainer/handlers may also mistake fear-related aggression for dominance or attempts to achieve "alpha" status. As is usually the case, misinterpreting fear- or anxiety-related behavior as an assertion of dominance leads to harsh efforts to change the behavior. Although positive punishment can momentarily inhibit aggression, the motivation for the behavior remains either unchanged or intensified (sensitized) the next time the dog is exposed to the stimulus.

Furthermore, punishment does not necessarily have to cause pain or even fear in order to meet the criteria of aversiveness, immediacy and consistency. For some dogs, the well-timed *removal of a desirable stimulus* (e.g. food) can effectively reduce the frequency of a behavior. Such negative punishment, along with positive reinforcement, can shape behavior without causing fear, intimidation or pain. And, again, even positive punishment – for example, the motion-detector spray – can work without pain or fear, depending upon the individual dog's sensitivity, although highly motivated dogs might override the spray's effects, while anxious dogs might become significantly frightened and avoid the vicinity as well as the spray.

"Balanced" training is a recently coined term implying that both positive reinforcement and positive punishment are needed for optimal training results, but the evidence is that mixed training techniques may, in fact, be least effective (Hiby *et al.*, 2004) and result in a higher prevalence of behavior problems (Blackwell *et al.*, 2008). The term itself is seen by some as masking a reliance on positive punishment and dominance-based handling of dog behavior (Brad, 2011).

Box 11.1 The shock-collar controversy

Electric shock devices, which typically work by delivering an electric shock to the dog's neck, are emblematic of the philosophical differences between "positive" and "aversive" trainers. The controversy of shock collar use is illustrated by popular euphemisms for electric shock, such as "static correction or stimulation" (misleading, because such collars work via alternating current and do not deliver static shock),[3] "e-Touch," "tap" and "tingle."[4] Used as tools for positive punishment (P+, a consequence of undesirable behavior) or negative reinforcement (R−, discontinued upon performance of desirable behavior), collars are widely available in three types: (1) one that delivers a shock (P+) when the dog barks, without human intervention; (2) one that works with an electric fence and is triggered when the dog approaches within a certain distance of the fence (P+), again without human intervention; (3) one triggered by the trainer/handler via remote control (either P+ or R−), sometimes called a "remote collar."

Proponents of shock collars assert that they are effective and produce fast results. Dogs can be punished by the owner/trainer from a long distance, and thus the contention that they are indispensible for correcting a dog's behavior without need for the owner's proximity (remote collars) or even the owner's presence (bark and fence collars). Users claim that a quick electric shock is preferable to the (incorrect) use of a choker or other aversive stimulus as positive punishment for an undesirable behavior, presumably because an effective punishment will obviate the need for ongoing punishment in the dog's lifetime and is therefore more humane in the long-term (Blackwell & Casey, 2006).

Shock is considered by its proponents to be especially useful for punishment of unwanted predatory behavior, as well as snake aversion and other avoidance training. Snake aversion training is currently a subject of debate between advocates and those who argue that its effectiveness has not been confirmed, and that its application compromises the welfare of both dogs and snakes (Cadelago, 2012). In a study of shock collar training to stop sheep predation in dogs, investigators found no owner-reported negative behavioral effects on the dogs (Christiansen et al., 2001). However, repeated shock was sometimes necessary, contradicting the claim that shock is brief and effective. Shock collars have been used successfully to train wolves to avoid baited sites (Gehring et al., 2006) and, in a relatively small sample of dogs, to reduce self-licking in dogs with acral lick dermatitis (Eckstein & Hart, 1996). No measurable differences in plasma cortisol, a physiological indicator of stress, were observed between dogs wearing shock collars, citronella collars (both of which work on the principle of positive punishment), or controls (no collar) to control excessive barking (Steiss et al., 2007).

While correctly applied electric shock meets the three criteria – immediacy, aversiveness, consistency – for positive punishment, there are both "soft" (welfare-based) and "hard" (evidence-based) arguments against its use in dog training. Critics contend that shock collars are an animal welfare issue simply because they function by causing pain (Schilder & van der Borg, 2004). Evidence of pain and fear has been reported both immediately at the time of shock, and as an enduring conditioned response in association with the handler or other stimuli afterwards (Schilder & van der Borg, 2004). The use of shock has been linked to increased salivary cortisol and heart rate in dogs, both indicators of stress (Schalke et al., 2007). Furthermore, shock can be misused so that animals are intentionally or unintentionally traumatized or develop some degree of learned helplessness. Learned helplessness may be induced when an animal cannot escape from repeated punishment (e.g. shock). When the animal is later

---

[3] Petsafe™ (Radio Systems Corporation), http://store.petsafe.net/training-behavior/remote-trainers

[4] www.internationaldogschool.com/index.php?option=com_virtuemart&view=productdetails&virtuemart_product_id=8&virtuemart_category_id=1 www.sitmeanssit.com/dog-training-videos/dog-training-video-teaching-with-a-remote-dog-training-collar/; www.dobermanpinscherpuppies.org/doberman-pinscher-training/anti-bark-collars-nothing-inhumane-about-them-at-all

punished but is given the option to escape, it does not (Maier & Seligman, 1976). For example, an inexperienced trainer might use a remote-control shock to correct a dog for ignoring a recall cue, but time it just as the dog turns towards the trainer. In this common scenario, the dog is punished both for "coming" and "not coming" and may subsequently stop offering behaviors of either type.

The controversy of shock collar use has led to several studies of the behavioral and physiological effects of shock-based training in dogs. Guard dogs trained using remote-control shock attempted to avoid the shock, yelped, showed tongue-flicking, lowered body postures and other behaviors consistent with fear (Schilder & van der Borg, 2004). Perhaps more surprisingly, longer-term signs of stress were noted even in a novel location in the absence of shock, when the dog was walked by the handler who had been present during the shock episodes (Schilder & van der Borg, 2004), indicating a classically conditioned association of the experience with the person who was present at the time. Conditioned fear is an important consideration in pet homes because shock can increase defensive or pain-related aggression in susceptible dogs (Herron *et al.*, 2009, Polsky, 2000). Dog owners or young children are thus paired with pain in the dog's mind, and might therefore become targets of unexpected aggression. Even underground fences can stimulate learned fear and defensive aggression at the yard boundaries where dogs were previously shocked, thereby increasing the risk of arousal and aggression when pedestrians walk past or children enter the yard to retrieve a ball (Polsky, 2000).

11.8   Conclusions

Controversy is to be expected when opinions are based in widely ranging views and cultures. There is more than one method that "works" in dog training, and this chapter has covered only the basics of the differences. The simple fact that a technique is effective does not make it ethical. Opinions differ even within the camps of "positive" and "intimidation" method trainers. It is ultimately up to the consumer – the person living with the dog – to decide which argument is more compelling.

Semantics and ambiguous language increase the confusion of inexperienced dog owners. For example, the concept of "leadership" itself is open to interpretation. On the one hand, there are positive trainers who have disavowed it on principle, because being a dog's "leader" is perhaps only one step away from being its hierarchical superior. Making the claim that dogs require leadership isn't that different, after all, from maintaining that humans should assert dominance over dogs. On the other hand, all dog owners want the ability to control their dogs' behavior; whether this is termed "leadership" or "teaching manners" or some other term may be irrelevant.

Dog owners these days have unprecedented access to information about training techniques and recommendations for dealing with behavior problems. Considering this large group of potential consumers, it is no surprise that the information available on the internet, on television, and in the popular press is widely disparate and often mistaken for expertise. In many cases, the advice given to pet owners is inappropriate, unsupported by learning principles and science, and may increase the risk of biting, anxiety or other behavior problems. The "disconnect" between reward- and punishment-based trainers and behaviorists appears to exist because of a lag between current knowledge and ethics on the one hand, and a dated view of dog behavior and corporeal control on the other.

The future of dog training may follow the trajectory of progressive reinforcement dog training (Larlham, 2014), coined to refer simply to pain-free, non-intimidation based training without the ambiguity of terms such as "positive training." Ultimately, training methods should continue to be based on the science of learning as well as the determination to do no harm.

References

American Academy of Pediatrics: Committee on Psychosocial Aspects of Child and Family Health (1998). Guidance for effective discipline. *Pediatrics*, 101: 723–8.

American Kennel Club. History of the American Kennel Club. [Online]. www.akc.org/about/history.cfm/ [accessed July 31, 2012].

American Pet Products Association (2012). *National Pet Owners' Survey 2011–2012*. [Online]. Available: www.americanpetproducts.org/press_industrytrends.asp [accessed July 25, 2012].

American Veterinary Society for Animal Behavior (2012). *How to Choose a Trainer* [Online], https://avsab.org/wp-content/uploads/2016/08/How_to_Choose_a_Trainer_AVSAB.pdf [accessed September 10, 2016].

Arhant, C., Bubna-Littitz, H., Bartels, A., Futschik, A. & Troxler, J. (2010). Behaviour of smaller and larger dogs: Effects of training methods, inconsistency of owner behaviour and level of engagement in activities with the dog. *Applied Animal Behaviour Science*, 123: 131–142.

Bark Busters Home Dog Training (2012). Common behavior issues: Bark Busters training techniques. [Online]. Available: www.barkbusters.com/page.cfm/ID/469/iNewsID/411/newsTypeID/23 [accessed September 7, 2012].

Batson, A. (2008). Global companion animal ownership and trade: project summary, June 2008. [Online]. Available: www.wspa.org.uk/Images/Pet ownership and trade – Global report_tcm9-10875.pdf [accessed November 24, 2013].

Beerda, B., Schilder, M., Van Hooff, J. & De Vries, H. (1997). Manifestations of chronic and acute stress in dogs. *Applied Animal Behaviour Science*, 52: 307–19.

Bekoff, M. (2012). Social dominance is not a myth: wolves, dogs and other animals. *Psychology Today*. [Online]. Available: www.psychologytoday.com/blog/animal-emotions/201202/social-dominance-is-not-myth-wolves-dogs-and [accessed November 10, 2013].

Bennett, P. & Rohlf, V. (2007). Owner-companion dog interactions: relationships between demographic variables and potentially problematic behaviors, training engagement and shared activities. *Applied Animal Behaviour Science*, 102: 65–84.

Berman, M. & Dunbar, I. (1983). The social behaviour of free-ranging suburban dogs. *Applied Animal Ethology*, 10: 5–17.

Blackwell, E., Bolster, C., Richards, G., Loftus, B. & Casey, R. (2012). The use of electronic collars for training domestic dogs: estimated prevalence, reasons and risk factors for use, and owner perceived success as compared to other training methods. *BMC Veterinary Research*, 8: 93.

Blackwell, E. & Casey, R. (2006). The use of shock collars and their impact on the welfare of dogs: A review of the current literature.

Blackwell, E., Twells, C., Seawright, A. & Casey, R. (2008). The relationship between training methods and the occurrence of behavior problems, as reported by owners, in a population of domestic dogs. *Journal of Veterinary Behavior*, 3: 207–217.

Brad, E. (2011). Dog training's latest buzzword – "Balance." [Online]. Available: http://lifeasahuman.com/2011/pets/dog-trainings-latest-buzzword-balance/ [accessed September 29, 2012].

Bradshaw, J., Blackwell, E. & Casey, R. (2009). Dominance in domestic dogs – useful construct, or bad habit? *Journal of Veterinary Behavior*, 4: 135–144.

Cadelago, C. (2012). Snake training for dogs in S.D. moves forward. *U-T San Diego* [Online]. Available: www.utsandiego.com/news/2012/sep/11/snake-training-for-dogs-in-sd-moves-forward/?page=2–article [accessed September 27, 2012].

Cafazzo, S., Valsecchi, P., Bonanni, R. & Natoli, E. (2010). Dominance in relation to age, sex, and competitive contexts in a group of free-ranging domestic dogs. *Behavioral Ecology*. http://doi:10.1093/beheco/arq001

Chorpita, B. F. & Barlow, D. H. (1998). The development of anxiety: the role of control in the early environment. *Psychological Bulletin*, 124: 3–21.

Christiansen, F., Bakken, M. & Braastad, B. (2001). Behavioural differences between three breed groups of hunting dogs confronted with domestic sheep. *Applied Animal Behaviour Science*, 72: 115–29.

Clark, G. & Boyer, M. (1993). The effects of dog obedience training and behavioral counseling upon the human-canine relationship. *Applied Animal Behaviour Science*, 37: 147–59.

Clayton, L. A. (2013). Applied behavior analysis: the science behind all that learning. *Association of Reptilian and Amphibian Veterinarians Twentieth Annual Conference, Indianapolis, IN*, pp. 44–8.

Curtis, P. (2002). *City Dog: Choosing and Living Well with a Dog in Town*, New York, NY: Lantern Books.

Daniels, T. J. (1983). The social organization of free-ranging urban dogs. I. Non-estrous social behavior. *Applied Animal Ethology*, 10: 341–63.

Derr, M. (2006). Pack of lies. *New York Times Op-Ed*, August 31.

Eckstein, R. & Hart, B. (1996). Treatment of canine acral lick dermatitis by behavior modification using electronic stimulation. *Journal of the American Animal Hospital Association*, 32: 225–230.

Fairfax, T. (1760). *The Complete Sportsman: or, Country Gentleman's Recreation*. London, Printed for J. Cooke. [Online]. Available: https://ia600408.us.archive.org/29/items/completesportsma00fair/completesportsma00fair.pdf

Fox, M. (2006). Arthur Haggerty, 74, master dog trainer, dies. *The New York Times* [Online]. Available: www.nytimes.com/2006/07/18/us/18haggerty.html?_r=0 [accessed January 11, 2014].

Gehring, T., Hawley, J., Davidson, S., Rossler, S., Cellar, A., Schultz, R., Wydeven, A. & Vercauteren, K. (2006). Are viable non-lethal management tools available for reducing wolf-human conflict? Preliminary results from field experiments. *Proceedings of the 22nd Vertebrate Pest Conference*. University of California, Davis, pp. 2–6.

Gershoff, E. (2002). Corporal punishment by parents and associated child behaviors and experiences: a meta-analytic and theoretical review. *Psychological Bulletin*, 128: 539–79.

Gershoff, E., Miller, P. & Holden, G. (1999). Parenting influences from the pulpit: religious affiliation as a determinant of parental corporal punishment. *Journal of Family Psychology*, 13: 307–20.

Griggs, R. A. (2012). *Psychology: A Concise Introduction*, New York, NY: Worth Publishers.

Haverbeke, A., Laporte, B., Depiereux, E., Giffroy, J.-M. & Diederich, C. (2008). Training methods of military dog handlers and their effects on the team's performances. *Applied Animal Behaviour Science*, 113: 110–22.

Herron, M., Shofer, F. & Reisner, I. (2009). Survey of the use and outcome of confrontational and non-confrontational training methods in client-owned dogs showing undesired behaviors. *Applied Animal Behaviour Science*, 117: 47–54.

Hiby, E., Rooney, N. & Bradshaw, J. (2004). Dog training methods: their use, effectiveness and interaction with behaviour and welfare. *Animal Welfare*, 13: 63–9.

Hutchinson, W. N. (1848). *Dog Breaking: The Most Expeditious, Certain and Easy Method, Whether Great Excellence or Only Mediocrity be Required, with Odds and Ends for Those who Love the Dog and the Gun*, 4th edition. London: John Murray.

Ingram, C. (2006). The biblical approach to spanking: seven steps to disciplining your child (Focus On The Family). [Online]. Available: www.focusonthefamily.com/parenting/effective_biblical_discipline/effective-child-discipline/biblical-approach-to-spanking.aspx [accessed November 27, 2013].

Jagoe, A. & Serpell, J. (1996). Owner characteristics and interactions and the prevalence of canine behavior problems. *Applied Animal Behaviour Science*, 47: 31–42.

Kilcommons, B. & Wilson, S. (1999). *Good Owners, Great Dogs*, New York, NY: Grand Central Publishing.

Kirn, T. (2009). Veterinary behaviorists question dominance theory in dogs. *VIN News Service* [Online]. Available: http://news.vin.com/VINNews.aspx?articleId=12230 [accessed September 28, 2012].

Koehler, W. (1984). *The Koehler Method of Dog Training: Certified Techniques by Movieland's Most Experienced Dog Trainer*. New York: Howell Book House.

Landsberg, G. (1991). The distribution of canine behavior cases at three behavior referral practices. *Veterinary Medicine*, 86: 1011–18.

Larlham, E. (2014). Progressive reinforcement training manifesto. [Online]. Available: http://dogmantics.com/progressive-reinforcement-training-manifesto/ [accessed January 11, 2014].

Laule, G., Bloomsmith, M. & Schapiro, S. (2003). The use of positive reinforcement training techniques to enhance the care, management, and welfare of primates in the laboratory. *Journal of Applied Animal Welfare Science*, 6: 163–73.

Littlefield, D. (2014) Why you need to be "Top Dog". Dog Breed Info Center. [Online]. Available: www.dogbreedinfo.com/topdog.htm [accessed January 11, 2014].

Luescher, A. (2014). Review of National Geographic's Dog Whisperer. [Online]. Available: www.animalbehavior.net/visitors/CesarMillan_Luescher.htm.

Luescher, A. & Reisner, I. (2009). Canine aggression toward familiar people: a new look at an old problem. *Veterinary Clinics of North America: Small Animal Practice*, 38: 1107–30.

Mace, F. C. (2010). Translational research in behavior analysis: historical traditions and imperative for the future. *Journal of the Experimental Analysis of Behavior*, 93: 293–312.

Mackenzie, M. J., Nicklas, E., Waldfogel, J. & Brooks-Gunn, J. (2013). Spanking and child development across the first decade of life. *Pediatrics*, 132: e1118–25

Maier, S. F. & Seligman, M. E. P. (1976). Learned helplessness: theory and evidence. *Journal of Experimental Psychology: General*, 105: 3–46.

Mech, D. (1981). *The Wolf: The Ecology and Behavior of an Endangered Species*, Minneapolis, MN: University of Minnesota Press.

Mech, L. (1999). Alpha status, dominance, and division of labor in wolf packs. *Canadian Journal of Zoology*, 77: 1196–203.

Millan, C. (2013). Dog behavior: understanding dog aggression. cesarsway.com. [Online]. Available: www.cesarsway.com/tips/problembehaviors/understanding-aggression [accessed January 11, 2014].

Monks of New Skete (2002). *How To Be Your Dog's Best Friend*. New York, NY: Little, Brown and Company.

Monks of New Skete (2011). *The Art of Raising a Puppy*. New York, NY: Little, Brown and Company.

Most, K. (2000). *Training Dogs: A Manual*, Wenatchee, WA, Dogwise Publishing.

Mugford, R. A. (1995). Canine behavioural therapy. In *The Domestic Dog: Its Evolution, Behaviour, and Interactions with People*, ed. J. A. Serpell, Cambridge: Cambridge University Press, pp. 140–52.

Overall, K. & Dunham, A. (2001). Frequency of nonspecific clinical signs in dogs with separation anxiety, thunderstorm phobia, and noise phobia, alone or in combination. *Journal of the American Veterinary Medical Association*, 219: 467–73.

Overall, K. L. & Love, M. (2001). Dog bites to humans – demography, epidemiology, injury, and risk. *Journal of the American Veterinary Medical Association*, 218: 1923–34.

Overmier, J. & Seligman, M. (1967). Effects of inescapable shock upon subsequent escape and avoidance responding. *Journal of Comparative and Physiological Psychology*, 63: 28–33.

Pathfinder & Dalziel, H. (1909). *Breaking and Training Dogs: Being Concise Directions for the Proper Education of Dogs Both for the Field and as Companions*. London: L. Upcott Gill.

Polsky, R. (2000). Can aggression in dogs be elicited through the use of electronic pet containment systems? *Journal of Applied Animal Welfare Science*, 3: 345–57.

Pryor, K. (1999). *Don't Shoot the Dog: The New Art of Teaching and Training*. New York: Bantam.

Rarey, J. (1859). *Horse-taming – Horsemanship – Hunting: A New Illustrated Edition of J.S. Rarey's Art of Taming Horses, with the Substance of the Lectures at the Round House, and Additional Chapters on Horsemanship and Hunting, for the Young and Timid*. London, Routledge, Warne, and Routledge.

Reisner, I., Erb, H. & Houpt, K. (1994). Risk factors for behavior-related euthanasia among dominant-aggressive dogs: 110 cases (1989–1992). *Journal of the American Veterinary Medical Association*, 205: 855–63.

Rooney, N. & Cowan, S. (2011). Training methods and owner-dog interactions: links with dog behaviour and learning ability. *Applied Animal Behaviour Science*, 132: 169–77.

Salman, M., Hutchinson, J., Ruch-Gallie, R. *et al.* (2000). Behavioral reasons for relinquishment of dogs and cats to 12 shelters. *Journal of Applied Animal Welfare Science*, 3: 93–106.

Schalke, E., Stichnoth, J., Ott, S. & Jones-Baade, R. (2007). Clinical signs caused by the use of electric training collars on dogs in everyday life situations. *Applied Animal Behaviour Science*, 105: 369–80.

Schenkel, R. (1947). Expression studies of wolves. *Behaviour*, 1: 81–129.

Schilder, M. & van der Borg, J. (2004). Training dogs with help of the shock collar: short and long term behavioural effects. *Applied Animal Behaviour Science*, 85: 319–34.

Shors, T. J. (2006). Stressful experience and learning across the lifespan. *Annual Review of Psychology*, 57: 55–85.

Skinner, B. (1958). Reinforcement today. *American Psychologist*, 13: 94–9.

Steiss, J., Schaffer, C., Ahmad, H. & Voith, V. (2007). Evaluation of plasma cortisol levels and behavior in dogs wearing bark control collars. *Applied Animal Behaviour Science*, 106: 96–106.

Stillwell, V. (2012). Why positive reinforcement (+R). [Online]. Available: http://positively.com/positive-reinforcement/why-positive-reinforcement/ [accessed September 7, 2012].

Strickland, W. (1966). *Expert Obedience Training for Dogs*. New York: The Macmillan Company.

Svartberg, K. (2005). Breed-typical behaviour in dogs: historical remnants or recent constructs? *Applied Animal Behaviour Science*, 96: 293–313.

Vacalopoulos, A. & Anderson, R. (1993). Canine behavior problems reported by clients in a study of veterinary hospitals [Abstract]. *Applied Animal Behaviour Science*, 37: 84.

Voith, V. & Borchelt, P. (1982). Diagnosis and treatment of dominance aggression in dogs. *Veterinary Clinics of North America: Small Animal Practice*, 12: 655–63.

Voith, V., Wright, J. & Danneman, P. (1992). Is there a relationship between canine behavior problems and spoiling activities, anthropomorphism, and obedience training? *Applied Animal Behaviour Science*, 34: 263–72.

12 | Dogs in today's society: The role of applied animal behavior

STEPHEN ZAWISTOWSKI AND PAMELA REID

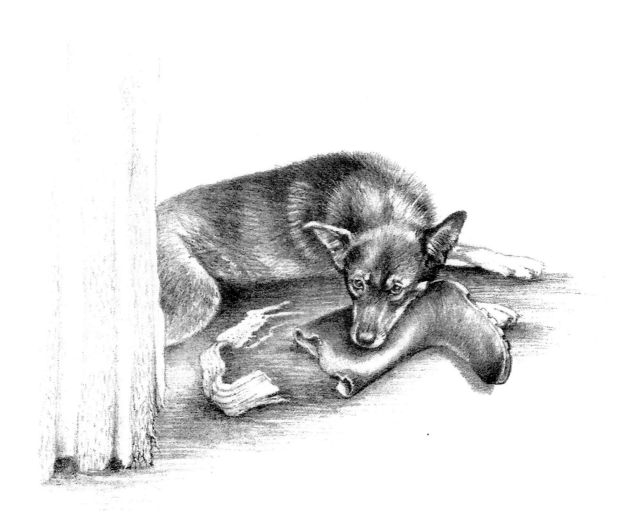

12.1   Introduction

It is likely that humans practiced applied animal behavior long before the development of formal studies of animal behavior. Hunters, herders and other early peoples depended on the careful observation of animal behavior and engaged in a wide range of practices to manage the animals in their care. Chief among these animals were the dogs that played so many different roles in human culture, as illustrated in this text's multiple chapters. In most cases, however, dogs in developed countries are no longer employed in their historic roles. When Americans are asked why they have a dog, a significant number respond that companionship is a primary reason (American Pet Products Association (APPA), 2012). Dogs are extremely popular; one-third of all American households have at least one. The estimated number of American pet dogs totals approximately 78 million (APPA, 2012), and similar rates of dog ownership have been reported elsewhere in the developed world (Dog News, 2011). This companionship between people and their dogs supports a substantial multibillion-dollar industry consisting of food, toys, equipment and pet-related services (Veterinary Practice News, 2010). Despite these investments, and the good intentions of dog owners, many millions of dogs suffer poor welfare, or end up homeless or relinquished to animal shelters each year. Applied animal behavior can play an important role in supporting the human–dog relationship and improving the lives of both pets and the people who own them.

12.2   The development of applied animal behavior

In many ways, the formal study of animal behavior can be traced to Charles Darwin and *The Expression of the Emotions in Man and Animals* (1965 [1872]). He was eventually followed by George Romanes (1970 [1881]) and many others. Important contributions to our understanding of learning in animals came from Ivan Pavlov (1927) and Edward Thorndike (1913). Pavlov's description of classical conditioning and Thorndike's elucidation of the "Law of Effect" and what we now call "instrumental conditioning" provided critical theoretical underpinnings for many of the interventions employed in applied animal behavior (Reid, 1996). John Watson (1959) and B. F. Skinner (1938) greatly expanded our understanding of instrumental conditioning, leading to the development of ever more sophisticated methods for influencing behavior. Much of this research was conducted in laboratories and was restricted to relatively few species, leading to some concern that the broader understanding of the underlying processes might be compromised (Beach, 1950). In the years after World War II, the discipline that came to be known as ethology began to focus more and more on the role the natural environment plays in the behavior of animals. A significant event in the recognition of animal behavior as a field of scientific study was the awarding of the 1973 Nobel Prize, shared by Konrad Lorenz, Nikko Tinbergen and Karl von Frisch, for work focused on the study of animals' natural behavior within an evolutionary context (Zawistowski, 2008). The specialization known as "applied animal behavior" emerged primarily to further study the behavior of captive and domesticated animals. With respect to pets, the birth of the field can be traced to the publication of "Animal clinical psychology: a modest proposal" by Tuber *et al*. (1974). The authors describe a basic approach that begins with (a) analysis of the pet's behavior problem, (b) training or intervention based on classical or instrumental conditioning principles, (c) instructing the pet owner on how to implement the procedures, and (d) follow-up to assess the efficacy of the intervention. As the field evolved in the ensuing years, it continued to integrate knowledge derived from laboratory studies of animal learning and behavior, ethology and psychopharmacology (Zawistowski, 2004).

12.3   Professional organizations

The application of applied animal behavior principles to evaluate and solve the behavior problems of pet dogs was practiced by a handful of intrepid scientists and veterinarians in the 1970s and 1980s. As additional people began to enter the field, thought was given to the training, qualifications and experience required to be an effective practitioner. The Animal Behavior Society formed a committee in 1990 to evaluate the field and recommend requirements for a certification program. The program was launched in 1990 with initial recognition for the first Certified Applied Animal Behaviorists (CAAB). Certification is based on academic training that includes a Ph.D. or Master's degree in animal behavior (with appropriate coursework and a research-based thesis), case studies that demonstrate competence, several years of experience in the field, and letters of reference. The American Veterinary Medical Association recognized the American College of Veterinary Behaviorists (ACVB) several years later in 1993. The Association for the Study of Animal Behavior also developed a certification scheme for clinical animal behaviorists working primarily in the United Kingdom (Association for the Study of Animal Behaviour, n.d.). The field is dynamic and there are other certifications available for professionals working with the behavior of companion animals (see for example: www.arpas.org). Evaluation of such programs should be based on the combination of both academic training and experience based on performance required for certification. The certification program should be independent of the educational institutions offering training to limit conflicts that might result when an institution is evaluating the credentials of its own students. A robust field of applied animal behavior requires the contributions of many disciplines and the cooperation of practitioners from various backgrounds. Academically trained behaviorists, veterinarians and dog trainers can all play important roles in the evaluation, analysis, treatment and management of behavior problems in dogs (see also Reisner, Chapter 11).

12.4   Significance of dog behavior problems

Dog behavior problems, real and perceived, are significant reasons why human–dog relationships fail. Behavior problems were given as a reason for relinquishment for 40% of dogs brought to 12 animal shelters in the United States (Salman *et al.*, 1998). The most common behaviors associated with relinquishment were aggression towards people or other animals and destructive behaviors, including chewing, digging and house soiling. These same problems are typically seen at veterinary behavior practices in North America (Landsberg, 1991) and in other countries (Fatjo *et al.*, 2006), and are consistent with the experience of the authors of this chapter. A survey of pet owners shows that the most frequent concerns are barking and damage to household furnishings. Aggression is a less frequent concern (APPA, 2012, p. 130). In our experience, it seems that many dog owners will tolerate a modest level of problem behavior and maintain a reasonable bond with their dogs.

However, there may be a threshold beyond which the behavior results in potential or real harm for household members or strangers. Likewise, owners may eventually decide that property damage has become a significant financial burden or that the presence of a pet with behavior problems jeopardizes living arrangements. Reaching such a threshold may move people to seek professional assistance or consider relinquishment or euthanasia of their dogs. It is not known how frequently behavior problems result in dogs being rehomed with friends or relatives, banished to outdoor living spaces, or simply discarded to roam as strays. Another concern is dogs who are subjected to punitive and abusive practices in a misguided effort by their owners to alter their behavior. It is clear that dogs exhibiting what are considered serious behavior problems are likely to experience premature mortality and/or reduced welfare.

Humans living with dogs with behavior problems also suffer reduced quality of life. Owners face the financial burden of replacing furniture, clothing or articles damaged by dogs. Damage and aesthetic costs associated with house-soiling also exist, and unruly or poorly behaved dogs can injure people by jumping on them or pulling on the leash. Dogs that vocalize or become destructive when left alone can jeopardize their owners' living arrangements. Aggressive dogs pose a significant risk to people or other animals. Owners of aggressive dogs may also risk losing their homeowners' insurance coverage. Finally, owners also suffer mental anguish when confronted with the need to rehome, relinquish or euthanize a dog (DiGiacomo *et al.*, 1998).

12.5   Common behavior problems

A comprehensive description of behavior problems reported in dogs is beyond the scope of this chapter. However, we can provide a general sense of the most common types of problems that confront applied animal behaviorists. When evaluating the behavior of an individual dog, it is helpful to keep in mind Tinbergen's now classic four questions about animal behavior: causation, function (or survival value), ontogeny and phylogeny (Tinbergen, 1963). In a general sense these questions are meant to elucidate the proximate and ultimate sources of a behavior. The proximate causes are those immediately associated with an individual animal. The initial causation or mechanism would include both the environmental stimuli that might have elicited the behavior and the underlying structural or physiological state or condition of the dog. For example, the reinforcement history of a dog's behavior would by definition have increased the frequency of those behaviors that have been reinforced, and decrease the frequency of those behaviors that have not been reinforced, or punished. For example, a dog that begged at the table and was rewarded with a bit of food, would beg more often. Unpredictable (or "partial") reinforcement would result in a more persistent behavior that is difficult to extinguish. A dog's health status will also impact its behavior. Obviously, neurological damage could result in a range of abnormal behaviors. It is also true that less severe health conditions might result in behaviors that are undesired. Orthopedic problems may result in pain-associated aggressive responses when dogs are touched or forced to move (Camps *et al.*, 2012). Behavioral development, or ontogeny, will also have an impact on a dog's behavior. Dogs that have limited or poor social experience while young may show a wide range of significant, lifelong behavior abnormalities (McMillan *et al.*, 2013; Serpell *et al.*, Chapter 6).

Ultimate causes of behavior are those that stem from selective advantage and phylogeny. The various breeds of dogs were often developed to preferentially express specific behaviors associated with the work they were tasked to perform. While highly valued and adaptive when still employed in

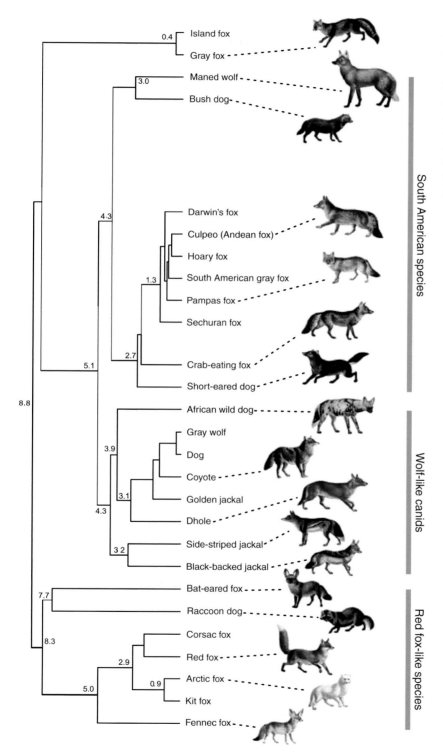

Figure 3.1 *Canidae* phylogeny with estimated dates of divergence in millions of years indicated on the branches. (Adapted by permission from John Wiley & Sons: *Journal of Evolutionary Biology* (Perini, F. A. *et al.*, The evolution of South American endemic canids, etc.), copyright 2009.) (A black and white version of this figure will appear in some formats.)

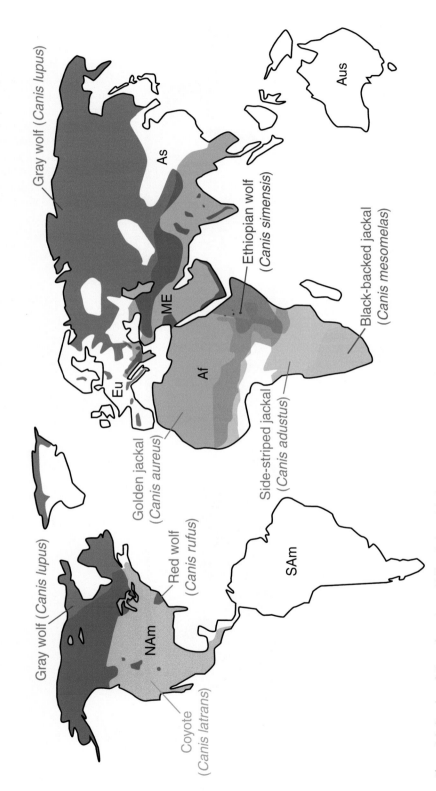

Figure 3.2 Species of *Canis* from the wolf-like clade and their current geographic distribution (IUCN, 2012). Distributions may overlap. Wolves were historically widespread across the Old and New Worlds, with current fragmentation a result of humans. Abbreviations: Af, Africa; As, Asia; Aus, Australia; Eu, Europe; ME, Middle East; NAm, North America; SAm, South America. (A black and white version of this figure will appear in some formats.)

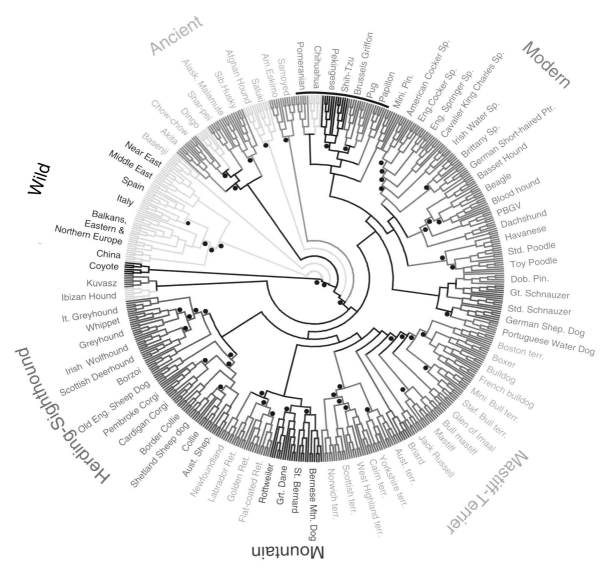

Figure 3.5 Breed phylogeny, where the colors of branches indicate a "functional" breed group: yellow, ancient breeds; brown, spitz breeds; black, toy breeds; blue, mastiff-like breeds; red, modern breeds; gray, wild canids; green, herding-sighthounds; purple, mountain breeds. Black bar indicates Toy breeds. Ancient breeds were as defined in vonHoldt *et al*. (2010) and Parker (2012). Dots on internal branches indicate >95% confidence. (Adapted from vonHoldt *et al*., 2010; Parker, 2012.) (A black and white version of this figure will appear in some formats.)

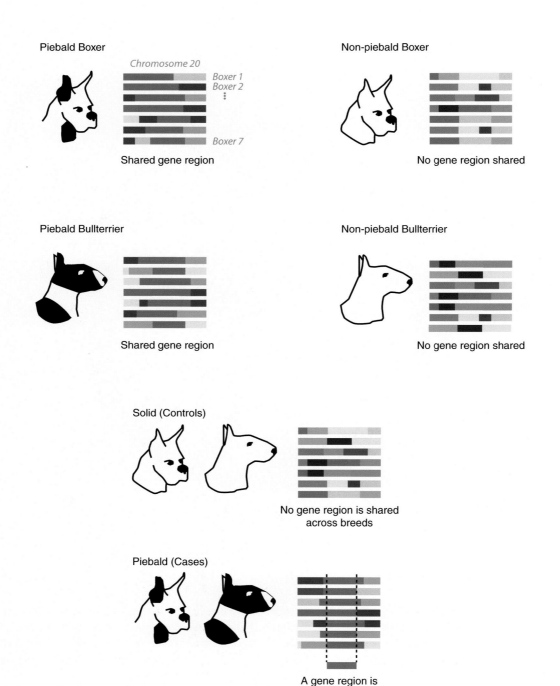

Figure 3.6 Conceptual framework of gene mapping through association. Here, the trait being mapped is piebald coloration across two breeds, the boxer and the bull terrier. Each colored segment is considered a different allele or variant on the chromosome. (Adapted by permission from Macmillan Publishers Ltd: *Nature Genetics* (Barsh, G.S., How the dog got its spots), copyright 2007.) (A black and white version of this figure will appear in some formats.)

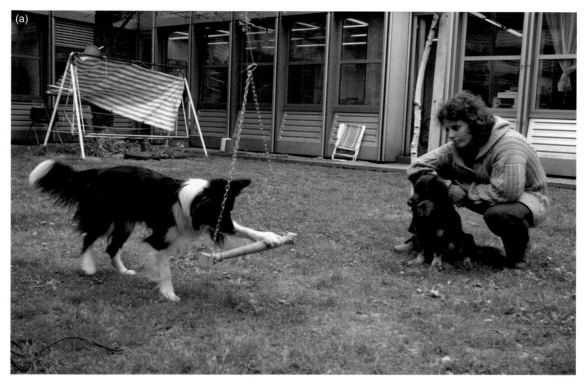

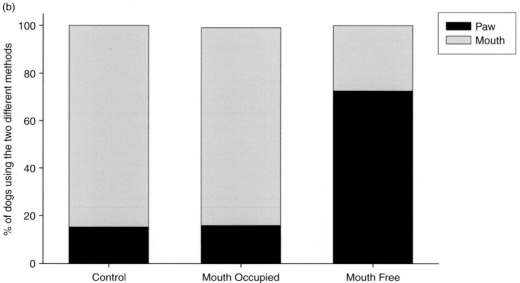

Figure 10.2 The procedure for a social learning experiment in which the "model" dog demonstrates the action (pushing the rod down with the paw), while the observer watches. After several demonstrations, the observer is allowed to try to manipulate the apparatus (a). The graph (b) depicts the proportion of dogs using their paw or only their mouth to manipulate the apparatus in the control group (left bar) and after watching the paw action used by the demonstrator dog under the two experimental conditions (middle bar, model had mouth occupied; right bar, model had mouth free), recorded in the first trial. Black, paw action was imitated; light grey, only mouth action was used. (© Friederike Range; Range *et al.*, 2007.) (A black and white version of this figure will appear in some formats.)

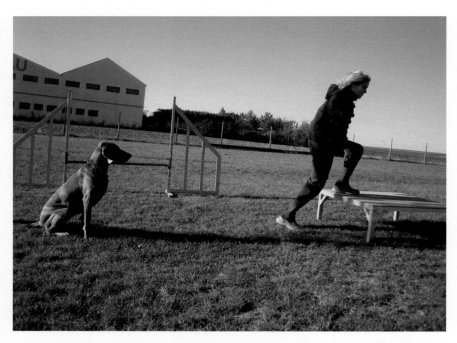

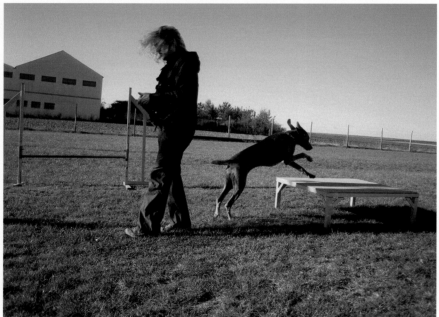

Figure 10.3 The "Do-As-I-Do" paradigm: The owner demonstrates an action (a), and then the owner tells the dog to "do-it." Here, the dog copies the correct action by jumping on the table (b), even though other possibilities were present e.g. jumping over the hurdle. (© Friederike Range.) (A black and white version of this figure will appear in some formats.)

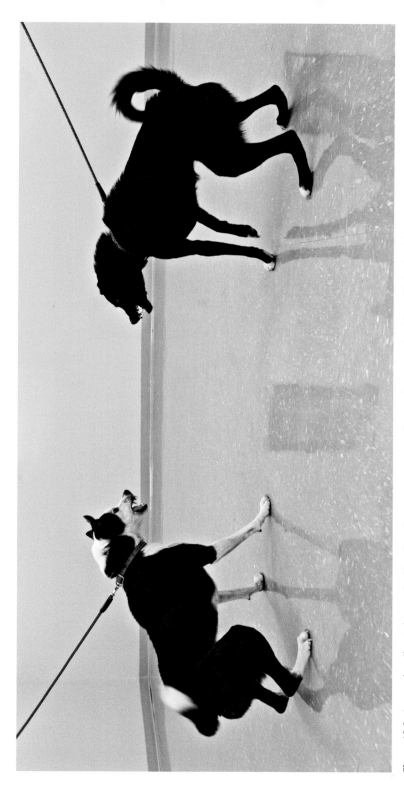

Figure 12.2 Aggression directed towards other dogs is a common reason for people to consult with applied animal behaviorists. (© Nick Burchell Photography, reprinted with permission.) (A black and white version of this figure will appear in some formats.)

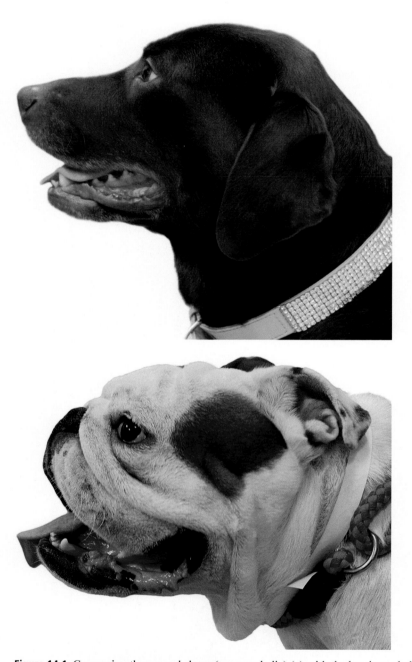

Figure 14.1 Comparing the normal shape (mesocephalic) (a) with the brachycephalic dog (b), the brachycephalic skull is severely shortened, particularly the muzzle, the eyes sockets are shallow and the jaw is deformed. (© Rowena Packer, reprinted with permission.) (A black and white version of this figure will appear in some formats.)

traditional roles of herding, guarding and coursing, among others, these behaviors may be maladaptive in the role of house pet. Understanding the history of a dog breed can help to explain the nature of the behavior to a bewildered owner, and suggest appropriate training, management and enrichment exercises to ensure that the behavior can be productively and safely directed. Finally, there is the question of phylogeny. Dogs are descended from wolves and this provides some understanding regarding the substrate that gave rise to their morphology and behavior. However, it is also true that the extent to which the social behavior of dogs is homologous to that of wolves has been overstated, frequently to the detriment of the welfare of dogs (Bradshaw, 2011; Bradshaw & Rooney, Chapter 8; Reisner, Chapter 11).

The types and frequency of behavior problems reported in dogs varies, depending on the methods used to collect the data, the location (e.g. animal hospital or animal shelter) or the sampling methods employed. Surveys of clinical practices have consistently listed aggression as one of the most common reasons for seeking professional consultation (Beaver, 1994; Landsberg, 1991; Voith, 1985). This frequent complaint has also been noted in some surveys of dog owners (González Martínez *et al.*, 2011), but not all (Duffy *et al.*, 2008). On the other hand, free consultation services, such as behavior helplines and online behavior help services, report that house-soiling, barking and household destructiveness are more commonly mentioned than aggression (Zawistowski, 2005). For example, the most common questions posed to the ASPCA's "Virtual Pet Behaviorist"[1] have been barking and house-soiling, although aggression ranked in the top three concerns as well. In a large study by Purina (2000), 97% of dog owners reported that their dogs were either fairly well behaved (37%) or well behaved (60%). However, additional follow-up questions revealed that 17% reported that their dogs barked or growled, 13% reported that their dogs jumped on people and 11% reported that their dogs begged for food. Aggression was reported by fewer than 4% of the people surveyed. The most common method of responding to a dog's undersired or unwanted behavior was to discipline or scold the dog. Eighteen percent of owners did nothing to correct or change the dog's behavior, and just 4% of owners enrolled in obedience classes with their dogs. Consulting with a professional applied animal behaviorist was not even mentioned as an option. Based on the experiences of the authors, the likelihood that an owner will seek professional help with a dog's behavior problem has less to do with the type of problem than with the severity of the problem. House-soiling and household destructiveness increase in importance when these behaviors result in significant expense to clean, repair or replace household items. Likewise, barking and destructive behaviors become critical when they may result in eviction from a domicile. Aggression poses obvious risks to dog owners, their friends and families, and members of the public, as well as to other dogs and animals in the household or the community. However, it is striking how long people are sometimes willing to continue living with a dog that has bitten multiple times before they decide to seek professional assistance, relinquishment or euthanasia. Dog owners often attempt several "home remedies" or employ advice from family and friends before consulting a professional. Owners may also opt to access the wide array of dog behavior information on the internet, which has varying levels of quality and is often contradictory, instead of seeking help from a behaviorist (see also Reisner, Chapter 11). Unfortunately, this choice sometimes results in the worsening of behavior problems. Financial considerations and the depth of the bond that owners have with their dogs play important roles in whether professional assistance is sought. In many cases, the "replacement cost" for acquiring a new dog is significantly less than consulting a qualified professional.

[1] www.aspca.org/Pet-care/virtual-pet-behaviorist

12.5.1 Anxiety and fear-related problems

Separation anxiety is one of the most common problems that prompt people to seek help for their dog. Separation anxiety typically manifests as attempts to escape, house-soiling, barking, whining and destructive behaviors when the dog is left alone (Figure 12.1). Dogs may also drool, tremble and show other signs of distress. These behaviors often commence when the owner prepares to leave and peak within 20 to 30 minutes after departure. The causes of separation anxiety are uncertain; however, it is thought that disruptions during early development may predispose dogs to this condition (see Serpell *et al.*, Chapter 6). There is some evidence that dogs that have been rehomed one or more times are more likely to exhibit separation anxiety (Takeuchi *et al.*, 2000).

The nature of this relationship is uncertain and it may be that separation anxiety was the cause of rehoming in the first place. It is important to recognize that many behaviors associated with separation anxiety may occur independent of distress associated with being separated from people. Even well-housetrained dogs may soil if the owner is away for an extended period of time that exceeds the length of time that they are able to retain their urine or feces. Puppies may not yet have developed complete bladder and bowel control so they may still have accidents. Puppies that are teething are also prone to chewing on items. Dogs may bark or howl in response to stimuli that occur outside the home or apartment and these stimuli may occur coincidentally when owners are away.

Phobias, especially those related to noises are a common concern reported by owners. Loud, percussive noises such as thunder, fireworks and gunshots are frequent triggers of intense fear reactions in dogs. The reactions may include intense attempts to escape, hiding, trembling, excessive salivation, urination and defecation. Anecdotal reports suggest that more dogs get lost or go missing during the American Fourth of July holiday than at any other time, presumably because fireworks are a common part of celebrations (Jakubczak, 2012). The causes for severe noise phobias vary. Some

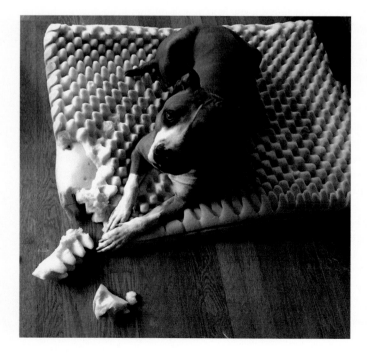

Figure 12.1 Dogs showing separation anxiety may cause significant damage to a household that may result in relinquishment to an animal shelter. (© Trish McMillan Loehr, reprinted with permission.)

dogs seem to have a particular sensitivity to loud sounds and this may be associated with a generalized fear response (Overall *et al.*, 2001). Other dogs may have a conditioned fear response due to trauma, either physical or psychological, associated with specific sounds (Dreschel & Granger, 2005; Shull-Selcer & Stagg, 1991). Dogs that suffer from fear and anxiety not only have a reduced quality of life, they may also have a reduced lifespan (Dreschel, 2010).

12.5.2 Compulsive behavior

Dogs can show a range of compulsive behaviors, including spinning, tail chasing, licking paws, legs or objects, flank-sucking, barking and fly-snapping. In some cases, the origin of compulsive behavior can be traced to an injury or trauma. A dog that has injured its paw or leg may initially lick it to heal and/or sooth itself. Over time, the licking can become more and more persistent, and even stereotyped in its form. This may inhibit healing of the original injury and, in some cases, lead to additional injury. In very severe cases, significant tissue damage may occur (Rappaport *et al.*, 1992).

Certain breeds may be predisposed to some forms of compulsive behaviors. Golden and Labrador retrievers seem more likely to lick, and Doberman pinschers are prone to flank-sucking (Luescher, 2000). Research has indicated that tail-chasing in bull terriers is a complex phenotype that is also associated with episodic aggression and trance-like states (Moon-Fanelli *et al.*, 2011). Because it has typically been observed in a subset of dogs, it may be a candidate for further genetic analyses (Spady & Ostrander, 2008). Detailed analysis of flank- and blanket-sucking in Doberman pinschers has identified a gene locus on canine chromosome 7 that is associated with the trait (Dodman *et al.*, 2010). Treatment and management of compulsive behaviors frequently requires a combination of drug therapy and behavior modification (Overall & Dunham, 2002).

12.5.3 Aggression

At gatherings of applied animal behaviorists who work with dog behavior problems, it is common to hear the concern that their practices are now dominated by aggression cases. Owners of aggressive dogs may be more likely to seek help than owners of dogs exhibiting other behavior problems. The danger an aggressive dog may pose to members of its household, as well as to other members of the community, along with concomitant concerns about liability, likely triggers the desire for professional assistance. In addition to consulting with owners about aggression issues with their dogs, applied animal behaviorists are frequently asked to serve as expert witnesses in legal cases resulting from dog bites. It is not unusual for both parties in a legal case to have a behavior expert ready to testify in court regarding the circumstances, motivation and cause of a dog bite or attack and future potential risk (Dog Bite Law, n.d.). While popular television personalities may posit that aggression is most frequently the result of dominance relationships in the "family pack," academically trained behaviorists now usually refrain from invoking dominance as an underlying cause for aggression (Bradshaw & Rooney Chapter 8; Reisner, Chapter 11). Television may also give pet owners an unrealistic expectation of how rapidly an aggression issue can be resolved. Duffy *et al.* (2008) evaluated aggression in a variety of breeds and distinguished between dog-directed aggression, stranger-directed aggression and owner-directed aggression. There were substantial differences between breeds. For example, some of the smaller breeds (Dachshunds, Chihuahuas and Yorkshire terriers) that showed higher levels of aggression towards strangers also tended to score high on measures of fear. At the same time, other breeds (Rottweilers, German shepherds, Doberman pinschers, Jack Russell terriers) were rated high on aggression to strangers but low on fear. The authors point out that different types of aggression may be mediated through different mechanisms. Within-breed variation compels caution when evaluating the behavior of an individual dog; breed alone should not be used as the explanation for aggressive behavior.

There is also an uncertain relationship between aggression and the neuter status of dogs (Hsu & Serpell, 2003). It is interesting to note, for example, that in a study of 103 dogs that had a record of biting a child, 93% had been sterilized (Reisner *et al.*, 2007). It is also striking that 66% of the dogs had attended or completed formal obedience training classes, a substanially higher rate than that typically reported for dogs in general. Eighty-one percent of the dogs had a previous history of biting a person. It is possible that the dogs in this study were sterilized or enrolled in obedience training because of previous bite histories, as these are two commonly recommended methods to deal with dogs showing aggression. Fear related aggression (87%), resource guarding (51%) and territorial defense (51%) were the most common assessments of these dogs. Podberscek & Serpell (1996) also found that neutering was not useful as a preventive measure against aggression in English cocker spaniels. These data may suggest that simple recommendations to sterilize dogs and attend obedience classes are not adequate responses to problems of dog aggression. A complete evaluation of a dog exhibiting aggressive behavior, including its medical condition should be performed, and a behavior modification and management plan based on the results of that evaluation ought to be developed for individual dogs.

12.5.4   Miscellaneous behaviors

It is not unusual to hear an applied animal behaviorist remark that, "I spend more time dealing with people problems than I do with animal problems." In other words, there are many cases in which unrealistic expectations or lack of knowledge of normal species-typical behavior causes the owner to believe that there is something wrong with the dog. There are also cases where the owner's own behavior may exacerbate the situation. Common examples include puppy house-soiling and chewing. People who have limited experience with dogs may not realize that puppies need to be trained to eliminate outdoors and learn to direct their chewing behavior towards appropriate toys or objects. In other cases, people may fondly remember a dog they had as a child but recall only the well-behaved adult dog – not the more mischievous puppy stage. More difficult cases occur when a family has acquired a dog that does not fit well into their living circumstances. Owners who enjoy sedentary lifestyles may be shocked by the demands that a high-activity dog, such as a Border collie, makes on them. Failing to provide such a dog with adequate exercise and mental stimulation often results in a range of destructive behaviors in the home. These types of problems are most common when the selection of a dog is based on appearance, with limited attention paid to its behavioral profile. One of the authors (SZ) dealt with a case in which an apartment-dwelling family in New York City purchased a Jack Russell terrier puppy at a riding stable they frequented. The dog came from a breeding line still used for its original purpose of rodent control in the barn. Needless to say, managing the dog in an apartment was a struggle to begin with, but it was a disaster when a mouse wandered into the apartment. When the owners returned home, they were greeted by a dog that had behaved perfectly according to its heritage but which had destroyed a significant part of the family's living room furniture before subduing its prey.

12.6   Assessing behavior problems

The causes of common behavior problems are multidimensional. Assessing a behavior problem demands an understanding of dog ethology, learning theory, and human behavior. In addition, a part of an initial assessment should always include information on the dog's medical history. Behavior problems are sometimes caused or exacerbated by medical conditions, so ideally the dog's owners should first consult with a veterinarian about their pet's behavior. If the owners were referred to the behaviorist by a veterinarian, the behaviorist can feel reasonably confident that medical problems have been ruled out as a cause of the problem behavior. If not, the behaviorist may need to advise the dog's owners that additional medical testing would be helpful. At the conclusion of the consultation, it is appropriate that the behaviorist offer to provide the dog's veterinarian with a summary of the assessment, including whether the problem behavior appears to be aberrant or if it is a manifestation of "normal" behavior, as well as recommendations for intervention.

Prior to a consultation, the behaviorist is typically presented with a basic description of the problem behavior, such as "the dog is defecating in the house" or "the dog is destroying the window blinds," and it is the task of the behaviorist to figure out why the dog is behaving this way. Perhaps the dog is defecating in the house because it is afraid of going outside or because it is experiencing distress when left alone (separation anxiety). A significant component of a behavior consultation involves questioning the owner about the dog and the circumstances under which the problematic behavior occurs (Voith & Borchelt, 1996). This is where training in the scientific method becomes especially beneficial. The behaviorist formulates alternative hypotheses for why the dog is exhibiting the problem behavior and generates methods for collecting the relevant evidence. Most behaviorists rely on some type of form or questionnaire to guide them while collecting basic demographic data and taking a history of the problem. An important aspect of this assessment process is for the behaviorist to explore the parameters of the misbehavior. Does the dog only react to unfamiliar people when they make eye contact, or simply whenever in close proximity to a stranger? Is the dog afraid of babies in general or is it afraid only when a baby vocalizes? Does the dog bark at other dogs even when they are across the street or specifically when another dog approaches on the same sidewalk? In some cases, the behaviorist can more accurately assess the problem by viewing video footage or even creating circumstances that elicit the problem behavior, assuming it is not harmful to do so. Many of the details should be factored into the behavior modification plan.

It's not uncommon for owners to simply misunderstand a dog's behavior. A dog that frightens its owner because it "shows its teeth" may turn out to be a submissive dog that grins as part of its appeasement display. An "aggressive" puppy that leaves its owner's hands scratched and raw may be exhibiting play biting that is normal for the puppy's developmental stage. Knowing that the dog is exhibiting normal behavior may be all the owner needs to feel comfortable living with the dog. Alternatively, the owner may need guidance from the behaviorist in how to channel these normal behaviors so that they are not problematic.

When faced with situations that involve aggressive behavior, the responsible behaviorist should assess the risks associated with working with the dog. There may be significant dangers to the family, members of the community, other pets or even the dog itself (Figure 12.2). In general, dealing with aggression is best attempted when: (1) the bites cause little to no damage; (2) the dog provides plenty of warning before biting; (3) the triggers that spark aggression are predictable and

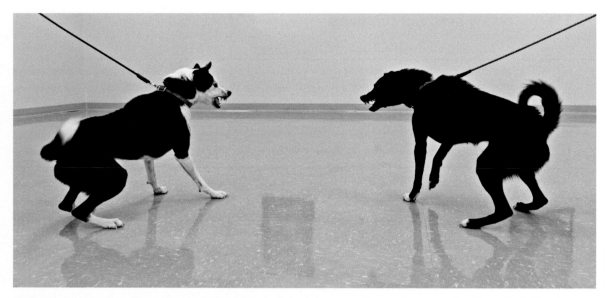

Figure 12.2 Aggression directed towards other dogs is a common reason for people to consult with applied animal behaviorists. (© Nick Burchell Photography, reprinted with permission.) (A black and white version of this figure will appear in some formats. For the color version, please refer to the plate section.)

manageable; (4) very young or elderly people or animals are not at risk; and (5) all members of the family are committed to, and capable of, implementing the behaviorist's recommendations. If these conditions are met, the behaviorist can, in good conscience, proceed with designing a treatment regimen.

The behaviorist should identify motivating events for the dog. Most behavioral interventions involve enticements for the dog to change its response to a triggering stimulus. For pet dogs, those enticements typically take the form of rewards (reinforcers), such as food treats, play or attention from the owner. A dog might be highly motivated to eat chicken but only mildly interested in praise from the owner, so it's important for the behaviorist to assess the dog's hierarchy of rewards (Vicars *et al.*, 2014). Likewise, if aversive stimuli are to be incorporated, these should be tailored to the specific dog. Excessive barking in one dog might be curbed by a scolding voice, whereas another dog might only be discouraged by the spray of a citronella collar. By determining the relative value of these stimuli for the dog, the behaviorist can maximize the effectiveness of behavior modification procedures.

Behaviorists are of two minds about the value of a label for the problem behavior. Some argue for a straightforward description of behavior in order to avoid inferences about the dog's emotional state. "Stranger-directed Aggression" is certainly a more objective and descriptive classification than is "Protective Aggression." Other behaviorists feel there is value in using labels, especially those that encompass a suite of behaviors such as "Separation Anxiety" or "Dominance Aggression." Indeed, an owner might feel better about his or her pet knowing that there is a commonly accepted name for the unwanted behavior. This implies that other dogs also exhibit the behavior, so the owner is not alone in this situation. Also, by describing their dogs as "anxious" or "compulsive," owners may be able to rid themselves of the idea that their dogs are "bad" or "defective."

12.7   Applied animal behavior approaches

Programs designed to change behavior usually consist of two primary components: management and behavioral conditioning (commonly termed "behavior modification"). Because behavior is multidimensional, an effective intervention plan often encompasses input from multiple specialists, including the animal behaviorist, the veterinarian, the trainer and, in some cases, a veterinary behaviorist. Consequently, adjunct interventions can be used in conjunction with management and behavior modification or, occasionally, in isolation. These include exercise, dietary change, hormonal manipulation, pheromone exposure, homeopathy and psychopharmacology.

12.7.1   Behavioral interventions – management

The purpose of management is to reduce opportunities for the dog to engage in unwanted behavior. In some cases, behavior problems can even be resolved with a simple change in the environment or in the owner's behavior. If the dog only soils in the basement, perhaps he's developed a preference for that location or the specific substrate, and restricting access to the basement may be all that's required to help the dog change. A house-soiling problem that stems from the owner's unwillingness to walk a strong dog that pulls on the leash can be resolved by providing appropriate walking equipment.

Management is also important as an adjunct to behavior modification. If the objective is for the dog to learn a new behavior or an association in response to a triggering stimulus, a critical aspect of successful behavior change involves ensuring that the animal does not continue to experience arousal or distress when exposed to the stimulus. For instance, alleviating separation anxiety typically involves conditioning the dog to relax and, perhaps, even enjoy brief periods alone. Accomplishing this is seriously hindered if the dog is occasionally left alone for substantial amounts of time, during which it endures severe distress. In such a case, making other arrangements, such as bringing in a sitter, avoids exposing the dog to repeated negative experiences.

Management is also important for empowering owners with simple strategies that they can implement right away. While a behavior modification regimen is designed to produce long-lasting behavior change, it can often take considerable time. By managing the situation, both owner and dog can enjoy some degree of respite from the problematic behavior until the behavior modification has an opportunity to work.

12.7.2   Behavior modification

The interventions most commonly used to accomplish behavior change in dogs have their origins in basic animal learning theory. The objective is to teach the dog new associations that will prompt changes in its response to specific stimuli. This can take the form of response substitution: training the dog to inhibit the problematic behavior and instead perform acceptable behaviors; and/or counter conditioning: setting up conditions so that the dog perceives the triggering stimuli differently and so emits different responses. For instance, a dog that jumps up on strangers in a threatening manner could be trained to go into a crate and stay there when guests come into the home. Alternatively, the dog could be conditioned to expect especially tasty treats in the presence of strangers. With sufficient pairings of strangers and treats, the dog comes to associate the two stimuli. It enjoys guests coming into the home and, instead of exhibiting threatening behavior, it now responds favorably. Both procedures can be equally effective, although some behaviorists argue that changing the dog's emotional response to a stimulus is more durable and more humane than simply changing its behavior (Wright *et al*., 2005). The dog that has learned to stay in a crate still dislikes strangers and, if the training degrades, the unacceptable behavior of jumping up would presumably resume. The most effective approach is to implement procedures that accomplish changes in both emotion and behavior.

12.7.3 Desensitization and counterconditioning (DSCC)

The mainstay of most behavior modification techniques is a form of classical conditioning called desensitization and counterconditioning (DSCC) (Wright *et al*., 2005). DSCC works to change an animal's response to a triggering stimulus by repeatedly presenting the stimulus at such a low level that the animal's arousal is kept to a minimum, thereby setting the animal up to not respond (or "desensitize") to the stimulus. At the same time, the stimulus is also paired with a second stimulus – a stimulus that elicits responses that are incompatible with the problematic response. The problematic response that was originally elicited by the stimulus is "countered" by this new and very different association.

Treating thunder phobia is a classic example of DSCC in applied animal behavior. First, the dog is presented with recordings of thunder at a volume sufficiently low that the dog does not become frightened. While this is going on, the dog is fed especially tasty food so that it learns the new association of thunder and food. Anticipation of the food elicits pleasant emotions and responses that are incompatible with fear, such as approach and relaxation. These responses eventually come to replace the original phobic response. Next, the intensity of the stimulus is increased – the volume of the thunder recordings is raised – but at such a gradual progression that the dog's arousal remains low. Fearful responses continue to decline while behaviors associated with the anticipation of food become more firmly established. The goal is for the dog to eventually tolerate, even enjoy, the sound of thunder at realistic volumes without becoming afraid. Typically DSCC is implemented over a series of sessions, often spanning weeks or months, in order to achieve reliable behavioral change.

Both desensitization and counterconditioning can be implemented separately, although, theoretically, one would not expect these single procedures to be as efficacious as implementing both in harmony (Wright *et al*., 2005). Desensitization alone consists of repeatedly exposing the dog to the triggering stimulus at low intensity, without any explicit pairing of a pleasant stimulus. For instance, the thunder recordings are played at a low volume until the dog learns to ignore the sounds. Gradually, the volume is increased and, with sufficient exposure, the hope is that the dog habituates. Counterconditioning alone involves presenting the triggering stimulus at full intensity, in association with a second stimulus that elicits incompatible responses. Typically, counterconditioning is used alone when there is no feasible way to lower the intensity of the stimulus, such as when a dog must be treated for fear of flying in an airplane. One of the authors (PR) counterconditioned her own dog to enjoy going to the veterinary clinic by pairing visits to the clinic with sessions on a water treadmill. At first, the dog had to be carried into the clinic. She was visibly frightened: her tail was tucked, her ears were flattened back, and she cowered and trembled. Once on the treadmill, she relaxed and played in the water. After several repetitions, the dog's overall demeanor changed. Her tail was up, her ears were forward, she pulled on her leash and appeared excited at the prospect of entering the clinic.

12.7.4   Response substitution

Response substitution, also known as operant counterconditioning, has its basis in instrumental conditioning (Wright *et al.*, 2005). The goal is to condition a new, typically incompatible behavior in response to the triggering stimulus. While at first glance this procedure sounds identical to DSCC, in actuality it is quite different. Here, the focus is on teaching the dog to perform a new behavior, even though the dog may still be experiencing negative emotions in response to the triggering stimulus. Proponents of this technique argue that as the new behavior becomes established, changes in the animal's emotional state ensue. A detailed distinction of classical DSCC and operant counterconditioning, as well as a discussion of the merits of one versus the other can be found in Wright *et al.* (2005).

Take, for example, a dog that behaves aggressively toward strangers. In close proximity to an unfamiliar person, the dog lunges forward and attempts to bite. In a response substitution protocol, the dog is first trained, in the absence of strangers, to adopt specific postures, such as "sit" and "down." The training is accomplished through positive or negative reinforcement procedures. The behaviors are taught to such a high degree of reliability that the dog remains in position regardless of what is going on in the environment, including the approach of a stranger. The learned behaviors "sit" and "down" are physically incompatible with lunging forward. In addition, the dog may be taught to hold an object, such as a stick, in its mouth to a similar high degree of reliability. Holding the stick in its mouth is physically incompatible with biting. At the completion of treatment, the new behaviors are substituted for the original problematic responses of lunging and biting.

Recently, it has become popular to effect a merging of desensitization and response substitution. Specific techniques that utilize a graded presentation of stimuli combined with negative and positive reinforcement have been branded Constructional Aggression Treatment (CAT) (Rosales-Ruiz & Snider, 2007) and Behavior Adjustment Training (BAT™) (Stewart, 2012).

12.7.5   Positive punishment

The objective of most behavior interventions is to diminish or eliminate unwanted behavior. By definition, positive punishment involves applying an aversive stimulus contingent upon the target behavior. In other words, when the dog misbehaves, something unpleasant happens, so the dog learns to inhibit the behavior in order to avoid the punishment (Reid, 2007). While infrequently recommended as a first choice for humane reasons, methods that rely on positive punishment can be very effective when applied correctly (Domjan, 2003).

However, the correct application of punishment turns out to be tricky at best (Reid, 2007). The punishing event needs to occur immediately after each and every instance of the unwanted behavior. Otherwise, the dog is unable to connect the punisher with the targeted behavior. This can be difficult if the owner is sometimes absent when the behavior occurs. The punishing stimulus also needs to be of an appropriate intensity to have the desired effect. If it is too weak, the target behavior is not suppressed or the effect is only temporary. If it is too strong, the dog becomes frightened, stressed and may cease all ongoing behavior. Despite the risk of generalized behavior suppression, it is best to start strong and decrease the stimulus intensity rather than to start with a low level of intensity. If the intensity has to be increased, the dog may develop a tolerance and end up needing a stronger punishment than it would have had the behaviorist not started with a lower level of intensity. Either way, it's an ethical dilemma just deciding on a starting point. Finally, the punishment should not become associated with the person delivering it or the circumstances surrounding the delivery. Otherwise, the dog may come to fear the person or other people, other animals or objects present at the time. For instance, if a dog that barks and excitedly lunges forward when it sees other dogs is only punished in the presence of other dogs, the dog could form an aversion to dogs and develop an even more serious behavior problem.

Punishing events that are orchestrated to come from the environment turn out to be the most effective (Hetts, 1999). The dog that surfs the kitchen counters to steal food can be discouraged if something frightening happens each time it places its paws on the counter. Placing upside-down mousetraps or a mat that delivers a mild static charge (e.g. the Scat Mat™) on countertops can prove extremely effective. The dog that sneaks off to urinate in the guest room might completely give up that behavior if, every time it enters the room, an avalanche of empty soda cans rains down noisily from the top of the door frame.

Positive punishment is always more effective when the animal is provided with other appropriate means for obtaining the same reinforcement (Herman & Azrin, 1964). For instance, a program that punishes the dog for chasing cars is likely to fail unless the dog is provided an alternative means for obtaining exercise, such as playing fetch or running leashed alongside a bicycle. A dog that is punished for jumping up to gain the owner's attention may well adopt other undesirable behaviors, such as barking or mouthing, unless it is taught acceptable ways to engage the owner.

Automated anti-bark collars work on the principle of positive punishment. Each time the dog barks, the collar automatically delivers a noxious stimulus, such as a spray of citronella or a brief pulse of electric shock. Because the collars are automated, the punishment is delivered in a timely manner and is strong enough to suppress the behavior in many dogs (Juarbe-Diaz & Houpt, 1996). Steiss et al. (2007) demonstrated that anti-bark collars were effective in suppressing alarm barking, with little to no impact on the dogs' activity levels or stress levels.

There is no question that correctly applied punishment can be effective in resolving certain behavior problems. Whether or not to use punishment, however, is probably the biggest ethical dilemma the behaviorist faces (see also Reisner, Chapter 11). Some behaviorists are never comfortable recommending it as an intervention. Some suggest it after reward-based methods have been tried and have failed. Others will resort to it only in dire situations, such as an owner facing an eviction notice because of a barking dog. Still others view positive punishment as a viable teaching tool to be used when appropriate, in conjunction with reward-based methods. A structured decision tree for making objective determinations about the use of punishment appears in Delta Society's *Professional Standards for Dog Trainers* (2001).

12.8   Adjunct treatments

A comprehensive approach to dealing with behavior problems often involves input from other disciplines, most notably veterinary medicine. Behavior management and modification can be facilitated by adjunct treatments that are intended to alter behavior by impacting the dog's physiology.

12.8.1   Dietary change

Altering the dog's diet to decrease protein has been demonstrated to have beneficial effects on aggression (Dodman et al., 1996). Providing a diet high in fiber can sometimes resolve problems stemming from hunger, such as food stealing or food-soliciting behaviors. Certain dietary supplements, such as tryptophan, can reduce aggressive tendencies and anxiety-related behaviors (DeNapoli et al.,

2000; Kato *et al*., 2012), and commercially prepared additives, such as Forbid™, are designed to discourage coprophagia.

12.8.2 Hormonal manipulation

Castration is often recommended for reducing a variety of behavior problems, including aggression (Borchelt & Voith, 1996). However, neutering male dogs has been shown to impact only sex-related behaviors, such as urine marking, roaming and fighting between male dogs (Neilson *et al*., 1997). Even then, the effect is limited. The older the dog is at the time of neutering, the less likely it is that behavior will change (Neilson *et al*., 1997). Spaying female dogs, which lessens estrogen and progesterone, in order to reduce aggression may actually have the reverse effect. Kim *et al*. (2006) found that spayed female German shepherd dogs were more reactive to strangers than intact females. Indeed, increasing progesterone with medication was, at one time, a common approach for lowering aggression in male dogs (Hart, 1981). As alternative medications have become available, these drugs have fallen out of favor due to the possible negative side effects of the hormones (Knol & Egbink-Alink, 1989; Overall, 1997). Palmer *et al*. (2012) have in fact questioned the ethics of routine neutering of companion animals, especially male dogs, in light of the limited impact it may have on undesired behaviors, and potential increased risks of some diseases.

12.8.3 Pheromone therapy

Dog Appeasing Pheromone™ (DAP) is a synthesized version of a pheromone naturally released by female dogs after parturition. The pheromone is believed to facilitate bonding between dam and puppies. DAP, which can be administered as a spray, through a diffuser, or via a collar, is promoted as a generalized stress reducer (Paget & Gaultier, 2003). Numerous studies report beneficial effects (Frank *et al*., 2010; Mills *et al*., 2006; Sheppard & Mills, 2003).

12.8.4 Homeopathy and other natural substances

A variety of homeopathic and naturopathic products claim to have beneficial effects on behavior, although few have received rigorous scientific study. Melatonin, which is thought to induce sleepiness, is sometimes suggested for dogs that exhibit nighttime restlessness and that suffer from anxiety and fear (Chang, 2009). Herbal mixtures, such as Rescue Remedy™, are purported to calm dogs, and, in doing so, help decrease aggression and anxiety. Shen Calmer™, traditionally known as modified Tian Wang Bu Xin Dan, is an herbal formula used to treat anxiety in dogs (Wrubel & Innis, 2011). Supplements that are believed to alter the neurochemical balance in the brain have been recommended as remedies for various behavior problems. Tryptophan, for example, is given in an effort to increase serotonin levels and thereby reduce aggressive tendencies. These substances are available over the counter or through consultation with a holistic veterinarian.

12.8.5 Psychopharmacology

Psychotropic medications can sometimes induce beneficial changes in behavior. Drugs such as Clomicalm® (Clomipramine HCl) and Reconcile® (Fluoxetine) have been approved for veterinary use and are marketed explicitly for the treatment of behavior problems in dogs (Horwitz, 2000; Simpson *et al.*, 2007). Many other drugs are used "off label" to treat various behavior problems. In the authors' experience, the impact can be quite dramatic in some cases and no further intervention is necessary. In most cases, however, the drug functions to alter the dog's physiology so that the animal is more receptive to behavioral interventions. For instance, a dog that is too fearful to accept treats in the presence of a frightening stimulus could be prescribed a benzodiazapine to reduce its overall anxiety and increase its appetite. More detailed discussions of psychopharmacological interventions for dogs are provided by Marder & Posage (2005) and Landsberg *et al.* (2012).

12.9 Conclusion

As the role of dogs continues to evolve in modern societies, ever greater attention will be paid to their behavior, including aspects of behavior that people find appealing and those they find objectionable. The human desire for dogs to function as members of harmonious households will at times put them in situations where skilled intervention is needed to ensure positive outcomes. Applied animal behaviorists are able to work along with veterinarians, veterinary behaviorists and dog trainers to facilitate these positive outcomes. It is important to ensure that applied animal behavior remains grounded in sound science as the field continues to grow and evolve.

References

American Pet Products Association (APPA) (2012). *National Pet Owners' Survey 2011–2012*. Greenwich, CT: American Pet Products Association.

Association for the Study of Animal Behaviour (n.d.) Certification Scheme. Association for the Study of Animal Behaviour. [Online]. Available: http://asab.nottingham.ac.uk/accred/cert.php [accessed September 28, 2012].

Beach, F. A. (1950). The snark was a boojum. *American Psychologist*, 5: 115–24.

Beaver, B. (1994). Owner complaints about dog behavior. *Journal of the American Veterinary Medical Association*, 204: 1953–5.

Borchelt, P. L. & Voith, V. L. (1996). Dominance aggression in dogs. In *Readings in Companion Animal Behavior*, eds. V. L. Voith & P. L. Borchelt. Trenton, NJ: Veterinary Learning Systems, pp. 230–9.

Bradshaw, J. (2011). *Dog Sense*. New York: Basic Books.

Camps, T., Amat, M., Mariotti, V. M., LeBrech, S. and Manteca, X. (2012). Pain related aggression in dogs: 12 clinical cases. *Journal of Veterinary Behavior*, 7: 99–102.

Chang, F-C. (2009). Minireview: Canine insomnia. *Journal of Veterinary Clinical Sciences*, 2: 100–7.

Darwin, C. (1965 [1872]). *The Expression of the Emotions in Man and Animals*. Chicago, IL: Chicago University Press (originally published 1872).

Delta Society (2001). *Professional Standards for Dog Trainers: Effective, Humane Principles*. Renton, WA: Delta Society.

DeNapoli, J. S., Dodman, N. H., Shuster, L., Rand, W. M. & Gross, K. L. (2000). Effects of dietary protein content and trypophan supplementation on dominance aggression, territorial aggression, and hyperactivity in dogs. *Journal of the American Veterinary Medical Association*, 217: 1012.

DiGiacomo, N., Arluke, A. & Patronek, G. (1998). Surrendering pets to shelters: the relinquisher perspective. *Anthrozoös*, 11: 41–51.

Dodman, N. H., Reisner, I., Shuster, L., Rand, W., Luescher, U. A., Robinson, I. & Houpt, K. A. (1996). Effect of dietary protein content on behavior in dogs. *Journal of the American Veterinary Medical Association*, 208: 376–9.

Dodman, N. H., Karlsson, E. K., Moon-Fanelli, A. Galdzicka, M., Perloski, M., Shuster, L., Lindblad-Toh, K. & Ginns, E. I. (2010). A canine chromosome 7 locus confers compulsive disorder susceptibility. *Molecular Psychiatry*, 15: 8–10.

Dog Bite Law (n.d.). The use of experts in dog bite cases: Canine issues. [Online]. Available: www.dogbitelaw.com/use-of-experts-in-dog-bite-cases/canine-issues.html [accessed October 1, 2012].

Dog News (2011). UK pet owner statistics. *Dog News*, March 28. [Online]. Available: www.dognews.co.uk/uk-pet-ower-statistics/ [accessed October 1, 2012].

Domjan, M. (2003). *The Principles of Learning and Behavior*, 5th edition. Belmont, CA: Wadsworth/Thomson.

Dreschel, N. A. & Granger, D. G. (2005). Physiological and behavioral reactivity to stress in thunderstorm phobic dogs and their caregivers. *Applied Animal Behaviour Science*, 95: 153–68

Dreschel, N. A. (2010). The effects of fear and anxiety on health and lifespan of pet dogs. *Applied Animal Behaviour Science*, 125: 157–62.

Duffy, D. L., Hsu, Y. & Serpell, J. A. (2008). Breed differences in canine aggression. *Applied Animal Behaviour Science*, 114: 441–60.

Fatjo, J., Ruiz-del-la-Torre, J. L. & Manteca, X. (2006). The epidemiology of behavioural problems in dogs and cats: a survey of veterinary practitioners. *Animal Welfare*, 15: 179–85.

Frank, D., Beauchamp, G. & Palestrini, C. (2010). Systematic review of the use of pheromones for treatment of undesirable behavior in cats and dogs. *Journal of the American Veterinary Medical Association*, 236: 1308–16.

González Martinez, Á., Pernas, G. S., Casalta, F. J. D., Rey, M. L. S. & Palomino, L. F. (2011). Risk factors associated with behavioral problems in dogs. *Journal of Veterinary Behavior*, 6: 225–31.

Hart, B. L. (1981). Progestin therapy for aggressive behavior in male dogs. *Journal of the American Veterinary Medical Association*, 178: 1070–1.

Herman, R. L. & Azrin, N. H. (1964). Punishment by noise in an alternative response situation. *Journal of the Experimental Analysis of Behavior*, 7: 185–8.

Hetts, S. (1999). *Pet Behavior Protocols (What to Say, What to Do, When to Refer)*. Lakewood, CO: American Animal Hospital Association Press.

Horwitz, D. F. (2000). Diagnosis and treatment of canine separation anxiety and the use of clomipramine hydrochloride (clomicalm). *Journal of the American Animal Hospital Association*, 36: 107–9.

Hsu, Y. & Serpell, J. A. (2003). Development and validation of a questionnaire for measuring behavior and temperament traits in pet dogs. *Journal of the American Veterinary Medical Association*, 223: 1293–300.

Jakubczak, M. (2012). Afraid of the 4th, keeping pets safe. *Pet Amber Alert*. [Online]. Available: www.petamberalert.com/blog/july-4th-fireworks-keeping-your-pet-safe [accessed September 28, 2012].

Juarbe-Diaz, S. V. & Houpt, K. A. (1996). Comparison of two antibarking collars for treatment of nuisance barking. *Journal of the American Animal Hospital Association*, 32: 231–5.

Kato, M., Miyaji, K., Ohtani, N. & Ohta, M. (2012). Effects of prescription diet on dealing with stressful situations and performance of anxiety-related behaviors in privately owned anxious dogs. *Journal of Veterinary Behavior*, 7: 21–6.

Kim, H. H., Yeon, S. C., Houpt, K. A., Lee, H. C., Chang, H. H. & Lee, H. J. (2006). Effects of ovariohysterectomy on reactivity in German shepherd dogs. *Veterinary Journal*, 172: 154–9.

Knol, B. W. & Egbink-Alink, S. T. (1989). Treatment of problem behaviour in dogs and cats by castration and progestagen administration: a review. *The Veterinary Quarterly*, 11: 102–7.

Landsberg, G. (1991). The distribution of canine behavior problem cases at three behavioral referral practices. *Veterinary Medicine*, 86: 1081–9.

Landsberg, G., Hunthausen, W. & Ackerman, L. (2012). *Behavior Problems of the Dog and Cat*, 3rd edition. Edinburgh: Elsevier Saunders.

Luescher, A. (2000). Compulsive behavior in companion animals. In *Recent Advances in Companion Animal Behavior Problems*, ed. K. A. Houpt. Ithaca, NY: International.

Marder, A. R. & Posage, J. M. (2005). Treatment of Emotional Distress and Disorders – Pharmacologic Methods. In *Mental Health and Well-Being in Animals*, ed. F. D. McMillan. Ames, IA: Wiley-Blackwell, pp. 159–66.

McMillan, F. D., Serpell, J. A., Duffy, D. L., Masaoud, E. & Dohoo, I. R. (2013). Differences in behavioral characteristics between dogs obtained as puppies from pet stores and those obtained from non-commercial breeders. *Journal of the American Veterinary Medical Association*, 242: 1359–63.

Mills, D. S., Ramos, D., Estelles, M. G. & Hargrave, C. (2006). A triple blind placebo-controlled investigation into the assessment of the effect of Dog Appeasing Pheromone (DAP) on anxiety related behavior of problem dogs in the veterinary clinic. *Applied Animal Behaviour Science*, 98: 114–26.

Moon-Fanelli, A. A., Dodman, N. H., Famula, T. R. & Cottam, N. (2011). Characteristics of compulsive tail chasing and associated risk factors in Bull Terriers. *Journal of the American Veterinary Medical Association*, 238: 883–9.

Neilson, J. C., Eckstein, R. A. & Hart, B. L. (1997). Effects of castration on problem behaviors in male dogs with reference to age and duration of behavior. *Journal of the American Veterinary Medical Association*, 211: 180–2.

Overall, K. L. (1997). *Clinical Behavioral Medicine for Small Animals*. St Louis, MO: Mosby.

Overall, K. L., Dunham, A. E. & Frank, D. (2001). Frequency of non-specific clinical signs in dogs with separation anxiety, thunderstorm phobia and noise phobia, alone or in combination. *Journal of the American Veterinary Medical Association*, 19: 467–73.

Overall, K. L. & Dunham, A. E. (2002). Clinical features and outcomes in dogs and cats with obsessive-compulsive disorder: 126 cases (1989–2000). *Journal of the American Veterinary Medical Association*, 221: 1445–52.

Paget, P. & Gaultier, E. (2003). Current research in canine and feline pheromones. *Veterinary Clinics of North America: Small Animal Practice*, 33: 201–8.

Palmer, C, Corr, S. & Sandøe, P. (2012). Inconvenient desires: should we routinely neuter companion animals. *Anthrozoös*, 25 (Supplement): S153–72.

Pavlov, I. (1927). *Conditioned Reflexes* (translated by G. V. Anrep). London: Oxford University Press.

Podberscek, A. L. & Serpell, J. A. (1996). Environmental influences on the expression of aggressive behavior in English Cocker Spaniels. *Applied Animal Behaviour Science*, 52: 215–27.

Purina. (2000). *The State of the American Pet: A Study Among Pet Owners*. St. Louis, MO: Ralston Purina.

Rappaport, J. L., Ryland, D. H. & Kriete, M. (1992). Drug treatment of canine acral lick: an animal model of obsessive-compulsive disorder. *Archives of General Psychiatry*, 49: 517–21.

Reid, P. J. (2007). Learning in dogs. In *The Behavioural Biology of Dogs*, ed. P. Jensen. Wallingford, UK: CAB International, pp. 120–44.

Reid, P. J. (1996). *Excel-erated Learning*. Berkeley, CA: James and Kenneth Publishers.

Reisner, I. R., Shofer, F. S. & Nance, M. L. (2007). Behavioral assessment of child-directed canine aggression. *Injury Prevention*: 13: 348–51.

Romanes, G. (1970 [1881]). *Animal Intelligence*. London: Gregg International Publishers (originally published 1881).

Rosales-Ruiz J & Snider K. (2007). *Constructional Aggression Treatment (CAT) – Shaping Your Way Out of Aggression* (DVD, 3rd edition). Eagle, ID: Tawzer Dog Videos.

Salman, M. D., New, J. C., Kass, P. H., Hetts, S. & Ruch-Gallie, R. (1998). Human and animal factors related to the relinquishment of dogs and cats in 12 selected animal shelters in the USA. *Journal of Applied Animal Welfare Science*, 1: 207–26.

Sheppard, G. & Mills, D.S. (2003). Evaluation of dog appeasing pheromone as a potential treatment of dogs fearful of fireworks. *Veterinary Record*, 152: 432–6.

Shull-Selcer, F. A. and Stagg, W. (1991). Advances in the understanding and treatment of noise phobias. *Veterinary Clinics of North America: Small Animal Practice*, 21: 353–67.

Simpson, B. S., Landsberg, G. M., Reisner, I. R., Ciribassi, J. J., Horwitz, D., Houpt, K. A. *et al.* (2007). Effects of Reconcile (fluoxetine) chewable tablets plus behavior management for canine separation anxiety. *Veterinary Therapeutics: Research in Applied Veterinary Medicine*, 8: 18–31.

Skinner, B. F. (1938). *The Behavior of Organisms: An Experimental Analysis*. New York: Appleton Century Crofts.

Spady, T. C. & Ostrander, E. A. (2008). Canine behavioral genetics: pointing out the phenotypes and herding up the genes. *The American Journal of Human Genetics*, 82: 10–18.

Steiss, J. E., Schaffer, C., Ahmad, H. A. & Voith, V. L. (2007). Evaluation of plasma cortisol levels and behavior in dogs wearing bark control collars. *Applied Animal Behaviour Science*, 106: 96–106.

Stewart, G. (2012). *Behavior Adjustment Training (BAT for Fear, Frustration, and Aggression in Dogs)*. Wanatchee, WA: Dogwise Publishing.

Takeuchi, Y., Houpt, K. A. & Scarlett, J. M. (2000). Evaluation of treatments for separation anxiety in dogs. *Journal of the American Veterinary Medical Association*, 217(3): 342–5.

Thorndike, E. (1913). *The Psychology of Learning*. New York: Teachers College.

Tinbergen, N. (1963). On the aims and methods of ethology. *Zeitschrift für Tierpsychologie*, 20: 410–63.

Tuber, D. S., Hothersall, D. & Voith, V. L. (1974). Animal clinical psychology: a modest proposal. *American Psychologist*, 29: 762–6.

Veterinary Practice News (2010). America's spending on pets continues to increase, APPA says. *Veterinary Practice News*, February 9. [Online]. Available: www.veterinarypracticenews.com/vet-breaking-news/2010/02/09/americas-spending-on-pets-continues-to-increase.aspx [accessed October 1, 2012].

Vicars, S. M., Miguel, C. F. & Sobie, J. L. (2014). Assessing preference and reinforcer effectiveness in dogs. *Behavioural Processes*, 103; 75–83.

Voith, V. L. & Borchelt, P. L. (1996). History taking and interviewing. In *Readings in Companion Animal Behavior*, eds. V. L. Voith & P. L. Borchelt. Trenton, NJ: Veterinary Learning Systems, pp. 42–7.

Voith, V. (1985). Attachment of people to companion animals. *Veterinary Clinics of North America: Small Animal Practice*, 2: 289–95.

Watson, J. (1959). *Behaviorism*. Chicago, IL: Chicago University Press.

Wright, J. C., Reid, P. J. & Rozier, Z. (2005). Treatment of emotional distress and disorders – non-pharmacologic methods. In *Mental Health and Well-Being in Animals*, ed. F. D. McMillan. Ames, IA: Wiley-Blackwell, pp. 145–57.

Wrubel, K. M. & Innis, B. (2011). The effects of Tian Wang Bu Xin Dan on situational and generalized anxiety in dogs and cats. Presentation at the Interdisciplinary Forum on Applied Animal Behavior Conference, New Orleans, LA.

Zawistowski, S. (2004). Applied animal behavior. In *Encyclopedia of Animal Behavior*, ed. M. Bekoff. Westport, CT: Greenwood Press, pp. 138–42.

Zawistowski, S. (2005). Effects of environmental enrichment on pet well-being. In *Iams Pediatric Care Symposium, The North American Veterinary Conference*, pp. 5–8. Dayton, OH: The Iams Company.

Zawistowski, S. (2008). *Companion Animals in Society*. Clifton Park, NY: Thomson Delmar Learning.

Part III

Dog–human interactions

13 Dogs as helping partners and companions for humans

LYNETTE A. HART AND MARIKO YAMAMOTO

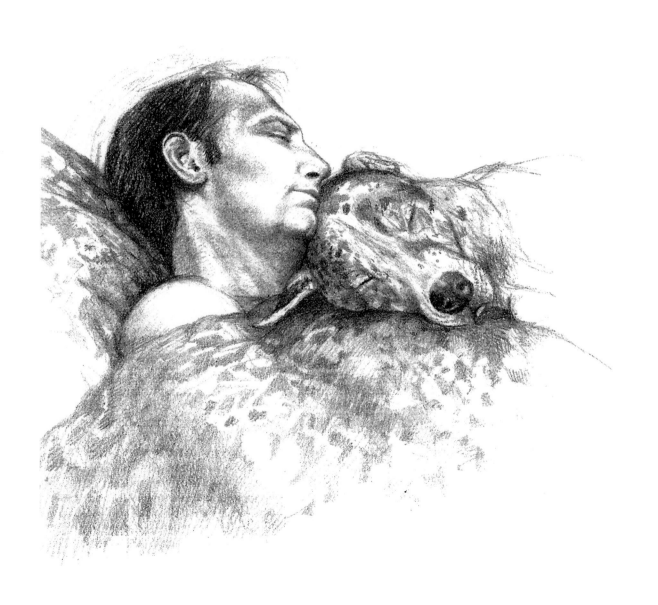

13.1   Introduction

Currently in the United States, about 78 million dogs reside in households (American Pet Products Association (APPA), 2011; American Veterinary Medical Association (AVMA), 2012). Relationships between humans and dogs continue to change, with pet dogs often referred to as companions and family members, and a growing number serving in assisting or supportive roles. Reflecting the changing status of dogs, sometimes terms such as "caregivers," "guardians" or "handlers" are used rather than "owners." Dogs are everywhere people live and play, providing partnership in all aspects of human life, including hunting, herding, sledding, guarding, military activities, law enforcement, assisting, and for therapeutic purposes. The dog is the only domestic species that plays such diverse roles for humans, as companions and increasingly as working partners (Hart et al., 2000; Kuhl, 2008; Lane et al., 1998). People go walking, hiking, running, and even camping with their dogs. Some enjoy sport competitions for dogs, such as agility contests, frisbee, and dog-dancing (Kobelt et al., 2003). TV advertisements include dogs in the scenes with families. Dog walking for improved public health is a topic of focused research interest (Ham & Epping, 2006), and many studies report beneficial physiological, psychological and social effects of dogs for humans (Hart, 2010). Training "service dogs" for working tasks to assist and aid people with disabilities is a growing enterprise in the US. The legal framework regarding public access for people with disabilities and their service dogs rapidly evolves. In the US, dogs (and other species) with no special training are even accorded special legal status in regards to housing and transportation as "emotional support animals" (ESAs). This chapter emphasizes the rapid changes currently occurring with dogs' status in their assistive, supportive, and therapeutic roles for people with disabilities.

13.2   Dogs as a special species

13.2.1   Comparisons with other species

Among companion animals, dogs are exceptional. Over a century ago, a large survey of children's school essays about pet animals had already demonstrated the dog's outstanding popularity (Bucke, 1903). These children emphasized the highly personalized attention provided by their dogs with phrases such as "he likes me," "guards me," "follows me," "protects me," "barks when I come home from school," and "is good to me." The children appreciated the dog's ability to express love and affection by jumping up, running around, wagging its tail and soliciting play. Many mentioned how the dog kept them company and played with them when they were feeling lonely or sad. More recent studies have confirmed these early observations.

In a telephone survey of 436 Rhode Island residents, for example, Albert & Bulcroft (1987, 1988) found that dogs were the most popular type of pet. Sixty percent of pet owners had at least one dog, and dogs were the most desired pets among non-owners. Owners who selected dogs as their favorite pets reported feeling more attached to their pets than did people whose favorite pets were cats or other animals. The dog owners spent more time actively interacting with their pets – grooming them, walking them, giving them special treats – than did cat owners. Dog owners were also more willing to spend any amount on veterinary treatment than were cat owners. Yet, a later study pointed to the specific qualities of dogs and cats, and the nature of interactions with owners, and criticized facile comparisons of attachment to dogs and cats when the activities with each are so different (Zasloff, 1996).

In observations of people and their pets interacting at home, Miller & Lago (1990) found that interactive behavior, such as whining, begging, making noise, obeying and being near the owner, occurred at far greater frequency with dogs than with cats. Dogs also interacted actively with unfamiliar persons whereas cats tended to be avoidant and aloof. Owners much more frequently issued orders to their dogs than their cats. However, owners told an average of 1.87 stories about their cats but only 1.32 stories about dogs. Earlier, Lago *et al.* (1983) had reported higher levels of both behavioral and physical intimacy between dogs and their owners than between cats and their owners, although some cat owners were also extremely attached to their pets. Overall, dogs seem to excel at adjusting their interactions to the owner's demands. Dogs exhibit highly coordinated behavior: standing, moving and sitting in synchrony with their owners to an extent rarely observed in cats.

13.2.2   Comparisons with human companions

People commonly feel close to their dogs, and grieve for them when they are gone (Kurdek, 2008), sometimes inconsolably. Studying the nature of young peoples' and adults' attachment to dogs more specifically, Kurdek (2009a, 2009b) learned that for most people dogs are not their most preferred "safe haven." College-aged people were more likely to seek out mothers, friends, and romantic partners than dogs in times of distress, yet they went for comfort to pets before fathers and brothers (Kurdek, 2009a). By adulthood, only romantic partners outranked pet dogs as a safe haven, especially for males, widowers, those highly involved in caring for the dog, and those uncomfortable with self-disclosure (Kurdek, 2009b). Pets are a consistent source of attachment and security; relationships with dogs are scored as more secure than those with partners on several measures (Beck & Madresh, 2008).

One study assessed the relative closeness that dog owners felt towards their dogs by asking them to represent their significant relationships pictorially using a technique known as the Family Life Space Diagram. More than one-third of these owners placed the dog closer to themselves than to any other family member (Barker & Barker, 1988), suggesting that for some owners, the dog's importance ranks close to the human members of their family. Occasionally people assign their pet dogs a priority above that of other humans. In a study exploring whether pets functioned as family members, a majority of 16 participants sometimes would have given a scarce drug to their pet in preference to a person outside the family (Cohen, 2002). The dog may better provide for its owner in areas where humans are lacking, and vice versa. Humans were found to be more effective in offering instrumental aid, affection, and admiration, whereas dogs were better at providing companionship, opportunities for nurturance, and reliable alliance, according to 90 informants (Bonas *et al.*, 2000).

Children derive a variety of benefits from their dogs, including exchanging interactions, enduring affection, self-enhancing affection, and exclusivity of relationship (Bryant, 1990). They understand that only their own pet provides love and reliable friendship (Bryant, 1985, 1986). Counterbalancing the benefits are potential costs, such as distress stemming from the pet's death or rejection, dissatisfaction with the pet's needs, worry about the pet's safety, getting into trouble in situations involving the pet, and distress when unable to help the pet.

The ascribed value of dogs varies with the person's life stage and circumstances. Albert & Bulcroft's (1987, 1988) Rhode Island study revealed the paradox of high rates of pet ownership being associated with low rates of pet attachment. Attachment to pets was highest among people living alone, and among couples who did not have children living at home. A longitudinal study of older people (a population that experiences increasing losses) found that persons who stayed at home and spent more time with the animal also became more attached and formed a stronger relationship with it (Lago *et al.*, 1985).

Dogs seem to satisfy more of the needs of widowed, separated and divorced people than those of people at other stages of life (Salmon & Salmon, 1983). Apparently, for people living in situations where a family network is lacking, social needs can be fulfilled by dogs. The dog was more of a close friend, more like a child, made them feel safer, and provided them with greater opportunity for exercise than it did for people living with intact families. Among older childless couples, 73% believed that walking the dog had encouraged conversations with people, as compared with only 48% of people at other stages of life.

The foregoing studies suggest that the mutual attachment between dogs and humans tends to increase with time spent together. For people who form close attachments, a dog may become a central focus of attention and love when the person's other social contacts are diminished.

13.3   Why dogs are special

13.3.1   Displays of affection

Many behavior patterns of dogs seem especially designed to elicit attachment. Dogs are naturally affectionate, a trait that is more characteristic of some breeds than others (Hart & Hart, 1988), and they can even be instructed to provide affection. From the earliest training of service dogs, it has been standard practice to teach a verbal command for them to provide displays of affection to the person using a wheelchair (Mader *et al.*, 1989); this command is commonly a favorite among service dog users (Figure 13.1).

Darwin (1969 [1873]) described specific behavior patterns dogs use to express affection. These include: lowering the head and whole body with the tail extended and wagging from side to side, drawing the ears back alongside the head, rubbing up against the owner, and attempting to lick the owner's hands, face or ears. These ritualized greeting signals indicate to owners that the dog is pleased to see them. Dogs seek out their owners for mutual contact, and provide affection that is not

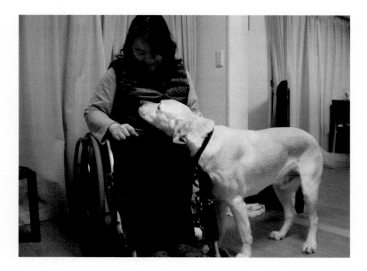

Figure 13.1 Assistance dogs freely offer affection and also provide it upon request. (© Yuki Nagaoka, reprinted with permission.)

contingent upon the owner's success or appearance. The unconditional nature of the dog's affection may also allow owners to direct or redirect anger at the dog without putting the entire relationship at risk (see Serpell, Chapter 15).

13.3.2   Loyalty and devotion

Certain traits make dogs ideally suited to be human companions. Dogs develop specific attachments for individuals, and remain near or in physical contact with their owners as if attached by an invisible cord (Serpell, 1996a). Even adult dogs can form these attachments quickly to a new person (Gácsi *et al.*, 2001). They also tend to be active during the daytime when people are active and, with appropriate training, they defer to people as the leading social partners. More important, however, are dogs' extraordinary powers of non-verbal expression by which they signal their love and regard for humans.

In order to assess the satisfaction of dog owners with various aspects of their pets' behavior, Serpell (1983) invited 57 urban dog owners to rate both their own pets and a hypothetical "ideal" dog on 22 different behavioral traits. The traits with the highest ratings and the least variability between owners included expressiveness, enjoyment of walks, loyalty/affection, welcoming behavior and attentiveness. These were the same items corresponding with the owners' "ideal" ratings. A larger scale study with 877 participants in Australia (King *et al.*, 2009) also showed that affection towards the owners is an important behavioral component of an ideal dog. In this study, 44 statements relating to dog behavior were rated as measures of an ideal dog by the participants. Five subscales were extracted using Principal Components Analysis: calm/compliant; social/healthy; energetic/faithful/protective; socially acceptable; non-aggressive. Among them, "social/healthy," which consists of behavior statements such as "my ideal dog shows affection toward me," "my ideal dog enjoys being cuddled and hugged," and "my ideal dog enjoys being petted," obtained the highest mean scores.

Like other pets, a major asset of dogs is that, despite their intimate involvement with humans, they lack the power of speech and are therefore unable to offer advice, judgment or criticism. Because dogs are affectionate and empathic, their friendship tends to be seen as sincere, reliable and trustworthy, while lacking many of the threats potentially associated with human friendship (Serpell, 1996a).

13.3.3   Physical and tactile interactions: Play and touch

Almost all dog owners in a US study reported playing often with their dogs (Stallones *et al.*, 1988). Similarly, when asked to respond to the statement, "the dog gives me an outlet for playfulness," 80% of 259 Swedish dog-owners agreed (Adell-Bath *et al.*, 1979). In another study involving observations of people walking their dogs, some type of game with the dog was observed on 36% of walks (Messent, 1983). In general, more fetch-type games were played with medium-sized to large dogs than with small ones. Bowing or lunging toward a dog stimulates more interactive play for owners seeking to escalate the playtime (Bradshaw & Rooney, Chapter 8; Rooney *et al.*, 2001). Surprisingly little is known about the amount of time people spend playing with their animal companions but one survey of Swiss pet owners found that owners reported spending an average of 17.5 hours per week interacting with their dogs (Turner, 1985).

In an analysis of 1105 photographs of dogs or cats in a family setting submitted to a national photographic contest, Katcher & Beck (1985) found that 97% of the pictures illustrated people and animals touching each other, generally with the heads of the animal and human close together. Over 92% showed a dyadic relationship, with one person and one animal occupying the center of the photograph. Touching was also a primary mode of interaction with a dog in a study of nursing home residents (Neer *et al.*, 1987). Of the nine different types of interaction recorded involving the dog, grooming and petting or touching were the two most commonly employed by residents. A study of long-term care facilities found that animal-assisted therapy (AAT) induced significantly higher rates of touching behavior among the people when compared to those involved in arts and crafts or "snack bingo" (Bernstein *et al.*, 2000).

13.4   Dogs as helping partners

In the US in particular, dogs have recently been further incorporated into roles as helping partners. Assistance/service dogs and emotional support dogs have special legal status to support people with disabilities, an aspect of assuring them "reasonable accommodation" (US Equal Employment Opportunity Commission (USEEOC), 2002). Therapy dogs accompany their handlers to work at facilities such as hospitals and elementary schools for various interventions – for example, with patients or school children. However, therapy dogs in the US lack special legal status for public access.

Some assistive tasks that dogs perform for disabled people may have existed before the concept of service or assistance dogs was formalized and publicized (Serpell, 2012). Dogs are the animals that live closest and are most attentive to humans, and are able to communicate with and respond to humans. People have realized many benefits through their interactions with dogs and continue to draw on canine abilities even more with various new relationships evolving. People are imagining new roles for dogs, followed closely by the creation of additional kinds of assistance dogs and animal-assisted interventions (AAIs).

13.4.1   Definitions and nomenclature

The use of assistive dogs has evolved through history, and a certain amount of confusion exists regarding nomenclature, and the legal status and historical conventions concerning the uses of these animals (Parenti *et al.*, 2013). Guide dogs and hearing dogs for people with visual and hearing impairments, respectively, are longstanding examples of dogs providing special assistance to people with disabilities. In the 1970s, Canine Companions for Independence began training and placing "service dogs" to assist people using wheelchairs for mobility. Assistance Dogs International (ADI), established in 1987, evolved into an umbrella coalition primarily comprising organizations that train and place service and hearing dogs, as well as other assistive dogs. Reflecting the ADI usage, "assistance dogs" became an inclusive term encompassing all types of specially trained dogs helping people with disabilities. This inclusive term is used in Europe, and also the state of California, where some of the new roles for dogs emerged. In fact, California issues "assistance dog tags" to any owner or trainer of a canine that qualifies as a guide, signal (for hearing disability), or service dog; these tags are free and supplant the need for a dog license (California Animal Control Directors Association, 2013). The applicant signs an affidavit concerning the dog's status that is subject to the penal code; fraudulent representation is a misdemeanor. The number of dogs has increased sharply over the past decade, along with the range of breeds and body sizes of dogs, and the tasks they perform (Yamamoto *et al.*, 2015).

The basis of a person's right to have a service dog is an attempt to assure "reasonable accommodation" for someone with a disability. The advent of psychiatric service dogs included an emphasis on essential tasks the dogs perform, hence the stress on the term "service." Since the 1980s, dogs termed "assistance dogs" have helped people with a wide range of disabilities. However, the US Department of Justice in 2011 (DOJ, 2011) formalized a shift in nomenclature with regulations that endorsed a broad array of disabilities (USEEOC, 2008) that could qualify a person for a service dog, so long as the dog had special training in specific tasks related to the disability. It was also required that the dog be on a leash at all times and exhibit appropriate behavior with obedience training. With this document the US adopted an inclusive use of the term "service dogs" as representing all dogs assisting with disabilities. These clarifications in 2011 were necessitated by the unbridled expansion of assistance animals in the United States. Lacking clear regulations, people had tried to claim snakes, geese, ducks, cats, and other species as assistance animals. Despite the detailed US regulations, there is little mechanism for enforcing the requirements or limiting cases of "imposter" service dogs of people who lack disabilities. This gap in enforcement arises because, in the US, protecting the privacy of the person with the disability is paramount. To assure privacy, only two questions may legally be asked by someone, such as a restaurant owner, of the person pertaining to the dog: Is this a service dog? What tasks has the dog been trained to perform?

The expansion in assisting roles for dogs was fueled by the return of US veterans from the wars in Iraq and Afghanistan, often with post-traumatic stress disorder, as well as other mental disabilities, homelessness and suicide. Dogs in helping roles gained wider acceptance by the general US public as Americans became aware of so many veterans with severe problems. This social change and the broader acceptance of assistance or service dogs was reflected in the US DOJ 2011 ruling on service dogs.

Countries in Europe and Japan have proceeded cautiously with acceptance of service dogs, requiring well-defined, centralized training and certification processes for the dogs. In contrast, the US has never adopted a centralized standardized system for training or certifying guide, service, or hearing dogs. Thus, the US offers a creative but largely unregulated cauldron for experimentation and expansion of personalized training where many new roles of dogs are tailored to assist people with their specific needs.

13.4.2   Legislative and regulatory frameworks

The US legal foundations pertaining to assistance or emotional support animals were laid down in the 1990 Americans with Disabilities Act (ADA, 1990), assuring "reasonable accommodation" to persons with disabilities. The revised definition of disabilities comprises a long list that includes any impairment that limits at least one major life activity (Americans with Disabilities Act Amendment Act of 2008; USEEOC, 2008). Although government agencies such as the US Department of Justice (2010, 2011; US Government Printing Office, 2010), US Department of Housing and Urban Development (HUD, 2004, 2008) and the US Department of Transportation (DOT, 2008) have issued their own differing regulations regarding service/assistance and emotional support animals, all regulations pertaining to these animals are based on a common goal of assuring "reasonable accommodation" to persons with disabilities.

Service/assistance dogs

Persons with a disability are entitled to acquire a service animal that performs tasks that support the person, mitigating the disability. With this comes the right of public access with the specially trained dog. In most cases, the person with the disability is the handler of the dog and assumes responsibility for its care and management. But when an autistic child or person with Alzheimer's disease is involved, it is acceptable for other family members to assume primary responsibility for managing the dog.

Emotional support animals

To make things more complicated, the US Department of Housing and Urban Development (HUD, 2008) has taken a broader position in defining animals acceptable for people with disabilities. While still seeking "reasonable accommodation" for those with disabilities, HUD operates under the Fair Housing Act and the Rehabilitation Act of 1974, Section 504, assuring a person's "opportunity to use and enjoy a dwelling." HUD (2008) recognizes the value of an "emotional support animal" for someone with a disability. Such an animal requires no special training because its very nature can be therapeutic, so long as there is a "nexus" between the disability and the person's relationship with the animal. The HUD regulations stipulate that emotional support animals (not only dogs) "have an innate ability to heal their human partner without training." For example, without any special training, emotional support dogs can naturally give psychiatric comfort and reduce anxiety for their partners with disabilities who are entitled to live with their emotional support animals. Only the landlord can request medical evidence of the person's disability.

DOT (2008) similarly takes a broader stance to allow emotional support animals as well as service dogs accompanying handlers on air transport, and, as with HUD, DOT personnel can request medical verification of the person's disability. DOT requires no special training for emotional support animals. In the case of psychiatric service dogs (viewed by DOJ as service dogs) and emotional support animals, the DOT can require a note providing medical verification of the person's disability. The letter from a physician or counselor affirms the significant role of the dog for the person's treatment, but need not reveal the nature of the disability.

These legal provisions have special importance in the US, where landlords often stipulate that pets are not allowed. Special status is accorded people with disabilities and their service dogs or their emotional support animals. Elderly people in certain government-assisted housing situations are allowed to keep companion animals. This limited access to companion animals contrasts with many European countries, where elderly people often have the right to live with their dogs or cats in their apartments. As the roles of dogs expand, along with the understanding and expectation of the public toward the benefits from such dogs, the lines between service, emotional support, therapy and pet dogs become more blurred.

In the US, the expansion of service dogs has occurred quickly with no centralized process for certification or effective regulatory mechanisms to assure compliance with the regulatory requirements. No one is in a position to effectively enforce the requirements. The situation allows for creative opportunities to explore new helping roles for dogs, but also opens the door to "impostor" service dogs and irresponsible exploitation of the ill-defined and poorly enforced regulations.

Thus, some people take advantage of the broad market for new types of assistance dogs. For example, seizure alert dogs are appealing when they actually provide advance warning of seizures (Brown & Goldstein, 2011; Ortiz & Liporace, 2005), but prospective handlers probably do not realize that this is a natural ability of some dogs, not a behavior that is reliably trained. Media report that some dog trainers exploit the economic market, selling dogs that are not fully trained as assistance dogs; these trainers often do not provide adequate team training and follow-ups with the handlers (FOX 31 Investigates, 2010; The Examiner, 2013). These problems are emerging as unwanted side effects of the increased popularity of assistance and emotional support dogs. Moreover, even assistance dogs that were trained by well-established training organizations can be unsuccessful in their pairings with people with disabilities. Some people return their dogs because of behavior problems and/or poor matching with the dogs (Batt *et al.*, 2010; Burrows *et al.*, 2008; Hart *et al.*, 1995; Lloyd *et al.*, 2008).

Gullible acceptance of untrained service dogs creates problems. However, the dramatic increase in assistance dogs in the US reveals the high expectations among the general public. Among recent fast-moving developments, economic constraints have become a major factor limiting the dissemination of assistance dogs. The Department of Veterans Affairs (VA) pays for service dogs assigned to veterans who have impaired vision, hearing, or mobility, but in a 2012 ruling, the VA (2012) cut payments for psychiatric service dogs, due to "lack of evidence of mental health service dog efficacy." Most recently, a new ruling was passed, and the VA now allows all service dogs to enter VA facilities (US Department of Veterans Affairs, 2015).[1]

Further, the US Army has implemented a policy regarding dogs on army bases (Moss, 2012). These dogs can be provided only through organizations that are approved by Assistance Dogs International. The soldier must first seek approval for a service dog from his or her commander, and then the soldier's eligibility for a dog must be reviewed by a panel of healthcare professionals. This new policy was adopted following the death of a 6-year-old boy who was killed near a US Army base by a service dog belonging to a soldier. Certain bases have set additional specific requirements, e.g. at Fort Bliss, a doctor's statement must indicate that the dog can perform at least three tasks to assist with a specific disability. Specific details of this new policy are now detailed in Army Directive 2013–01, Guidance on the Acquisition and Use of Service Dogs by Soldiers (US Department of Defense, 2013). The Directive does not allow emotional support or psychiatric service dogs.

Local pushback relating to assistance dog tags is evident in California. Service dogs accompanying handlers are required to wear a California assistance dog tag at one Veterans Administration hospital (personal communication). Registrations of service dogs assisting with seizures are sometimes reported to the California Department of Motor Vehicles (personal communication).

13.4.3   Dogs helping people with physical and psychological disabilities or aging

Specific tasks are generally associated with the work of each type of service dog. Guide dogs assist in avoiding obstacles: for example, alerting their partners with visual impairments to stairs or corners. Mobility service dogs for people with mobility impairments pick up dropped items, turn switches on or off, bring things that are out of reach, and call for help when needed. Hearing (or signal) dogs alert their hearing-impaired owners to sounds such as doorbells, telephones, and fire alarms.

The roles of assistance dogs recently have widened to encompass more than their well-known guide, service, and hearing dog functions. Diabetes alert dogs signal hypoglycemia episodes for their diabetic partners (O'Connor *et al.*, 2008; Rosenthal, 2010). Seizure dogs alert to forthcoming seizures and/or respond to seizures by staying at the epileptic partner's side to calm him/her down or call for help (Dalziel *et al.*, 2003; Strong *et al.*, 1999; Strong *et al.*, 2002). Service dogs for children with autism work to calm the partnering child and assure his/her safety (Burrows *et al.*, 2008; Viau *et al.*, 2010). Psychiatric service dogs support partners with psychiatric disorders such as post-traumatic stress disorder, panic disorder, and depression (Esnayra, 2007; Smith *et al.*, 2003).

With expanding roles of assistance dogs, many breeds with various body sizes have become assistance dogs. Some tasks do not require large body sizes. Even some very small breeds under 11 lbs

[1] Fed Regist. 2015 Aug 17; 80(158): 49157–64.

(5 kg) such as Chihuahuas, miniature pinschers, and miniature poodles support their partners with disabilities, along with the conventional breeds such as Labrador and golden retrievers (Yamamoto *et al.*, 2015). Lacking governmental laws obligating people to certify or label their dogs as assistance dogs, such as the dog wearing a labeled vest, it is sometimes impossible to distinguish between assistance dogs and well-behaved pet dogs. Some people have given up living with dogs due to concerns regarding adequate dog care because of health problems and/or housing problems, such as the apartment size and the inconvenient environment for taking care of the dog. The new trend to employ dogs of various body sizes gives people with disabilities more incentives and choices for living with the most appropriate type of assistance dog, and will likely lead to a further expansion of their roles.

The primary task of dogs for people with mobility limitations is retrieving – picking up dropped items. This task can easily be taught to dogs of various sizes, and could help many people. For example, elderly people with a small dog living in an apartment could benefit from a companion dog that was trained to retrieve. Already, in multi-story apartments in Japan, most people prefer small dogs, and many find it most feasible to toilet the dog in the apartment. Dogs are trained to use special products such as diaper pads on the floor, rather than taking an elevator down 20+ stories, three times a day, to go outdoors where there may be little space for walking dogs.

Assistance dogs mainly provide various functional supports to their partners with disabilities. With this support, the human partners can conduct some of their daily tasks without requiring human assistance and are therefore more independent, regardless of their disabilities (Davis *et al.*, 2004; Fairman & Huebner, 2001; Rintala *et al.*, 2008; Valentine *et al.*, 1993; Whitmarsh, 2005; Zee, 1983). Additionally, assistance dogs' partners report psychological benefits from their dogs, including increased confidence, feelings of safety, relaxation, improved self-esteem, decreased anxiety and stress, and reduced feelings of loneliness (Allen & Blascovich, 1996; Camp, 2000; Fairman & Huebner, 2001; Guest *et al.*, 2006; Hart *et al.*, 1996; Lane *et al.*, 1998; Rossignol & Barardi, 2007; Valentine *et al.*, 1993; Whitmarsh, 2005; Zee, 1983).

Social benefits are also reported. Strangers are less likely to avoid, and more likely to engage in social interactions with, a disabled person when he or she is accompanied by a dog (Hart *et al.*, 1987; Mader *et al.*, 1989; Winkle *et al.*, 2012). With dogs present, more people give smiles and talk to persons with disabilities than when they are without dogs (Eddy *et al.*, 1988). Of course, these benefits are not caused solely by the assistance dogs' practical assistance but by the dogs themselves as living creatures.

People with disabilities may tend to be ignored by others or sometimes feel a sense of emotional isolation. These stigmatizing experiences are perhaps the most scalding aspect of the disability that people with disabilities of various ages and types of disabilities and their family members report (Bedini, 2000; Cooney *et al.*, 2006). Mothers of children with disabilities particularly experience the pain of stigma (Gray, 1993; Green *et al.*, 2005). The dog has no concept of stigma, and people view the disabled person differently due to the capacity to control and manage the dog. Since dogs work as "icebreakers" and increase their partners' social interactions, the dogs can mitigate these effects and provide some relief. After acquiring their assistance dogs, most people describe emotional and social improvements in their lives (Fairman & Huebner, 2001; Figure 13.2a and b).

People with disabilities assume responsibility for oversight of the dog's care, feeling that they are needed by the dog. This contrasts with their typical experience of always being recipients of care, thus increasing their self-esteem, confidence and dignity. In one study, new service and hearing dog recipients reduced their dependence on other persons, in contrast to control persons awaiting their dogs (Rintala *et al.*, 2008). These benefits show that being assisted by and providing for an assistance dog is crucial for many people with disabilities. A study of parents of 12 children who had recently acquired hearing dogs showed that their levels of concern across all areas of their children's

(a)

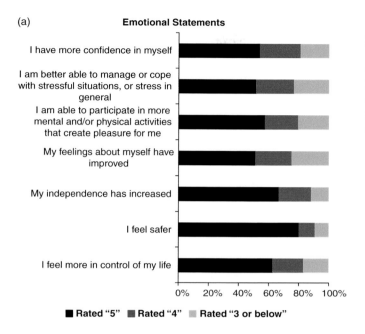

Emotional Statements

I have more confidence in myself

I am better able to manage or cope with stressful situations, or stress in general

I am able to participate in more mental and/or physical activities that create pleasure for me

My feelings about myself have improved

My independence has increased

I feel safer

I feel more in control of my life

0% 20% 40% 60% 80% 100%

■ Rated "5" ■ Rated "4" ▨ Rated "3 or below"

Figure 13.2 Most of 202 assistance dogs' partners surveyed felt their emotional and social status had greatly improved after acquiring their dogs. Ninety-four percent of the participants had physical disabilities and the remainder had emotional or hearing, or combined disabilities. Rate 5: definitely true; rate 1: definitely false. (After Fairman & Huebner, 2001.)

(b)

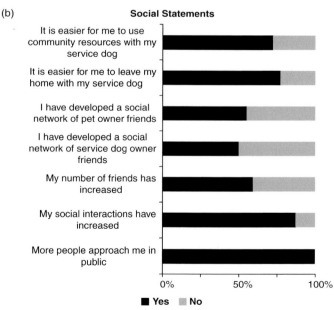

Social Statements

It is easier for me to use community resources with my service dog

It is easier for me to leave my home with my service dog

I have developed a social network of pet owner friends

I have developed a social network of service dog owner friends

My number of friends has increased

My social interactions have increased

More people approach me in public

0% 50% 100%

■ Yes ▨ No

lives fell dramatically after their children acquired the dogs (Hearing Dogs for Deaf People, 2012; Figure 13.3). Assistance dogs play a significant role in the positive development of children as well as offering functional daily life supports.

The levels of attachment between people and their pets influence the psychological and physical effects of keeping companion animals (Boldt & Dellmann-Jenkins, 1992; Garrity et al., 1989). To maximize the supportive abilities of animals, optimizing their relationships with their owners is important (Boldt & Dellmann-Jenkins, 1992; Friedmann, 1995). The maximum gain from the

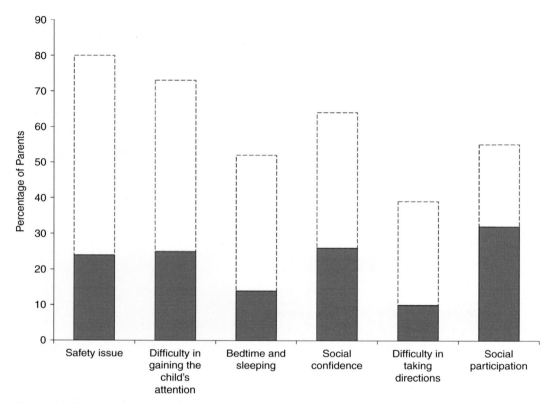

Figure 13.3 The percentage of parents with concerns for their children with hearing disabilities (*n* = 12) declined after the children acquired hearing dogs. Dashed boxes: before the acquisition of a hearing dog; solid boxes: after acquisition. (After Hearing Dogs for Deaf People, 2012.)

assistance dog occurs when the relationship with the human partner is functional and positive. The additional variability of a living assistant cannot be expected to produce only positive results, as it is not as consistent as other non-living medical assistive technologies.

With a growing number of dogs having special status and increased public access, it is important to consider the negative impacts of introducing dogs to public spheres, such as dog allergies, dog phobias, and vulnerabilities to being knocked over. Accommodating societal interests includes protecting people who are uncomfortable or fearful around dogs so they are able to welcome the assistance dogs passing by, or at least see them without experiencing great anxiety. Benefiting from dogs depends on the person's past experiences and preferences (Friedmann *et al.*, 1993, 2000). While many people have high expectations of benefits from dogs, not everyone benefits or has favorable perceptions of these animals.

13.4.4   Therapy dogs used in animal-assisted interventions (AAIs)

Starting originally with the introduction of dogs into nursing homes, AAIs have since expanded in new directions. While some dogs are bred for use in these types of interventions, most "therapy dogs" are companion dogs that have received some training with their owners. Nationwide therapy

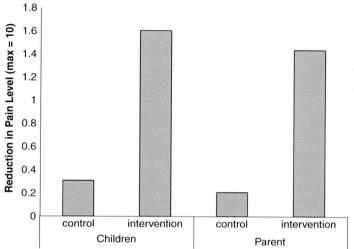

Figure 13.4 Both the parents and their children in an acute care pediatric setting that received a 15–20 min AAT session with dog and handler reported a reduction in pain level for the child; the pain reduction was greater than with children not receiving the AAT intervention. No pain: 0; worst pain: 5. (After Braun *et al.*, 2009.)

organizations, such as Pet Partners® and Therapy Dogs International (TDI®) certify companion animals and have 11 000 and 24 750 therapy animal (mainly dogs) teams, respectively (Pet Partners®, 2012; TDI®, 2013). These dogs have no special legal access because the handlers lack a disability. AAIs range from various recreational activities to therapy. Therapy dogs interact with patients to fulfill certain therapeutic objectives outlined by the medical professionals for animal-assisted therapy (AAT). For example, AAT has been used as a pain-relieving intervention for children (Braun *et al.*, 2009; Figure 13.4). Reducing the stress and pain of aversive medical treatments is a rapidly expanding application of AAT now being studied with more scrutiny (Marcus *et al.*, 2012; Sobo *et al.*, 2006). Using a therapy dog to relieve the stress for children giving forensic interviews is another growing application of AAT (Courthouse Dogs, 2013). These "courthouse dogs" are trained by ADI accredited organizations to a standard equivalent to ADI-trained service dogs, and they sometimes are called "facility dogs."

In animal-assisted activities (AAA), which do not require the oversight of medical professionals, the goals focus on recreational activities, often involving dogs visiting nursing homes, hospitals, and schools. Interventions specifically for children teach them empathy and improve their social cohesion while also creating more favorable classroom learning environments through the interactions with dogs (Kotrschal & Ortbauer, 2003); these interventions are sometimes referred to as animal-assisted education (AAE).

One standardized program that has become popular throughout the USA and beyond is the Reading Education Assistance Dogs (R.E.A.D®) program. By reading to a dog, a favorable environment is created for the children to read books and improve communication skills (Intermountain Therapy Animals, 2012). Shannon (2007) surveyed 51 parents or guardians whose children participated in programs reading to dogs, and most of the participants reported their children displaying beneficial behaviors, such as being more willing to read aloud and showing increased confidence regarding reading.

Dog training programs have also spread to many prison and juvenile facilities, which now offer programs for inmates: over 160 sites offer prison-based animal programs throughout the USA (Furst, 2006; Strimple, 2003). In some programs, inmates train shelter dogs to be adopted into the community as pets, or assistance dogs for people with disabilities. Fournier *et al.*'s (2007) study indicates that inmates who participated in dog training programs showed improvements in institutional infractions, level of treatment for psychosocial functioning, and social skills. For handlers in prisons participating in training programs, the dogs served as their own "therapy dogs." In other programs, veterans train dogs in a similar way to be placed with other veterans. There is concern for the effect that giving up the dog may have on the inmate or veteran, and whether a longer relationship with the dog would be more efficacious. However, we are not aware of any research on this question.

With the rapid expansion of roles for therapy dogs, the scientific studies of efficacy of their use, though numerous, do not follow the conventions that would be routine for clinical trials of a new drug. Often the persons seeking the AAI therapy are self-selected, and administration of the therapy is neither blinded nor randomized. A recent systematic review of randomized controlled trials of animal-assisted therapy found only 11 studies meeting the specified criteria, and these were extremely heterogeneous, involving eight different species of animals. A meta-analysis could not be performed (Kamioka et al., 2014). Nonetheless, the results suggested that AAT may be effective for mental and behavioral disorders such as depression, schizophrenia, and alcohol/drug addictions. In another review study, Marino (2012) investigated components of validity in studies of AAA and AAT to answer the question "how important is the animal in animal therapy?" by reviewing two meta-analyses and 28 single empirical studies. She pointed out methodological weaknesses in the AAT and AAA literature, and was unable to answer the question of whether a live animal is necessary for a therapeutic effect. As these systematic review studies emphasize, it is necessary to provide objective outcomes of AAT and AAA by conducting rigorous experimental studies. However, in contrast to drug trials, people's perceptions and past experiences highly affect the outcomes of interacting with animals (Friedmann et al., 1993, 2000). Many variables could provide unexpected benefits depending on recipients: types of animals, breeds, colors, hair length and sizes of animals, behavior of the animals, and even spontaneous interactions between humans and animals. Therefore, the more we attempt to control the study environments, the more the benefits of animals may be limited. Future studies of AAT and AAA may benefit from focusing on which types of populations benefit most, and what kinds of programs produce the best outcomes, as well as generalizing the outcomes of AAA and AAT through the use of controlled trials.

13.5   Dogs as companions

13.5.1   Socialization effects of dogs for people

The social value of canine companionship and partnership is most obvious with persons who use wheelchairs and have service dogs (Hart, 1999). Retrospective and prospective studies revealed that wheelchair-bound adults with service dogs received more social acknowledgments from passers-by than those without dogs (Eddy et al., 1988; Hart et al., 1987; Lane et al., 1998). McNicholas & Collis (2000, p. 61) showed the robust effect of dogs as catalysts for social interactions in an experimental observation: the number of people interacting with the handler was increased by a dog over tenfold or about eightfold (depending on whether the handler dressed smartly or sloppily). They concluded that, "although there were significantly more interactions when he was smartly dressed, the greatest effect was between the Dog Present and No Dog conditions irrespective of the handler's dress." A dog can therefore normalize social responses toward individuals who are often ignored or avoided due to a disability, shyness or physical unattractiveness.

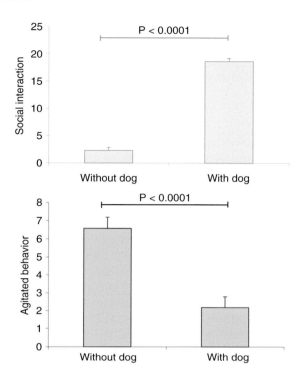

Figure 13.5 Elderly people with dementia in long-term care responded to the presence of AAT with a therapy dog by increasing their social interaction and reducing their agitated behavior. The four phases of the study included a baseline condition without AAT, an AAT treatment condition, a second baseline, and a second AAT treatment. Social interaction: social behavior observation checklist; agitation behavior: Agitation Behavior Mapping Instrument. (After Sellers, 2006.)

Dogs seem to display an inexhaustible willingness to form and sustain partnerships with humans, as dramatically illustrated by the partnership between service dogs and people in wheelchairs. Dog and owner become a team to other people, more predictably together than any mother and child, marital couple, or pair of siblings: a closeness made evident to both the owner and to onlookers by the dog's alert attention and responsiveness to the owner's commands.

When children were asked in another study to rate their own social competence, their self-ratings were positively associated with the number of pets in the family and most felt that their pets had helped them to make friends (Serpell, 1986). Paul & Serpell's (1996) prospective study showed that children who obtained a new dog had more friends visiting them than non-dog owning children.

In addition to many studies that have explored the therapeutic role of visiting or residential dogs in nursing home settings, there is increasing interest in the possible social effects for staff and/or patients. One early Australian study reported that patients spent less time alone following the introduction of a resident dog than previously (Hogarth-Scott *et al.*, 1983). Ninety-one percent of patients appreciated that the dog was something to talk about, and 86% of staff felt that the dog was something they could share with patients. Studies investigating the effect of therapy dogs on elderly people with dementia at nursing homes have shown significant increases in social interaction and decreases in agitated behavior as a consequence of animal-assisted therapy (Richeson, 2003; Sellers, 2006; Figure 13.5).

Dogs serve as social companions as well as primers for human social interactions by providing a topic of relaxed and entertaining conversation. Since social contact is the mechanism for nurturing self-esteem in people, the socializing effects of dog companionship are among the most important indirect benefits of these interactions.

13.5.2   Physical and psychological benefits of canine companionship

In addition to somewhat commonplace observations regarding animals' contributions to calming and human health, scientists have conducted formal studies into the psychological, physiological and therapeutic impact of relationships with dogs.

Developmental benefits

Dogs provide significant companionship for children as well as for adults. They respond to demands and offer uncritical sympathy; they may serve as transitional objects and sources of security for a young child venturing away from the mother (Triebenbacher, 1998). Children commonly use their pets for comfort when they are feeling bored, lonely or unhappy. The fact that children reveal their empathic concerns for pets supports the notion that children may sometimes learn how to care for others from their experiences with animals (see Melson, 1990). Some evidence suggests that children who lack younger siblings may compensate by spending more time with animals. Children who lack younger siblings seem to perceive their pets with more positive emotion than children with younger siblings (Bryant, 1986; Paul & Serpell, 1992). Children with pets also appear to be better informed about how adult animals care for their young than do non-pet owning children (Melson & Fogel, 1989). When Melson (1988) interviewed mothers of young school children, she found that children without younger siblings played more with their pets. Evidence that children adjust their involvement with animals according to their family structure was also found in a French study; children without siblings showed more frequent and longer interactions with a dog than children with siblings (Filiatre et al., 1985, 1986).

In a study of kindergarten and day-care children, Nielsen & Delude (1989) used a variety of animals to capture children's attention including a tarantula, a cockatiel, two breeds of rabbits, two breeds of dog, and various toy animals. Only the dogs elicited displays of intimacy, with 21% of the children hugging or kissing them, three times as much by boys as by girls. When dogs direct enthusiastic affection toward someone, that person is likely to feel accepted and viewed as a good person by the dog. In a study of twenty-two 10–12 year-olds, 65% of the children believed that the dog thought the child was a wonderful person (Davis, 1987). This positive reflected appraisal provided by the dog would tend to support the development of a stronger and more positive self-concept. Especially for adolescents, a clear and consistent message that they matter helps them infer that they are significant (Rosenberg & McCullough, 1981).

Psychological benefits

Therapists often find that emotionally disturbed children or adults who have been hurt in their relationships with people relate more easily to animals than the therapist (Levinson, 1969). If the disturbed person first opens up to an animal, the animal may then facilitate acceptance for the associated therapist, making it possible to establish a connection much sooner (Lapp, 1991). This has been the anchor philosophy for residential treatment of highly disturbed children at Green Chimneys, a farm in New York that affords exposure to many different animals to initiate trust, comfort, and a feeling of safety (Mallon, 1998). Psychological benefits of farm animal-assisted interventions are also reported among adults with clinical depression (Pedersen et al., 2012). Twelve weekly sessions of AAI significantly decreased the participants' depression and increased their self-efficacy, while no significant changes were found in the control group.

In a study of elderly people at nursing homes, the participants showed a significant positive change in mood when they received visits from volunteers with a dog compared to volunteers without a dog (Lutwack-Bloom et al., 2005). A study of three aphasia patients found no differences in subsequent language function for the patients following the traditional sessions and the AAT sessions (Macauley, 2006). However, the patients believed they had improved more during the AAT sessions. Further, they were more motivated to attend the therapy during AAT than during traditional therapy, and enjoyed the AAT sessions more.

For both children and elderly adults, the opportunity to care for an animal may have value by providing an experience of mattering to another. Melson's (1988) study of preadolescent children found a substantial correlation between caretaking and their emotional engagement. In a study of nursing home patients with Alzheimer's disease, more than 25% of the patients showed some behavioral improvements during twice-weekly visits from trained dogs and their volunteer handlers (Schultz, 1987). In an eight-week study at a psychiatric facility where puppies and handlers made weekly visits, Francis (1985) reported improvements in patients' social interaction, psychosocial function, life satisfaction, mental function, depression, social competence and psychologic well-being. Dogs may also have particular value in assuring people that they are secure from harm. People frequently obtain a dog to serve as a watchdog, and a prospective study of new cat and dog owners found that, among dog owners, a lasting and statistically significant reduction occurred in fear of crime (Serpell, 1990).

Physiological health

Several studies have documented the immediate physiological effects on humans of canine companionship (see reviews in Baun *et al.*, 1991; Friedmann, 1990). While the effect of the presence of a dog on cardiovascular function is possibly the most extensively studied aspect of human–animal interactions, the findings are difficult to interpret and there is no evidence to prove that petting a dog induces beneficial health effects over the long-term. What has been demonstrated in several studies is a reduction in blood pressure for normotensive or hypertensive persons when they pet a dog, with a stronger effect for hypertensive individuals (Katcher *et al.*, 1983). An exploratory study of insecurely attached children showed that their salivary cortisol level was significantly lower in the presence of a real dog than in conditions with a toy dog or a friendly person during a stressful task (Beetz *et al.*, 2011). In another study, pet owners who had suffered a heart attack were found to show improved survivorship after one year, as compared with those who did not have a pet (Friedmann *et al.*, 1980). This finding was subsequently replicated with a larger sample size in a study that found that having a dog and/or human social support were associated with improved survivorship (Friedmann & Thomas, 1995). A randomized study of patients hospitalized with heart failure consisting of three groups of volunteer-dog visit, volunteer visit, and no visit found the volunteer-dog group showing significantly greater decreases in cardiopulmonary pressures, neurohormone levels, and anxiety than the other two control groups (Cole *et al.*, 2007).

Touch may play a major role in the lowering of blood pressure while petting a dog (see Vormbrock & Grossberg, 1988). Interestingly, the dog may share the person's feeling of calmness associated with petting or being with a dog. A dog's heart rate drops when being petted by a person (Lynch & McCarthy, 1969). One study also reported that mutual physiological changes, including increased concentration of oxytocin (also called the "happiness hormone"), were shown in dogs as well as dog lovers during positive interaction between the two (Odendaal & Meintjes, 2003). Women (but not men) in one study showed increases in oxytocin levels after interacting with their dogs (Miller *et al.*, 2009). In another study, engaging with their dogs' gaze was associated with heightened urinary oxytocin of owners during social interactions (Nagasawa *et al.*, 2009). These studies are just a few of many suggesting that the oxytocin system plays a key role in the psychophysiological effects of human–animal interactions (Beetz *et al.*, 2012).

Physical and general health

Dramatic increases in walking were found among new dog owners in England in a prospective study of dog and cat adoption (Serpell, 1991), providing strong support for the view that dogs can benefit owners by increasing the amount of exercise they take. Serpell's study also found that dog owners developed a heightened sense of security and self-esteem, and improvements in general health that continued through 10 months following adoption. Many studies focus on the physical activities, especially dog-walking, facilitated by dogs. Cutt et al. (2007) reviewed papers related to dog ownership and owners' health and physical activity, and concluded that, "there is increasing evidence to suggest that dog owners are more physically active (primarily through walking their dog) than non-owners." Although results from studies on physical and general health caused by dog ownership are not consistent, there are interesting findings. Thorpe et al. (2006) examined the physical activity of elderly people with follow-up research. The participants consisted of two basic groups: dog owners and non-dog owners. These two groups were divided into walking and non-walking subgroups depending on whether they walked at least three times per week or not. Walking speeds were measured for all participants, at usual and rapid walking rates. At baseline, walkers (both dog owners and non-owners) had faster usual and rapid walking speeds than non-walkers. Three years later, the four groups of participants declined in their usual and rapid walking speeds at similar rates, but dog owning and non-owning walkers maintained their initial advantage over the owning and non-owning non-walkers, emphasizing the benefits of walking, whether with or without a dog. Another experimental study on elderly people also revealed the benefits of dog walking from a different perspective by examining autonomic nervous activity (Motooka et al., 2006). Parasympathetic neural activity was significantly higher during episodes of walking with a dog than without a dog. The authors concluded that walking a dog would have potentially greater health benefits as a buffer against stress in elderly people than walking without a dog.

Further evidence for effects on general health was reported in a United States study of 938 Medicare enrollees, where pet owners reported fewer doctor visits during a one year period than non-owners (Siegel, 1990). Generally, people experiencing stressful life events increased their number of doctor visits, but respondents with pets were less likely to increase their doctor visits during stressful events. Dog owners spent more time outdoors with their pets, more time talking to their pets and more time overall with their pets than other people they knew. They felt more attached to their dogs, and the positive aspects of dog ownership strongly outweighed the negative ones compared with owners of other pets. Dog owners were more likely to mention that their pets made them feel secure and provided entertainment.

13.6   Conclusions

Dogs fill a growing variety of roles, sometimes performing assisting tasks, even as they also contribute psychosocial benefits such as improving mood, offering comfort, relieving depression, exerting a calming effect, and relieving stigma. Considering their special roles and their legal and regulatory status, dogs can be categorized as companion, therapy, emotional support, or service dogs, as depicted in Figure 13.6. Although therapy dogs lack any special legal status or access, they participate in animal-assisted interventions conducted in settings such as hospitals, schools, libraries, courtrooms, and residential facilities. Emotional support dogs for people with disabilities are afforded access in the US to housing and air transportation; service dogs perform assisting tasks and have full public access.

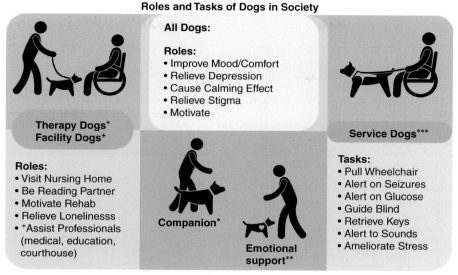

Figure 13.6 Roles and tasks of dogs in human society. Companion, therapy, emotional support, and service dogs can all offer similar psychosocial roles, offering comfort, calming, relief from depression and stigma, and motivation. Therapy dogs assist their handlers in providing animal-assisted interventions to help people in facilities such as hospitals, schools, courtrooms, prisons, or residential facilities, but these dogs have no special legal status for public access. A person with a disability is allowed an emotional support dog, with access to housing and air transport; no tasks are required of the dog. A person with a disability is allowed full public access with a service dog that is trained to perform tasks related to the disability. Emotional support and service dogs are required to exhibit appropriate behavior. (© Lynette Hart and Mariko Yamamoto.)

Some pushback against the broad expansion of service dogs has arisen in specific contexts. We anticipate that the variety of service dogs and their roles and tasks will continue to proliferate, with an increasing number of smaller dogs serving these roles.

Acknowledgments

Financial support for preparation of this chapter was provided by a grant (##2009-36-F) from the Center for Companion Animal Health, School of Veterinary Medicine, at the University of California, Davis. Pfizer/Zoetis also provided generous financial support toward preparation of this chapter. Abigail Gallaher Thigpen and Martha Bryant provided outstanding editing and technical assistance. We appreciate Yuki Nagaoka allowing use of her photographs. We thank Justin Ross for creating the artistic design and icons for Figure 13.6.

References

Adell-Bath, M., Krook, A., Sandqvist, G. & Skantze, K. (1979). *Do We Need Dogs? A Study of Dogs' Social Significance to Man.* Gothenburg: University of Gothenburg Press.

Albert, A. & Bulcroft, K. (1987). Pets and urban life. *Anthrozoös*, 1: 9–23.

Albert, A. & Bulcroft, K. (1988). Pets, families, and the life course. *Journal of Marriage and the Family*, 50: 543–52.

Allen, K. & Blascovich, J. (1996). The value of service dogs for people with severe ambulatory disabilities: a randomized controlled trial. *The Journal of the American Medical Association*, 275: 1001–6.

American Pet Products Association (APPA) (2011). *2011/2012 APPA National Pet Owners Survey.* [Online]. Available: www.americanpetproducts.org/pubs_survey.asp

American Veterinary Medical Association (AVMA) (2012). *U.S. Pet Ownership: Demographics Sourcebook.* Schaumburg, IL: AVMA.

Americans with Disabilities Act (ADA) (1990). 42 USC §§ 12181–12189. Title III. 28 CFR Part 36.

Americans with Disabilities Act Amendments Act of 2008 (2008). PL 110–325 (S 3406). [Online]. Available: www.eeoc.gov/laws/statutes/adaaa.cfm

Barker, S. B. & Barker, R. T. (1988). The human–canine bond: closer than family ties? *Journal of Mental Health Counseling*, 10: 46–56.

Batt, L., Batt, M., Baguley, J. & McGreevy, P. (2010). Relationships between puppy management practices and reported measures of success in guide dog training. *Journal of Veterinary Behavior*, 5: 240–6.

Baun, M. M., Oetting, K. & Bergstrom, N. (1991). Health benefits of companion animals in relation to the physiologic indices of relaxation. *Holistic Nursing Practice*, 5: 16–23.

Beck, L. & Madresh, E. A. (2008). Romantic partners and four-legged friends: an extension of attachment theory to relationships with pets. *Anthrozoös*, 21: 43–56.

Bedini, L. A. (2000). Just sit down so we can talk: perceived stigma and the pursuit of community recreation for people with disabilities. *Therapeutic Recreation Journal*, 34: 55–68.

Beetz, A., Kotrschal, K., Turner, D. C., Hediger, K., Uvnäs-Moberg, K. & Julius, H. (2011). The effect of a real dog, toy dog and friendly person on insecurely attached children during a stressful task: an exploratory study. *Anthrozoös*, 24: 349–68.

Beetz, A., Uvnäs-Moberg, K., Julius, H. & Kotrschal, K. (2012). Psychosocial and psychophysiological effects of human-animal interactions: the possible role of oxytocin. *Frontiers in Psychology*, 3:234. http://doi:10.3389/fpsyg.2012.00234

Bernstein, P L., Friedmann, E. & Malaspina, A. (2000). Animal-assisted therapy enhances resident social interaction and initiation in long-term care facilities. *Anthrozoös*, 13: 213–24.

Boldt, M. A. & Dellmann-Jenkins, M. (1992). The impact of companion animals in later life and considerations for practice. *The Journal of Applied Gerontology*. 11: 228–39.

Bonas, S., McNicholas, J. & Collis, G. M. (2000). Pets in the network of family relationships: an empirical study. In *Animals and Us: Exploring the Relationships between People and Pets*, eds. A. L. Podberscek, E. S. Paul & J. A. Serpell. Cambridge: Cambridge University Press, pp. 209–36.

Braun, C., Stangler, T., Narveson, J. & Pettingell, S. (2009). Animal-assisted therapy as a pain relief intervention for children. *Complementary Therapies in Clinical Practice*, 15: 105–9.

Brown, S. W. & Goldstein, L. H. (2011). Can seizure-alert dogs predict seizures? *Epilepsy Research*, 97: 236–42.

Bryant, B. (1985). The neighborhood walk: sources of support in middle childhood. *Monographs of the Society for Research in Child Development*, 50(3): Serial No. 210.

Bryant, B. (1986). The relevance of family and neighborhood animals to social-emotional development in middle childhood (Abstract). *Living Together: People, Animals, and the Environment*, p. 68. Renton, WA: Delta Society.

Bryant, B. K. (1990). The richness of the child-pet relationship: a consideration of both benefits and costs of pets to children. *Anthrozoös*, 3: 253–61.

Bucke, W. F. (1903). Cyno-psychoses. Children's thoughts, reactions, and feelings toward pet dogs. *Pedagogical Seminary*, 10: 459–513.

Burrows, K. E., Adams, C. L. & Millman, S. T. (2008). Factors affecting behavior and welfare of service dogs for children with autism spectrum disorder. *Journal of Applied Animal Welfare Science*, 11: 42–62.

California Animal Control Directors Association (2013). Assistance tags. [Online]. Available: www.cacda.org/home/documents/Assistance_Tags_CACDA.doc

Camp, M. M. (2000). The use of service dogs as an adaptive strategy: A qualitative study. *The American Journal of Occupational Therapy*, 55: 509–17.

Cohen, S. P. (2002). Can pets function as family members? *Western Journal of Nursing Research*, 24: 621–38.

Cole, K. M., Gawlinski, A., Steers, N. & Kotlerman, J. (2007). Animal-assisted therapy in patients hospitalized with heart failure. *American Journal of Critical Care*, 16: 575–88.

Cooney, G., Jahoda, A., Gumley, A. & Knott, F. (2006). Young people with intellectual disabilities attending mainstream and segregated schooling: perceived stigma, social comparison and future aspirations. *Journal of Intellectual Disability Research*, 50: 432–44.

Courthouse Dogs (2013). [Online]. Available: http://courthousedogs.com/

Cutt, H., Giles-Corti, B., Knuiman, M. & Burke, V. (2007). Dog ownership, health and physical activity: a critical review of the literature. *Health & Place*, 13: 261–72.

Dalziel, D. J., Uthman, B., McGorray, S. P. & Reep, R. L. (2003). Seizure-alert dogs: a review and preliminary study. *Seizure*, 12: 115–120.

Darwin, C. (1969 [1873]). The *Expression of the Emotions in Man and Animals*. New York: Greenwood Press (originally published 1873).

Davis, J. H. (1987). Preadolescent self-concept development and pet ownership. *Anthrozoös*, 1: 90–4.

Davis, B. W., Nattrass, K., O'Brien, S., Patronek, G. & MacCollin, M. (2004). Assistance dog placement in the pediatric population: benefits, risks, and recommendations for future application. *Anthrozoös*, 17: 130–45.

Eddy, J., Hart, L. A. & Boltz, R. P. (1988). The effects of service dogs on social acknowledgements of people in wheelchairs. *Journal of Psychology*, 122: 39–45.

Esnayra, J. (2007). Help from man's best friend: psychiatric service dogs are helping consumers deal with the symptoms of mental illness. *Behavioral Healthcare*, 27, 30–2.

Fairman, S. K. & Huebner, R. A. (2001). Service dogs: a compensatory resource to improve function. *Occupational Therapy in Health Care*, 13: 41–52.

Filiatre, J. C, Millot, J. L. & Montagner, H. (1985). New findings on communication behavior between the young child and his pet dog. In *The Human–Pet Relationship*. Vienna: IEMT, pp. 51–7.

Filiatre, J. C, Millot, J. L. & Montagner, H. (1986). New data on communication behaviour between the young child and his pet dog. *Behavioral Processes*, 12: 33–44.

Fournier, A. K., Geller, E. S. & Fortney, E. V. (2007). Human-animal interaction in a prison setting: impact on criminal behavior, treatment progress, and social skills. *Behavior and Social Issues*, 16: 89–105.

FOX 31 Investigates (2010). Untrained service dogs. [Online]. Available: www.dailymotion.com/video/xfviv1_fox31-investigates-untrained-service-dogs_news

Francis, G. M. (1985). Domestic animal visitation as therapy with adult home residents. *International Journal of Nursing Studies*, 22: 201–6.

Friedmann, E. (1990). The value of pets for health and recovery. In *Pets, Benefits and Practice*, Waltham Symposium 20, ed. I. H. Burger. London: BVA Publications., pp. 8–17

Friedmann, E. (1995). The role of pets in enhancing human well-being: physiological effects. In *The Waltham Book of Human-Animal Interaction: Benefits and Responsibilities of Pet Ownership*, ed. I. Robinson. Oxford: Pergamon Press, pp. 33–5.

Friedmann, E., Katcher, A. H., Lynch, J. J. & Thomas, S. A. (1980). Animal companions and one year survival of patients after discharge from a coronary care unit. *Public Health Reports*, 95: 307–12.

Friedmann, E., Locker, B. Z. & Lockwood, R. (1993). Perception of animals and cardiovascular responses during verbalization with an animal present. *Anthrozoös*, 6: 115–34.

Friedmann, E. & Thomas, S. A. (1995). Pet ownership, social support, and one-year survival after acute myocardial infarction in the cardiac arrhythmia suppression trial (CAST). *American Journal of Cardiology*, 76: 1213–17.

Friedmann, E., Thomas, S. A. & Eddy, T. J. (2000). Companion animals and human health: physical and cardiovascular influences. In *Companion Animals & Us: Exploring the Relationships between People & Pets*, eds. A. L. Podberscek, E. S. Paul & J. A. Serpell. Cambridge: Cambridge University Press, pp. 125–42.

Furst, G. (2006). Prison-based animal programs: a national survey. *The Prison Journal*, 86: 407–30.

Gácsi, M., Topál, J., Miklósi, A., Dóca, A. & Czányi, V. (2001). Attachment behavior of adult dogs (*Canis familiaris*) living at rescue centers: forming new bonds. *Journal of Comparative Psychology*, 115: 423–31.

Garrity, T. F., Stallones, L., Marx, M. B. & Johnson, T. P. (1989). Pet ownership and attachment as supportive factors in the health of the elderly. *Anthrozoös*, 3: 35–44.

Gray, D. E. (1993). Perceptions of stigma: the parents of autistic children. *Sociology of Health & Illness*, 15: 102–20.

Green, S., Davis, C., Karshmer, E., Marsh, P. & Straight, B. (2005). Living stigma: the impact of labeling, stereotyping, separation, status loss, and discrimination in the lives of individuals with disabilities and their families. *Sociological Inquiry*, 75: 197–215.

Guest, C. M., Collis, G. M. & McNicholas, J. (2006). Hearing dogs: a longitudinal study of social and psychological effects on deaf and hard-of-hearing recipients. *Journal of Deaf Studies and Deaf Education*, 11: 252–61.

Ham, S. A. & Epping, J. (2006). Dog walking and physical activity in the United States. *Preventing Chronic Disease*, 3, 1–6. [Online]. Available: www.cdc.gov/pcd/issues/2006/apr/05_0106.htm

Hart, B. L. & Hart, L. A. (1988). *The Perfect Puppy: How to Choose your Dog by Its Behavior*. New York: W. H. Freeman.

Hart, L. A. (1999). Psychosocial benefits of animal companionship. In *Handbook on Animal-Assisted Therapy*, ed. A. H. Fine. Amsterdam: Elsevier, pp. 59–78.

Hart, L. A. (2010). Positive effects of animals for psychosocially vulnerable people: a turning point for delivery. In *Handbook on Animal-Assisted Therapy*, 3rd edition, ed. A. H. Fine. Amsterdam: Elsevier, pp. 59–84.

Hart, L. A., Hart, B. L. & Bergin, B. (1987). Socializing effects of service dogs for people with disabilities. *Anthrozoös*, 1: 41–4.

Hart, L. A., Zasloff, R. L. & Benfatto, A. M. (1995). The pleasures and problems of hearing dog ownership. *Psychological Reports*, 77: 969–70.

Hart, L. A., Zasloff, R. L. & Benfatto, A. M. (1996). The socializing role of hearing dogs. *Applied Animal Behaviour Science*, 47: 7–15.

Hart, L. A., Zasloff, R. L., Bryson, S. & Christensen, S. L. (2000). The role of police dogs as companions and working partners. *Psychological Reports*, 86: 190–202.

Hearing Dogs for Deaf People (2012). Special hearing dogs are changing deaf children's lives. [Online]. Available: www.hearingdogs.org.uk/news/latest-news/special-hearing-dogs-are-changing-deaf-childrens-lives

Hogarth-Scott, S., Salmon, I. & Lavelle, R. (1983). A dog in residence. *People–Animals–Environment*, 1: 4–6.

Intermountain Therapy Animals (2012). *Bibliography: Selected R.E.A.D.® and reading articles*. [Online]. Available: www.therapyanimals.org/Read_in_the_News_files/R.E.A.D.%20Bibliography%202013.pdf

Kamioka, H., Okada, S., Tsutani, K. *et al*. (2014). Effectiveness of animal-assisted therapy: a systematic review of randomized controlled trials. *Complementary Therapies in Medicine*. http://doi:0.1016/j.ctim.2013.12.016

Katcher, A. H. & Beck, A. M. (1985). Safety and intimacy: physiological and behavioral responses to interaction with companion animals. In *The Human–Pet Relationship*, ed. Institut für Interdisziplinäre Erforschung der Mensch-Tier-Beziehung. Vienna: IEMT, pp. 122–8.

Katcher, A. H., Friedmann, E., Beck, A. M. & Lynch, T. (1983). Looking, talking, and blood pressure: the physiological consequences of interaction with the living environment. In *New Perspectives on Our Lives with Companion Animals*, eds. A. H. Katcher & A. M. Beck. Philadelphia, PA: University of Pennsylvania Press, pp. 351–62.

King, T., Marston, L C. & Bennett, P. C. (2009). Describing the ideal Australian companion dog. *Applied Animal Behaviour Science*, 120: 84–93.

Kobelt, A. J., Hemsworth, P. H., Barnett, J. L. & Coleman, G. J. (2003). A survey of dog ownership in suburban Australia – conditions and behaviour problems. *Applied Animal Behaviour Science*, 82: 137–48.

Kotrschal, K. & Ortbauer, B. (2003). Behavioral effects of the presence of a dog in a classroom. *Anthrozoös*, 16: 147–59.

Kuhl, G. (2008). Human-sled dog relations: what can we learn from the stories and experiences of mushers? Unpublished Master's thesis, Lakehead University, Thunder Bay, Ontario.

Kurdek, L. A. (2008). Pet dogs as attachment figures. *Journal of Social and Personal Relationships*, 25: 247–66.

Kurdek, L. A. (2009a). Pet dogs as attachment figures for adult owners. *Journal of Family Psychology*, 23: 439–46.

Kurdek, L. A. (2009b). Young adults' attachment to pet dogs: findings from open-ended methods. *Anthrozoös*, 22: 359–69.

Lago, D. J., Connell, C. M. & Knight, B. (1985). The effects of animal companionship on older persons living at home. In *The Human–Pet Relationship*, ed. Institut für Interdisziplinäre Erforschung der Mensch-Tier-Beziehung. Vienna: IEMT, pp. 34–46.

Lago, D. J., Knight, B. & Connell, C. (1983). Relationships with companion animals among the rural elderly. In *New Perspectives on Our Lives with Companion Animals*, eds. A. H. Katcher & A. M. Beck. Philadelphia, PA: University of Pennsylvania Press, pp. 329–40.

Lane, D. R., McNicholas, J. & Collis, G. M. (1998). Dogs for the disabled: benefits to recipients and welfare of the dog. *Applied Animal Behaviour Science*, 59: 49–60.

Lapp, C. A. (1991). Nursing students and the elderly: enhancing intergenerational communication through human–animal interaction. *Holistic Nursing Practice*, 5: 72–9.

Levinson, B. M. (1969). *Pet-Oriented Child Psychotherapy*. Springfield, IL: Charles C. Thomas.

Lloyd, J. K. F., La Grow, S., Stafford, K. J. & Budge, R. C. (2008). The guide dog as a mobility aid, Part 1: perceived effectiveness on travel performance. *International Journal of Orientation & Mobility*, 1: 17–33.

Lutwack-Bloom, P., Wijewickrama, R. & Smith, B. (2005). Effects of pets versus people visits with nursing home residents. *Journal of Gerontological Social Work*, 44: 137–59.

Lynch, J. J. & McCarthy, J. F. (1969). Social responding in dogs: heart rate changes to a person. *Psychophysiology*, 5: 389–93.

Macauley, B. L. (2006). Animal-assisted therapy for persons with aphasia: a pilot study. *Journal of Rehabilitation Research and Development*, 43: 357–66.

Mader, B., Hart, L. A. & Bergin, B. (1989). Social acknowledgements for children with disabilities: effects of service dogs. *Child Development*, 60: 1529–34.

Mallon, G. P. (1998). After care, then where? Outcomes of an independent living program. *Child Welfare*, 77: 61–78.

Marcus, D. A., Bernstein, C. D., Constantin, J. M., Kunkel, F. A., Breuer, P. & Hanlon, R. R. (2012). Animal-assisted therapy at an outpatient pain management clinic. *Pain Medicine*, 13: 45–57.

Marino, L. (2012). Construct validity of animal-assisted therapy and activities: How important is the animal in AAT? *Anthrozoös*, 25: S139–151.

McNicholas, J. & Collis, G. M. (2000). Dogs as catalysts for social interactions: robustness of the effect. *British Journal of Psychology*, 91: 61–70.

Melson, G. F. (1988). Availability of an involvement with pets by children: determinants and correlates. *Anthrozoös*, 2: 45–52.

Melson, G. F. (1990). Fostering inter-connectedness with animals and nature: the developmental benefits for children. *People, Animals, Environment*, 8: 15–17.

Melson, G. F. & Fogel, A. (1989). Children's ideas about animal young and their care: a reassessment of gender differences in the development of nurturance. *Anthrozoös*, 2: 265–73.

Messent, P. R. (1983). Social facilitation of contact with other people by pet dogs. In *New Perspectives on Our Lives with Companion Animals*, eds. A. H. Katcher & A. M. Beck. Philadelphia, PA: University of Pennsylvania Press, pp. 37–46.

Miller, S. C., Kennedy, C., DeVoe, D., Hickey, M., Nelson, T. & Kogan, L. (2009). An examination of changes in oxytocin levels in men and women before and after interaction with a bonded dog. *Anthrozoös*, 22: 31–42.

Miller, M. & Lago, D. (1990). Observed pet-owner in-home interactions: species differences and association with the pet relationship scale. *Anthrozoös*, 4: 49–54.

Moss, L. (2012). New Army policy makes it harder for soldiers to obtain service dogs. *Mother Nature Network*, June 6.

Motooka, M., Koike, H., Yokoyama, T. & Kennedy, N. L. (2006). Effect of dog-walking on autonomic nervous activity in senior citizens. *Medical Journal of Australia*, 184: 60–3.

Nagasawa, M., Kikusui, T., Onaka, T. & Ohta, M. (2009). Dog's gaze at its owner increases owner's urinary oxytocin during social interaction. *Hormones and Behavior*, 55: 434–41.

Neer, C. A., Dorn, C. R. & Grayson, I. (1987). Dog interaction with persons receiving institutional geriatric care. *Journal of the American Veterinary Medical Association*, 191: 300–4.

Nielsen, J. A. & Delude, L. A. (1989). Behavior of young children in the presence of different kinds of animals. *Anthrozoös*, 3: 119–29.

O'Connor, M. B., O'Connor, C. & Walsh, C. H. (2008). A dog's detection of low blood sugar: a case report. *Irish Journal of Medical Science*, 177: 155–7.

Odendaal, J. S. J. & Meintjes, R. A. (2003). Neurophysiological correlates of affiliative behavior between humans and dogs. *The Veterinary Journal*, 165: 296–301.

Ortiz, R. & Liporace, J. (2005). "Seizure-alert dogs": observations from an inpatient video/EEG unit. *Epilepsy and Behaviour*, 6: 620–22.

Parenti, L., Foreman, A., Meade, B. J. & Wirth, O. (2013). A revised taxonomy of assistance animals. *Journal of Rehabilitation Research & Development* 50: 745–56.

Paul, E. S. & Serpell, J. A. (1992). Why children keep pets: the influence of child and family characteristics. *Anthrozoös*, 5: 231–44.

Paul, E. S. & Serpell, J. A. (1996). Obtaining a new pet dog: effects on middle childhood children and their families. *Applied Animal Behaviour Science*, 47: 17–29.

Pedersen, I., Martinsen, E. W., Berget, B. & Braastad, B. O. (2012). Farm animal-assisted intervention for people with clinical depression: a randomized controlled trial. *Anthrozoös*, 25: 149–60.

Pet Partners® (2012). *Interactions*, 30. Spring/Summer. [Online]. Available: www.petpartners.org/document.doc?id=1079

Richeson, N. E. (2003). Effects of animal-assisted therapy on agitated behaviors and social interactions of older adults with dementia. *American Journal of Alzheimer's Disease and Other Dementias*, 18: 353–8.

Rintala, D. H., Matamoros, R. & Seitz, L. L. (2008). Effects of assistance dogs on persons with mobility or hearing impairments: a pilot study. *Journal of Rehabilitation Research & Development*, 45: 489–504.

Rooney, N. J., Bradshaw, J. W. S. & Robinson, I. H. (2001). Do dogs respond to play signals given by humans? *Animal Behaviour*, 61: 715–22.

Rosenberg, M. & McCullough, B. C. (1981). Mattering: inferred significance and mental health among adolescents. *Research in Community and Mental Health*,

Vol. 2, ed. R. G. Simmons. Greenwich: JAI Press, pp. 163–82.

Rosenthal, M. (2010). Diabetes alert dogs. *Diabetes Self Management*, 27: 23–6.

Rossignol, A. & Barardi, A. M. (2007). Beneficial effects of guide dogs in the visually-impaired. *The 11th International Conference on Human-Animal Interactions*. IAHAIO, Tokyo, Japan, September, p. 56.

Salmon, P. W. & Salmon, I. M. (1983). Who owns who? Psychological research into the human–pet bond in Australia. In *New Perspectives on Our Lives with Companion Animals*, eds. A. H. Katcher & A. M. Beck. Philadelphia, PA: University of Pennsylvania Press, pp. 244–65.

Schultz, D. J. (1987). Special design considerations for Alzheimer's facilities. *Contemporary Long Term Care*, 10(November): 48–56, 112.

Sellers, D. M. (2006). The evaluation of an animal assisted therapy intervention for elders with dementia in long-term care. *Activities, Adaptation & Aging*, 30: 61–77.

Serpell, J. A. (1983). The personality of the dog and its influence on the pet-owner bond. In *New Perspectives on Our Lives with Companion Animals*, eds. A. H. Katcher & A. M. Beck. Philadelphia, PA: University of Pennsylvania Press, pp. 57–63.

Serpell, J. A. (1986). Social and attitudinal correlates of pet-ownership in middle childhood (Abstract). *Living Together: People, Animals, and the Environment*. Renton, WA: Delta Society, p. 127.

Serpell, J. A. (1990). Evidence for long-term effects of pet ownership on human health. In *Pets, Benefits and Practice*, Waltham Symposium 20, ed. I. H. Burger. London: BVA Publications, pp. 1–7.

Serpell, J. A. (1991). Beneficial effects of pet ownership on some aspects of human health and behaviour. *Journal of the Royal Society of Medicine*, 84: 717–20.

Serpell, J. A. (1996a). *In the Company of Animals*, 2nd edition. Cambridge: Cambridge University Press.

Serpell, J. A. (1996b). Evidence for an association between pet behavior and owner attachment levels. *Applied Animal Behaviour Science*, 47: 49–60.

Serpell, J. A. (2012). Animal-assisted interventions and human health: an historical overview. *European Journal of Companion Animal Practice*, 23: 1–9.

Shannon, M. (2007). The benefits of children reading to dogs in public libraries and after school centers: an exploratory study. MLS thesis, Queens College of the City University of New York. [Online]. Available: http://readtothedogs.org/READthesis.pdf

Siegel, J. M. (1990). Stressful life events and use of physician services among the elderly: the modifying role of pet ownership. *Journal of Personality and Social Psychology*, 58: 1081–6.

Smith, M. J., Esnayra, J. & Love, C. (2003). Use of a psychiatric service dog. *Psychiatric Services*, 54: 110–11.

Sobo, E. J., Eng, B. & Kassity-Krich, N. (2006). Canine visitation (pet) therapy: pilot data on decreases in child pain perception. *Journal of Holistic Nursing*, 24: 51–7.

Stallones, L., Marx, M., Garrity, T. F. & Johnson, T. P. (1988). Attachment to companion animals among older pet owners. *Anthrozoös*, 2: 118–24.

Strimple, E. O. (2003). A history of prison inmate-animal interaction programs. *American Behavioral Scientist*, 47: 70–8.

Strong, V., Brown, S. W. & Walker, R. (1999). Seizure-alert dogs – fact or fiction? *Seizure*, 8: 62–5.

Strong, V., Brown, S., Huyton, M. & Coyle, H. (2002). Effect of trained Seizure Alert Dogs® on frequency of tonic-clonic seizures. *Seizure*, 11: 402–5.

The Examiner (2013). Court battle over $20,000 dog will stay in Beaumont. *The Examiner*. [Online]. Available: http://theexaminer.com/stories/news/court-battle-over-20000-dog-will-stay-beaumont

Therapy Dogs International (2013). About TDI. [Online]. Available: www.tdi-dog.org/About.aspx

Thorpe, R. J., Simonsick, E. M., Brach, J. S., Ayonayon, H., Satterfield, S., Harris, T. B. *et al.* (2006). Dog ownership, walking behavior, and maintained mobility in late life. *Journal of the American Geriatrics Society*, 54: 1419–24.

Triebenbacher, S. L. (1998). Pets as transitional objects: their role in children's emotional development. *Psychological Reports*, 82, 191–200.

Turner, D. C. (1985). The human–cat relationship: methods analysis. In *The Human–Pet Relationship*, ed. Institut für Interdisziplinäre Erforschung der Mensch-Tier-Beziehung. Vienna: IEMT, pp. 147–52.

US Department of Defense (2013). *Army Directive 2013–1, Guidance on the acquisition and use of service dogs by soldiers.* [Online]. Available: www.apd.army.mil/pdffiles/ad2013_01.pdf

US Department of Housing and Urban Development (HUD). Office of Fair Housing and Equal Opportunity (2004). *Joint Statement of the Department of Housing and Urban Development and the Department of Justice. Reasonable accommodations under the Fair Housing Act.* 42 U.S.C. § 3604(f)(3)(B). [Online]. Available: www.hud.gov/offices/fheo/library/huddojstatement.pdf

US Department of Housing and Urban Development (HUD) (2008). *24 CER Part 5. Pet ownership for the elderly and persons with disabilities: Final rule.* [Online]. Available: www.hud.gov/offices/fheo/FINALRULE/Pet_Ownership_Final_Rule.pdf

US Department of Justice (DOJ) (2010). Title II. Nondiscrimination on the basis of disability in state and local government services (as amended by the final rule published on September 15, 2010). [Online]. Available: www.ada.gov/regs2010/titleII_2010/titleII_2010_withbold.htm

US Department of Justice (DOJ) (2011). ADA 2010 revised requirements. Service dogs. [Online]. Available: www.ADA.gov

US Department of Transportation (DOT) (2008). Disability issues: DOT rule (Part 382). [Online]. Available: http://airconsumer.ost.dot.gov/ACAAcomplaint.htm

US Department of Veterans Affairs (VA) (2012). *38 CFR Part 17. Service Dogs.* [Online]. Available: www.gpo.gov/fdsys/pkg/FR-2012-09-05/pdf/2012-21784.pdf

US Department of Veterans Affairs (VA) (2015). New regulation updates VA policy on service dogs at VA facilities. [Online]. Available: www.blogs.va.gov/VAntage/22300/new-regulation-updates-va-policy-on-service-dogs-at-va-facilities/

US Equal Employment Opportunity Commission (USEEOC) (2002). Enforcement guidance: reasonable accommodation and undue hardship under the Americans with Disabilities Act. [Online]. Available: www.eeoc.gov/policy/docs/accommodation.html

US Equal Employment Opportunity Commission (USEEOC) (2008). ADA Amendments Act of 2008. [Online]. Available: www.eeoc.gov/laws/statutes/adaaa.cfm

US Government Printing Office (2010). Regulation on nondiscrimination on the basis of disability by public accommodations and in commercial facilities. Revised Title III rule. 28 C.F.R. § 36

Valentine, D. P., Kiddoo, M. & LaFleur, B. (1993). Psychosocial implications of service dog ownership for people who have mobility or hearing impairments. *Social Work in Health Care*, 19: 109–25.

Viau, R., Arsenault-Lapierre, G., Fecteau, S., Champagne, N., Walker, C. D. & Lupien, S. (2010). Effect of service dogs on salivary cortisol secretion in autistic children. *Psychoneuroendocrinology*, 35: 1187–93.

Vormbrock, J. K. & Grossberg, J. M. (1988). Cardiovascular effects of human–pet dog interactions. *Journal of Behavioral Medicine*, 11: 509–17.

Whitmarsh, L. (2005). The benefits of guide dog ownership. *Visual Impairment Research*, 7: 27–42.

Winkle, M., Crowe, T. K. & Hendrix, I. (2012). Service dogs and people with physical disabilities partnerships: a systematic review. *Occupational Therapy International*, 19: 54–66.

Yamamoto, M., Lopez, M. T. & Hart, L. A. (2015). Registrations of assistance dogs in California for identification tags: 1999–2012. *PLoS ONE*. http://doi10.1371/journal.pone.0132820

Zasloff, R. L. (1996) Measuring attachment to companion animals: a dog is not a cat is not a bird. *Applied Animal Behaviour Science*, 47: 43–8.

Zee, A. (1983). Guide dogs and their owners: assistance and friendship. In *New Perspectives on Our Lives With Companion Animals*, eds. A. H. Katcher & A. M. Beck. Pennsylvania, PA: University of Pennsylvania Press, pp. 473–83.

14 The welfare of dogs in human care

ROBERT HUBRECHT, STEPHEN WICKENS AND JAMES KIRKWOOD

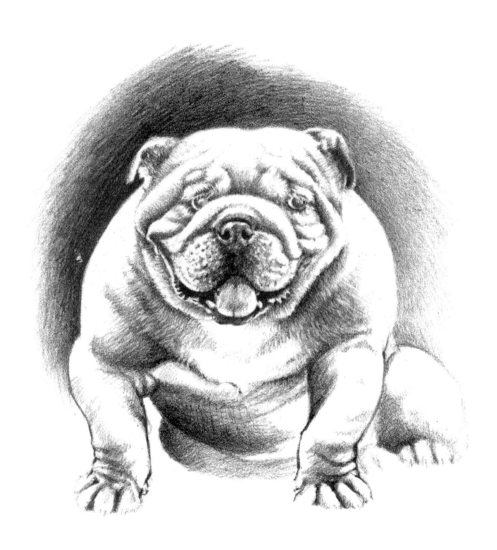

14.1   Introduction

The majority of domestic dogs in Western countries are companion or pet animals. However, dogs are also used as working and laboratory animals, and may live alongside human society in feral or free-roaming populations. In each of these different types of relationship, situations arise in which dog welfare may be compromised. Most people would agree that we have a duty of stewardship to the dogs that we own, and that we have some responsibility for the welfare of dogs that become ownerless, or which have suffered or are likely to suffer harm as a result of human actions. For all these dogs we need to make decisions on their care, housing, methods of transport, medical care, euthanasia, and other issues, and these decisions should be based on the best available evidence.

This chapter provides a brief introduction to the subject of welfare and its assessment. It focuses on some of the welfare issues that affect dogs (genetic welfare problems, issues relating to dogs as companions and their housing and care), discusses their causes, and indicates how some of these problems might be alleviated.

14.2   What do we mean by welfare?

Welfare scientists have not always agreed as to how welfare should be defined (Fraser *et al.*, 1997). Our view is that what matters to the animal, and hence what should matter most to us, is that it is healthy and generally feeling a range of positive and pleasurable feelings rather than negative experiences such as pain, boredom, frustration, and so on (Dawkins, 1980, 2004; Duncan, 1993; Kirkwood, 2006).

14.2.1   How good can it get?

Many of the traditional concerns about animal welfare have been about correcting states of poor welfare resulting, for example, from poor husbandry or cruelty. However, those who care for dogs often want to do more, wishing to provide a "good life" full of positive experiences and good feelings. Some animal welfare scientists and regulatory agencies are beginning to give thought to ideas such as "quality of life" and "a life worth living" (e.g. Farm Animal Welfare Council, 2009; Grandin & Johnson, 2009, p. 5; Taylor & Mills, 2007; Yeates, 2011; Yeates & Main, 2009). These concepts are not, however, simple. It is not clear, for example, whether it is possible or even desirable to live in a state of permanent positive affect, and if not, how long or how positive a state, or what balance of positives and (unavoidable) negatives one should be aiming for. Moreover, if one is thinking of using legal sanctions, what should owners reasonably be required to do to ensure their animal is experiencing these positive states? Finally, an animal's wants, e.g. for food treats may not always be in its best long-term interests.

14.3   Assessing welfare

We do not have access to any but our own minds and have no way to measure objectively the mental experiences that constitute an animal's welfare. We can only assess or judge the intensity of feelings, such as pain and anxiety, indirectly from clinical, pathological and behavioral signs. This is a fundamental difficulty in animal welfare and in animal welfare science, as it is in the case of humans who, because of age, infirmity, injury or disease, are unable to speak or use signs to report how they feel. However, as the brain states that give rise to mental states interact with physiology and behavior, it is possible to use these (preferably in combination) to inform the assessment of animal welfare (see e.g. Fraser, 2008; Hawkins, 2002; Latham, 2010; Rooney et al., 2007).

Whatever measures or techniques are used, their interpretation invariably involves a degree of subjectivity (Mason & Mendl, 1993). The process is therefore a two-stage one: careful review of the observable, measurable physical and behavioral changes, followed by judgement about the feelings they are likely to reflect. The difficulties of the second, subjective stage of the process can be minimised by making the bases of the inferences as explicit as possible (Kirkwood et al., 1994).

14.3.1   Behavioral measures of welfare

Animals use behavior to respond rapidly to changes in their environment, to avoid stressors, and to express preferences. As such, behavior can be a sensitive and non-invasive indicator of welfare.

Performance of natural behavior

The behavior of animals in the wild can provide clues to their needs in captivity (Dawkins, 1980). However, the domestic dog has been subjected to a minimum of 10 000 years of artificial selection (vonHoldt & Driscoll, Chapter 3). As a result, its behavior differs significantly from that of its ancestor, *Canis lupus*, and it is unclear what a natural environment for a dog might be. It is even arguable whether we can treat the domestic dog as a single entity with respect to its welfare. We have selected for a wide range of dog breeds that differ in size, shape and behavior, and which may have different welfare needs. Despite this caveat, all dogs share some characteristics that can inform husbandry decisions, such as sociality, neophilia (Kaulfuß & Mills, 2008), and may range over large areas when free-roaming (Nesbitt, 1975).

Behavior under different husbandry regimens

Observations of behavior under different husbandry regimens can be used to make comparative assessments of welfare, and to assess the quality of various housing and husbandry regimens, including enrichment options. An initial approach may be to study the overall pattern of behavior by drawing up so-called "time, or activity, budgets" that quantify the time animals spend performing various behaviors. Another approach is to record specific behaviors of interest, such as the prevalence of desirable behaviors (e.g. play, social behavior, use of enrichment items, etc.), as well as undesirable behaviors considered to be indicative of poor welfare (Table 14.1). Although laborious, collection of these kinds of data is relatively straightforward. Interpretation of the results is much harder. For example, is increased activity following an attempt to improve husbandry a good or a bad thing? Some types of behavior are generally accepted as cause for concern. Dogs may develop stereotyped/repetitive behavior such as circling, wall-bouncing or repetitive jumping; or self-injurious behavior such as flank-sucking or excessive self-grooming when kept in poor or restrictive housing conditions for long periods. Stereotypies can be signs of a serious welfare insult to the animal and some stereotypies have been linked with deficits in the functioning of the brain's basal ganglia that could affect other aspects of the animal's behavior (Garner & Mason, 2002). However, while stereotypies can be a warning signal that something bad has happened, they are

Table 14.1 Some responses of dogs to acute and chronic stressors.	
Acute (e.g. sudden loud noise)	**Chronic (e.g. austere housing)**
Low posture	Low posture
Body shaking	Increased auto grooming
Crouching	Paw lifting
Oral behaviors (tongue out, licking muzzle, swallowing, etc.)	Vocalising
	Repetitive behavior
Restlessness	Coprophagy
Yawning	Elevated cortisol/creatine ratio
Heart rate changes	Increased catecholamines
Elevated cortisol	Increased acute phase proteins
Peripheral leukocytosis	Decreased immune response (neutrophil/ lymphocyte ratio)
	When stimulated:
	High levels of locomotor activity
	Increased levels of change of active state
	Body shaking
	Yawning
	Ambivalent postures
	Displacement behavior
	Hypervigilance

Sources: Beerda *et al*. (1997, 1998, 1999a, 1999b, 2000); Siracusa *et al*. (2008).

not always good indicators of current welfare status as stereotypies may persist when the animal is placed in better conditions (Mason, 1991).

Experimental behavioral studies

A number of experimental techniques have been used to assess the value that animals place on particular resources such as social contacts, environmental enrichment, and other aspects of their husbandry and care. Choice or preference tests can be used to rank motivation to use or obtain certain resources (e.g. Pullen *et al*., 2010), but such studies only indicate that the animal prefers one resource or environment to another, not how much more the animal wants it. Operant studies, in which the animal has to work to obtain access to a resource, have been used to assess animals' desires for various resources (see e.g. Kirkden & Pajor, 2006 for review) but, to our knowledge, there are no published studies of this sort that address aspects of dog husbandry.

In humans, expectations about the future are biased by affective state; depressed patients being more likely to predict a negative outcome than normal patients. These kinds of "cognitive biases" have been demonstrated in a variety of species including dogs (Mendl *et al*., 2010) and their measurement may represent a useful approach to assessing animals' responses to various husbandry regimes. Increased sensitivity to reward loss (Burman *et al*., 2008) and the development of anhedonia (Willner *et al*., 1987) may also provide insights into animals' affective states, and anticipatory behavior has been suggested as a way of distinguishing between the value of different housing and husbandry systems (van der Harst *et al.*, 2003; van der Harst & Spruijt, 2007), but we are not aware that these methods have been tried with dogs.

14.3.2   Physiological measures of welfare

Animals use a combination of physiological and behavioral coping mechanisms to respond to stressful situations (Moberg & Mench, 2000). For other species, see National Research Council (NRC), 2008; Latham, 2010), there are a number of physiological parameters that have been, or could be, used to assess responses to stressors in dogs. These include body weight and heart rate (Beerda *et al.*, 1998; Newton & Lucas, 1982), cortisol (Beerda *et al.*, 1999a; Hennessy *et al.*, 1997; Hiby *et al.*, 2006; Hubrecht, 1993; Rooney *et al.*, 2007; Tuber *et al.*, 1996), prolactin, adrenalin (epinephrine) and various measures of immune response.

Physiological measures, like behavioral measures, need to be interpreted with care. Responses vary depending on the stressor and whether it is chronic or acute (Table 14.1). Concentrations of cortisol vary with time of day so samples need to be taken at a fixed time. Also, the link with welfare is not always clear (Rooney *et al.*, 2007). Measures of cortisol, for example, do not tell you whether the animal's mental state is positive or negative, as they can rise in response to general activity as well as to long-term unpleasant stressors. Care should also be taken regarding the sampling procedure as the sampling techniques themselves may be stressful. Samples must be taken quickly before hormone levels have a chance to rise either due to the procedure or anticipation of the procedure. On ethical grounds the least invasive techniques for collecting samples should be used; so salivary, urinary or fecal samples may be preferable to using blood.

14.4   Genetic welfare problems

During the process of domestication of the dog from the wolf, humans have gradually taken over from natural selection in deciding which individuals should survive and breed. Depending on what their keepers required of them, dogs were selected variously for strength, size, speed, shepherding ability, and many other physical and behavioral characteristics (Lord *et al.*, Chapter 4). More recently, selection for more apparently whimsical preferences, such as coat length, quality and colour; facial morphology; tail and ear carriage, and many other aspects of appearance has become prevalent. The result is that, in a very short time in evolutionary terms, the wolf's descendants have become hundreds of distinct breeds of dogs.

This transformation of the wolf into the Chihuahua, the Great Dane and everything else in between, was not the result of some overall plan or breeding strategy. It just happened as a result of countless owners around the world pursuing their own breeding interests and preferences. The process has become a little more formalised in some parts of the world in the last two centuries with the development of the idea of breed standards, which often continue to reflect arbitrary preferences (or unconscious biases) about aspects of appearance. In these ways, humans have, wittingly or unwittingly, been opening up new niches for wolves and their descendants to exploit – from hill farms or greyhound race-tracks to urban sitting rooms. Evolution has taken the opportunities presented to it, and yielded a diversity of animals to fill these roles. The outcome of selection on the animals has remained evolutionary fitness, but this "fitness" has come to be largely about how closely animals match arbitrary human preferences.

Only very recently has there been any interest in the welfare consequences of the changes that we have brought about to the biology of the animals. In 2006, the UK Companion Animal Welfare Council (CAWC) stated in its report on Breeding and Welfare in Companion Animals:

In contrast to the considerable attention given to, and concern expressed about, the welfare of farmed animals and about animals used in scientific procedures, society's tolerance of the scale and severity of the welfare risks inherent in selection for arbitrary traits in companion animals seems rather surprising. It appears that the subject has been, to a large extent, overlooked. (CAWC, 2006)

This was not the first time that concerns had been raised – the problem had been commented upon several times in previous decades. However, this time it appeared to "strike a chord" and, following the publication of the CAWC report, and stimulated especially by Jemima Harrison's (2008) powerful BBC television documentary *Pedigree Dogs Exposed*, there has been evidence of greater awareness and growing concern about the subject all around the world.

In the UK, further reviews were undertaken (Associate Parliamentary Group for Animal Welfare (APGAW), 2009; Bateson, 2010), and these also concluded that concerted efforts were necessary to address the problems. In 2010, breed-related health issues among dogs and cats were among the top three concerns voiced by veterinarians and veterinary nurses surveyed by the People's Dispensary for Sick Animals (PDSA and YouGov, 2011).

14.4.1   What are the problems?

Genetic welfare problems tend to arise in one of two ways: first, as consequences of deliberate selection for accentuated anatomical features. For example, the breathing difficulties of pugs and bulldogs are caused by their having been bred for an abnormal, short-muzzled (brachycephalic) head shape (Figure 14.1). In these animals, the shortening of the bone structure of the muzzle is not matched by corresponding reduction in the soft tissues of the mouth, nose and throat, so the airways are narrowed and obstructed (Brown and Gregory, 2005). And second, when a rare, chance, harmful genetic mutation becomes prevalent in a breed because of inbreeding.[1] For example, Dalmatians very commonly have a recessive gene that affects the normal breakdown of body protein resulting in high levels of uric acid in the urine (Bannasch *et al.*, 2008). This tends to crystallise out in the urine causing uric acid calculi (stones) to form in the bladder. These calculi can cause severe and painful disease if they pass into the urethra and block the passage of urine.

While the nature of the problem will dictate the best approaches to tackling it, this distinction between the ways in which genetic welfare problems arise is neither very clear nor necessarily useful. Basically the problem is the same in both cases: selection for, or maintenance of, arbitrary features has resulted in some form of disease that affects the animals' welfare. In both cases, the adverse welfare consequences were unintended and, in both cases, the problems (high uric acid levels and restricted airways) are due to the effects of genes. Hundreds of hereditary conditions that affect health and welfare have been recognized in dogs (Gough and Thomas, 2010; Lindblad-Toh *et al.*, 2005; Universities Federation for Animal Welfare (UFAW), 2011). Some are common (e.g. the various respiratory and ocular problems associated with brachycephalic head shape – see the UFAW Genetic Welfare Problems website[2]) and some are rare.

[1] Inbreeding has been a very common practice in many breeds of domestic dogs resulting in the effective population sizes of some breeds becoming very limited (Calboli *et al.*, 2008).

[2] www.ufaw.org.uk

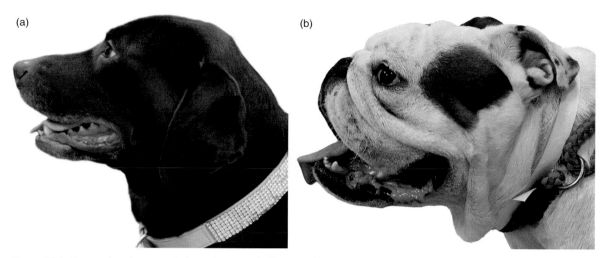

(a)   (b)

Figure 14.1 Comparing the normal shape (mesocephalic) (a) with the brachycephalic dog (b), the brachycephalic skull is severely shortened, particularly the muzzle, the eyes sockets are shallow and the jaw is deformed. (© Rowena Packer, reprinted with permission.) (A black and white version of this figure will appear in some formats. For the color version, please refer to the plate section.)

14.4.2   How do genetic changes affect welfare?

Most genetic changes (mutations) are minor and arise, not because of the complete loss or addition of numerous genes, but through slight changes to one. A change to a gene may result in it producing a (usually, very slightly) different protein. Depending on the role of the protein – what it does and when, from conception to old age, and under what circumstances it is triggered to do it – the change may have no wider effects at all or it may, at the other end of the spectrum, be catastrophic. Some proteins perform relatively minor and limited functions; others play key roles throughout the body and throughout life. For these reasons, it is usually very difficult or impossible to predict what selection for one characteristic – for example, an aspect of behavior or coat colour – may also have on other aspects of the biology of the descendants.

14.4.3   Assessment of the welfare effects of genetic conditions and diseases

Although the welfare effects of some genetic diseases and conditions are relatively mild, it is thought that some conditions, such as syringomyelia, can cause severe and prolonged pain or discomfort (Rusbridge, 2007). How are such welfare effects assessed? Where efforts have been made to assess the welfare effects of genetic conditions and diseases (e.g. UFAW, 2011), these have been based on knowledge of the nature and severity of the pathology caused, the changes in behavior that they cause, and on knowledge or inferences about how such pathology feels in humans.

14.4.4   What can be done to address the problems?

The high prevalence of genetic welfare problems in dogs has arisen as a side-effect of anthropogenic (human) selection. In principle, it should be possible and, in many cases, relatively simple, to tackle these problems and minimise or eliminate them merely by breeding from unaffected animals (i.e. not breeding from affected animals even if the entire breed is affected – except perhaps to outcross with unaffected animals of other breeds as part of a program to eliminate the condition whilst retaining some characteristics of the original breed). Many genetic welfare conditions could be consigned to history in this way in a very short time.

This is likely to happen in cases where, as a result of development of genetic tests, animals that carry mutations resulting in serious diseases can be detected and prevented from breeding. For example, the discovery by Farias *et al.* (2010) of the mutation that underlies the cause of primary lens luxation (displacement of the lens within the eye), seen in various terrier breeds, has led to the development of a genetic test that should enable elimination of this painful condition (Animal Health Trust, 2011).

However, in practice, there can be several difficulties in tackling these genetic diseases and conditions. Care must be taken to ensure that selective breeding to eliminate one disease does not worsen or inadvertently cause another. Such complications are a serious problem in some breeds (e.g. Cavalier King Charles spaniel) in which various genetic disorders are highly prevalent (e.g. Forman *et al.*, 2012).

A more fundamental difficulty is that abnormalities that some people see as diseases that need to be tackled are perceived by others, not as diseases at all, but as desirable features. We might include abnormalities such as brachycephalic head shape, excessive skin folding, and floppy ears in some breeds as examples of such cases. Progress in preventing genetic welfare diseases will depend, to a great extent, on public understanding of the need to tackle the problems. There are indications of the beginnings of a change in attitudes to companion animal breeding, with much greater emphasis being put on health and welfare. This and the development of new genetic tests and efforts to put in place coordinated breeding strategies for health, will, we hope, lead quite rapidly to huge welfare improvements.

14.5   Dogs as companions

Despite a worldwide increase in urban living – a lifestyle often assumed to militate against the keeping of dogs – the popularity and demand for dogs as pets is at an all time high. One estimate placed the worldwide dog population in 2003 at 283 million.[3] Nonetheless, the popularity of dogs as indicated by dog ownership per household, varies quite considerably by nation (Australian Companion Animal Council (ACAC), 2010; Japan Pet Food Associationa (JFPA), 2010; Perrin, 2009; Scarlett, 2008; The European Pet Food Industry Federation (FEDIAF), 2010).

The domestication process has included selection for behavior that makes dogs suitable as companions, including a propensity to bond with humans (Nagasawa *et al.*, 2009). Most dogs kept as companions probably lead relatively contented lives in which they are housed in comfort, adequately fed and exercised, and cared for when sick. Unfortunately, for some dogs problems arise as a result of unsuitable owners and/or inadequate resources. Problems may be precipitated when the dog–human relationship breaks down, resulting in rejection of the dog by the owner/carer, which can in turn lead to neglect, abandonment or relinquishment to a shelter and, in some cases, overt abuse or cruelty.

Relationship breakdowns may occur because the dog fails to adapt adequately to its role, or because the owner/carer makes unrealistic demands on the dog that it is unable to meet. Commonly,

[3] Carodog. *Science Law and Policy, Dog Ownership and Canine Overpopulation.* [Online]. Available: www.carodog.eu [accessed August 28, 2013].

unreasonable demands are founded on anthropomorphic beliefs that dogs experience human emotions and motivations, such as guilt and revenge, despite little evidence that they are capable of such feelings (see Range & Viranyi, Chapter 10). Dog owners, for example, may misinterpret a dog's anxious behavior after house-soiling or damage as a sign of guilt, when in fact the behavior results from the anticipation of punishment or disapproval (Horowitz, 2009; Overall, 1997; Weng et al., 2006).

Even when countries have effective animal protection legislation, poor welfare and cruelty to dogs (and other animals) still occurs. While in some cases there is deliberate cruelty most cases of poor welfare are a result of owner ignorance, inactivity, or a lack of concern that may result from weak or broken owner–dog bonds. Conversely, in exceptional cases, poor welfare results from the owner's pathologically strong attachment to the dogs in their care, as is the case with animal hoarders (Patronek & Nathanson, 2009).

Poor welfare can result from neglect; for example, through a failure to provide adequate shelter; access to a regular supply of clean, fresh water; through poor nutrition; keeping the dog in insanitary conditions, or tied up or confined for extended periods. Neglect may result in poor body and coat condition, pressure sores and urine scalding of the feet, over-long nails, poor oral health and severe infestation with parasites such as fleas, which may be sufficient to cause skin allergies and hair-loss. In addition, undesirable or problematic behaviors may develop such as a loss of house-training, excessive barking, repetitive spinning or circling.

The veterinary surgeon is in the front line to spot and correct neglect and poor welfare when dogs are brought into the clinic. Accordingly, many national veterinary associations now provide their members with guidance about handling these situations (e.g. Arkow et al., 2011). Government departments and NGOs have also provided codes of practice that set out owners' duty of care (e.g. Department of the Environment, Food and Rural Affairs (Defra), 2009) or through provision of general advice on care and management from organizations such as the American Society for the Prevention of Cruelty to Animals (ASPCA), PDSA and The Royal Society for the Prevention of Cruelty to Animals (RSPCA).

14.5.1   Socialization, habituation and training

The dog's early social and physical environment affects its ability to cope with subsequent environments, the bond it forms with humans and so its long-term welfare (Scott & Fuller, 1965; Serpell & Jagoe, 1995; Serpell et al., Chapter 6). The period of 3–14 weeks of age (the socialization period) is particularly important (Scott and Fuller, 1965). During this period, familiarization to animals or humans (socialization), and exposure to environmental stimuli and objects such as loud noises, traffic and household appliances (habituation) reduce the chances of the dog developing fear, aggression, or anxiety-related behavioral problems (see later section).

Dogs reared in conditions of social deprivation are antagonistic when greeted by humans and exhibit agonistic behavior in response to human approach (Feddersen-Petersen, 1994). Similarly, dogs reared in non-domestic maternal environments for longer than the first 12 weeks of life are significantly more likely to show avoidant behavior and aggression towards unfamiliar people than those homed earlier (Appleby et al., 2002). People are far more likely to see behaviors that directly affect humans, such as aggression, as severe and problematic compared to those that primarily affect the dog, such as fearfulness. So, aggressive dogs are more likely to have their freedom of movement and exercise opportunities restricted and are at a higher risk of relinquishment or of euthanasia, while owners of fearful dogs are less likely to seek help (Shore et al., 2008). It is worth noting that dogs with non-social fear and separation anxiety are more likely to develop skin problems, suggesting a compromised immune system, while dogs that show stranger-directed fear have a significantly decreased lifespan (Dreschel, 2010).

The need to adequately socialize and habituate puppies to improve their quality of life and acceptability to owners is now well recognized (Overall, 1997) and regarded as standard practice for commercial breeding establishments (Australian Veterinary Association (AVA), 2012). Many veterinary practices run socialization classes where puppies play with each other in a controlled manner, resulting in sociable dogs with a reduced tendency to develop problematic behaviors (Blackwell et al., 2008; Thompson et al., 2010). However, some authors (Seksel et al., 1999) have questioned whether this extra level of socialization makes a significant beneficial difference to puppies that have already experienced some level of socialization.

It is now generally accepted that responsible dog owners should ensure that their animals are well trained and obedient (AVA, 2012; Defra, 2009). Although training has advantages for the dog that include reducing problem behaviors and improving the bond between the dog and owner (Arhant et al., 2010; Bennett & Rohlf, 2007; Jagoe & Serpell, 1996; Lefebvre et al., 2007), the choice of training method can have an impact on welfare (see Reisner, Chapter 11; Zawistowski & Reid, Chapter 12).

14.5.2 Separation anxiety

In response to separation from humans, which may only be short term, some dogs show a range of separation-related behaviors indicating that they are not coping (Podberscek et al., 1999; Serpell et al., Chapter 6). Bradshaw et al. (2002) concluded that around 50% of dogs, at some stage of their life, show behavior indicating that they find separation from their owner distressing. Dogs that exhibit high levels of separation related behaviors also show "pessimistic" cognitive bias (Mendl et al., 2010), which might suggest that such individuals have a more negative emotional state.

As separation-related behaviors are shown in the absence of the owner or carer, it is difficult to assess the number of dogs that suffer, or the degree of severity. Most owners are only aware of the behaviors because of evidence on their return – commonly inappropriate elimination or destruction of household objects – or because of the reports of people living close by of repetitive and prolonged incidents of barking or howling. The UK's Association of Pet Behaviour Counsellors (APBC) reports that on average between 10–15% of owners who contact them for advice on problem behaviors are seeking guidance on behaviors associated with separation distress, most frequently problems of inappropriate elimination (APBC, 2014). Dogs with separation problems may be more likely to be relinquished to rescue shelters, which may help to account for the predisposition to separation problems in dogs obtained from these establishments (Serguson et al., 2005). Interestingly Diesel et al. (2010a) found that over 40% of the dogs relinquished in their study had spent, on average, four or more hours left alone, and 20% spent six or more hours alone in a day.

It has been hypothesized that dogs with hyper-attachment to their owner are more likely to suffer separation distress (APBC, 2014; Flannigan & Dodman, 2001), but others disagree, arguing that dogs with separation distress differ in the style of attachment (Parthasarathy & Crowell-Davis, 2006). The length of time that they are left also has an impact on their behavior (Rehn & Keeling, 2011). One study of dogs with separation distress (Palestrini et al., 2010) found that behaviors fell into four categories – exploratory behavior (e.g. pacing), object play, destructive behavior (6% of total observed time) and vocalization (23% of total observed time). These behaviors were cyclical and most frequently shown on initial separation, becoming less frequent with time. Panting (14% of observed time) and excessive salivation were also seen. Elimination was only observed infrequently despite this being one of the primary indicators for owners that their dog may have a problem. Events such as delivery of mail or the barking of a dog outside could trigger the cycle of behavior again. Frustration caused by separation from the owner, which leads to arousal and increased fear, seems to be the cause of the behavior rather than boredom (Lund & Jørgensen, 1999).

Separation anxiety is treatable, and systematic desensitization has proved successful. This involves gradually accustoming the dog to being left alone (Blackwell *et al.*, 2006; Butler *et al.*, 2011). However, it is preferable to avoid the problem by ensuring that the dog has experienced socially diverse environments between 6–12 months of age (Bradshaw *et al.*, 2002; Thompson *et al.*, 2010, see also Serpell *et al.*, Chapter 6).

14.5.3 Obesity

Canine obesity is an increasing cause of concern in many countries. It has been suggested that in Europe, for example, around 50% of all dogs are overweight.[4] The main cause of obesity is over-feeding with energy-rich food and treats, although lack of exercise and medical illness contribute to the problem (Anderson, 1973; Bland *et al.*, 2009; Courcier *et al.*, 2010). Some breeds, such as Labrador retrievers, also seem genetically predisposed to obesity. Associated health problems include joint problems, cardiac, circulatory and liver diseases, diabetes, skin complaints and respiratory difficulties. Obesity also decreases life span (German, 2006) and can exacerbate inherent breed health problems.

Better owner education about dietary and exercise needs is the only way to address this concern (Bland *et al.*, 2010; Robertson, 2003), but some owners are reluctant to change their behavior as they enjoy feeding their animal (Carciofi *et al.*, 2005; Kienzle *et al.*, 1998) and may be ambivalent or even positively disposed to them being overweight (Rohlf *et al.*, 2010). Others have cited difficulties in exercising their dog properly, including a lack of access to places where dogs can be exercised "off-leash."

14.5.4 Abandonment/relinquishment

For various reasons, dogs may be abandoned and/or enter a shelter, following which they are either reclaimed, rehomed or euthanized (Table 14.2). Reliable data are hard to obtain but it appears that about 1–4% of the dog population in the countries shown in the table may be at risk of being abandoned and/or of entering a shelter each year. During this process dogs are likely to experience poor welfare whether as a stray, if their accommodation does not meet their needs, or while they adapt to changes in circumstances and the shelter environment (Hennessy *et al.*, 1997; Stephen & Ledger, 2005).

The majority of dogs entering shelters are strays as opposed to having been given up by owners for rehoming (although some strays may have been deliberately abandoned by their owners). The fate of stray dogs is heavily influenced by the culture of the country. In Japan, very few strays are reclaimed or rehomed, the majority being euthanized. This contrasts with the situation in the UK and Australia where reclaiming rates for stray dogs are high (nearly 50% in the UK) and where the reported percentage of euthanized dogs is lower.

---

[4] International Federation for Animal Health – Europe (2011). *Companion Animal Health in Europe: Factsheet*. [Online]. Available: www.carodog.eu/data/pet_health_fact_sheet_january_2011.pdf [accessed August 29, 2013].

Table 14.2 Numbers and fates of dogs entering shelters

Country	Population of companion dogs (Millions)	Number of dogs entering animal shelters per year	Proportion of strays vs. relinquished	Percentage of dogs that are reclaimed/returned to their owners	Rehomed	Euthanized
USA	77.5 (ACAC, 2010)	2 329 978[5]	63% / 27%	25–50%	25–50%	50–56%
UK	9.4 (Asher *et al.*, 2011)	126 176 (stray) Unknown number of dogs relinquished – 17 500 dogs to the RSPCA alone	88% / 12%	48%	Wardens rehome 6% of stray dogs, 25% are passed on to rescue shelters. The RSPCA reports that they rehome 90%+ of the animals they receive.[6]	7.3% of stray dogs (~ 5–6% RSPCA)
Australia	3.4 (ACAC, 2010)	157 094	84% / 15%	35.4%	27.2%	29%
Canada	6 (Perrin, 2009)	57 277		25.50%	42.70%	23%
Japan	11.8 (JFPA, 2010)	173 777	75% / 25%	9%	8%	58%
Spain	4.7 (FEDIAF, 2010)	98 000 (estimated as 2% of national population)				

Sources for columns other than population: USA (The Humane Society of the United States (HSUS), 2009; ASPCA, 2011; National Council on Pet Population Study and Policy (NCPPSP), 2012); UK (RSPCA, 2010; Brickell, 2011); Australia (RSPCA Australia, 2011); Canada (Canadian Federation of Humane Societies, 2011); Japan (ALIVE, 2009); Spain All Life in Viable Environment (Houpt *et al.*, 2007).

[5] The NCPPSP study which reports these data only provided figures from those shelters that responded to its survey, so the figures for number of animals admitted to shelters may be underestimates. The report warns that, "It is not possible to use these statistics to estimate the numbers of animals entering animal shelters in the United States, or the numbers euthanized on an annual basis."

[6] NB The RSPCA study reports figures for the number of all species handled (e.g. dogs, cats, reptiles, small mammals, etc.). Also, the proportion of animals euthanized is reported only for those regarded as healthy. As such, those that are ill or regarded as being unsuitable for rehoming due to problem behaviors such as excessive aggression have been excluded from the data.

Behavioral problems are a significant cause of relinquishment. Approximately 34–40% of dogs relinquished to shelters were reported by their owner as having one or more unwanted or problematic behaviors, of which aggression (to animals or people), hyperactivity, destructive behaviors, and inappropriate elimination in the house are the most consistently cited (Marston *et al.*, 2004; New *et al.*, 2002; Patronek *et al.*, 1996; Salman *et al.*, 2000). The real incidence of behavior problems may be even higher if owners know that dogs are less likely to be rehomed when the owner gives the dog's behavior or health as a reason (DeLeeuw, 2011), and that dogs with behavior problems, particularly aggression, are more likely to be euthanized (55% of the 19 583 dogs euthanized by the Australian RSPCA in 2010–11 were killed because of behavioral problems; RSPCA Australia, 2011).

New owners often report that their dog shows one or more problem behaviors, the most common being fearfulness (Wells & Hepper, 2000b). Fearfulness may indicate that the shelter/rehoming experience has some detrimental impact on welfare, even if this is transient.[7] Other problem behaviors shown in the new home can be more difficult for owners to cope with and problems with aggression, house-soiling and barking are the main reasons given for returning dogs to shelters (Christensen *et al.*, 2007; Diesel *et al.*, 2008; Marston *et al.*, 2004; Wells & Hepper, 2000a). Return rates as high as 18.8% were reported in one study (Patronek *et al.*, 1995).

Reducing the incidence of owner–dog relationship breakdown should reduce the numbers of animals that experience the stresses of abandonment and rehoming. Measures include ensuring that the dog behaves acceptably, through basic training and appropriate socialization and habituation at an early age, and swift resolution of any problematic behaviors (see Askew, 1996; Overall, 1997; Thompson *et al.*, 2010; Zawistowski & Reid, Chapter 12). Some authors have suggested that the largest reduction in risk of future unsuccessful ownership could be achieved by preventing owners with a previous history of unsuccessful dog ownership from acquiring a dog in the future (Weng *et al.*, 2006). Others argue that more attention needs to be devoted to the identification and selective breeding of dogs with behavioral traits that make them good companions (King *et al.*, 2012).

14.5.5 Animal hoarding

Some people develop a pathological hyperattachment to their animals and become animal hoarders (Patronek, 2008). One estimate placed the total number of animals that died as a result of inappropriate husbandry in the USA in 2010 at 23 758, of which the largest category (12%) were due to the actions of animal hoarders (Pet-Abuse.Com, 2011).

Animal hoarding is generally recognized by the following criteria:

- Having more than the typical number of companion animals.
- Failing to provide even minimal standards of nutrition, sanitation, shelter, and veterinary care, with this neglect often resulting in illness and death from starvation, spread of infectious disease, and untreated injury or medical condition.
- Denial of the inability to provide this minimum care and the impact of that failure on the animals, the household, and human occupants of the dwelling (The Hoarding of Animals Research Consortium (HARC), 2011).

---

[7] This is despite the fact that some shelters euthanize fearful dogs rather than trying to rehome them (Marston *et al.*, 2004). Temperament tests used to discriminate between dogs and decide what should happen to them on entry to a shelter – e.g. put up for rehoming or euthanized – are commonly unvalidated or unreliable (see Christensen *et al.*, 2007; Mornement *et al.*, 2010).

The homes of animal hoarders, or the places where they keep the animals, are often squalid and insanitary. Hoarders refuse to acknowledge this and are reluctant to seek or act on offers of help or advice to ensure that their animals are adequately cared for (Patronek, 2008). Hoarders often become isolated which worsens the problems, and unlike others that have been prosecuted for committing deliberate acts of wanton cruelty, are very likely to commit the offence again given the opportunity (Patronek, 2008). The act of animal hoarding has been likened to an obsessive-compulsive disorder similar to those who hoard inanimate objects. However, Mataix-Cols *et al.* (2010) suggest that animal hoarding should be regarded as a new disorder within the spectrum of obsessive-compulsive behaviors.

14.5.6   Non-essential "cosmetic" surgery

A number of non-therapeutic surgical procedures are carried out on dogs, such as marking or to modify dogs towards some arbitrary ideal (see also genetic welfare problems). Young (1976) regarded all such surgical procedures, including castration, spaying, declawing, teeth-cutting and ear implants, as "mutilations" and as morally unacceptable, but a more balanced approach is to consider the justification for each procedure and to weigh up the harms and benefits to the animals involved.

Some consider that there is little justification for mutilations done solely for aesthetic reasons, but arguments for some procedures, such as tail-docking and removal of dewclaws, have been made on welfare as well as aesthetic grounds. Those who support docking, for example, variously argue that, for some breeds, it is established custom, forms part of the breed standard, prevents possible damage to the tail or that, in long-haired dogs, it reduces the accumulation of fecal matter around the tail area. Others have raised significant welfare concerns. Noonan *et al.* (1996) reported that puppies vocalise strongly at the time of the amputation and that the more vocalizations made, the longer the pup took to settle in the recovery period. They concluded that although it was difficult to objectively quantify the stress experienced by puppies, they apparently experienced pain, albeit short-lived. Tail-docking has also been associated with an increased risk of long-term pain from neuromas, although others dispute this (Bennett and Perini, 2003; Defra, 2002). With respect to the welfare benefits, these seem to be limited given the risks of acute and possibly chronic pain. A recent UK study found that docking reduced the risk of injury by 12% and that the number of dogs that would need to have their tail docked to prevent one tail injury was 500 dogs (Diesel *et al.*, 2010b).

In a number of countries – e.g. Sweden, France, the Netherlands, the UK, Belgium, Australia and New Zealand – docking and ear-cropping are now prohibited or restricted, and dogs that have experienced either procedure cannot participate in dog shows. Elsewhere, veterinary and other organizations, such as the American Veterinary Medical Association (AVMA), Canadian Veterinary Medical Association (CVMA) and European convention for the protection of pet animals, have issued position statements against routine cosmetic surgery (AVMA, 2012; CVMA, 2005; Rehn & Keeling, 2011). Removal of dewclaws is, however, less proscribed.

Debarking, or devocalization, is a procedure in which the vocal folds are partially or totally removed under anaesthesia. Dogs that have undergone the procedure can still vocalise but the bark subsequently sounds like a "husky" cough. Potential harms include the risks associated with the surgery itself, possible infection, pain and bleeding and later risk of scar tissue occluding the throat. In addition, the procedure does not address the issue of the dog's motivation to bark, which may be caused by another welfare issue (Lund & Jørgensen, 1999). It has been suggested that debarking is only justified if the procedure is carried out as a last resort, when other approaches such as behavioral modification to reduce excessive barking have failed (Butler *et al.*, 2011; Overall, 1997), and the dog is faced with euthanasia (AVMA, 2012; CVMA, 2012; Houpt *et al.*, 2007).

Some elective procedures such as sterilization are more widely supported. Carried out under anaesthetic, the small amount of suffering inflicted during and after the procedure can be balanced against the reduction in unwanted puppies and some health benefits (Houpt *et al.*, 2007). Sterilized animals are at a reduced risk of some diseases such as testicular tumour, hormone-dependent anal gland neoplasia, avoid pyometra later in life and live significantly longer than intact animals (Dreschel, 2010). Opponents of routine sterilization point to weight increase, possible urinary incontinence and change in temperament. In addition, some contend that sterilization takes away some essential part of what it is to be a dog – a concept called "telos" by Rollin (2007). Early sterilization can be part of a strategy to rid a population of genetic health problems, but could also result in the loss of genes from individuals that are free of genetic health problems. Nonetheless, for the reasons outlined, most veterinary associations now support or positively encourage the routine sterilization of dogs (e.g. AVA, 2012; AVMA, 2012; British Small Animal Veterinary Association (BSAVA), 1999a, 1999b; CVMA, 2005, 2012).

14.6   Housing and husbandry

Examples of dog housing that may be used for some or all of a dogs life include: breeding establishments, rescue shelters, quarantine kennels, boarding kennels, racing kennels, training establishments for assistance dogs, kennels for hunt dogs, kennels for police, security and military working dogs, and breeding and research units for dogs used in biomedical or pet food research. In all these circumstances poor housing and husbandry can result in behavioral abnormalities that increase in prevalence the longer dogs are housed in these conditions (Hubrecht *et al.*, 1992; Mertens & Unshelm, 1996).

There are reasons other than welfare to provide high standards. Many people value dogs highly (Driscoll, 1995), and consequently expect good quality dog housing. For rescue shelters, rehoming is improved if enclosures look good and contain objects that are thought to improve the dogs' welfare (Wells & Hepper, 1992, 2000b). For animals used in research, inadequate environments result in stress, affecting a range of physiological and behavioral measures that may bias or otherwise invalidate experimental outcomes (Garner, 2005; Poole, 1997).

Good general approaches are to provide complexity and choice within the dog's environment, and to build kennelling that is relatively easy and inexpensive to modify in response to changing needs and better understanding of dog biology and requirements. The sections that follow highlight some of the major issues that need to be considered by anyone managing a kennel facility (see also Anon, 2003; Hubrecht & Buckwell, 2004; Joint Working Group on Refinement, 2004; MacArthur-Clark & Pomeroy, 2010; Wells, 2004).

14.6.1   Space allowances

Most codes of practice specify minimum areas and stocking densities. However, there is little agreement between different jurisdictions on these minimum space allowances. The United States Code of Federal Regulations[8] requires that the minimum floor space for dogs should be calculated by

---

[8] Code of Federal Regulations Title 9 – Animals and Animal Products § 2.31 Volume: 1 Date: 2009–01-01. Institutional Animal Care and Use Committee (IACUC). d(1). [Online]. Available: www.gpo.gov/fdsys/pkg/CFR-2009-title9-vol1/xml/CFR-2009-title9-vol1-chapI-subchapA.xml [accessed August 29, 2013].

finding the mathematical square of the sum of the length of the dog in inches (measured from the tip of its nose to the base of its tail) plus 6 inches, divided by 144. The regulations also require an interior enclosure height at least 6 inches higher than the head of the tallest dog in the enclosure when in a normal standing position. These dimensions would seem to be just sufficient to allow a single dog to turn and lie down. In 1996 the National Research Council (NRC) *Guide for the Care and Use of Laboratory Animals* (NRC, 1996) provided weight-dependent minimum floor area space requirements for dogs ranging from 0.74 m^2 for dogs under 15 kg through 1.1 m^2 for dogs up to 30 kg and $\geq$ 2.2 m^2 for over 30 kg. The Guide was revised in 2010 and, although the minimum space allowances were not changed, the new Guide promoted the use of social housing which, if implemented, would at least double the space available to each dog (NRC, 2010).

The 2010 NRC space allowances are similar to those specified in Appendix A of the Council of Europe's 1986 Convention for the Protection of Vertebrate Animals Used For Experimental and other Scientific Purposes (ETS 123), and Annex II of The 1986 European Directive 86/609/EEC. However, the UK has for some time required considerably larger space allowances for dogs used for research (4.5 m^2 for a pair of average-size adult beagles (Home Office, 1989, 1995), and these allowances have also been adopted in New South Wales, Australia (NSW Agriculture Animal Research Panel, 1999). Both the European Convention and the European Directive have now been updated, to provide a minimum of 4.0 m^2 for one or two average-sized beagles with the aim of encouraging social housing.

Recommendations for space allowances in other types of dog accommodation also vary. The UK Chartered Institute of Animal Health (1995) guidance for dog boarding kennels specifies a sleeping area of 1.9 m^2 and an exercise area of 2.46 m^2 for medium-sized dogs (total area 4.67 m^2), although the maximum number of dogs that can be housed in this area is not specified. The UK Government has published a voluntary Code of Practice on the welfare of dogs and cats in quarantine premises[9] that suggests a suitable size for a medium-sized dog is a sleeping area of at least 1.4 m^2 with a run at least 5.5 m^2 (total area 6.9 m^2). On the other hand, the British Veterinary Association (2000) guidance for breeding establishments gives no specific space recommendations, other than a minimum height of 1.8 m (to allow access by kennel staff), instead suggesting that dogs should be provided with an adequate sleeping area, and that adequate exercise areas must be provided for all kennels. In New South Wales, Australia, the code of practice for assistance dogs in correctional centers specifies a minimum floor space of 3.5 m^2, with an exercise yard of at least 8 m^2 per dog (total area 12.5 m^2).[10]

There is a link between space provided and the physical activity possible. It is often suggested that dogs need exercise, but in very small enclosures dogs do not, or cannot run (Hubrecht *et al.*, 1992). The United States Regulations require exercise programs for dogs, but Clark *et al.* (1991) showed little fitness benefit from a treadmill regime. For a dog the value of a walk lies in more than physical activity. Some dogs may enjoy exercise, but most probably derive more from exploring, examining and adding to the various scents on the way.

Variability in regulatory space requirements reflects the fact that there have been few studies on the subject for dogs (see Beerda *et al.* 1999a; Hetts *et al.*, 1992; Hubrecht *et al.*, 1992). Moreover, interpretation of research is difficult as space is often confounded with other factors such as social vs. single housing and stocking density. Realistically, it is unlikely that science will ever provide precise minimum dimensions for animal housing. Much depends on the shape of the space and what is provided within it, and it is always possible to argue that a few centimetres less or more would

---

[9] https://www.gov.uk/pet-travel-quarantine#premises [accessed August 29, 2013].

[10] www.dpi.nsw.gov.au/agriculture/livestock/animal-welfare/general/dogs-horses [accessed August 29, 2013].

not make any difference to the animal. Animals' needs may also vary depending on age, gender or individual differences. Nonetheless, there are grounds for believing that some published minimum space allowances may be too small:

1. All of the minimum space allowances are comparatively small when considering the natural behavior of dogs. Feral dogs have been recorded with home ranges of 3–10 ha to 28.5 km^2 (Nesbitt, 1975; Nakada *et al.*, 1996; Pal *et al.*, 1998). The propensity of carnivores to show stereotyped behavior in zoos is correlated positively with home range size (Clubb & Mason, 2003), and may result from frustration of various motivations involved in the use of natural home ranges (Clubb & Vickery, 2006).
2. The dog is a social animal, and should, therefore, normally be housed socially (see Social needs, Section 14.6.2 below). Minimum space allowances that only provide space sufficient for one dog are, therefore, inappropriate.
3. Small cages or pens may not allow the dog to control its social contacts with other dogs within the enclosure.
4. Small cages or pens do not allow a functional division of space.
5. Small cages or pens do not provide sufficient room for enrichment items.
6. Small cages or pens restrict the dogs' opportunities to express their normal behavioral repertoire.
7. Even in current UK laboratory housing with 4.5 m^2 floor space, some dogs develop behavioral abnormalities (Hubrecht, 1995a). Moreover there are some indications that dogs in very restricted housing show chronic signs of stress.

A sensible approach to space requirements is to ask what functional resources the animals need (social and environmental, see below), and then to decide on the space required to accommodate them, taking into account the animals' activity whilst using them.

14.6.2 Social needs

As discussed earlier, dogs reared with human contact are likely to be motivated to interact with people. Human social contact reduces the cortisol stress response of dogs to stressors (Coppola *et al.*, 2006a; Hennessy *et al.*, 1998; Tuber *et al.*, 1996). It follows that human social contact and dog–human as well as dog–dog socialization time are important considerations in management routines. In the past, socialization time with humans was often very limited in kennels (Hubrecht *et al.*, 1992; Hubrecht, 1995b), but periods of socialization, during which dogs are allowed to run together and to interact with a caregiver, are now an established part of kennel routines in research establishments in the UK. Human contact can, however, be difficult and expensive to provide for any great duration. It is therefore important to consider how social needs can be addressed by housing dogs in groups while bearing in mind that a dog's motivation for human socialization might differ to that for dog socialization.

A social partner within the kennel provides more complexity, interest and variability than any non-animate provision. Nonetheless, the need for social housing is sometimes still questioned and so it is useful to briefly provide some justification. First, although the dog's social behavior differs from that of the grey wolf in several respects (Bradshaw & Rooney, Chapter 8), it remains a highly social animal, and a range of guides and regulations accept that social animals should normally be housed in compatible social groups (e.g. Annex III to European Directive 2010/63/EU; Bradshaw, 2011). Secondly, as previously discussed, many dogs kept as companion animals find it hard to cope with separation, seeming to experience fear, frustration and negative cognitive bias. Thirdly, dogs housed singly in institutions seem to be more prone to develop abnormal behavior (Hetts *et al.*, 1992; Hubrecht *et al.*, 1992).[11]

Social housing is probably now the norm, but for various reasons, for example, for the dogs' safety, or for health or experimental reasons, dogs may be housed singly. However, experience shows that in many cases social housing for at least part of the day is a viable option. Dogs used in toxicology testing used to be housed singly throughout the day on the grounds that it was necessary to prevent the dogs from eating each others food, and to prevent dogs from eating test substances in another's faeces or vomit. However, as a result of the experience of better laboratories, European legislation now specifies 4 hours as the maximum, beyond which authorization should be sought.

There are few data to guide decisions regarding optimum group size in kennels. The natural social group size of feral dogs may be about 3–10 animals (Pal *et al.*, 1998). However, Hubrecht (1993) found that there was little difference in the time spent socializing between dogs housed in pairs, and dogs housed in larger groups, suggesting that pair housing may be an acceptable way of meeting dogs' conspecific social requirements. It is now common practice to allow dogs exercise and social-ization periods with other dogs, and dogs seem to enjoy this, but it is not a compensation for inade-quate housing. For example, Clark *et al.* (1997) found that three 20-minute periods of socialization in a week were not enough to compensate for single housing in cages measuring $1.37 \times 0.82 \times 0.92$ m.

Social housing and aggression

Social housing is usually a viable option, even in shelter environments where there is considerable turnover and the history of the dogs is not always known. Mertens & Unshelm (1996) showed that socially housed dogs settled 91% of their confrontations without aggression, and that social housing increased sociability. Nonetheless, aggression can result in serious injuries or death, so appropriate management strategies are necessary, and staff should understand the causes of aggression.

Like other animals, dogs fight as a result of fear or when competing for limited or especially valuable resources. Aggression is also more likely at times when the dogs' abilities or physiolog-ical status are changing, such as when reaching sexual maturity or prior to oestrus. Suggestions to avoid aggression include: ensuring that dogs are well socialized with other dogs, giving dogs opportunities to get to know each other before housing them together, ensuring that there are suffi-cient high-value resources (e.g. toys, chews, food bowls, etc.) for all the animals in the enclosure, and avoiding providing high-value items when the dogs are already excited (Hubrecht & Buckwell, 2004). Good kennel design should allow dogs to be separated when necessary. Pop-holes between adjacent enclosures allow this, and have the additional benefit that dogs can be allowed access to empty enclosures when the kennels are not full, increasing the size and complexity of the space available to them. Where dogs must be housed singly, then it may be beneficial to allow them visual contact with a conspecific. Single-housed dogs in shelters move to the front of their pens to observe other dogs, when this is possible (Wells & Hepper, 1998), although their motivation for seeking this visual contact is unclear.

14.6.3   Enhancing the enclosure for welfare

The design of dog enclosures varies widely, from racked cages, to pens, to pens with access to indoor or outdoor runs. Generally, larger enclosures give the animals more choice, permit adequate enrich-ment, and allow staff to enter the enclosure to socialize with the animals. It is beneficial to design

[11] In Hubrecht's study, social housing was counfounded with more available space, so both may have been important.

dog enclosures so that staff can easily socialize with the dogs from both within and from outside the enclosure. It is considered better to encourage socialization at the dog's level rather than forcing the dog to jump up, as might happen if the access is over a barrier or low door.

Enclosures should be designed to allow the dog a degree of choice and control. The enclosure should have areas where the dog can retreat to feel safe, and for different functions (e.g. sleeping, activity, elimination, etc.). Visual barriers or structures, or linked pens enable the dog to exert some control over its social interactions, but dogs should also have clear lines of sight out of the pens to provide them with some predictability. If this is not provided, then dogs at the far ends of rooms will often jump repetitively when personnel enter or pass the room, showing their motivation to see out. Vision can be improved by using horizontal rather than vertical bars (taking care to ensure that they cannot be used by the dogs as a ladder), or by using glass between enclosures (Figure 14.2).

Platforms

Platforms within pens are a useful way of providing better sightlines out of the pen and have the added advantage of providing increased complexity and choice within the pen as well as opportunities for play and exercise (Hubrecht, 1993) (Figure 14.3). Dogs make extensive use of them, and they have now been widely adopted by the research industry. In cases where dogs may fail to use them, it may be that the dogs cannot easily access and negotiate the ramp or stairs due to their size, age or health. Although platforms may provide more usable space within a pen, it is our view that the platform area should not be used in calculations of pen area when complying with minimum space allowances.

Outdoor runs

Outdoor runs provide dogs with a more varied environment giving more choice of location, viewpoint, access to odors, etc. On the other hand, increased risk of disease through contact with wildlife, may rule them out in some circumstances. External runs may also be noisier as the dogs respond to events outside the run (Sales *et al.* 1997). Unfortunately, there has been little research on the benefits

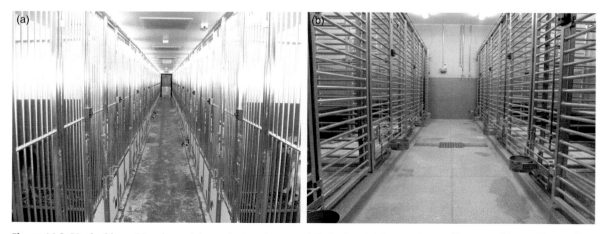

Figure 14.2 Vertical bars (a) reduce vision out of enclosure, while horizontal bars and a smaller room (b) provide much better visibility into and out of the pens. (© Robert Hubrecht.)

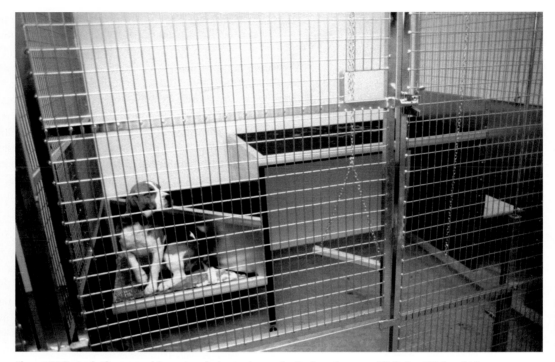

Figure 14.3 A platform provides extra choice and complexity in a dog pen. (© Robert Hubrecht.)

of access to the outdoors. Spangenberg *et al*. (2006) found that dogs increased their activity when provided with an outside run; however, this may have been simply due to the increased space available. If dogs are housed entirely indoors, it seems reasonable to argue that greater attention should be given to providing them with an interesting and stimulating environment.

Toys and chews

Toys and chews provide dogs with something that they can manipulate and interact with. A variety of types are commercially available, some of which can be used in play but may also be used for chewing or destruction. Indeed, destructible toys seem to be preferred to more robust ones (Pullen *et al*. 2010). Flavour and presentation may matter. DeLuca & Kranda (1992) found that beagles, but not hounds, lost interest in ham-flavoured chews after a couple of day. However, another study found that suspended chews, particularly those tasting of food, such as ham-flavoured chews or those made of rawhide, were extensively used by beagles in research establishments, and this continued over periods of months (Hubrecht, 1993, 1995a). Suspension of the chews so that they could be chewed on the ground in a normal fashion but spring off the floor when the dog had finished, proved successful as the chews were used, remained clean, did not block the drains and could not be monopolized by individual dogs.

Studies of dogs in shelters suggest that in this context toys are less useful (Pullen *et al*., 2010; Wells, 2004; Wells & Hepper, 1992), perhaps because shelter dogs differ from dogs used in research (stress levels, breed, age, experience, duration of stay, etc.), or because of methodological differences. In the shelter studies, the toys were necessarily presented to the dogs for a much shorter period than for the dogs used in research so there would have been less time for them to become familiar with the items. There were also differences in toy type and presentation. Pullen *et al.* (2010) found that dogs in shelters and at nutrition research establishments preferred toys placed on the floor rather than those suspended. However, these toys were chosen specifically not to taste of food, were presented for short periods rather than being permanently available, and were suspended at collar height rather than in a more natural chewing position.

Although the terms "toy" and "chew" are often used interchangeably, it is best to look at toys and chews as different categories. Available evidence suggests that toy items are not greatly used by dogs in kennels, but dogs, and particularly young dogs, are motivated to chew objects. Indeed, if dogs are not provided with suitable items they may chew undesirable items of the enclosure or its furniture. Hence, if the goal is to satisfy a dog's motivation to chew, and to occupy its time, then chewable, appropriately suspended items remain a good option that can be used in many circumstances. Care should be taken to choose chews that are as far as possible safe, i.e. non-toxic and not likely to cause choking or obstruction. Chews can be provided for dogs used in toxicology studies as long as a certificate of analysis is available. Other items that can be included in dog housing include water baths, ropes and pulls (Loveridge, 1998), but there is a general need to evaluate and validate many of the enrichment items and devices used with dogs (Hubrecht & Buckwell, 2004; Pullen *et al.*, 2010).

14.6.4   Relating husbandry provisions to the dog's sensory world

Vision
Many commercial dog toys are brightly coloured. The dog generally has good vision (Miller and Murphy, 1995) but like many other mammals it is dichromatic, probably giving it colour vision very similar to that of a human suffering from deuteranopia[12] (Jacobs *et al.*, 1993; Neitz *et al.*, 1989). People with this form of colour blindness have difficulty in distinguishing red, orange, yellow and green, so the use of these colours on dog toys has more to do with human preferences than considerations of their attractiveness to dogs. Television has been suggested as enrichment for some captive animals but, when this was tried in a shelter, television proved to have only marginal value for the dogs, though perhaps worth providing on the grounds that it might encourage rehoming (Graham *et al.*, 2005a).

Olfaction
Dogs are macro-osmatic, capable of detecting substances 1000 to 100 000 000 times lower in concentration than humans can detect (reviewed in Thorne, 1995). We micro-osmatic humans may, therefore, underestimate the importance of olfactory stimuli with respect to dog housing, and we do not know how odors of disinfectants, air fresheners, scents and perfumes could affect dogs. Odors are used in social communication by dogs both between dogs and when they interact with humans (Bradshaw & Nott, 1995; Bradshaw & Rooney, Chapter 8; Filiatre *et al.*, 1991; Millot, 1994; Millot *et al.*, 1987; Sommerville & Broom, 1998). Odors may be detected directly from the other animal, or from marks or other traces in the environment. There is some evidence that housing dogs in groups as small as two increases the attention that dogs pay to odors left on the substrate (Hubrecht *et al.*, 1992), and this may help keep the dogs occupied. Therefore, while hygiene is important, unnecessary removal of scent marks should be avoided.

[12] A colour vision deficiency for which one cause is lack of, or poorly functioning, green retinal photoreceptors.

There has been very limited work on olfaction as enrichment. Graham *et al.* (2005b) found that lavender and chamomile odors decreased barking and increased resting behavior, whilst rosemary and peppermint heightened activity. Other more pungent smells might well be of more interest to dogs, but probably for aesthetic reasons there has been no research on these. Dog appeasing pheromone (DAP) is a synthetic odor, based on fatty acids produced by sebaceous glands in the intermammary sulci of post-partum female dogs. Mills *et al.* (2006) have shown that DAP reduces fear in dogs at veterinary surgeries, and Levine *et al.* (2007) found that DAP, used in conjunction with a desensitization CD, reduced fear responses to fireworks. These results suggest that DAP might also be useful in other areas of dog husbandry.

Hearing and noise

Dogs have much more acute hearing than humans and can hear sounds up to four times quieter than humans can detect (Fay, 1988) and of much higher frequency (up to 50 kHz.) They are most sensitive to noise between 1 and 20 kHz and the maximum energy of a dog's bark is within this region (between 500 Hz and 16 kHz). Dog kennels can be extremely noisy places, and as noise is a stressor for humans and other species, it is a potential problem for dog and human hearing and stress levels within kennels (Coppola *et al.*, 2006b; Hubrecht *et al.*, 1997; Sales *et al.*, 1997). The dogs themselves produce much of the noise, but metal cages, latches, and tools such as pressure washers can also be significant sources. Dog kennels are often built using durable materials that are also very efficient sound reflectors. This results in slow decay of sound, so increasing exposure.

Noise levels in kennels can be reduced by appropriate design and management techniques (see Hubrecht & Buckwell, 2004). Sound absorbing materials are important, as is limiting the numbers of dogs in any particular room within a building. Eight pairs of dogs to a room may be about the right number to keep noise levels low and limit the spread of barking. Consideration should also be given to avoiding activities that stimulate barking (leading a dog past other pens often leads to noise). Music is often played within kennels, as much for the staff's as for the animals' benefit, although it is often reported that background noise helps to prevent animals being startled by sudden sounds. There has been little research on music or other sound as enrichment for dogs; Wells *et al.* (2002) found that classical music appeared to relax dogs in shelters.

14.7   Transport

Knowledge of the hazards of transport is important. Welfare organizations mount periodic campaigns warning of the risks of leaving dogs in cars in the sun, and draw attention to the importance of belts for dogs in cars. When dogs are shipped or transported commercially there is a potential for undetected welfare problems. The International Air Transport Association (IATA) provides regularly updated regulations pertaining to the transport of live animals by air and further guidance relating to all forms of transport are provided in Swallow *et al.* (2005) and White *et al.* (2010). The guidance in these latter publications is specifically for the transport of laboratory animals but many of the general principles apply to the transport of dogs for other purposes.

The increased transport of companion dogs subjects them to greater risks of infectious diseases (e.g. heart worm and rabies). Controls may include vaccination or quarantine, of which the latter may have welfare consequences due to separation from the owner and prolonged housing in kennels (see Housing section).

14.8   Conclusion

Since the publication of the first edition of this book there has been considerable growth in scientific interest in animal welfare, and some of this has benefited the dog. Nonetheless, despite the dog's special status, and remarkable new research on its cognitive abilities (Range and Viranyi, Chapter 8), and genetics (van den Berg, Chapter 5), the dog is still under-represented in welfare research when compared with farm animals and other species such as rodents used in research. As we have seen, there are major welfare issues that affect many dogs (see also Buckland *et al.*, 2014) and there is a need for further study of these problems and how they can be addressed.

References

ALIVE (2009). *Companion Animals ALIVE Research: Dogs and Cats Destroyed in Japan in 2007*. [Online]. Available: www.alive-net.net/english/en-companion/dog&cat2009-1 .html [accessed December 11, 2011].

American Society for the Prevention of Cruelty to Animals (ASPCA) (2011). Pet statistics. [Online]. Available: www.aspca.org/about-us/faq/pet-statistics.aspx [accessed October 2011].

American Veterinary Medical Association (AVMA) (2012). Animal welfare policy statements. [Online]. Available: www.avma.org/issues/animal_welfare/policies.asp [accessed January 30, 2012].

Anderson, R. S. (1973). Obesity in the dog and cat. *Veterinary Annual*, 14: 182–6.

Animal Health Trust (2011). Canine genetics success stories. [Online]. Available: www.aht.org.uk/cms-display/genetics_ success.html [accessed August 29, 2013].

Anon (2003). *Working Party for The Preparation of The Fourth Multilateral Consultation of Parties to The European Convention for The Protection of Vertebrate Animals Used for Experimental and Other Scientific Purposes (ETS 123). Species specific provisions for dogs: Background information for the proposals presented by the Group of Experts on dogs and cats. PART B*. [Online]. Available: www.felasa.eu/about-us/library/ [accessed August 29, 2013].

Appleby, D. L., Bradshaw, J. W. S. & Casey, R. A. (2002). Relationship between aggressive and avoidance behaviour by dogs and their experience in the first six months of life. *Veterinary Record*, 150: 434–8.

Arhant, C., Bubna-Littitz, H., Bartels, A., Futschik, A. & Troxler, J. (2010). Behaviour of smaller and larger dogs: effects of training methods, inconsistency of owner behaviour and level of engagement in activities with the dog. *Applied Animal Behaviour Science*, 123: 131–42.

Arkow, P., Boyden, P. & Patterson-Kane, E. (2011). *Practical Guidance for the Effective Response by Veterinarians to Suspected Animal Cruelty, Abuse and Neglect*. American Veterinary Medical Association. Available: www .avma.org

Asher, L., Buckland, E. L., Phylactopoulos, I. C., Whiting, M., Abeyesinghe, S. & Wathes, C. (2011). Estimation of the number and demographics of companion dogs in the UK. *BMC Veterinary Research*, 7: 1–12.

Askew, H. R. (1996). General treatment principles. In *Treatment of Behaviour Problems In Dogs And Cats: A Guide for the Small Animal Veterinarian*, H. R. Askew (ed.): Blackwell Science, pp. 77–96.

Association of Pet Behaviour Counsellors (APBC) (2014). *Data from the APBC Annual Review of Cases, 1994–2005*. I. MacKeller. [Online]. Available: www.apbc.org .uk/apbc/data [accessed February 21, 2014].

Associate Parliamentary Group for Animal Welfare (APGAW) (2009). *Pedigree Dog Report*. Associate Parliamentary Group for Animal Welfare. [Online]. Available: www.apgaw.org [accessed August 29, 2013].

Australian Companion Animal Council (ACAC) (2010). *Contribution of the Pet Care Industry to the Australian Economy*, 7th edition. [Online]. Available: www.acac .org.au/pdf/ACAC Report 0810_sm.pdf [accessed August 29, 2013].

Australian Veterinary Association (AVA) (2012). Policies and position statements. [Online]. Available: www .ava.com.au/about-us/policy-and-positions-1 [accessed March 21, 2013].

Bannasch, D., Safra, N., Young, A., Karmi, N., Schaible, R. S. & Ling, G. V. (2008). Mutations in the SLC2A9 gene cause hyperuricosuria and hyperuricemia in the dog. *PLoS Genetics*, 4: e1000246.

Bateson, P. (2010). Independent inquiry into dog breeding. [Online]. Available: www.dogbreedinginquiry.com [accessed April 22, 2010].

Beerda, B., Schilder, M. B. H., Bernadina, W., Van Hooff, J. A. N., De Vries, H. W. & Mol, J. A. (1999a). Chronic stress in dogs subjected to social and spatial restriction. II. Hormonal and immunological responses. *Physiology & Behavior*, 66: 243–54.

Beerda, B., Schilder, M. B. H. & van Hooff, J. (1997). Manifestations of chronic and acute stress in dogs. *Applied Animal Behaviour Science*, 52: 307–19.

Beerda, B., Schilder, M. B. H., van Hooff, J. A. R. A. M., de Vries, H. W. & Mol, J. A. (1998). Behavioural, saliva cortisol and heart rate responses to different types of stimuli in dogs. *Applied Animal Behaviour Science*, 58: 365–81.

Beerda, B., Schilder, M. B. H., Van Hooff, J. A. R. A. M., De Vries, H. W. & Mol, J. A. (1999b). Chronic stress in dogs subjected to social and spatial restriction. I. Behavioral responses. *Physiology & Behavior*, 66: 233–42.

Beerda, B., Schilder, M. B. H., van Hooff, J., De Vries, H. W. & Mol, J. A. (2000). Behavioural and hormonal indicators of enduring environmental stress in dogs. *Animal Welfare*, 9: 49–62.

Bennett, P. C. & Perini, E. (2003). Tail docking in dogs: a review of the issues. *Australian Veterinary Journal*, 81: 208–18.

Bennett, P. C. & Rohlf, V. I. (2007). Owner-companion dog interactions: relationships between demographic variables, potentially problematic behaviours, training engagement and shared activities. *Applied Animal Behaviour Science*, 102: 65–84.

Blackwell, E., Casey, R. A. & Bradshaw, J. W. S. (2006). Controlled trial of behavioural therapy for separation-related disorders in dogs. *Veterinary Record*, 158: 551–4.

Blackwell, E. J., Twells, C., Seawright, A. & Casey, R. A. (2008). The relationship between training methods and the occurrence of behavior problems, as reported by owners, in a population of domestic dogs. *Journal of Veterinary Behavior*, 3: 207–17.

Bland, I. M., Guthrie-Jones, A., Taylor, R. D. & Hill, J. (2009). Dog obesity: Owner attitudes and behaviour. *Preventive Veterinary Medicine*, 92: 333–40.

Bland, I. M., Guthrie-Jones, A., Taylor, R. D. & Hill, J. (2010). Dog obesity: veterinary practices' and owners' opinions on cause and management. *Preventive Veterinary Medicine*, 94: 310–15.

Bradshaw, J. (2011). *In Defence of Dogs*. London, Allen Lane.

Bradshaw, J. W. S., McPherson, J. A., Casey, R. A. & Larter, I. S. (2002). Aetiology of separation-related behaviour in domestic dogs. *Veterinary Record*, 151: 43–6.

Bradshaw, J. W. S. & Nott, H. M. R. (1995). Social and communication behaviour of companion dogs. In *The Domestic Dog: Its Evolution, Behaviour, and Interactions with People*, ed. J. Serpell. Cambridge: Cambridge University Press, pp. 116–30.

Brickell, E. (2011). *Stray Dog Survey 2011*. Dogs Trust; GfK NOP Social Research: 58.

British Small Animal Veterinary Association (BSAVA) (1999a). *Policy Statement No. 24 (Spaying of bitches)*. [Online]. Available: www.bsava.com/Advice/PolicyStatements/SpayingofBitches/tabid/159/Default.aspx [accessed January 30, 2012].

British Small Animal Veterinary Association (BSAVA) (1999b). *Policy Statement No. 25 (Castration of dogs)*. [Online]. Available: www.bsava.com/Advice/PolicyStatements/CastrationofDogs/tabid/160/Default.aspx [accessed January 30, 2012].

British Veterinary Association (2000). *Breeding of Dogs Acts 1973 and 1991. Breeding and Sale of Dogs (Welfare Act 1999). Guidance for local authorities and their authorised officers and veterinary inspectors*. London: BVA Publications.

Brown, D. & Gregory, S. (2005). Brachycephalic Airway Disease. In *BSAVA Manual of Canine and Feline Head, Neck and Thoracic Surgery*, eds. D. Brockman & D. Holt. Cheltenham: British Small Animal Veterinary Association, p. 84.

Buckland, E. L., Corr, S. A., Abeyesinghe, S. M. & Wathes, C. M. (2014). Prioritisation of companion dog welfare issues using expert consensus. *Animal Welfare*, 23: 39–46.

Burman, O. H. P., Parker, R. M. A., Paul, E. S. & Mendl, M. (2008). Sensitivity to reward loss as an indicator of animal emotion and welfare. *Biology Letters*, 4: 330–3.

Butler, R., Sargisson, R. J. & Elliffe, D. (2011). The efficacy of systematic desensitization for treating the separation-related problem behaviour of domestic dogs. *Applied Animal Behaviour Science*, 129: 136–45.

Calboli, F. C. F., Sampson, J., Fretwell, N. & Balding, D. J. (2008). Population structure and inbreeding from pedigree analysis of purebred dogs. *Genetics*, 179: 593–601.

Canadian Federation of Humane Societies (2011). Comparison of shelter statistics, 1993–2008. [Online]. Available: http://cfhs.ca/files/cfhs_comparison_of_animal_shelter_statistics_1993_2008_1.pdf [accessed August 29, 2013].

Canadian Veterinary Medical Association (CVMA) (2005). Dog and cat spay/castration. [Online]. Available: http://canadianveterinarians.net [accessed January 30, 2012].

Canadian Veterinary Medical Association (CVMA) (2012). Animal welfare position statements. [Online]. Available: http://canadianveterinarians.net [accessed January 30, 2012].

Carciofi, A. C., Gonçalves, K. N. V., Vasconcellos, R. S., Bazolli, R. S., Brunetto, M. A. & Prada, F. (2005). A weight loss protocol and owners participation in the treatment of canine obesity. *Ciência Rural*, 135: 1331–8.

Chartered Institute of Animal Health (1995). *Model Licence Conditions and Guidance for Dog Boarding Establishments*. London: Chameleon Press Ltd.

Christensen, E. L., Scarlett, J., Campagna, M. & Houpt, K. A. (2007). Aggressive behavior in adopted dogs that passed a temperament test. *Applied Animal Behaviour Science*, 106: 85–95.

Clark, J. D., Calpin, J. P. & Armstrong, R. B. (1991). Influence of type of enclosure on exercise fitness of dogs. *American Journal of Veterinary Research*, 49: 1298–301.

Clark, J. D., Rager, D. R., Crowell-Davis, S. & Evans, D. L. (1997). Housing and exercise of dogs: effects on behavior, immune function, and cortisol concentration. *Comparative Medicine*, 47: 500–10.

Clubb, R. & Mason, G. (2003). Animal welfare: captivity effects on wide-ranging carnivores. *Nature*, 425: 473–4.

Clubb, R. & Vickery, S. (2006). Locomotory stereotypies in carnivores: does pacing stem from hunting, ranging or frustrated escape? In *Stereotypic Animal Behaviour: Fundamentals and Applications to Welfare*, eds. G. Mason and J. Rushen. Wallingford: CABI, pp. 58–85.

Companion Animal Welfare Council (CAWC) (2006). *Breeding and Welfare in Companion Animals: Welfare Aspects of Modifications, through Selective Breeding or Biotechnological Methods, to the Form, Function, or Behaviour of Companion Animals*. London: Companion Animal Welfare Council.

Coppola, C. L., Enns, R. M. & Grandin, T. (2006b). Noise in the animal shelter environment: building design and the effects of daily noise exposure. *Journal of Applied Animal Welfare Science*, 9: 1–7.

Coppola, C. L., Grandin, T. & Enns, R. M. (2006a). Human interaction and cortisol: can human contact reduce stress for shelter dogs? *Physiology & Behavior*, 87: 537–41.

Courcier, E. A., Thomson, R. M., Mellor, D. J. & Yam, P. S. (2010). An epidemiological study of environmental factors associated with canine obesity. *Journal of Small Animal Practice*, 51: 362–7.

Dawkins, M. S. (1980). *Animal Suffering: The Science of Animal Welfare*. London: Chapman and Hall.

Dawkins, M. S. (2004). Using behaviour to assess animal welfare. *Animal Welfare*, 13 (Supplement 1): 3–7.

Defra (2002). *Information On Dog Tail Docking Provided For The Animal Welfare Division: A Review of the Scientific Aspects and Veterinary Opinions Relating to Tail Docking in Dogs*. [Online]. Available: www.cdb.org/defra/awbillconsulttaildocking.pdf [accessed February 6, 2011].

Defra (2009). *Code of Practice for the Welfare of Dogs*. [Online]. Available: www.defra.gov.uk/publications/files/pb13333-cop-dogs-091204.pdf [accessed February 6, 2011].

DeLeeuw, J. L. (2011). Animal shelter dogs: factors predicting adoption versus euthanasia. Unpublished Ph.D., Wichita State University.

DeLuca, A. M. & Kranda, K. C. (1992). Environmental enrichment in a large animal facility. *Lab Animal (USA)*, 21: 38–44.

Diesel, G., Brodbelt, D. & Pfeiffer, D. U. (2010a). Characteristics of relinquished dogs and their owners at 14 rehoming centers in the United Kingdom. *Journal of Applied Animal Welfare Science*, 13: 15–30.

Diesel, G., Pfeiffer, D. U. & Brodbelt, D. (2008). Factors affecting the success of rehoming dogs in the UK during 2005. *Preventive Veterinary Medicine*, 84: 228–41.

Diesel, G., Pfeiffer, D., Crispin, S. & Brodbelt, D. (2010b). Risk factors for tail injuries in dogs in Great Britain. *Veterinary Record*, 166: 812–17.

Dreschel, N. A. (2010). The effects of fear and anxiety on health and lifespan in pet dogs. *Applied Animal Behaviour Science*, 125: 157–62.

Driscoll, J. W. (1995). Attitudes toward animals: species ratings. *Society and Animals*, 3(2), 139–50.

Duncan, I. J. H. (1993). Welfare is to do with what animals feel. *Journal of Agricultural and Environmental Ethics*, 6 (Supplement 2): 8–14.

Farias, F. H. G., Johnson, G. S., Taylor, J. F., Giuliano, E., Katz, M. L., Sanders, D. N. *et al.* (2010). An ADAMTS17 splice donor site mutation in dogs with primary lens luxation. *Investigative Ophthalmology & Visual Science*, 51: 4716–4721.

Farm Animal Welfare Council (2009) *Farm Animal Welfare in Great Britain: Past, Present and Future*. London: Farm Animal Welfare Council. [Online]. Available: www.gov.uk/government/publications/fawc-report-on-farm-animal-welfare-in-great-britain-past-present-and-future

Fay, R. (1988). *Hearing in Vertebrates: A Psychophysics Data Book*. Illinois: Hill-Fay Associates.

Feddersen-Petersen, D. (1994). Some interactive aspects between dogs and their owners: are there reciprocal influences between both inter- and intraspecific communication? *Applied Animal Behaviour Science*, 40: 78.

FEDIAF (2010). *FEDIAF Facts & Figures 2010*. European Pet Food Industry Federation. Available: www.fediaf.org/facts-figures/ [accessed January 30, 2012].

Filiatre, J. C., Millot, J. L. & Eckerlin, A. (1991). Behavioural variability of olfactory exploration of the pet dog in relation to human adults. *Applied Animal Behaviour Science*, 30: 341–50.

Flannigan, G. & Dodman, N. H. (2001). Risk factors and behaviors associated with separation anxiety in dogs. *Journal of the American Veterinary Medical Association*, 219: 460–6.

Forman, O. P., Penderis, J., Hartley, C., Hayward, L. J., Ricketts, S. L. & Mellersh, C. S. (2012). Parallel mapping and simultaneous sequencing reveals deletions in BCAN and FAM83H associated with discrete inherited disorders in a domestic dog breed. *PLoS Genetics*, 8: e1002462.

Fraser, D. (2008). *Understanding Animal Welfare: The Science in its Cultural Context*. Oxford: Wiley-Blackwell.

Fraser, D., Weary, D. M., Pajor, E. A. & Milligan, B. N. (1997). A scientific conception of animal welfare that reflects ethical concerns. *Animal Welfare*, 6: 187–205.

Garner, J. P. (2005). Stereotypies and other abnormal repetitive behaviors: potential impact on validity, reliability, and replicability of scientific outcomes. *ILAR Journal*, 46: 106–17.

Garner, J. P. & Mason, G. J. (2002). Evidence for a relationship between cage stereotypies and behavioural disinhibition in laboratory rodents. *Behavioural Brain Research*, 136: 83–92.

German, A. J. (2006). The growing problem of obesity in dogs and cats. *The Journal of Nutrition*, 136: 1940S–1946S.

Gough, A. & Thomas, A. (2010). *Breed Predispositions to Disease in Dogs and Cats*. Oxford: Wiley-Blackwell.

Graham, L., Wells, D. L. & Hepper, P. G. (2005a). The influence of visual stimulation on the behaviour of dogs housed in a rescue shelter. *Animal Welfare*, 14: 143–8.

Graham, L., Wells, D. L. & Hepper, P. G. (2005b). The influence of olfactory stimulation on the behaviour of dogs housed in a rescue shelter. *Applied Animal Behaviour Science*, 91: 143–53.

Grandin, T. & Johnson, C. (2009). *Making Animals Happy: Creating the Best Life for Animals*. London: Bloomsbury.

HARC (2011). The Hoarding of Animals Research Consortium. [Online]. Available: www.tufts.edu/vet/hoarding/abthoard.htm [accessed November 24, 2011].

Hawkins, P. (2002). Recognizing and assessing pain, suffering and distress in laboratory animals: a survey of current practice in the UK with recommendations. *Laboratory Animals*, 36: 378–95.

Hennessy, M. B., Davis, H. N., Williams, M. T., Mellott, C. & Douglas, C. W. (1997). Plasma cortisol levels of dogs at a county animal shelter. *Physiology & Behavior*, 62: 485–90.

Hennessy, M. B., Williams, M. T., Miller, D. D., Douglas, C. W. & Voith, V. L. (1998). Influence of male and female petters on plasma cortisol and behaviour: can human interaction reduce the stress of dogs in a public animal shelter? *Applied Animal Behaviour Science*, 61: 63–77.

Hetts, S., Derrell Clark, J., Calpin, J. P., Arnold, C. E. & Mateo, J. M. (1992). Influence of housing conditions on beagle behaviour. *Applied Animal Behaviour Science*, 34: 137–55.

Hiby, E. F., Rooney, N. J. & Bradshaw, J. W. S. (2006). Behavioural and physiological responses of dogs entering re-homing kennels. *Physiology & Behavior*, 89(3): 385–391.

Home Office (1989). *Code of Practice for the Housing and Care of Animals used in Scientific Procedures*. London: HMSO.

Home Office (1995). *Code of Practice for the Housing and Care of Animals used in Designated Breeding and Supplying Establishments*. London: HMSO.

Horowitz, A. (2009). Disambiguating the "guilty look": salient prompts to a familiar dog behaviour. *Behavioural Processes*, 81: 447–52.

Houpt, K. A., Goodwin, D., Uchida, Y., Baranyiová, E., Fatjó, J. & Kakuma, Y. (2007). Proceedings of a workshop to identify dog welfare issues in the US, Japan, Czech Republic, Spain and the UK. *Applied Animal Behaviour Science*, 106: 221–33.

HSUS (2009). HSUS pet overpopulation estimates. [Online]. Available: www.humanesociety.org/issues/pet_overpopulation/facts/overpopulation_estimates.html [accessed January 30, 2012].

Hubrecht, R. C. (1993). A comparison of social and environmental enrichment methods for laboratory housed dogs. *Applied Animal Behaviour Science*, 37: 345–61.

Hubrecht, R. C. (1995a). Enrichment in puppyhood and its effects on later behavior of dogs. *Laboratory Animal Science*, 45: 70.

Hubrecht, R. (1995b). *Housing Husbandry and Welfare Provision for Animals used in Toxicology Studies: Results of a UK Questionnaire on Current Practice 1994*. Wheathampstead, Hertfordshire: UFAW.

Hubrecht, R. C. & Buckwell, A. (2004). The welfare of laboratory dogs. In *The Welfare of Laboratory Animals*, ed. E. Kaliste. Dordrecht; London: Kluwer Academic, pp. 245–73.

Hubrecht, R., Sales, G., Peyvandi, A., Milligan, S. & Shield, B. (1997). *Noise in Dog Kennels: Effects of Design and Husbandry*. Animal Alternatives Welfare and Ethics: Developments in Animal and Veterinary Sciences 27. Utrecht: Elsevier Science B.V.

Hubrecht, R. C., Serpell, J. A. & Poole, T. B. (1992). Correlates of pen size and housing conditions on the behaviour of kennelled dogs. *Applied Animal Behaviour Science*, 34: 365–83.

Jacobs, G. H., Deegan, J. F., Crognale, M. A. & Fenwick, J. A. (1993). Photopigments of dogs and foxes and their implications for canid vision. *Visual Neuroscience*, 10: 173–80.

Jagoe, A. & Serpell, J. (1996). Owner characteristics and interactions and the prevalence of canine behaviour problems. *Applied Animal Behaviour Science*, 47: 31–42.

JFPA (2010). Results of the 2010 nationwide survey of dog and cat ownership. [Online]. Available: www.petfood.or.jp/topics/1216.shtml [accessed March 19, 2012].

Joint Working Group on Refinement (2004). Refining dog husbandry and care: Eighth report of the BVAAWF/FRAME/RSPCA/UFAW Joint Working Group on Refinement. *Laboratory Animals*, 38 (Supplement 1): 1–94.

Kaulfuß, P. & Mills, D. S. (2008). Neophilia in domestic dogs (*Canis familiaris*) and its implication for studies of dog cognition. *Animal Cognition*, 11: 553–56.

Kienzle, E., Bergler, R. & Mandernach, A. (1998). A comparison of the feeding behavior and the human–animal relationship in owners of normal and obese dogs. *The Journal of Nutrition*, 128: 2779S–2782S.

King, T., Marston, L. C. & Bennett, P. C. (2012). Breeding dogs for beauty and behaviour: why scientists need to do more to develop valid and reliable behaviour assessments for dogs kept as companions. *Applied Animal Behaviour Science*, 137: 1–12.

Kirkden, R. D. & Pajor, E. A. (2006). Using preference, motivation and aversion tests to ask scientific questions about animals' feelings. *Applied Animal Behaviour Science*, 100: 29–47.

Kirkwood, J., Sainsbury, A. W. & Bennett, P. M. (1994). The welfare of free-living wild animals: methods of assessment. *Animal Welfare*, 3: 257–73.

Kirkwood, J. K. (2006). The distribution of the capacity for sentience in the animal kingdom. In *Animals, Ethics and Trade: The Challenge of Animal Sentience*, eds. J. Turner & J. D'Silva. London: Earthscan, pp. 12–26.

Latham, N. (2010). Brief introduction to welfare assessment: a "toolbox" of techniques. In *The UFAW Handbook on the Care and Management of Laboratory and Other Research Animals*, eds. R. Hubrecht & J. Kirkwood. Oxford: Wiley-Blackwell, pp. 76–91.

Lefebvre, D., Diederich, C., Delcourt, M. & Giffroy, J.-M. (2007). The quality of the relation between handler and military dogs influences efficiency and welfare of dogs. *Applied Animal Behaviour Science*, 104: 49–60.

Levine, E. D., Ramos, D. & Mills, D. S. (2007). A prospective study of two self-help CD based desensitization and counter-conditioning programmes with the use of Dog Appeasing Pheromone for the treatment of firework fears in dogs (*Canis familiaris*). *Applied Animal Behaviour Science*, 105: 311–29.

Lindblad-Toh, K., Wade, C. M., Mikkelsen, T. S., Karlsson, E. K., Jaffe, D. B., Kamal, M. *et al*. (2005). Genome sequence, comparative analysis and haplotype structure of the domestic dog. *Nature*, 438: 803–19.

Loveridge, G. G. (1998). Environmentally enriched dog housing. *Applied Animal Behaviour Science*, 59: 101–13.

Lund, J. D. & Jørgensen, M. C. (1999). Behaviour patterns and time course of activity in dogs with separation problems. *Applied Animal Behaviour Science*, 63: 219–36.

MacArthur Clark, J. & Pomeroy, J. (2010). The laboratory dog. In *The UFAW Handbook on the Care and Management of Laboratory and Other Research Animals*, eds. R. Hubrecht & J. Kirkwood. Oxford: Wiley-Blackwell, pp. 432–52.

Marston, L. C., Bennett, P. C. & Coleman, G. J. (2004). What happens to shelter dogs? An analysis of data for 1 year from three Australian shelters. *Journal of Applied Animal Welfare Science*, 7, 27–47.

Mason, G. J. (1991). Stereotypies: a critical review. *Animal Behaviour*, 41: 1015–1037.

Mason, G. & Mendl, M. (1993). Why is there no simple way of measuring animal welfare? *Animal Welfare*, 2: 301–19.

Mataix-Cols, D., Frost, R. O., Pertusa, A., Clark, L. A., Saxena, S., Leckman, J. F. *et al.* (2010). Hoarding disorder: a new diagnosis for DSM-V? *Depression and Anxiety*, 27: 556–72.

Mendl, M., Brooks, J., Basse, C., Burman, O., Paul, E., Blackwell, E. *et al.* (2010). Dogs showing separation-related behaviour exhibit a "pessimistic" cognitive bias. *Current Biology*, 20: R839–40.

Mertens, P. A. & Unshelm, J. (1996). Effects of group and individual housing on the behavior of kennelled dogs in animal shelters. *Anthrozoos*, 9: 40–51.

Miller, P. E. & Murphy, C. J. (1995). Vision in dogs. *Journal of the American Veterinary Medical Association*, 207: 1623–4.

Millot, J. L. (1994). Olfactory and visual cues in the interaction systems between dogs and children. *Behavioural Processes*, 33: 177–88.

Millot, J. L., Filiatre, J. C., Eckerlin, A., Gagnon, A. C. & Montagner, H. (1987). Olfactory cues in the relations between children and their pet dogs. *Applied Animal Behaviour Science*, 19: 189–95.

Mills, D. S., Ramos, D., Estelles, M. G. & Hargrave, C. (2006). A triple blind placebo-controlled investigation into the assessment of the effect of Dog Appeasing Pheromone (DAP) on anxiety related behaviour of problem dogs in the veterinary clinic. *Applied Animal Behaviour Science*, 98: 114–26.

Moberg, G. P. & Mench, J. A. (2000). *The Biology of Animal Stress: Basic Principles and Implications for Animal Welfare*. Wallingford: CABI Publishing.

Mornement, K. M., Coleman, G. J., Toukhsati, S. & Bennett, P. C. (2010). A review of behavioral assessment protocols used by Australian animal shelters to determine the adoption suitability of dogs. *Journal of Applied Animal Welfare Science* 13: 314–29.

Nagasawa, M., Mogi, K. & Kikusui, T. (2009). Attachment between humans and dogs. *Japanese Psychological Research*, 51: 209–21.

Nakada, A., Tetsuya, F. & Hideo, S. (1996). A case study of home range use and habitat use in 3 free-ranging dogs: effects of past histories. *Journal of Ethology*, 14: 139–43.

NCPPSP (2012). National Council Research. [Online]. Available: www.petpopulation.org/research.html [accessed January 30, 2012].

Neitz, J., Geist, T. & Jacobs, G. H. (1989). Color vision in the dog. *Visual Neuroscience*, 3: 119–25.

Nesbitt, W. H. (1975). Ecology of a feral dog pack on a wildlife refuge. In *The Wild Canids: Their Systematics, Behavioral Ecology, and Evolution*, ed. M. Fox. New York: Van Nostrand Reinhold, pp. 391–5.

New, J. C., Salman, M. D., Scarlett, J. M., Kass, P. H., King, M. & Hutchison, J. M. (2002). Shelter relinquishment: characteristics of shelter-relinquished animals and their owners compared with animals and their owners in U.S. pet owning households. *Journal of Applied Animal Welfare Science*, 3: 179–201.

Newton, J. E. O. & Lucas, L. A. (1982). Differential heart-rate responses to person in nervous and normal pointer dogs. *Behavior Genetics*, 12: 379–93.

Noonan, G. J., Rand, J. S., Blackshaw, J. K. & Priest, J. (1996). Behavioural observations of puppies undergoing tail docking. *Applied Animal Behaviour Science*, 49: 335–42.

NRC (National Research Council) (1996). *Guide for the Care and Use of Laboratory Animals*. Washington, DC: National Academy Press.

NRC (National Research Council) (2008). *Recognition and Alleviation of Distress in Laboratory Animals*. Washington, DC: National Academies Press.

NRC (National Research Council) (2010). *Guide for the Care and Use of Laboratory Animals*. Washington, DC: National Academies Press.

NSW Agriculture Animal Research Panel (1999). *Guidelines for the Care and Housing of Dogs in Scientific Institutions*, Guideline 14, 1 March 1999.

Overall, K. L. (1997). *Clinical Behavioural Medicine for Small Animals*. St. Louis, MO: Mosby.

Pal, S. K., Ghosh, B. & Roy, S. (1998). Agonistic behaviour of free-ranging dogs (*Canis familiaris*) in relation to season, sex and age. *Applied Animal Behaviour Science*, 59: 331–348.

Palestrini, C., Minero, M., Cannas, S., Rossi, E. & Frank, D. (2010). Video analysis of dogs with separation-related behaviors. *Applied Animal Behaviour Science*, 124: 61–7.

Parthasarathy, V. & Crowell-Davis, S. L. (2006). Relationship between attachment to owners and separation anxiety in pet dogs (*Canis lupus familiaris*). *Journal of Veterinary Behavior*, 1: 109–20.

Patronek, G. J. (2008). Animal hoarding. In *The International Handbook of Animal Abuse and Cruelty: Theory, Research and Application*, ed. F. R. Ascione. Purdue University Press, pp. 206–46.

Patronek, G. J., Glickman, L. T., Beck, A. M., McCabe, G. P. & Ecker, C. (1996). Risk factors for relinquishment of dogs to an animal shelter. *Journal of the American Veterinary Medical Association*, 209: 572–81.

Patronek, G. J., Glickman, L. T. & Moyer, M. R. (1995). Population Dynamics and the Risk of Euthanasia for Dogs in an Animal Shelter. *Anthrozoös*, 8: 31–43.

Patronek, G. J. & Nathanson, J. N. (2009). A theoretical perspective to inform assessment and treatment strategies for animal hoarders. *Clinical Psychology Review*, 29: 274–81.

PDSA and YouGov (2011). *The State of Our Pet Nation: Animal Wellbeing Report 2011*. [Online]. Available: www.pdsa.org.uk [accessed January 20, 2012].

Podberscek, A. L., Hsu, Y. & Serpell, J. A. (1999). Evaluation of clomipramine as an adjunct to behavioural therapy in the treatment of separation-related problems in dogs. *Veterinary Record*, 145: 365–9.

Perrin, T. (2009). The business of urban animals survey: the facts and statistics on companion animals in Canada. *Canadian Veterinary Journal*, 50: 48–52.

Pet-Abuse.Com (2011). [Online]. Available: www.pet-abuse.com [accessed November 15, 2011].

Poole, T. (1997). Happy animals make good science. *Laboratory Animals*, 31: 116–24.

Pullen, A. J., Merrill, R. J. N. & Bradshaw, J. W. S. (2010). Preferences for toy types and presentations in kennel housed dogs. *Applied Animal Behaviour Science*, 125: 151–6.

Rehn, T. & Keeling, L. J. (2011). The effect of time left alone at home on dog welfare. *Applied Animal Behaviour Science*, 129: 129–35.

Robertson, I. D. (2003). The association of exercise, diet and other factors with owner-perceived obesity in privately owned dogs from metropolitan Perth, WA. *Preventive Veterinary Medicine*, 58: 75–83.

Rohlf, V. I., Toukhsati, S., Coleman, G. J. & Bennett, P. C. (2010). Dog obesity: can dog caregivers' (owners') feeding and exercise intentions and behaviors be predicted from attitudes? *Journal of Applied Animal Welfare Science*, 13: 213–36.

Rollin, B. E. (2007). Cultural variation, animal welfare and telos. *Animal Welfare*, 16 (Supplement 1): 129–33.

Rooney, N. J., Gaines, S. A. & Bradshaw, J. W. S. (2007). Behavioural and glucocorticoid responses of dogs (*Canis familiaris*) to kennelling: investigating mitigation of stress by prior habituation. *Physiology & Behavior*, 92: 847–54.

RSPCA (2010). *The Welfare State: Five Years Measuring Animal Welfare in the UK, 2005–2009*, RSPCA: 117.

RSPCA Australia (2011). *RSPCA Australia National Statistics 2010–2011*, RSPCA Australia. 2011: 9.

Rusbridge, C. (2007). Chiari-like malformation and Syringomyelia in the Cavalier King Charles spaniel. Unpublished Ph.D. thesis, University of Utrecht.

Sales, G., Hubrecht, R., Peyvandi, A., Milligan, S. & Shield, B. (1997). Noise in dog kennelling: is barking a welfare problem for dogs? *Applied Animal Behaviour Science*, 52: 321–9.

Salman, M. D., Hutchison, J., Ruch-Gallie, R., Kogan, L., New, J. C., Kass, P. H. & Scarlett, J. M. (2000). Behavioral reasons for relinquishment of dogs and cats to 12 shelters. *Journal of Applied Animal Welfare Science*, 3: 93–106.

Scarlett, J. M. (2008). Interface of epidemiology, pet population issues and policy. *Preventive Veterinary Medicine*, 86: 188–97.

Scott, J. P. & Fuller, J. L. (1965). *Genetics and the Social Behavior of the Dog*. Chicago & London: University of Chicago Press.

Seksel, K., Mazurski, E. J. & Taylor, A. (1999). Puppy socialization programs: short and long term behavioural effects. *Applied Animal Behaviour Science*, 62: 335–49.

Serguson, S. A., Serpell, J. A. & Hart, B. A. (2005). Evaluation of a behavioural assessment questionnaire for use in the characterization of behavioural problems of dogs relinquished to animal shelters. *Journal of the American Veterinary Medical Association*, 227: 1755–61.

Serpell, J. & Jagoe, J. A. (1995). Early experience and the development of behaviour. In *The Domestic Dog: Its Evolution, Behaviour and Interactions with People*, ed. J. Serpell. Cambridge: Cambridge University Press, pp. 79–102.

Shore, E. R., Burdsal, C. & Douglas, D. K. (2008). Pet owners' views of pet behavior problems and willingness to consult experts for assistance. *Journal of Applied Animal Welfare Science*, 11: 63–73.

Siracusa, C., Manteca, X., Cerón, J., Martínez-Subiela, S., Cuenca, R., Lavín, S., Garcia, F. et al. (2008). Perioperative stress response in dogs undergoing elective surgery: variations in behavioural, neuroendocrine, immune and acute phase responses. *Animal Welfare*, 17: 259–73.

Sommerville, B. A. and Broom, D. M. (1998). Olfactory awareness. *Applied Animal Behaviour Science*, 57: 269–86.

Spangenberg, E. M. F., Björklund, L. & Dahlborn, K. (2006). Outdoor housing of laboratory dogs: effects on activity, behaviour and physiology. *Applied Animal Behaviour Science*, 98: 260–76.

Stephen, J. M. & Ledger, R. A. (2005). An audit of behavioral indicators of poor welfare in kenneled dogs in the United Kingdom. *Journal of Applied Animal Welfare Science*, 8: 79–95.

Swallow, J., Anderson, D., Buckwell, A. C., Harris, T., Hawkins, P., Kirkwood, J. et al. (2005). Guidance on the transport of laboratory animals. *Laboratory Animals*, 39: 1.

Taylor, K. D. & Mills, D. S. (2007). Is quality of life a useful concept for companion animals? *Animal Welfare*, 16 (Supplement 1): S55–65.

Thompson, K. F., McBride, E. A. & Redhead, E. (2010). Training engagement and the development of behavior problems in the dog: a longitudinal study. *Journal of Veterinary Behavior: Clinical Applications and Research*, 5: 57.

Thorne, C. (1995). Feeding behaviour of domestic dogs and the role of experience. In *The Domestic Dog: Its Evolution, Behaviour and Interactions with People*, ed. J. Serpell. Cambridge: Cambridge University Press, pp. 103–14.

Tuber, D. S., Hennessy, M. B., Sanders, S. & Miller, J. A. (1996). Behavioral and glucocorticoid responses of adult domestic dogs (*Canis familiaris*) to companionship and social separation. *Journal of Comparative Psychology*, 110: 103–8.

UFAW (2011). Genetic welfare problems of companion animals: an information resource for prospective pet owners and breeders. [Online]. Available: www.ufaw.org.uk

van der Harst, J. E., Baars, A. M. & Spruijt, B. M. (2003). Standard housed rats are more sensitive to rewards than enriched housed rats as reflected by their anticipatory behaviour. *Behavioural Brain Research*, 142: 151–6.

van der Harst, J. E. & Spruijt, B. M. (2007). Tools to measure and improve animal welfare: reward-related behaviour. *Animal Welfare*, 16 (Supplement 1): S67–73.

Wells, D. L. (2004). A review of environmental enrichment for kennelled dogs, Canis familiaris. *Applied Animal Behaviour Science*, 85: 307–17.

Wells, D. L., Graham, L. & Hepper, P. G. (2002). The influence of auditory stimulation on the behaviour of dogs housed in a rescue shelter. *Animal Welfare*, 11: 385–93.

Wells, D. & Hepper, P. G. (1992). The behaviour of dogs in a rescue shelter. *Animal Welfare*, 1: 171–86.

Wells, D. L. & Hepper, P. G. (1998). A note on the influence of visual conspecific contact on the behaviour of sheltered dogs. *Applied Animal Behaviour Science*, 60: 83–8.

Wells, D. L. & Hepper, P. G. (2000a). Prevalence of behaviour problems reported by owners of dogs purchased from an animal rescue shelter. *Applied Animal Behaviour Science*, 69: 55–6.

Wells, D. L. & Hepper, P. G. (2000b). The influence of environmental change on the behaviour of sheltered dogs. *Applied Animal Behaviour Science*, 68: 151–62.

Weng, H.-Y., Kass, P. H., Hart, L. A. & Chomel, B. B. (2006). Risk factors for unsuccessful dog ownership: an epidemiologic study in Taiwan. *Preventive Veterinary Medicine*, 77: 82–95.

White, W. J., Chou, S. T., Kole, C. B. & Sutcliffe, R. (2010). Transportation of laboratory animals. In *The UFAW Handbook on the Care and Management of Laboratory and Other Research Animals*, eds. R. Hubrecht and J. Kirkwood. Oxford: Wiley-Blackwell, pp. 169–82.

Willner, P., Towell, A., Sampson, D., Sophokleous, S. & Muscat, R. (1987). Reduction of sucrose preference by chronic unpredictable mild stress, and its restoration by a tricyclic antidepressant. *Psychopharmacology*, 93: 358–64.

Yeates, J. W. (2011). Is "a life worth living" a concept worth having? *Animal Welfare*, 20: 397–406.

Yeates, J. & Main, D. (2009). Assessment of companion animal quality of life in veterinary practice and research. *Journal of Small Animal Practice*, 50: 274–81.

Young, M. (1976). The mutilation of pet animals. In *The Mutilation of Animals: Proceedings of the 2nd Symposium Sponsored by the Farm Livestock Committee RSPCA*, pp. 109–13.

15 From paragon to pariah: Cross-cultural perspectives on attitudes to dogs

JAMES SERPELL

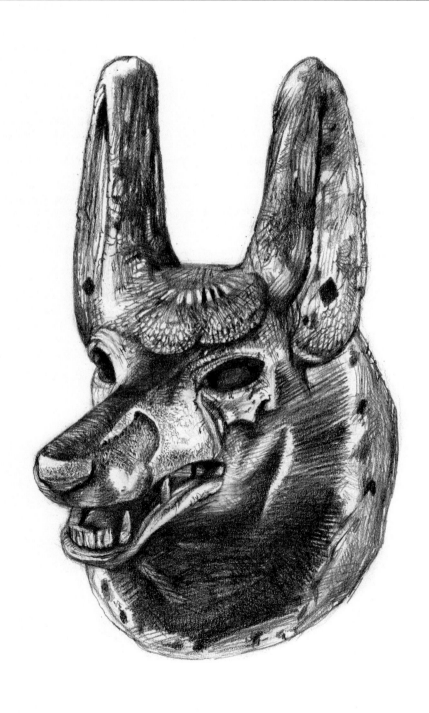

15.1 Introduction

Human attitudes to non-human animals (henceforth "animals") are influenced by a variety of factors. For example, animals that are perceived to be economically or instrumentally beneficial to human interests are generally, though not invariably, viewed more positively than those that are seen to be detrimental. Thus, honey bees that make honey and pollinate crops are regarded more positively than cockroaches, even though bees can sting – sometimes fatally – and cockroaches cannot. Certain animals may also possess inherent characteristics of appearance or behavior that humans find appealing or repellant on a purely emotional level, independent of the animal's instrumental value. Butterflies, for instance, tend to be liked for purely aesthetic reasons, while snakes are commonly loathed, despite the latter playing an important role in the control of agricultural pests. Animals are also "culturally constructed" in the sense that they acquire a wealth of symbolic and metaphorical associations and meanings that are peculiar to particular cultural settings. For example, the "sacred" status of cows in India is a cultural construct derived from Hindu religion that contrasts markedly with attitudes to cattle in, say, Europe or North America (Serpell, 1996, 2004).

Western attitudes to animals are colored by a strong sense of human exceptionalism that has its roots in the traditional Judaeo-Christian worldview. According to this perspective, humans and other animals were produced by separate acts of divine creation; the former to rule over the latter, and the latter to serve the exclusive interests of the former (Midgley, 1983; Serpell, 1996, 2005; Thomas, 1983). Despite such traditions, it is nonetheless clear that the distinction between human and non-human can become blurred under certain circumstances, such as when human victims of political or racial oppression find themselves summarily reclassified as "animals" preparatory to having their legal and moral rights ignored or denied (see e.g. Arluke & Sax, 1992). Occasionally, the barrier can also be penetrated from the opposite direction. Just as people are sometimes classified as animals, so animals – for one reason or another – may be categorized and treated as persons. In the Middle Ages, dangerous animals and vermin were occasionally tried, tortured and executed for committing "crimes," as if they were guilty of malicious intent and, like people, could be held morally accountable for their actions (Dinzelbacher, 2002; Evans, 1906; Girgen, 2003). Conversely, animals may also acquire many of the benefits and privileges normally reserved for human beings, usually by becoming the objects of strong emotional attachments.

In theory, any animal can attain quasi-human status in this way but, in practice, only two domestic species, the dog and cat, appear to have done so with any degree of permanence. And while cats often tend to behave like temporary lodgers, retaining the ability to come and go as they please (Serpell, 2013), dogs are now so thoroughly assimilated into the human domain that it is hard to imagine them flourishing outside of this context. Indeed, as several chapters in this book suggest, the lives of feral or free-roaming dogs are typically short and uncomfortable (see Macdonald & Carr, Chapter 16; Boitani et al., Chapter 17; Hiby & Hiby, Chapter 19). Dogs and cats are also the only domestic animals that do not require physical barriers – walls, cages, fences or tethers – to enforce their association with people. But whereas cats are generally more tied to places than to people, many dogs behave as if permanently attached to their humans by invisible bonds. Given the opportunity, these dogs will accompany their owners everywhere, and exhibit obvious signs of distress when separated involuntarily (Serpell, 1996). Moreover, this form of separation-related anxiety may become so exaggerated that the animal will howl, bark, whine, defecate, urinate, or chew up and destroy household furniture and fittings whenever it is left alone (Appleby & Pluijmakers, 2003; Podberscek et al., 1999).

Although dogs may form these strong attachments for people at any age, the process tends to occur more readily in early development during the so-called "socialization period." At this time, from roughly 3 to 12 weeks of age, puppies establish their primary social relationships (see Scott, 1963; Serpell *et al.*, Chapter 6). The process of primary socialization not only determines who or what the puppy will respond to in a positive social manner, it also effectively defines the species to which it belongs. Cross-fostering experiments have shown that if a puppy is reared exclusively with cats and kittens during this period, it will grow up to regard cats as conspecifics rather than dogs (Fox, 1967). It is also apparent that, if a young dog is exposed to the attentions of two different species within the socialization period, it will readily form attachments to both.

A further important aspect of early socialization is that it appears to occur independent of rewards and punishments. Scott (1963) was able to show that while puppies, like all animals, react positively to rewarding stimuli and negatively to aversive ones, the process of primary socialization will proceed irrespective of the quality of the accompanying stimulus. In other words, if exposed to their company at the appropriate age, a dog will develop a strong affinity for humans, regardless of whether it is rewarded or punished for doing so.

This tendency to voluntarily ally itself with humans – this capacity to form strong interspecific attachments, even in the face of rejection or punishment – places the dog in an unusual position relative to most other animals. With the possible exception of some non-human primates (see Dawkins, 1993; Diamond, 1993), no other species comes as close to us as the dog in affective or symbolic terms, and, by the same token, no other species makes a stronger claim to be treated as human. Yet, far from making the dog the object of universal affection and respect, this unusual "closeness" or affinity seems to provoke a puzzling degree of psychological tension and ambivalence. The purpose of this chapter is to explore the nature and sources of this tension in our relations with the domestic dog across a range of different cultural contexts.

15.2 Dogs as hunting partners

Before joining forces in the late Palaeolithic, both humans and wolves lived in cooperative societies that specialized, at least to some extent, in hunting large game animals. Scott (1968) suggested that, in this respect, wolves and humans were already pre-adapted for life in a combined social group, and Downs (1960) has argued that the original domestication of the wolf may have arisen out of a kind of mutually beneficial hunting symbiosis between the two species. While Downs' theory is no longer widely accepted, it is clear from the archaeological record that the use of dogs for hunting was one of the earliest economic functions for this species (Clutton-Brock, Chapter 2; Hole & Wyllie, 2007).

Given the longevity and mutual compatibility of this partnership, and the fact that humans hunting with dogs tend to have more success than humans hunting alone (Ikeya, 1994; Koster, 2008, 2009; Lee, 1979), it is not surprising to find widespread respect and affection for hunting dogs throughout the world, especially in cultures where hunting forms a primary mode of subsistence.

Among the Onges, a hunter-gatherer group from the Andaman Islands, dogs were first acquired in 1857 and are now frequently employed for hunting wild pig. Since the Onges formerly subsisted mainly on fish and shellfish, the advent of dogs has revolutionized their economy. As a result, according to one authority, the Onges have developed a "somewhat unbalanced affection" for these animals (Cipriani, 1966, pp. 80–1). The same author goes on to state that this "inordinate love of dogs has allowed the animals to become a pest. They already outnumber the human population; families of only three or four people may have ten or twelve dogs," and this despite the fact that the Onges suffer from constant flea infestations, are frequently bitten by their canine friends, and are kept awake at night by their continuous barking and howling. Similar intense affection for hunting dogs has also been reported among the Punan Dyaks of Malaysian Borneo (Harrison, 1965), the Matinen of eastern Indonesia (Broch, 2008), the Vedda people of Sri Lanka (Seligmann & Seligmann, 1911), the Dorobo of Kenya (Huntingford, 1955), the Panaré, an Amerindian group from Venezuela (Dumont, 1976), and the Jívaro and Shipibo from Ecuador and Peru, respectively (Roe, 1993).

Some of the most extreme cases of devotion to hunting dogs come from early accounts of Australian Aborigines. During a visit to Stradbroke Island off the coast of Queensland in 1828, Lockyer remarked that the "attachment of these people to their dogs is worthy of notice." When he attempted to purchase one from its owner in exchange for a small axe, "his companions urged him to take it, and he was about to do so, when he looked at the dog and the animal licked his face, which settled the business. He shook his head and determined to keep him" (quoted in Bueler, 1974, p. 102). Similarly, the Swedish explorer Carl Lumholtz (1989, p. 179) observed that the Aborigines treated these animals:

with greater care than they bestow on their own children. The dingo is an important member of the family; it sleeps in the huts and gets plenty to eat, not only of meat but also of fruit. Its master never strikes, but merely threatens it. He caresses it like a child, eats the fleas off it, and then kisses it on the snout … When hunting, sometimes it refuses to go any further, and its owner has then to carry it on his shoulders, a luxury of which it is very fond.

Although it is difficult to think of any sensible reason why anyone should harbor equivocal feelings about such a useful companion, hunting dogs are (or were) nevertheless regarded with considerable ambivalence in a number of other societies. For example, the Nuala, a group from the Indonesian island of Seram, obtain much of their food from hunting and make effective use of dogs for this purpose. Unlike other domestic animals, individual hunting dogs are given proper names – although not the same names as people – are allowed to sleep in the family house, are provided with human food to eat, especially as puppies, and are generally admired. Striking someone's dog is also considered a serious offense, and killing one is viewed as an abomination. Despite this high regard for dogs, however, the Nuala word for dog, *asu*, is a common term of abuse, and any dog that fails to succeed as a hunter, whether through old age, injury or lack of talent, is likely to be routinely abused and/or neglected and forced to fend for itself. Thus, the Nuala appear to differentiate between individual hunting dogs that earn the right to be treated as quasi-persons by virtue of their positive contribution to the domestic economy, and dogs in general – the ones that live outside and don't serve any useful purpose. To justify the distinction, the Nuala point to the socially unacceptable behavior performed by latter, such as their overt sexual promiscuity and their practice of eating human waste (Ellen, 1999).

Among the Yurok Indians of California, dogs were also valued highly, especially for hunting deer, which they were trained to drive towards awaiting hunters. Yurok folklore recounts tales of men becoming obsessively devoted to their dogs although, in the real world, such intimacy was considered taboo. Dogs, for example, were not allowed into human habitations, and they were never named or spoken to in the belief that they might answer back, thus upsetting the natural order and provoking general catastrophe. Nevertheless, dogs that died were provided with ceremonial burial, and it was also believed that when a man died the spirit of his dog preceded him to the underworld as a guide and protector, even though the dog itself remained alive. This oddly cautious approach to dogs apparently arose, not because dogs were considered ceremonially unclean,[1] but because they

---

[1] Some social anthropologists would argue that the dog's liminality, its closeness to the border between human and non-human, is sufficient reason in itself for regarding the species as potentially unclean or polluting (see e.g. Douglas, 1966).

were too close to humans. Dogs were a potential menace because the critical psychological line that distinguished humans from animals was constantly in danger of being erased by their presence (Elmendorf & Kroeber, 1960). Rather similar beliefs have also been described among the Ruma, an indigenous group from the upper Amazon region of Ecuador (Kohn, 2007).

James Jordan (1975) provides a further account of similar ambivalent attitudes to dogs within a small, white, rural community in the southern US state of Georgia. Here dogs serve a variety of functions, but are valued primarily for hunting. Ownership of a good hunting dog carries with it considerable social prestige, and southern males are intensely proud of their dogs and their abilities. Yet the overall care and treatment of dogs is both callous and frequently cruel:

On the one hand [says Jordan] the dog is highly esteemed for his various abilities in hunting, tracking, guarding, and providing companionship and trustworthy fidelity. On the other hand, the dog is used as a low-status marker within the same cultural context: to label a human a dog, to suggest that a human is the offspring of a female dog, or to liken a human as being in any way similar to a dog is to insult the human deeply … The dog is treated as though it is useful *and* useless; the dog is referred to as symbolically valuable *and* worthless; the dog is employed as a standard of excellence *and* of baseness. (Jordan, 1975, p. 245)

Jordan offers a variety of possible explanations for such apparently inconsistent attitudes. He suggests that economic constraints may be a factor and that indifference to canine welfare may simply reflect the hardships experienced by people in such communities. He also proposes that the masculine ethos of violence and toughness that enables people to endure such conditions of life is applied equally to dogs, and that the maintenance of shallow, ambivalent attachments to dogs, and seeming indifference to their well being, may represent an unconscious defence against unpredictable losses due to frequent accidents or disease. Finally, he suggests that the dog, because of its quasi-human but subordinate status, may serve as a "whipping-boy"; an outlet for the exercise of dominance, power and displaced anger in a community where men tend to feel dispossessed and powerless themselves (Jordan, 1975).

A somewhat similar theory has also been applied to the BaMbuti Pygmies of Zaire, who display such excessive cruelty and violence towards their hunting dogs, that it led one observer to remark: "I thank God we are not pygmies. I thank Him still more that we are not pygmy women, and even still more again that we are not pygmy dogs" (see Singer, 1978, p. 271). Once again, paradoxically, the BaMbuti value these dogs highly as hunting aides, and most authorities agree that it would be difficult, if not impossible, for these people to track down certain types of game successfully without their canine assistants. In an attempt to explain this contradictory behavior, the anthropologist Singer (1978) postulated that dogs serve an important function as scapegoats in these communities. The BaMbuti believe that overt demonstrations of aggression between people are extremely distasteful. The dog, however, serves as a convenient and socially acceptable outlet for repressed anger, and is a particularly suitable victim in this respect because of its closeness to humans.

Among the Matinen, an indigenous group from the Indonesian island of Tanimbar, ambivalent, love–hate attitudes to hunting dogs are divided strictly along gender lines. Matinen men are self-consciously proud of their reputation as hunters of wild pig and buffalo, a skill for which they rely heavily on the assistance of dogs. Perhaps not surprisingly, Matinen men are also "generously fond of their dogs" (Broch, 2008, p. 67). Men and boys habitually carry dogs and puppies around, fondling them and talking endlessly about their different colors and personalities, and even taking them to bed with them at night. In contrast, Matinen women and girls express intense dislike of dogs, and consider them filthy animals that should neither be touched nor petted. Indeed, any dog that is unlucky enough to be caught skulking around the family kitchen is likely to be kicked or beaten, at least when there are no men around to intervene. As with the BaMbuti, it seems that Matinen dogs provide a convenient outlet for the expression of latent hostility, this time between Matinen women and their menfolk. The roots of this conflict may lie in the fact that young women marry into their husband's households and are therefore dispossessed and relatively powerless (Broch, 2008).

In short, despite its almost universal value for hunting certain types of game, the dog's affinity with humans seems to be able to inspire suspicion, denigration and hostility as well as devotion and respect.

15.3 Dogs for dinner

The concept of slaughtering and eating dogs is utterly abhorrent to the majority of Europeans and North Americans. As the anthropologist, Marshall Sahlins, noted more than 30 years ago, the practice of keeping dogs as family pets tends to render their slaughter and consumption beyond the pale:

> Dogs and horses participate in American society in the capacity of subjects. They have proper personal names, and indeed we are in the habit of conversing with them as we do not talk to pigs and cattle … But as domestic cohabitants, dogs are closer to men than are horses, and their consumption is more unthinkable: they are one of the family. Traditionally horses stand in a more menial, working relationship to people; if dogs are as kinsmen, horses are as servants and nonkin. Hence the consumption of horses is at least conceivable, if not general, whereas the notion of eating dogs understandably evokes some of the revulsion of the incest tabu. (Sahlins, 1976, p. 174)

Few taboos are more universal than the proscription against harming (let alone consuming) members of one's own social group or family. For this reason, people socialized to cultural norms that view and treat dogs as family members find the notion of killing and eating them morally repugnant (Haidt, 2001; Serpell, 2009).

Opposition to dog-eating is also widespread among many other cultural groups. For example, dog is one of the 10 types of meat specifically proscribed by Buddhist scriptures, along with human, elephant, horse, snake, tiger, leopard, bear and hyena (Tambiah, 1969). While some Buddhist sources attribute the dog-eating taboo to the positive view that dogs are man's best friend and eating them is therefore tantamount to cannibalism, others take a different perspective. Theravada Buddhists in Thailand and Mahayana Buddhists in central Vietnam agree that dogs are humanlike, but that they are also disgusting and therefore inedible because they openly violate two fundamental human taboos: incest and the consumption of excrement. In other words, paradoxically, Buddhists seem to refrain from eating dogs because they both like them and despise them (Avieli, 2011; Tambiah, 1969).

Despite these widespread reservations, dogs are – or at least were until recently – exploited as food items in many other societies around the world, including China and Korea, Southeast Asia and Indochina, North and Central America, sub-Saharan Africa, and the islands of the Pacific (Avieli, 2011; Beier, 1959; Burkardt, 1960; Driver & Massey, 1957; Frank, 1965; Ishige, 1977; Olowo Ojoade, 1990; Podberscek, 2009; Simoons, 1996; Titcomb, 1969). Archaeological evidence suggests that, during the Neolithic and Bronze Age, the practice of dog-eating was also widespread in Europe (Bökönyi, 1974), as it was among the Preclassic (1200 BCE–AD 250) Maya of Belize (Clutton-Brock, 1994).

When humans slaughter and eat dogs they are, in a purely practical sense, treating them no different than any other kind of domestic food animal. Theory would predict that, in these circumstances, people would exercise detachment and attempt to distance themselves emotionally from those animals destined for consumption (see Serpell, 1996; Thomas, 1983). In practice, however, dog-eating is often associated with more complex psychological contortions.

In present day West Africa, Korea and the Philippines, where edible dogs are still produced and reared on a commercial scale, attitudes towards them may tend, superficially, to resemble our own relatively detached, Western attitudes to domestic livestock, such as pigs or chickens. But even in these circumstances, views on dog-eating appear somewhat ambivalent. Some people regard the practice as abhorrent, others only eat dog's flesh for special medicinal purposes, and it is not uncommon for people to refuse to slaughter and devour their own dogs, although evidently happy to kill and consume someone else's (Olowo Ojoade, 1990; Osgood, 1951, 1975). In South Korea where keeping dogs as pets is growing in popularity, edible dogs and pet dogs tend to belong to different breeds or physical types, and where they are sold alongside each other in markets, the pets are distinguished by housing them in pink cages (Podberscek, 2009). In parts of West Africa, the true origins of dog meat may be disguised through the use of euphemistic terminology (Olowo Ojoade, 1990), and in central Vietnam, men who privately admit to eating and enjoying dog meat will publicly condemn the practice due to its shameful associations with criminal behavior and illicit sex (Avieli, 2011).

In many other societies where dogs are or were traditionally eaten, the practice is associated with more overt expressions of ambivalence and is generally performed within the context of a sacramental ritual. For example, according to George Catlin, a famous nineteenth-century explorer, the Sioux Indians were devoted to their dogs:

The dog is more valued than in any part of the civilized world. The Indian has more time to devote to his company, and his untutored mind more nearly assimilates that of his faithful servant. He keeps his dog closer company, and draws him nearer to his heart. They hunt together and are equal sharers in the chase. Their bed is one. On rocks and on their coats of arms they carve his image as the symbol of fidelity. (in Mooney, 1975)

Yet to celebrate Catlin's arrival in their camp, the Indians promptly slaughtered a large number of their dogs and served them up as a wholesome canine stew which Catlin himself had the greatest difficulty eating, in spite of it being "well-flavored and palatable." Rather than reflecting callous indifference, however, this dog-feast apparently constituted a form of ultimate sacrifice; a solemn and binding gesture of friendship. Catlin goes on to explain:

the feast of venison or buffalo meat is due to anyone who enters an Indian's wigwam, it conveys but passive or neutral evidence of friendship and counts for nothing … Yet the Indian will sacrifice his faithful follower to seal a sacred pledge of friendship … I have seen the master take from the bowl the head of his victim and talk of its former affection and fidelity with tears in his eyes. And I have seen civilized men by my side jesting at Indian folly and stupidity. I have said in my heart they never deserved a name as honourable as that of the animal whose bones they were picking. (in Mooney, 1975)

Interestingly, the Sioux still eat dogs and, notwithstanding Catlin's somewhat overblown depiction of "noble savagery," it is clear that the practice is still associated with considerable ritual solemnity. According to a more recent study, the Oglala Sioux consider the dog to be a kind of human with an individual personality of its own. Dogs are sometimes named and, significantly, named dogs are never eaten or, stated more accurately, dogs that are destined for the stewpot are never named. Dogs are invariably slaughtered in a ritual way, and the sacrifice is performed by a medicine man with two female assistants. Before striking the death blow, the medicine man extols the virtues of the victim, calling it "my friend" and announcing to all those assembled how difficult it is for him to sacrifice such a worthy and faithful creature. The two female assistants then put nooses round the dog's neck and draw them abruptly tight, while the medicine man strikes the dog on the head with a blunt instrument from behind. According to the Oglala, this manner of slaughter ensures that the dog's spirit will be released to travel west as a messenger to the mythical Thunder People, to whom it will plead on behalf of humanity.[2] The dog is the most suitable animal to perform this spiritual function precisely because it *is* man's best friend (Powers & Powers, 1986). Similar dog sacrifices and dog feasts have also been described among the Cherokee, as well as the Ojibwa, Cree, and other Algonquian-speaking tribes around the Great Lakes region of North America. Archaeological evidence further suggests that such practices may be of great antiquity (James, 2006; Oberholtzer, 2002).

In pre-colonial Hawaii, and other parts of Polynesia, attitudes to dogs and dog-eating were even more intricate. Roast dog cooked in the traditional earth-oven was considered a delicacy, and was sampled and apparently relished by Captain Cook and his officers during an early visit to Tahiti. At the same time, however, the Polynesians also developed extraordinary affections for pet dogs: "Men, women and children, of all social ranks, fondled, pampered, and talked to their pets, named them, and grieved when death or other circumstances separated them" (Luomala, 1960, p. 203). Grief over a dog might be expressed through tears and poetical eulogies, and a favourite pet was sometimes given special burial as a further token of its owner's high esteem. This curious double standard provoked George Jesse (1866, p. 299) to remark that it was, "strange that this gentle and manly race of beings should not have had their sympathies more entwined with the creatures so much partaking of their character. That mothers should suckle an animal [Polynesian women frequently nursed puppies at the breast], and yet allow that same race to become an item of food, is a singular contradiction in feeling."

In her lengthy and detailed analysis of Polynesian attitudes to dogs, the anthropologist Katherine Luomala (1960) made no attempt to explain this apparent contradiction, although she did mention that the owners of such dogs were frequently overcome with sorrow when the animal was taken away to be slaughtered. Also, according to one of Titcomb's informants, breast-fed puppies were never eaten: "Close physical association would rule out the animal as a creature to kill, for it had taken on some of the 'being' of the nourisher" (Titcomb, 1969, p. 10). It is also clear that Polynesian dog-eating was usually, if not invariably, performed as a part of a sacrificial ritual and this may, in some way, have helped to alleviate the inevitable anxieties associated with killing and eating social companions (see Serpell, 1996), as it evidently does among the Sioux. In addition, and despite their value both as pets and as food, dogs were not necessarily always regarded in a positive light. On the contrary, according to Luomala, "identifying a man as a dog or as being in any way like one presented the creature most dramatically as the symbol of the pariah, the degraded outcast of human society." The comparison damaged the ego because it was believed that:

the dog originated from a human being whose social misbehavior was punished by his human appearance being modified into that of a dog's, his power of speech removed and replaced by a howl, and his status reduced to that of a social inferior of the group which then granted him occasional favours and let him indulge, as best he could, the traits which had led to his social rejection. (Luomala, 1960)

In ideological terms the dog was not a gregarious, wild animal that had flatteringly attached itself to human society. It was, "a transformed human being ostracized by human society and tolerated as a hanger-on of its lowest fringes" (Luomala, 1960, p. 218). Perceiving dogs in such a disparaging

---

[2]This idea of dogs acting as messengers or intermediaries between this world and the next is an extremely widespread and ancient one, exemplified by the early Egyptian canine psychopomp, Anubis, who guided and protected the souls of the dead on their journey to the Underworld. This conception of the dog also conforms with its status as a liminal creature living on the edges of the human domain. White (1991) also notes that, in folklore and mythology, the doorway or threshold of the house (*domus*) is universally associated with the dog, "whose relationship with humans has always located it on the boundary between wildness and domesticity."

light perhaps made it easier to slaughter and devour them with a clear conscience, although, as noted earlier, exactly the same disparaged traits can also render them inedible in other cultural and normative contexts (Avieli, 2011).

15.4   Dogs as scavengers

Since prehistoric times, the waste products of human society have provided an important source of nourishment for canine scavengers. Many countries and cultures still harbor large populations of unemployed, free-roaming dogs, some of which are truly ownerless or feral, while the majority maintain loose associations with people but receive little if any care or consideration in return (see e.g. Boitani *et al.*, Chapter 17; Hiby & Hiby, Chapter 19; Ortolani *et al.*, 2009; Smith & Litchfield, 2009). Such dogs are usually expected to fend for themselves, scavenging off carrion and human waste, and even their habit of barking vociferously at visitors or intruders is commonly regarded as something of a mixed blessing. As is often the case with animals that eat carrion, garbage, or human excrement, one might reasonably expect people's attitudes towards such dogs to be uniformly negative rather than ambivalent (Menache, 1997). But, once again, when we look at the relationship in detail, a more complex picture emerges.

Throughout much of southern Asia, for example, religious proscriptions specifically designate free-roaming street dogs or "pariahs" as *unclean* or *untouchable* (Menache, 1997). Yet, in these same areas, there is also a widespread reluctance to kill surplus dogs, which in some cases amounts to a religious taboo. Although there have been few detailed studies of attitudes to dogs among such communities, the few that exist describe often quite elaborate mythological reasons for exercising tolerance.

One particularly revealing and ancient example is contained in the Hindu legend of Yudhishthira. In the final scene of the Mahabharata Epic, the hero Yudhishthira approaches Heaven after a lengthy mountain pilgrimage during which his queen and his four brothers have all perished. His only surviving companion at this stage is a dog that has followed him faithfully since he set out on his journey. Suddenly, Indra, the King of Heaven, appears in a blaze of light and invites Yudhishthira to complete his journey in a heavenly chariot. Yudhishthira happily accepts and stands aside to allow the dog to enter the chariot, whereupon Indra objects strenuously on the grounds that dogs are unclean and that the animal's presence would defile Heaven itself. Yudhishthira, however, is unmoved and says that he cannot imagine happiness, even in Heaven, while haunted by the memory of casting off such a devoted, loyal and loving companion. A heated argument then ensues until Yudhishthira finally announces that he cannot conceive of a crime that would be more heinous than to leave the dog behind. At this point, all is revealed. By refusing Heaven for the sake of a dog, Yudhishthira has passed his final test. The dog is suddenly transformed into Dharma, the God of Righteousness, and Yudhishthira is carried off to Heaven amidst the acclamation of radiant multitudes (Nivedita & Coomaraswamy, 1913).

The Lisu, a mountain tribe from Thailand, provide a more contemporaneous example of how tolerant attitudes to dogs are reinforced by myth. Among the Lisu, non-working village dogs are tolerated because, in their mythology, the dog is a culture hero who once saved humanity from starvation by stealing rice seeds from God's paddy fields. Also, according to Lisu folklore, humans were once inconvenienced by a copulatory tie, so they petitioned God for his help. God responded by exchanging their genitals with those of dogs – perhaps in retaliation for stealing his rice – and now only dogs are inconvenienced in this way. This is not regarded as a problem, however, because dogs have no work to do (Durrenburger, 1977).

Among the Kenyah people of Kalimantan (Indonesian Borneo) large numbers of dogs are tolerated around the villages and houses, and they are occasionally fed with rice, although the majority serve no useful purpose. No Kenyah will ever kill a dog, but the animals are shown no respect or affection and children are discouraged from playing with them. When asked why these dogs were tolerated, one Kenyah informant merely stated that dogs, "are like children, and eat and sleep together with men in the same house" (Hose & McDougall, 1912). The authors of this study point out that the Kenyahs believe that all animals are potentially capable of thinking like humans and of understanding human speech: "Their objection to killing their troublesome and superfluous dogs seems to be due to a somewhat similar feeling – a recognition of intelligence and emotions not unlike their own."

Among the Beng people, an ethnic group from the Ivory Coast, the corpus of myths concerning dogs is both elaborate and revealing. As with the Lisu or the Kenyah, the Beng tolerate dogs but never feed them or show them any overt affection. Indeed, when the husband of the American anthropologist, Alma Gottlieb, attempted to pet one of these animals, "both the dog and its owner looked at him in surprise – it had clearly never occurred to anyone, canine or human, that such a thing should or even could be done" (Gottlieb, 1986, p. 478). On the other hand, the Beng name their dogs (although they invariably employ foreign rather than Beng names for this purpose), and make sincere efforts to nurse them back to health when they become sick or injured. This inconsistency in the way the Beng treat their dogs is reflected in the ambiguous role that dogs play in Beng folklore. According to one legend, for instance, the dog was responsible for the origin of death. The story recounts how when death first appeared, the people sent a dog and cat as messengers to the Sky to plead for immortality on their behalf. On the way, however, the dog found some bones and became so engrossed with these that the cat, who was too stupid to understand the message correctly, reached the Sky first and relayed the wrong instructions. As a result, everyone now dies and, once dead, cannot be revived. Interestingly, the Beng do not hold cats responsible for this unfortunate outcome because they regard them as too unintelligent to have known any better. Instead, the dog is blamed for allowing his own base gluttony to bring the worst possible calamity down on the heads of humanity.

In another myth, however, the dog redeems itself by forming an alliance with humans against the other animals. In this story, the dog discovers an egg containing the primordial human couple, which it secretly hides and protects from the other animals. When the egg hatches, the first man begins killing the other animals for food, so the latter call a meeting at which they decide to launch a surprise attack on the humans to destroy them. The dog, however, betrays these plans to the man who then ambushes the animals and scatters them all over the world (Gottlieb, 1986). In other words, the dog is portrayed as both an ally of humans against animals, and a potential traitor to both humans and animals; a Jekyll and Hyde character who simultaneously embodies both craven *animal* instincts and laudable *human* virtues.

15.5   Dogs as friends

In much of Europe and North America, the dog's unconditional allegiance to humanity has, justifiably, earned it the title "Man's best friend" and secured it the admiration and affection of countless millions of dog owners. Like Indian pariahs, the vast majority of dogs in the West serve no significant economic or practical function, yet their owners cherish and pamper them to an unprecedented degree. The Western stereotype of the dog is that of the loyal and faithful companion who shares our homes, our lives and, not infrequently, our food and furniture as an equal or near-equal member of the family. Dogs are given personal names – often the same names we give to people – we pet them, hug them, play with them, groom them and ensure that they receive all the exercise, social contact and medical attention they need to keep them happy and healthy (Serpell, 1996). And, in exchange for all this care and attention, pet dogs appear to make a beneficial contribution to their owner's overall health and wellbeing (see Hart & Yamamoto, Chapter 13; Julius *et al.*, 2012).

Despite the mutually beneficial nature of this friendship between people and dogs, it would be a mistake to imagine that the relationship is entirely harmonious. In the United States alone, an estimated 3.9 million dogs enter animal shelters each year, of which approximately 1.3 million are euthanized (ASPCA, 2014). Humane society statistics also reveal that dogs are among the most common animal victims of human negligence and abuse (see Hubrecht *et al.*, Chapter 14). By moulding dogs to fit our own curious notions of canine beauty, we condemn many of them to chronic pain or poor health through the propagation of physical disabilities and inherited disease (Arman, 2007; Asher *et al.*, 2009; Summers *et al.*, 2010). In various ways we also limit their ability to lead normal lives. By altering their height, the carriage of their ears and tail, and the length of their fur we prevent them from communicating effectively with each other (see Bradshaw & Rooney, Chapter 8). And although we indulge them in some respects, we still deny them the freedom to express much of their natural behavior (Beck & Katcher, 1996). The truth is that much of the dog's normal behavioral repertoire – its appetite for garbage, sexual promiscuity, olfactory preoccupations, toilet habits, and occasional naked hostility towards strangers and visitors – can be a source of disgust or embarrassment to many owners. And even the dog's characteristic loyalty, its fawning eagerness to please, appears to be the subject of mixed feelings. On the one hand, it is one of the things that make dogs so appealing. On the other, it can also be construed as sycophantic, servile and obsequious; the sort of behavior we associate with toadies, lovesick fools and cringeing cowards.[3]

This sort of cultural ambivalence towards certain aspects of canine personality is nicely illustrated by what happened in Britain back in 1989, when an 11-year-old girl was attacked and killed on a Scottish beach by two Rottweilers. Over the ensuing months, this incident, together with four or five other less serious Rottweiler attacks, ignited a wave of hysteria that swept the country. A senior government minister was obliged to issue a public statement on the subject, as if to avert a national crisis. An eminent criminologist reported that, for the first time ever, public fears concerning dogs had surpassed every other social issue, including crime, unemployment and racial harassment. And, in one bizarre incident, a young police officer was hailed as a national hero when he strangled some-one's Rottweiler to death after it attacked and killed two pet rabbits. The tide of panic was further exacerbated by a veritable flood of purple prose from the tabloid press. Rottweilers were branded as "Devil Dogs" and "Canine Terrorists" while newspaper columnists across the country vied with each other for the most arresting headlines. One report in *The Sunday Times* (June 4, 1989) began with the words: "They used to be our best friends. Now dogs, traditionally beloved by the British, have become a fang-bearing, mouth-frothing national nightmare." The price of Rottweiler puppies plummeted, animal rescue shelters were inundated with disowned and abandoned pets, and innocent Rottweiler-owners were harangued in the street for merely taking their dog for a walk. Before long, government ministers were calling for a blanket ban on Rottweilers and, indeed, any breed of large or potentially dangerous dog. In the words of one government official, "If people are going to keep wild beasts, they must be made criminally responsible for their actions."

---

[3]These various less appealing aspects of canine behavior are, of course, implicit in vernacular usage where the word "dog," and its female equivalent "bitch," has few positive connotations. When used to describe people it is almost invariably insulting or disparaging and, when applied as a prefix to things, it denotes spuriousness, baseness or inferiority, as in doggerel, dog-Latin, doghouse, dog-end, dogfish, dog rose and so on (see Paulson, 1979).

As it happens, drastic government action was avoided on this occasion, and the furore gradually died down. However, it re-emerged with a vengeance in the spring and summer of 1991 following two savage, and apparently unprovoked, attacks on people by pit bull terriers. This time the public and media reaction was so intense that the Government was forced to act. After the briefest possible consultation with appropriate authorities (many of whose recommendations were ignored) new legislation was swiftly drafted, and the Dangerous Dogs Act 1991 came into being. The Act imposed a ban on the breeding, sale or exchange of all "dogs bred for fighting," which, in practice, encompassed pit bull terriers and one Japanese tosa[4] that had recently been imported as a puppy. Owners of these dogs were given the choice of having them euthanized (at taxpayer's expense) or of having them neutered, tattooed and registered with the authorities, as well as keeping them securely muzzled and leashed in public. Police were authorized to use "reasonable force" to enter premises suspected of harbouring unneutered and unregistered animals, and Magistrates were actually *required* to order the destruction of any dog whose owner failed to comply with the regulations, regardless of whether or not it had ever shown signs of aggressiveness. Unfortunately, these events in Britain seemed to trigger a global wave of breed-specific legislation that has yet to abate, despite growing evidence that breed bans and restrictions are an ineffective way to prevent dog attacks (Collier, 2006; Lockwood, Chapter 9; Patronek *et al.*, 2013).

Without in any sense minimizing the potential threat posed by large and powerful dogs, such as Rottweilers or pit bull terriers, or the frightful injuries inflicted on the individual victims of their attacks, it is clear that the spasms of horror and outrage generated by such incidents are generally out of proportion to the actual risks. In the USA, for example, a nation of 319 million people and approximately 80 million dogs – perhaps half of which are large and at least potentially dangerous – dog attacks account for roughly 20 human fatalities each year, substantially fewer than the average number of people killed by lightning strikes (Centers for Disease Control, 2014). So how, then, do we account for such extreme reactions?

For whatever reason, our culture has transformed the dog into a paragon of canine virtue. He is our loyal and faithful servant and companion; a sort of amiable culture-hero whose friendship is proverbially better than that of our fellow humans. That such a devoted and trusted admirer should suddenly turn and savage one of us is both frightening and disturbing. For not only does this behavior appear disloyal – a betrayal of trust – it could also be construed as grossly insubordinate. Dogs, furthermore, fulfill a childlike role in our society and, as perpetual children, we expect them to be forever innocent, playful and fun-loving (Beck & Katcher, 1996). A murderous dog, like a murderous child, is therefore nothing less than an abomination – a disturbance in the natural order – an unacceptable threat to the perceived security and stability of the entire community.

15.6   Discussion and conclusions

Some of our ambivalence towards the domestic dog arises from simple conflicts of interest. As our voluntary companion and ally, the dog, like a faithful human employee, presses moral claims upon us that are more strident and less easily ignored than those emanating from most other domestic species. This poses relatively few ethical problems when we ask dogs to perform enjoyable tasks,

[4]Somewhat mysteriously, two other breeds, the Fila Brasiliero and Dogo Argentino, were also banned, although neither existed in Britain at the time and neither was bred specifically for fighting. Rottweilers were not included in the ban, probably because they were too widely employed for security purposes.

such as hunting, herding livestock or providing us with company. Dogs seem to like doing these things anyway so their interests and ours, broadly-speaking, coincide. The proverbial friendliness and fidelity of dogs may, however, create a burdensome sense of guilt when we use these animals in ways that appear to betray their loyalty and affection. Where people are obliged to kill dogs either for food or to control their numbers, for example, or where they use them as beasts of burden or as experimental subjects in biomedical research, it is common to find that they either avoid affectionate contact with these animals, or employ complex psychological defence mechanisms to protect their consciences from conflict (Arluke, 1988, 1994; Serpell, 1985, 1996). Even when we make allowances for these relatively straightforward ethical dilemmas, however, it is clear that people's attitudes towards dogs remain strangely contradictory.

Constance Perin (1981) argued that Western ambivalence towards the dog arises from this animal's peculiar symbolic role as an archetypal attachment figure; an idealized provider of love who reawakens memories of the love we once received as infants from our mothers. According to her theory, the tension that exists in our relationships with dogs denotes the re-emergence of all those unresolved love–hate tensions of infancy associated with the process of separation and individuation from our parents. Although in some ways compelling, one problem with this idea is that it is too culture-specific. Ambivalence towards dogs appears to be almost universal, but it is difficult to see how Perin's theory could be applied to societies, such as the Beng, who display this ambivalence in the absence of any obvious affection.

Other authors (e.g. Beck & Katcher, 1983; Burt, 1988) have resorted to a more psychoanalytic interpretation, according to which animals, such as dogs, often represent unconscious aspects of "self" (Jung, 1959). From this perspective, our love–hate, tolerant–intolerant attitudes to dogs are simply a reflection of our own ambivalence about the *animal* within us – the Freudian "id" – the source of all those instinctual, impulsive, forbidden feelings and desires that we tend to keep so firmly repressed. This would certainly help to explain why we are often uncomfortable with the more unbridled aspects of our dogs' behavior, although it is possible to think of other reasons for diffidence in this respect. Dogs, after all, flatter us with their attention and devotion; we see ourselves magnified in their eyes. But the satisfaction we derive from this hero-worship is inevitably tempered by the behavior of the worshipper. To be loved by a paragon is one thing, to be adored by a creature that eats shit, sniffs genitals, and bites people is quite another.

In some respects, however, all of these theories may miss the point. As the Yurok Indians recognized, the real danger posed by the domestic dog is that its friendship threatens to dissolve or undermine the psychological barrier that distinguishes human from animals (Elmendorf & Kroeber, 1960). By adopting us and treating us as conspecifics, even in the absence of any positive encouragement to do so, the dog unwittingly represents the thin end of the wedge; a demanding and insistent reminder of the feelings, interests and moral claims not only of dogs, but of animals in general (Serpell & Paul, 1994).

In symbolic terms, the domestic dog exists precariously in the no-man's-land between the human and non-human worlds. It is an interstitial creature – neither person nor beast – forever oscillating uncomfortably between the roles of high-status animal and low-status human. As a consequence, the dog is rarely accepted and appreciated purely for what it is; a uniquely varied, carnivorous mammal adapted to a huge range of mutualistic associations with people. Instead, it has become a creature of metaphor, simultaneously embodying or representing a strange mixture of admirable and despicable traits. As a beast that voluntarily allies itself to humans, the dog often seems to lose its right to be regarded as a true animal. In many societies, it now occupies the role of a stateless refugee, tolerated and occasionally pitied as a hanger-on, but never properly assimilated or accepted. In others, it is viewed as the victim of its own depravity, a person transmogrified into a dog for engaging in immoral behavior, a creature unworthy of humane considerations and a suitable candidate for abuse, displaced anger or the cooking pot. Elsewhere, the dog's ambiguous or intermediate status has endowed it with supernatural powers, and the ability to travel as a spiritual messenger or psychopomp between this world and the next. Such beliefs may help to engender a certain respect or even reverence for dogs, but they can also provide a convenient justification for hastening the animal on its journey and then devouring its mortal remains. In our own culture, the dog has been granted temporary personhood in return for its unfailing companionship. But, as we have seen, this privilege is swiftly withdrawn whenever the dog reveals too much of its animal nature. In other words, we love dogs and invest them with quasi-human status, but only so long as they refrain from behaving like dogs.

Whether paragon or pariah, dogs confront us with essentially the same dilemma: the problem of deciding how far our moral responsibilities should extend beyond the taxonomic boundaries of our own species. Seen in this light, our ambivalence towards the dog is ultimately an expression of the profound uncertainty we humans feel concerning our assumed "right" to live at the expense of other sentient beings.

Acknowledgements

My thanks to Harriet Ritvo and Randall Lockwood for their valuable comments on the original version of this chapter.

References

American Society for the Protection of Animals (ASPCA) (2014). [Online]. Available: www.aspca.org/about-us/faq/pet-statistics [accessed November 19, 2014].

Appleby, D. & Pluijmakers, J. (2003). Separation anxiety in dogs: the function of homeostasis in its development and treatment. *Veterinary Clinics Small Animal Practice*, 33: 321–44.

Arluke, A. (1988). Sacrificial symbolism in animal experimentation: object or pet? *Anthrozoös*, 2: 98–117.

Arluke, A. (1994). Managing emotions in an animal shelter. In *Animals and Human Society: Changing Perspectives*, eds. A. Manning & J. A. Serpell. London: Routledge, pp. 145–65.

Arluke, A. & Sax, B. (1992). Understanding Nazi animal protection and the Holocaust. *Anthrozoös*, 5: 6–31.

Arman, K. (2007). A new direction for kennel club regulations and breed standards. *Canadian Veterinary Journal*, 48: 953–965.

Asher, L., Diesel, G., Summers, J. F., McGreevy, P. D. & Collins, L. M. (2009). Inherited defects in pedigree dogs. Part 1: Disorders related to breed standards. *The Veterinary Journal*, 182: 402–11.

Avieli, N. (2011). Dog meat politics in a Vietnamese town. *Ethnology*, 50: 59–78.

Beck, A. M. & Katcher, A. H. (1996). *Between Pets and People: The Importance of Animal Companionship*. West Lafayette, IN: Purdue University Press.

Beier, U. (1959). The Yoruba attitude to dogs. *Odu*, 7: 31–7.

Bökönyi, S. (1974). *History of Domestic Mammals in Central and Eastern Europe*. Budapest: Académiai Kaidó.

Broch, H. B. (2008). Gender and Matinen dogs. *Asian Anthropology*, 7: 57–77

Bueler, L. (1974). *Wild Dogs of The World*. London: Constable.

Burkardt, V. R. (1960). *Chinese Creeds and Customs*, vol. 3. Hong Kong: South China Morning Post Ltd.

Burt, M. R. (1988). The animal as Alter Ego: cruelty, altruism, and the work of art. In *Animals and People Sharing the World*, ed. A. N. Rowan. Hanover, NH: University Press of New England, pp. 117–35.

Centers for Disease Control (2014). [Online]. Available: http://emergency.cdc.gov/disasters/lightning/index.asp [accessed November 14, 2014].

Cipriani, L. (1966). *The Andaman Islanders*. London: Weidenfeld & Nicholson.

Clutton-Brock, J. (1994). Hot dogs: comestible canids in preclassic Maya culture at Cuello, Belize. *Journal of Archaeological Science*, 21: 819–26

Collier, S. (2006). Breed-specific legislation and the pit bull terrier: are the laws justified? *Journal of Veterinary Behavior*, 1: 17–22.

Dawkins, R. (1993). Gaps in the mind. In *The Great Ape Project*, eds. P. Cavalieri & P. Singer. London: Fourth Estate, pp. 80–7.

Diamond, J. M. (1993). The third chimpanzee. In *The Great Ape Project*, eds. P. Cavalieri & P. Singer. London: Fourth Estate, pp. 88–101.

Dinzelbacher, P. (2002). Animal trials: a multidisciplinary approach. *Journal of Interdisciplinary History*, 32: 405–421.

Douglas, M. (1966). *Purity and Danger: An Analysis of the Concepts of Pollution and Taboo*. New York: Routledge & Kegan Paul.

Downs, J. F. (1960). Domestication: an examination of the changing social relationships between man and animals. *Kroeber Anthropological Society Papers*, 22: 18–67.

Driver, H. E. & Massey, W. C. (1957). Comparative studies of North American Indians. *Transactions of the American Philosophical Society*, 42: 165–456.

Dumont, J. P. (1976). *Under the Rainbow: Nature and Supernature among the Panaré Indians*. Austin: University of Texas Press.

Durrenburger, E. P. (1977). Of Lisu dogs and Lisu spirits. *Folklore*, 88: 61–3.

Ellen, R. (1999). Categories of animality and canine abuse: Exploring contradictions in Nuala social relationships with dogs. *Anthropos*, 94: 57–68.

Elmendorf, W. W. & Kroeber, A. L. (1960). The structure of Twana culture with comparative notes on the structure of Yurok culture. *Washington University Research Studies*, 28(2). Pullman, WA: Washington State University.

Evans, E.P. (1906). *The Criminal Prosecution and Capital Punishment of Animals*. London: Heinemann.

Fox, M. W. (1967). Effects of early experience on the development of inter and intra-specific social relationships in the dog. *Animal Behaviour*, 15: 377–86.

Frank, B. (1965). *Die Rolle des Hunde im Africanischen Kulturen*. Wiesbaden: Franz Steiner Verlag.

Girgen, J. (2003). The historical and contemporary prosecution and punishment of animals. *Animal Law*, 9: 97–133.

Gottlieb, A. (1986). Dog: ally or traitor? Mythology, cosmology, and society among the Beng of Ivory Coast. *American Ethnologist*, 13: 447–88.

Haidt, J. (2001). The emotional dog and its rational tail: a social intuitionist approach to moral judgment. *Psychological Review*, 108: 814–34.

Harrison, T. (1965). Three "secret" communication systems between Borneo nomads (and their dogs). *Journal of the Malay Branch of the Royal Asiatic Society*, 38: 67–86.

Hole, F. & Wyllie, C. (2007) The oldest depictions of canines and a possible early breed of dog in Iran. *Paléorient*, 33: 175–85.

Hose, C. & McDougall, M. B. (1912). *The Pagan Tribes of Borneo*. London: Macmillan.

Huntingford, G. W. B. 1955. The economic life of the Dorobo. *Anthropos*, 50: 602–34.

Ikeya, K. (1994). Hunting with dogs among the San in the Central Kalahari. *African Study Monographs*, 15: 119–34.

Ishige, N. (1977). Roasting dog (or a substitute) in an earth oven: an unusual method of preparation from Ponape. In *The Anthropologist's Cookbook*, ed. J. Kuper. New York: Universe Books, pp. 204–5.

James, J. (2006). The dog tribe. *The Southern Anthropologist*, 32: 17–46.

Jesse, G.R. (1866). *Researches into the History of the British Dog*, vol. I. London: Robert Hardwicke.

Jordan, J. W. (1975). An ambivalent relationship: dog and human in the folk culture of the rural south. *Appalachian Journal*, Spring: 238–48.

Julius, H., Beetz, A., Kotrschal, K., Turner, D. C. & Uvnäs-Moberg, K. (2012). *Attachment to Pets*. New York: Hogrefe.

Jung, C. (1959). *The Archetypes and the Collective Unconscious*. New York: Pantheon.

Kohn, E. (2007). How dogs dream: Amazonian natures and the politics of transspecies engagement. *American Ethnologist*, 34: 3–24.

Koster, J. (2008). Hunting with dogs in Nicaragua: an optimal foraging approach. *Current Anthropology*, 49: 935–44.

Koster, J. (2009). Hunting dogs in the lowland tropics. *Journal of Anthropological Research*, 65: 575–610.

Lee, R. B. (1979). *The !Kung San: Men, Women and Work in a Foraging Society*. Cambridge: Cambridge University Press.

Lumholtz, C. (1989). *Among Cannibals*. London: John Murray.

Luomala, K. (1960). The native dog in the Polynesian system of values. In *Culture in History*, ed. S. Diamond. New York: Columbia University Press, pp. 190–240.

Menache, S. (1997). Dogs: God's worst enemies? *Society and Animals*, 5: 23–44.

Midgley, M. (1983). *Animals and Why They Matter*. Harmondsworth, Middlesex: Penguin Books.

Mooney, M. M. (1975). *George Catlin Letters and Notes on the North American Indians*. New York: Clarkson N. Potter.

Nivedita, The Sister & Coomaraswamy, A. K. (1913). *Myths of the Hindus and Buddhists*. London: Harrap & Co.

Oberholtzer, C. (2002). Fleshing out the evidence: from archaic dog burials to historic dog feasts. *Ontario Archaeology*, 73: 3–14.

Olowo Ojoade, J. (1990). Nigerian cultural attitudes to the dog. In *Signifying Animals: Human Meaning in the Natural World*, ed. R. G. Willis. London: Unwin Hyman, pp. 215–21.

Ortolani, A., Vernooij, H. & Coppinger, R. (2009). Ethiopian village dogs: behavioural responses to stranger's approach. *Applied Animal Behaviour Science*, 119: 210–18.

Osgood, C. (1951). *The Koreans and their Culture*. New York: Ronald Press.

Osgood, C. (1975). *The Chinese: A Study of a Hong Kong Community*. Tucson, AZ: University of Arizona Press.

Patronek, G.J., Sacks, J.J., Delise, K.M., Cleary, D.V. & Marder, A. R. (2013). Co-occurrence of potentially preventable factors in 256 dog bite-related fatalities in the United States (2000–2009). *JAVMA*, 243: 1726–36.

Paulson, R. (1979). *Popular and Polite Art in the Age of Hogarth and Fielding*. Notre Dame, IN: University of Notre Dame Press.

Perin, C. (1981). Dogs as symbols in human development. In *Interrelations between People and Pets*, ed. B. Fogle. Springfield, IL: Charles C. Thomas, pp. 68–88.

Podberscek, A. L. (2009). Good to pet and eat: the keeping and consuming of dogs and cats in South Korea. *Journal of Social Issues*, 65: 615–32.

Podberscek, A. L., Hsu, Y. & Serpell, J. A. (1999). Evaluation of clomipramine as an adjunct to behavioural therapy in the treatment of separation-related problems in dogs. *Veterinary Record*, 145: 365–9.

Powers, W. K. & Powers, M. N. (1986). Putting on the dog. *Natural History*, 2: 6–16.

Roe, P. G. (1993). The domesticated jaguar: dog symbolism in the lowlands. *Proceedings of the 15th International Congress on Caribbean Archaeology, San Juan, Puerto Rico*, pp. 2–42.

Sahlins, M. (1976). *Culture and Practical Reason*. Chicago, IL: Chicago University Press.

Scott, J. P. (1963). The process of primary socialization in canine and human infants. *Monographs of the Society for Research on Child Development*, 28: 1–49.

Scott, J. P. (1968). Evolution and domestication of the dog. *Evolutionary Biology*, 2: 243–75.

Seligmann, C. G. & Seligmann, B. A. (1911). *The Veddas*. Cambridge: Cambridge University Press.

Serpell, J. A. (1985). Best friend or worst enemy: cross-cultural variation in attitudes to the dog. In *The Human–Pet Relationship*. Vienna: IEMT – Institute for Interdisciplinary Research on the Human–Pet Relationship.

Serpell, J. A. (1996). *In the Company of Animals*, 2nd edition. Cambridge: Cambridge University Press.

Serpell, J. A. (2004). Factors influencing attitudes to animals and their welfare. *Animal Welfare*, 13: S145–51.

Serpell, J. A. (2005). Animals and religion: Towards a unifying theory. In *The Human-Animal Relationship*, eds. F. de Jong & R. Van den Bos. Assen, Netherlands: Royal Van Gorcum, pp. 9–22.

Serpell, J. A. (2009). Having our dogs and eating them too: Why animals are a social issue. *Journal of Social Issues*, 65: 633–44.

Serpell, J. A. (2013). Domestication and history of the cat. In *The Domestic Cat: The Biology of Its Behaviour*, 3rd edition, eds. D. C. Turner & P. P. G. Bateson. Cambridge: Cambridge University Press, pp. 83–100.

Serpell, J. A. & Paul, E. S. (1994). Pets and the development of positive attitudes to animals. In *Animals and Human Society: Changing Perspectives*, eds. A. Manning & J. A. Serpell. London: Routledge, pp. 127–44.

Simoons, F. J. (1996). Dogflesh eating by humans in sub-Saharan Africa. *Ecology of Food and Nutrition*, 34: 251–92.

Singer, M. (1978). Pygmies and their dogs: a note on culturally constituted defence mechanisms. *Ethos*, 6: 270–7.

Smith, B. P. & Litchfield, C. A. (2009). A review of the relationship between indigenous Australians, dingoes (*Canis dingo*) and domestic dogs (*Canis familiaris*). *Anthrozoös*, 22: 111–28.

Summers, J. F., Diesel, G., Asher, L. McGreevy, P. D. & Collins, L.M. (2010) Inherited defects in pedigree dogs. Part 2: Disorders that are not related to breed standards. *The Veterinary Journal*, 183: 39–45.

Tambiah, J. S. (1969). Animals are good to think and good to prohibit. *Ethnology*, 8: 423–59

Thomas, K. (1983). *Man and the Natural World: Changing Attitudes in England 1500–1800*. London: Allen Lane.

Titcomb, M. (1969). *Dog and Man in the Ancient Pacific with Special Attention to Hawaii*. Honolulu, HI: Bernice P. Bishop Museum Special Publications 59.

White, D. G. (1991). *Myths of the Dog-Man*. Chicago, IL: University of Chicago Press.

Part IV

Life on the margins

16 Variation in dog society: Between resource dispersion and social flux

DAVID W. MACDONALD AND GEOFFREY M. CARR

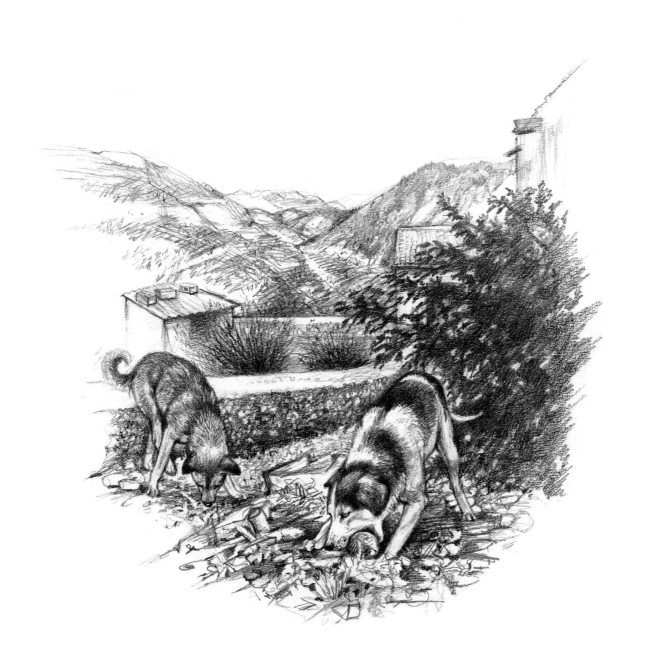

16.1 Introduction

Domestic dogs, *Canis familiaris*, live in various degrees of association with people. Extremes of this continuum range from the lap dog to those living in uninhabited areas (Young *et al.*, 2011) or islands (e.g. Kruuk & Snell, 1981). Dogs that are not strictly controlled by their owners might be expected to modify their behavior to match their ecological circumstances according to the same principles that affect wild Carnivora (e.g. Kruuk, 1975; Macdonald, 1983; Macdonald & Sillero-Zubiri, 2004) and free-ranging domestic ones such as cats, *Felis catus* (e.g. Daniels *et al.*, 2001; Liberg *et al.*, 2000; Macdonald *et al.*, 1987). Therefore, we would expect that free-roaming dogs studied under different conditions would behave differently, and that these differences would be adaptive (in so far as artificial selection had not compromised the traits in question). This prediction, however, has not been formally tested (three studies explored variation in behavior amongst different free-roaming dogs – Bonanni *et al.*, 2010a, 2010b; Mangalam & Singh, 2013). Studies of feral dogs in urban areas have tended to conclude that they form amorphous, and probably ephemeral associations (e.g. Beck, 1973; Daniels & Bekoff, 1989a). Furthermore, the questions of whether these associations are adapted to ecological circumstances and whether membership of groups has functional consequences have received little attention. Such questions have both theoretical and practical importance. The abundance, accessibility and potential manipulability of free-roaming dogs, combined with background knowledge of the genetic and physiological differences between breeds, make them strong candidates for testing ideas about canid socioecology. In addition, an understanding of dog behavior should help the design of control programs intended to counteract their potential as pests – whether as predators of stock or game, vectors of disease (e.g. rabies, distemper and *Echinococcus;* Bhunu, 2011; WHO, 1988), or as genetic contaminators of wild canid populations (see Boitani, 1983; Ginsberg & Macdonald, 1990; Hughes *et al.*, Chapter 18). Finally, free-roaming dog behavior is interesting because of the opportunity it affords for comparison between breeds and with the ancestral wolf (Boitani & Ciucci, 1995), *Canis lupus*, and as part of the study of domestication (Driscoll *et al.*, 2009; Scott & Fuller, 1965; Zimen, 1972).

We therefore compared the behavior of free-roaming dogs in contrasting ecological conditions in order to observe whether their social organization differed, and to determine whether their behavior matched predictions based on their ecology. Our approach was based on three general findings about the behavior of the Carnivora.

First, in addition to obvious inter-specific variation (e.g. Gittleman, 1989; Macdonald *et al.*, 2010), there is enormous intra-specific variation in the social organization of carnivores (Kruuk, 1975; Johnson *et al.*, 2002; Macdonald, 1983; Tallents *et al.*, 2012). A classic example is Kruuk's (1972) demonstration that populations of spotted hyaena, *Crocuta crocuta*, live in different sorts of societies depending on whether their prey are migratory or sedentary (see also Mills, 1990). A similar example, especially apposite to the case of the free-living dogs we studied, is Doncaster & Macdonald's (1991) finding that the spatial organization, group dynamics and reproductive behavior of red foxes, *Vulpes vulpes*, varied between an urban and an adjoining rural habitat (see also Macdonald, 1981, 1987; Macdonald *et al.*, 1999).

Second, intra-specific variation may be explained in terms of the pattern in which resources, such as food, are available. One idea, reviewed by Macdonald (1983), is called the Resource Dispersion Hypothesis (RDH) and stems from the proposition that groups may develop where resources are dispersed such that the smallest economically defensible territory for a minimum-sized social unit might also sustain additional animals. In a simple case, territory size would be determined by the dispersion of the minimum number of patches of food required to sustain an individual, whereas group size would be determined by the richness of those patches. A related concept is food security, which is the probability that a territorial occupant can satisfy its food requirements at any given time (Carr & Macdonald, 1986). The more variable the pattern in which food is available, the greater the resources that must be commandeered in a territory to achieve a given food security, and consequently the greater the opportunity for providing substantial food security to additional group members (Woodroffe & Macdonald, 1993 review this and related models – see also Johnson, 2003).

Third, the functional consequences of group membership vary between populations and between individuals even within one group. Amongst the many advantages that have been proposed for group-living carnivores (see reviews in Gittleman, 1989; and a general account in Macdonald, 1992), obvious candidate benefits that might apply to free-living domestic dogs include cooperative hunting, communal care of young, and corporate defence of food. Depending on the structure of groups, a vested interest in the survival of kin may be important, as elaborated in Lindstrom's (1986) Territory Inheritance Model (see also Blackwell & Bacon, 1993). The marginal contribution made by each additional group member to the fitness of each member will be one of the factors that determines whether the benefits of larger groups compensate for any expansionism necessary to provide adequate food security for their members (Macdonald & Carr, 1989 – see also Newman *et al.*, 2011).

16.2   The study

It was with these three points in mind that we designed our study. The fieldwork was carried out in Italy, where Boitani & Fabbri (1983) estimated that 10% of 80 000 free-roaming dogs lived independently of people. The study area was in the mountainous Abruzzo region of central Italy (42° N, 13° 30" E), which afforded the opportunity to compare dogs living in adjacent but different habitat types: small villages and open countryside. Preliminary observations suggested that the former depended on several food patches, each unpredictable in the time-table and abundance of food, whereas the latter depended mainly on a single very rich patch of food. (The RDH predicts that these differing patterns would have different consequences for group and territory sizes and social behavior.)

There was wide phenotypic variation between individual dogs, but no observable systematic differences in phenotype between those living in the different habitats. The dominant phenotypes were the traditional Abruzzese (pastore maremmano), and the more recently introduced German shepherd. The Abruzzese is a large, predominantly white breed, similar to the Pyrenean. Both types were once used to guard flocks of sheep against the depredations of wolves. The virtual elimination of wolves from the area has, according to local people, coincided with the establishment of the free-living dog population in the countryside. The phenotypic similarity of the village and country populations, the youth of the latter, and the proximity of the two habitats, permit the hope that any differences in their social and spatial organization result from different ecological circumstances, rather than selective differences (whether natural or artificial) between the populations involved.

Three dog populations were observed intermittently between 1981 and 1983; two of these were located in villages, and the third in open countryside:

- Rovere (Figure 16.1): This ancient village (population 225) occupies one side of a small hill (altitude 1413 m) and part of the surrounding plain. About half of the settlement is on the hill and consists of old terraced stone buildings and narrow streets. More modern houses, together with

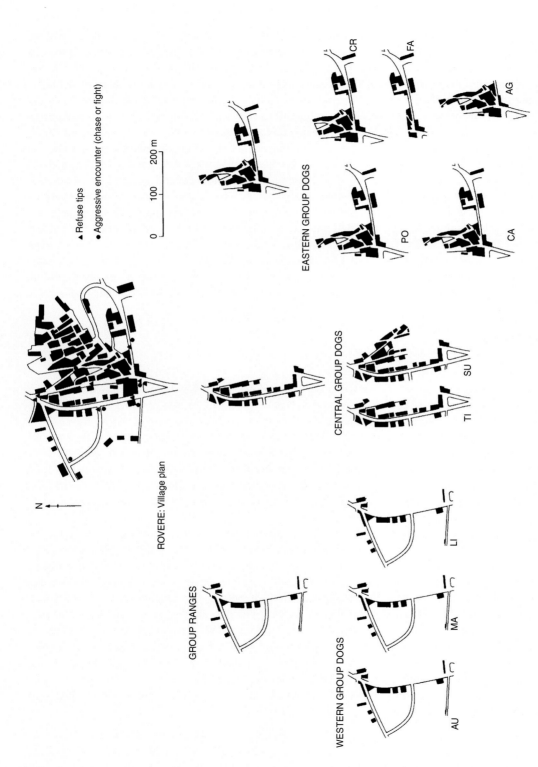

Figure 16.1 Plan of Rovere village indicating the locations of refuse tips from which village dogs largely fed, and of aggressive encounters observed during March 1981. The second tier of maps are those sections of the village used by each of three groups of dogs. The locations of these collective ranges can be fitted together, like segments of a jig-saw puzzle, by reference to the base map. The third tier of maps illustrates the ranges of individual members of the western group (Augustus, Marcello, Livia), central group (Tiberius, Sulla) and eastern group (Pompei, Crassus, Fabius, Caius, Aggrippina), each identified by a two letter code. The ranges are based on observations made intensively in March 1981 and sporadically during the following summer.

some larger farms, have spilled out onto the plain. These latter form a roughly triangular structure enclosing an open meadow.

- Sant'Iona (Figure 16.2): Another ancient settlement, similar to Rovere (population 142), but at lower altitude (969 m). A large (600 m²) open space is enclosed within the village, and there is an area of ruined buildings – the result of an earthquake in 1915. Sant'Iona has very little modern development, although some older houses have been renovated as holiday homes.
- Altopiano delle Rocche (Figure 16.3): This small upland plain (1340 m) formed the focus of the third study area. It is approximately elliptical, with major and minor axes of 4 km and 1.5 km, and

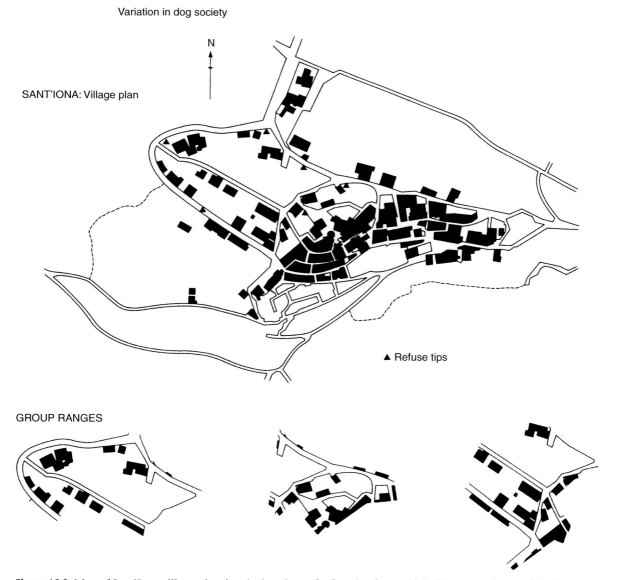

Figure 16.2 Map of Sant'Iona village, showing the locations of refuse tips from which village dogs largely fed. The second tier of maps are those sections of the village used by each of three groups of dogs (displayed as explained in Figure 16.1).

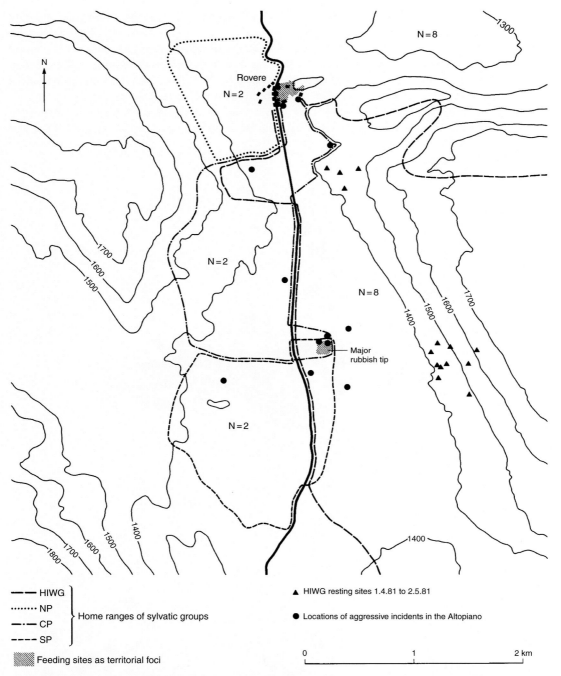

Figure 16.3 Map of the Altopiano delle Rocche showing the location of the village of Rovere and the major communal rubbish tip. The hand-drawn borders of home ranges are shown for northern, central and southern pairs of sylvatic dogs (group sizes indicated by: $N = 2$), and for the western edge of the HIWG's range. To the north ($N = 8$) no borders are plotted for the group that operated in the vicinity of the rubbish tip at Rocca di Mezzo. The HIWG (Hole in the Wall gang, named after their site of entry to Rovere village) rested in beech woodland on the valley walls, either south of Rovere or east of the rubbish tip (day-time resting sites of radio-tagged dogs indicated for spring 1981). The sites of aggressive encounters between resident sylvatic dogs and between them and unaccompanied non-residents are also shown, clustered particularly around the two important feeding sites.

is surrounded by mountains that rise to more than 2400 m. The plain is mainly meadowland, while the surrounding mountains are covered by beech woods interspersed with herbaceous grassland. Cattle, sheep and horses are grazed in the area. Near the middle of the plain is a large dump that receives the domestic refuse of nearby settlements and is replenished on a daily basis. Between 6 and 10 wolves occurred in the vicinity.

The nomenclature of free-living dogs has become somewhat confused (Daniels & Bekoff, 1989a; Nesbitt, 1975). We shall use three terms: any dog not living under the close control of a human being may be referred to as "free-living"; dogs living in the Altopiano, or similar habitats are "sylvatic"; dogs living in villages will simply be known as "village" dogs. We shall eschew the words "feral," "stray," etc.

16.3   Methods

Data on the sylvatic dogs were collected by a combination of observation (using image intensifying equipment at night) and radio-tracking. Candidates for radio-tracking were captured in baited cage traps and fitted with home-made radio-collars (173 kHz, following the construction described by Macdonald & Amlaner, 1980). Eight sylvatic individuals, weighing 20–30 kg, were collared during the course of the study, one of them twice. Radio-tracking was used to locate daytime resting places, and to follow movement at night. Fixes at night were taken *ad lib.*, according to circumstances. Radio data were collected on 175 days (approximately 2000 radio sweeps), principally during an intensive study between April and August 1981, and during occasional monitoring thereafter. For the purposes of this account, the spatial organization of dogs is adequately represented by hand-drawn boundaries of home ranges based on combined radio-location and direct observation (Macdonald *et al.*, 1980a).

Village dogs, being habituated to humans, could be watched at close quarters. Focal animals were selected each day and their behavior and exact location (based on a one metre grid) sampled once per minute, normally for a 4-hour observation period by day. Behavior was divided into three broad categories: sedentary, active and translocatory (i.e. moving from one place to another), and subdivided within these categories to allow for more detailed analysis. Dogs not selected for focal studies were scan-sampled regularly to record their locations, and thus their ranges. Eighty hours of focal observations were made in Rovere in March 1981, and 350 hours in Sant'Iona, of which 100 directly comparable hours recorded in March 1983 are used in direct comparisons with Rovere.

16.4   Results

16.4.1   Demography

The initial census for Rovere (February 1981) gave 10 dogs (8 male, 2 female); whilst Sant'Iona (March 1982) had 18 (13 male, 5 female). Both village populations were thus biased towards males (binomial test Rovere: $P = 0.055$; Sant'Iona: $P = 0.045$). The initial census of the Altopiano revealed 15 dogs (8 male, 7 female) living there. Table 16.1 shows how the composition of one Altopiano pack changed over the course of the study. In addition to these animals, a group of around eight sylvatic dogs lived to the north of the study area, apparently in conjunction with a second rubbish dump near the town of Rocca di Mezzo.

Table 16.1	Annual changes in the composition of the sylvatic dog pack (HIWG).		
	Summer 1981	**Summer 1982**	**Summer 1983**
Males			
Radio	P	D	D
Dark	P	D	D
Big White	P	P	P
Second White	P	P	P
Cream	P	P	P
Shaggy	P	D	D
Houdini[a]	–	P	P
Black[b]	–	–	P
Females			
1st Mama	P	P	P
2nd Mama	P	D	D
3rd Mama	P	P	P
Odd Mama	P	D	D
Noisy[b]	–	P	D
Pseudo Wolf[b]	–	–	P
Total	10	7	8
Sex ratio	6:4	4:3	5:3

P, Present; D, Died or Disappeared
[a]External recruit
[b]Matured pup

16.4.2 Village dog society

Casual observations in both villages suggested a rather amorphous society. Although certain dogs regularly kept one another company, there were no obvious packs. However, more detailed scrutiny identified discrete social groups. Tables 16.2(a) and 16.2(b) summarize the springtime patterns of amicable interaction (greeting, play, co-ordinated movement) between village dogs. Dogs varied in their amicability (percentage of observations in company varied between 5 and 70%) and often had preferred associates. But it is clear from the tables that they split up into mutually exclusive groups under this analysis. The converse is also true (Tables 16.3(a) and 16.3(b)): if social groups are provisionally erected on the basis of company keeping, hostile interactions are almost completely confined to encounters between dogs from different groups. Only about 2% of all hostile interactions were between group members. However, hostile encounters were not observed

Table 16.2   Pattern of amicable interactions between adult dogs in (a) Rovere and (b) Sant'Iona in March 1981 (80 hours) and 1983 (100 hours), respectively. The dogs are identified by two letter codes and sex (M/F), and are grouped on the tables in accordance with amicable ties as revealed by these data.

(a) Rovere

	AU(M)	MA(M)	LI(F)	SU(M)	TI(M)	CA(M)	CR(M)	FA(M)	PO(M)
AU(M)	–								
MA(M)	78	–							
LI(F)	139	93	–						
SU(M)	0		0	–					
TI(M)	0	0	0	11	–				
CA(M)	0	0	0	0	0	–			
CR(M)	0	0	0	0	0	116	–		
FA(M)	0	0	0	0	0	37	15	–	
PO(M)	0	0	0	0	0	152	98	24	–
AG(F)	3	0	0	0	0	74	47	3	43

This table shows the pattern of amicable interaction between dogs in the village of Rovere. The demographic make-up altered considerably at the end of this period. Dogs have been organized into social groups on the basis of amicable interactions (greetings, play, etc. and coordinated non-aggressive movement). Eighty hours of observations.

(b) Sant'Iona

	WH(M)	NI(M)	MA(M)	BL(M)	OE(F)	OP(F)	TP(F)	EY(M)	CH(M)	BI(M)
WH(M)	–									
NI(M)	49	–								
MA(M)	101	37	–							
BL(M)	13	0	0	–						
OE(F)	2	0	0	121	–					
OP(F)	0	0	0	35	33	–				
TP(F)	0	0	0	42	27	113	–			
EY(M)	0	0	0	0	0	0	0	–		
CH(M)	0	0	0	0	0	0	0	41	–	
BI(M)	0	0	0	5	2	0	0	48	92	–
NE(F)	0	0	0	0	0	0	0	77	63	69

This table shows the pattern of amicable interaction between dogs in the village of Sant'Iona in a comparable month to that shown elsewhere for Rovere. The dogs have again been organized into social groups on the basis of amicable interactions (greetings, play, etc. and coordinated non-aggressive movement). One hundred hours of observations.

Members of different sylvatic groups were never seen amicably in one another's company. Meetings between such animals were characterized by avoidance or aggression – one indication that, like their village counterparts, they were territorial.

Table 16.3 Pattern of aggressive interactions between adult dogs in (a) Rovere and (b) Sant'Iona in social groups defined from the results presented in Table 16.2.

(a) Rovere

	AU(M)	MA(M)	LI(F)	SU(M)	TI(M)	CA(M)	CR(M)	FA(M)	PO(M)
AU(M)	–								
MA(M)	0	–							
LI(F)	0	0	–						
SU(M)	5	2	2	–					
TI(M)	1	0	0	0	–				
CA(M)	3	0	0	4	1	–			
CR(M)	1	2	0	4	0	0	–		
FA(M)	0	0	0	0	0	0	0	–	
PO(M)	2	0	0	5	1	1	0	0	–
AG(F)	1	0	0	0	0	0	0	0	0

This table shows the pattern of hostile interactions between dogs in the village of Rovere. Hostilities were observed only once between members of social groups as previously defined.

(b) Sant'Iona

	WH(M)	NI(M)	MA(M)	BL(M)	OE(F)	OP(F)	TP(F)	EY(M)	CH(M)	BI(M)
WH(M)	–									
NI(M)	0	–								
MA(M)	0	0	–							
BL(M)	0	3	0	–						
OE(F)	1	0	0	0	–					
OP(F)	0	0	1	0	0	–				
TP(F)	0	0	1	0	0	0	–			
EY(M)	3	5	0	3	0	0	0	–		
CH(M)	0	2	1	1	0	0	0	0	–	
BI(M)	1	2	0	0	0	0	0	0	0	–
NE(F)	0	0	0	0	0	0	0	0	0	0

This table shows the pattern of hostile interactions between dogs in the village of Sant'Iona for a month comparable to that shown elsewhere for Rovere. No hostilities were observed between members of social groups as previously defined.

between all possible neighboring dyads, so mere lack of hostility is not a sufficient indicator of group membership.

Despite their not routinely accompanying one another, and, indeed, often spending time alone, it thus appears that village dogs do belong to social groups. These social groups also have a spatial dimension: they appear to be defending territories. The evidence for territoriality comes from two sources: their use of space, and the locations and nature of their hostile interactions with one another.

Figure 16.1 depicts the observed ranges of Roveresi dogs in spring 1981. The figure shows that the ranges of individual dogs formed three more or less exclusive clusters, which we shall refer to as the western, central and eastern (collective) ranges. Collective ranges averaged roughly 2 ha. Within two of these collective ranges, some dogs appeared to use the whole area, while others restricted most of their activities to a part of it (10 individual ranges are depicted in Figure 16.1). However, no dog's individual range was observed to straddle the border of a collective range to any significant degree.

There were, as Figure 16.1 indicates, two zones of overlap between collective ranges, of less than 5% of the range areas. These zones were the areas around two rubbish dumps at which the dogs fed.

A similar pattern of collective and largely exclusive ranges was found in Sant'Iona in spring 1983 (Figure 16.2). The village was divided into four such areas, averaging 0.25 ha. Because of the larger canine population of Sant'Iona, not all of its dogs were the objects of extended focal studies, though all were subjected to scan sampling to determine their ranges. Figure 16.2 shows three collective ranges as established from scan and focal sampling.

The overlap area of the Sant'Ionan collective ranges was somewhat larger than in Rovere but this overlap was mostly in the extensive open central area, which thus appeared to form a sort of "no dog's land" with few geographical features, where range boundaries were not clear cut (although it was the object of considerable scent marking activity).

Figures 16.1 and 16.2 also show the locations of one month's hostile interactions in the two villages. These were largely confined (45 of 59 observations in 180 hours) to the putative borders of the collective ranges, and were particularly concentrated around important feeding sites, further confirming the idea that these ranges are territories in the sense of being exclusive, defended areas. Another confirmation of this hypothesis came from the rare occasions when a dog trespassed in a neighboring range and was detected. In these cases, the trespasser would either leave immediately, or be chased out. On two occasions a trespasser was ejected by an individual it had itself ejected from its own range on a previous occasion, suggesting that location, rather than individual prowess was the deciding factor in such contests.

Village dogs were occasionally seen travelling, sometimes in company, to rubbish dumps in the vicinity and although we have no data on the frequency of these trips, Boitani *et al.* (Chapter 17) emphasize that such excursions provide an important opportunity to meet, and be recruited by, the sylvatic population.

16.4.3   Sylvatic dog society

Sylvatic dog society was different from that in the villages in one immediately noticeable respect. Sylvatic dogs were generally seen in company. It became clear during the course of the census that such associations regularly involved the same individuals, either pairs, or subsets of a single larger closed group. Four such units were identified at the beginning of the study, although, initially, one of these was actually a lone female, and two of the others were pairs.

There was a very strong tendency for these dogs to keep one another company, although nursing mothers were a partial exception to this rule. In April 1981, no sylvatic dog (apart from the female,

Nera, who was then the only animal in her range) was seen alone on more than 5% of observations. July 1981 presents a contrast. By July the females, First Mama, Second Mama and Third Mama, had all given birth (May 1981) and they were rarely seen in the company of their adult fellows.

Figure 16.3 shows the patterns of observed range-use of each of the four sylvatic social units between the summers of 1981 and 1982. The general level of separation between the groups' ranges is immediately clear. Equally clear is that there is one principal area of overlap. This is the communal dump that all sylvatic dogs used as a feeding site on a regular basis. A second "contested" area was the village of Rovere itself. This was regularly visited during the summer of 1981 by the largest group, known as HIWG, and also by dogs of the northern pair. Rovere had its own population of resident dogs (see above) and they fought the trespassing sylvatic dogs.

Fifteen aggressive incidents between members of different sylvatic groups were observed during 70 days of observation between April and August 1981 (Figure 16.3). They almost always occurred near the dump or village. Such aggression did not result in physical contact. In all 13 episodes involving the HIWG (2 vs. Nera, 4 vs. the southern pair, and 7 vs. the central pair) they were clearly victorious. When the large HIWG was involved, the other group always withdrew. In these cases, barking was often sufficient to drive off the opposition and, if this was not successful, the ensuing chase would do so. Indeed, aggression was rarely face to face: on all of seven occasions when the HIWG made a challenging bark from lying-up sites as far away as 1 km this was observed to clear the dump of rivals before any members of the group actually arrived. The remaining two encounters were between the northern and central pairs and the central and southern pairs. These encounters were confined to barking matches, and neither side forced a withdrawal by the other.

16.4.4   Food supply

Both sylvatic and village dogs depended heavily on human activity for their food. Village dogs fed mainly on domestic refuse, farmyard refuse and "handouts" from people. The distribution of refuse tips within the villages is shown in Figures 16.1 and 16.2. One dog (Livia; Rovere) was reported to have taken some live chickens. She was killed shortly afterwards by the farmer involved. Based on our observations of abundant garbage, there was no indication that the village dogs were limited by food availability. Only one dog (Video; Sant'Iona) was observed to cache food, although he did not do so on a regular basis.

In the countryside, dependence on human activity was almost as complete as in the villages. All the dogs of the Altopiano fed at the large refuse dump. Dogs belonging to HIWG scavenged from the carcasses of stock animals (two cattle and a horse) that had died within their range, although there was no evidence that the dogs had killed them (their observed interactions with horses, at least, were entirely playful). They also scavenged from Rovere and its surrounding farmyards, and broke into chicken coops on two occasions. Only once were sylvatic dogs in the study area seen to hunt a large animal. This was a red fox, and it successfully evaded them. However, two dogs, Blackwhite and Clone (who were putative father and son), were observed digging for small mammals in the banks of drainage ditches on a total of 18 occasions during the summer months of 1982 and 1983. The apparent lack of hunting in this area may be atypical – perhaps encouraged by the reliable sources of immobile food. Nearby sylvatic dogs apparently did take livestock: a pack 25 km away was reliably reported to kill foals until (illegally) poisoned. The pack of eight, occasionally observed at Rocca di Mezzo, was alleged, on two occasions, to have killed large numbers of sheep.

The dogs of HIWG seemed to decide where they would feed on a given night during the early hours of the previous morning. They visited their food sources, the dump and the village of Rovere, with approximately equal frequency during the spring and summer of 1981 and then spent the day resting in the mountains close to one or other of them. Irrespective of where they fed the previous night, if they spent the day close to Rovere they fed there by night, whereas if they slept close to the dump they fed there. On all nights when they were observed during this summer, HIWG fed at one of the two sites. During and after the winter of 1981–2, visits to Rovere became considerably rarer, but the pattern of traveling to a lying-up site adjacent to the next night's foraging site remained.

16.4.5 Reproductive behavior

A total of 17 litters whelped by nine different sylvatic bitches were recorded during the study period. Of these, 15 were born to HIWG and one each in the central and southern ranges. Village dog reproduction was subjected to considerable human interference. Only one litter was observed in Rovere (born to the female, Agrippina). This was destroyed almost immediately. Of three litters noted in Sant'Iona, one litter of five pups was allowed to live. Table 16.4 summarizes the details of sylvatic litters. Sylvatic females were generally dioestrus. Summer litters were born in May or June, winter litters in November or December. The two females that survived for the whole study period followed different patterns: Third Mama produced large litters in alternate breeding seasons and small litters or none at all in the intervals; First Mama produced median litters every season. Unfortunately, there are too few data to generalize from this observation.

Pregnant sylvatic females usually selected a rocky cleft or a tangle of exposed tree roots as a den for their pups (although, on one occasion, an underground burrow of unknown provenance was chosen). HIWG females chose sites more than 100 m above the level of the plain. For the first six

Table 16.4 The breeding pattern of HIWG sylvatic females during summers and winters 1981–3. The data are observed litter sizes.

Bitch	Season				
	S 81	W 81	S 82	W 82	S 83
1st Mama	5	5	5	?2	5
2nd Mama	9	0	D	D	D
3rd Mama	9	3	7	?2	6
Odd Mama	1	D	D	D	D
Noisy	–	9	0	D	D
New Mama	–	3	D	D	D
Pseudo Wolf	–	–	–	–	5
Total	24	20	12	?4	16
Mean pups/litter: 5.5					

D, indicates that the female died; – indicates that she had not entered the group (New Mama) or reached adult size (Pseudo Wolf and Noisy).

weeks, mothers remained with their pups unless disturbed or left for relatively short periods while feeding. In the two cases of non-HIWG sylvatic litters, the male and female of the pair stayed closely associated before and after the birth of the pups. The male slept in close proximity to the bitch and her litter and, when the pups became mobile, played with them, although in neither case was he observed to bring food to the den.

Pregnant HIWG females remained associated with the rest of the pack until they whelped. But once they had given birth, they led a semi-detached existence for several months. No dog other than the mother was seen to visit any HIWG litter, although females sometimes whelped in close proximity (within 100 m of each other on two occasions). For the first six weeks, or so, the only contact HIWG mothers appeared to have with other adult group members was when they met at feeding sites.

If the den site was approached while the mother was present, she would sometimes engage in what appeared to be a distraction display – exiting noisily from the site, and then circling quietly back to it. Such clearly detected approaches to dens sometimes resulted in a change of den site, while physical disturbance of the den, always did so. Den site changes were a significant cause of pup mortality (see below). However, two litters were apparently destroyed in their dens shortly after birth (by unknown agents – see below), so relocation may have been a less expensive option than staying put.

By the age of about 10 weeks, pups were relatively autonomous behaviorally and highly mobile. At this stage HIWG litters would move to a new site, usually still on the mountainside, but closer to a feeding site, though on two occasions such "base camps" were established in hedgerows on the plain. The two non-HIWG sylvatic litters stayed put. From 10 to 20 weeks mothers spent an increasing proportion of time away from their litters, and from about 14 weeks, surviving pups began to socialize with other adults from the group, and with any other surviving pups. Until the age of about 20 weeks, however, they continued to sleep at different sites from the other adults.

The mortality rate was high. Only 16% of 76 pups born survived to the age of 20 weeks. Identified causes of death were: adverse weather, getting left behind during den changes, getting lost when first mobile, and predation (two episodes of predation involved circumstantial evidence that the pups had been killed by a large canid, possibly a wolf or a dog). An additional hazard was the removal of pups by people seeking pets.

Of 12 pups surviving to 20 weeks over three years, four were observed to be recruited into their natal groups: three into HIWG (one male, two females) and one (male) into the central range. The fate of the remainder is unknown, but they did not disperse into other monitored packs.

16.4.6   Non-resident dogs and external recruitment

Accompanied dogs (sheepdogs with shepherds and their flocks, gun dogs with hunters, or pets with tourists) passed routinely through the area. More interesting was the arrival of unaccompanied dogs. These sometimes arrived by human agency (e.g. the reportedly common practice of releasing unwanted pets) but were, when first detected, free ranging. A dog was counted as an unaccompanied nonresident (UNR) if it was detected on two different days. Four such dogs were noted in Rovere, three in Sant'Iona and 20 in the Altopiano. Two of the Roveresi dogs were, when first detected, a mixed-sex pair. The Altopiano dogs included two groups, one of five individuals, and one of nine, and also a pair.

UNRs suffered one of four fates: some established themselves as residents, either by incorporating themselves into existing social groups, or establishing new ones. Some were killed by existing residents, and some, after remaining in the area for a few days, disappeared to an unknown fate.

Three of the four observed UNRs established themselves successfully in Rovere; two were a pair, who moved into the vacated western range six months after its occupants had been killed in April 1981. The third, a male, joined the eastern group a year after the beginning of the study. However, a fourth dog, also male, was killed shortly after his arrival in a nocturnal fight with members of HIWG on the edge of the village. Three male UNRs arrived in Sant'Iona in the summer of 1982.

The most notable UNRs in the Altopiano were the two large groups. These appeared in successive summers (1981, 1982), in each case first being spotted in the south of the area. The first group consisted of five individuals (three males, two females). They had two observed hostile encounters with HIWG, both lasting for around 15 minutes and involving barking and chasing, but no physical contact. In both of these encounters, the intruders were driven off by the residents. The last contact with this group was five days after the first. The second group consisted of nine beagle-like hounds. No interactions between this group and any residents were observed, and the period between first and last sightings was seven days.

Five UNRs were observed to establish themselves in the area. Two were a pair who took over the northern range four months after the last observation of the female, Nera. A third was a female who joined the pair occupying the central range, and the fourth a male who succeeded in becoming a member of HIWG. The fifth, the female, New Mama joined the HIWG in late summer of 1981, whelped three pups in autumn of which none survived, and herself died before the following spring. One UNR in the Altopiano was almost certainly killed by resident dogs of HIWG, although the fight was not observed.

All UNRs appeared during spring and summer. This reinforces Boitani et al.'s (Chapter 17) suspicion that dispersal from villages and recruitment to the sylvatic population is greatest during the mating season, perhaps involving the attraction of male village dogs to sylvatic females on heat.

16.5   Discussion and conclusions

In summary, free-living dogs in this part of Italy appear to adjust their behavior to their local circumstances. In the villages, they adopt a "fox-like" existence in which individuals live in loose social groups that defend a territory, but pursue a relatively solitary existence. In the countryside, sylvatic dogs adopt a more wolf-like lifestyle, generally operating as a pack, although individuals sometimes travel alone. Both village and sylvatic dogs were largely dependent for food on human activity and, in the villages at least, were subjected to significant human interference, a fact reflected in their sex ratios and the culled litters. That males are more tolerated by villagers than females was confirmed in conversations.

During 1981–3 population levels appeared stable, although recruitment from outside was important. No dog was observed to change group or to disperse. The groups of dogs clearly had social integrity: relationships within groups were largely amicable, those between groups were hostile, and fights could be fatal between neighboring groups and when resident dogs encountered itinerants.

Many of our observations agree with those made of other free-roaming dogs: male-biased sex ratios are common in free-roaming dogs (e.g. Daniels, 1983a, 1983b; Pal, 2001) and probably result from human interference with the population from which these dogs are drawn (but see Pal, 2003). The home range sizes we recorded are of the same order as those noted elsewhere, varying between 2–10 ha for urban dogs (e.g. Berman & Dunbar, 1983; Pal et al. 1998) and 4–10 km^2 (e.g. Scott & Causey, 1973) for rural dogs. From Alabama to Illinois, packs of "feral" dogs number 2–6 adults (e.g. Nesbitt, 1975; Scott & Causey, 1973) – compared with which the HIWG was rather large. We have few data on the breeding system of our dogs, but the association between pairs even within the HIWG is in accord with other observations (Daniels, 1983b). Multiple pairs breeding within larger packs of wild canids are uncommon, but have been recorded for coyotes (Camenzind, 1978), wolves (van Ballenberghe, 1983), African wild dogs (Creel *et al.* 1997) and, circumstantially, golden jackals (Macdonald, 1979). The behavior of Abruzzese free-roaming dogs is reviewed more fully by Boitani *et al.* (Chapter 17), and our observations fit within the general pattern of previous observations.

We will conclude by readdressing our three initial questions. First, how does the behavior of these free-living dogs relate to observations on other canids? Second, can the contrasting behavior of village and sylvatic dogs be interpreted within the framework of ideas on ecological pressures affecting carnivore society? Third, is it appropriate to seek adaptive explanations for the behavior of these dogs? In exploring these questions we have the great advantage of comparing our results with those gathered subsequently on the same population by our colleagues Boitani *et al.* (Chapter 17).

16.5.1   Inter-specific comparisons

While this is not the place for a comprehensive review of canid social systems, we note certain striking parallels between the behavior of these dogs and that of some other species.

The sylvatic dogs formed packs that have much in common with those described for wolves in many parts of their range (see review by Harrington *et al.*, 1982). Like wolves, these dogs apparently benefited from strength of numbers and, on occasion, killed rival conspecifics. Unlike wolves, they showed no evidence of co-operative care of young or of adoption, although these traits are widespread in wild canids (reviewed in Macdonald & Moehlman, 1982; see also Jennions & Macdonald, 1994). Nevertheless, these dogs were sympatric with the remnant wolf population of the Abruzzo, and actually traveled much smaller territories and behaved as a more coherent pack than is common amongst the local wolves (Boitani, 1983). In contrast, the village dogs displayed a social system that was strikingly similar to that of red foxes (Macdonald, 1981; Mela & Weber 1996) although their territories did not drift as do those of some urban foxes (Doncaster & Macdonald, 1991).

Out of this comparison the obvious question is why do foxes not form packs when feeding at superabundant rubbish tips, such as on the Altopiano. Indeed, red foxes did feed from that same tip, and from similar ones in the Abruzzo region (Macdonald *et al.*, 1980b). In these cases, even if a group used the tip, they never moved as a cohesive pack, although members of larger groups monopolized access and defeated members of smaller groups and occasionally joined forces to repel intruders (e.g. Macdonald, 1987, pp. 80–2). The ecological circumstances of tip-feeding foxes are so similar to those of the HIWG that the contrast is puzzling. Of course, in such cases, the foxes have larger competitors around (e.g. dogs and wolves), but so too the sylvatic dogs (though larger than foxes) were obliged to compete with wolves. Although it is an untestable hypothesis there seems little choice but to resort to a phylogenetic argument: packing is a behavior never observed amongst vulpine foxes, but frequently observed in lupine canids.

16.5.2   Ecological pressures acting on dog society

The refuse on which both village and sylvatic dogs depend is clearly defendable. Furthermore, a dog arriving at a rubbish site in the wake of an intruder could find the food gone. Territoriality is the general solution to safeguarding economically defendable resources. Range configurations and aggression between neighbors both indicated that village and sylvatic dogs were territorial.

The refuse tips, farmyard scraps, and food handouts on which the village dogs depended were unpredictable. Householders dumped food on an unpredictable schedule, in variable quantities, and it was collected erratically each week. It was obvious that no single dump would provide adequate food security for even one dog, and so we conclude that it was necessary for a village dog to configure its territory so as to encompass several potential feeding sites, thereby hedging its bets. Within such a territory, however, several dumps might be fruitful on a particular day, and sometimes a particular dump might be supplied with enough edible scraps to satisfy more than one dog. These are the circumstances that Macdonald (1981) proposed would lead to red foxes living in social groups – since empirically supported by a range of studies (e.g. Bino et al., 2010; Macdonald et al., 1999; Mela & Weber, 1996; Poulle et al., 1994) – and there is much in common between the behavior of the village dogs and that of foxes. If group size is limited by food (more probably it is limited, in this case, by human interference), the simplest prediction of the RDH would be a correlation between patch richness during periods of minimum food availability (bottleneck periods) and group size. Our data on food availability are inadequate to test this.

Assessment of the availability of food to village dogs is complicated because they had the opportunity to make excursions to nearby communal rubbish dumps. Such excursions led to a relatively predictable and abundant food source, but may have involved some danger in encounters with sylvatic dogs.

The sylvatic dogs depended on food scavenged from the Altopiano tip and throughout Rovere, sites separated by a distance of roughly 2.7 km. There is thus an association between patch dispersion and territory size, but this is complicated by the fact that sylvatic dogs also required access to safe refuges in the forest, and they may have visited villages in search of resources other than food (e.g. females). Why did group size in the villages vary between 2 and 5, whereas in the countryside it was between 1 and 10? We propose that the mean group size of 3.5 in seven village groups reflects the modest richness of the unpredictable dumps from which they fed. In contrast, food at the Altopiano dump was very abundant and possibly superabundant. The high maximum group size (10 adults, HIWG 1981) accords with this high patch richness. The great variance in group size of sylvatic dogs is explicable because all the other groups in the vicinity were subjugated by the HIWG, and thus had effectively reduced access to food. The eight adults using the Rocca di Mezzo dump were in analogous circumstances to those of the HIWG.

Why did the sylvatic dogs form packs? We found no evidence of co-operative hunting, none of communal pup care (nor adoption), but ample evidence of the benefits of strength of numbers. The success of the HIWG in driving smaller groups of sylvatic dogs (and itinerants) from the Altopiano dump, and from Rovere during raids, was conspicuous. Furthermore, it directly parallels observations on other canids in which larger packs prevail (e.g. coyotes, Bekoff & Wells, 1980, 1986; golden jackals, Macdonald, 1979; and jackals, Moehlman, 1989). It also parallels interspecific clashes, e.g. the capacity of larger groups of spotted hyaena to withstand piratical lions and vice versa (Cooper, 1991; Kruuk, 1972). Such advantages of co-operative defence are particularly marked amongst competing species of canids (Fanshawe & Fitzgibbon, 1993; Lamprecht, 1978; see also Macdonald & Sillero-Zubiri, 2004), making it interesting to know whether larger packs of sylvatic dogs fare better in encounters with wolves. It seems likely that wolves were a major factor affecting the sylvatic dogs, both as predators and competitors. Competition with coyotes affects the spatial organization of red foxes (Voigt & Earle, 1983), inter-specific competition may result in character displacement in canids (Dayan et al., 1989, 1992), and behavioral domination of smaller canids by larger sympatric species is widespread (Hersteinsson & Macdonald, 1992; Paquet, 1992; Sargeant & Allen, 1989; Tannerfeldt et al., 2002). Certainly, similarities in the niches of wolf and sylvatic dog in Italy indicate the potential for strong competition between them (Boitani, 1983). The movement patterns of sylvatic dogs and their tendency to travel as a pack may both have been affected by the likelihood of encounters with wolves. Indeed, the configuration of their territory may have tessellated between wolf ranges in just the way that red fox ranges squeeze between coyote territories (Voigt & Earle, 1983). The cohesiveness of the HIWG was forcefully illustrated on the occasion when one of them was snared and the remainder of the pack stayed at hand barking ferociously even when closely approached, in contrast to their normal timorousness. The advantages of strength of numbers would be predicted to lead to an arms race to recruit a larger group and perhaps even to expansionism (*sensu* Kruuk & Macdonald, 1985; see also Loveridge *et al.*, 2009).

It seems unsurprising that the sylvatic dogs packed together, but why then did the village dogs not do so as well? One possibility is that they did not need to: the small diameter (the largest, in Rovere, were less than 200 m across) of village territories meant that members of a collective group were invariably within earshot of each other. If the food available at any site was often likely to be insufficient for more than one dog then travelling in company could be disadvantageous. Equally, travelling singly might be the best way to intercept intruders, knowing that a bark can bring help within seconds. According to this scenario, greater patch dispersion, combined with large patch size, might favour packing to ensure that assistance was on hand.

16.5.3   The adaptive significance of dog behavior

The interpretation of the behavior of free-roaming domestic animals is complicated by effects of artificial selection. Insofar as behavior patterns may have been directly selected by humans, or may be pleiotropic corollaries of selection for other traits (e.g. see Belaev & Trut, 1975; Wiren *et al.*, 2009), it may be inappropriate to assume that domestic animals behave adaptively. This misgiving has been widely voiced in the interpretation of the behavior of free-roaming cats. However, Macdonald *et al.* (1987) and Kerby & Macdonald (1988) have argued that farm cats are sufficiently independent of humans that their behavior may plausibly be interpreted in functional terms. Nonetheless, Macdonald (unpublished) radio-tracked the ancestral *Felis silvestris lybica* and found that it persists in feeding solitarily around rubbish dumps at which free-ranging domestic cats form groups.

Is it sensible to consider free-living dogs as wolves, of which they are, by any genetical standard, merely a subspecies? There are some substantial differences, of which the wolf's 25% larger relative brain size is one (Coppinger & Schneider, 1995). Furthermore, there are behavioral anomalies. Kleiman & Malcolm's (1981) observation that domestic dogs are the only canids in which males show no paternal care may indicate either an adaptive departure, an artifact of domestication, or a dearth of observation. In comparison to domestic cats, it is far harder to argue that dogs have continued to be subject to natural selection throughout their association with humans. The anatomical consequences of selective breeding are obvious in the differences between domestic breeds, and behavioral differences are equally marked (Starling *et al.* 2013; Zimen, 1972). Lord *et al.*, Chapter 4, show intriguing ontogenetic differences in the behavior of puppies from livestock guarding and herding breeds of dog. The quality of play in these breeds is almost totally different from the age of 10 weeks. Breed differences have tangible physiological bases: the concentration of dopamine (a precursor of adrenal biosynthesis) in the brains of herding border collies is substantially greater than in the brains of the guarding maremmas from which our study population partly descended. The minimal exposure of most domestic dogs to natural selection, the extreme pressure of artificial selection, the scope for pleiotropic genetic effects, and the potential impact that breed differences might have on the behavior of a group of free-living dogs, all combine to sound a note of extreme caution in seeking too precise an adaptive interpretation to their behavior.

On the other hand, the speed of selective change is sometimes remarkable. Although the example is back to front, Belaev & Trut (1975) managed to breed placid, sociable foxes from hysterically nervous wild-types in just 20 generations (and this change coincided, pleiotropically, with the appearance of attractively piebald coat colours and dioestrous reproductive cycles). Furthermore, there is one overwhelmingly compelling line of evidence that our free-living dogs were behaving adaptively: as predicted on adaptationist arguments, individuals from the same population behaved quite differently when exposed to contrasting ecological circumstances.

The interpretation of village dog society is complicated, more than is that of sylvatic dogs, by the active involvement of people. Although the link may be tenuous, most of these dogs were notionally owned by somebody, and we cannot exclude the influence of this ownership during ontogeny as a factor shaping adult dog behavior and movements (as argued elsewhere by Daniels & Bekoff, 1989b). Furthermore, villagers may have affected group size directly, as they manifestly affected sex ratio and breeding success. Nonetheless, we were impressed by the autonomy of the village dogs and judge that it is fruitful to consider seriously the proposition that at least many aspects of their behavior have functional explanations.

16.5.4 The role of chance: the social flux model

Both sylvatic and village communities were subject to drastic density independent mortality at various ages. Pups were routinely killed *en masse* and females were selectively culled. In Rovere the seemingly stable organization described in 1981 was shattered by the violent deaths of several dogs (shot, hit by cars, etc.), and the composition of groups was affected by recruitment of immigrants into existing groups and by immigrants occupying vacant territories. The sylvatic dogs were shot and poisoned, their pups were stolen as pets, killed by storms and by other canids. Between 1981 and 1983 the HIWG recruited three pups born into the pack, and two apparently unrelated immigrants. We conclude that groups of free-living dogs suffer frequent changes in composition and in kinship structure. Stochastic events may determine the balance of kin versus outside recruits in the pack at any given time.

This state of affairs leads to two observations. First, immigration of unrelated outsiders into groups where individuals of the same sex are already present occurs in some wild carnivore societies (e.g. dwarf mongoose, Rood, 1987; red foxes, Zabel, 1986) including wolves (Lehman *et al.*, 1992). Therefore, the commonly reported presence of immigrants in dog groups (e.g. Daniels & Bekoff, 1989b; Pal, 2001; Scott & Causey, 1973) does not make them qualitatively different from other carnivore groups, although they may be unusual in the high frequency of immigration. Recruitment into sylvatic groups may be associated with some social turmoil, particularly if it tends to occur in the mating season. Second, many canid societies are largely based on kin groups, and kin selection is frequently invoked as a contributor to their behavior (e.g. Macdonald & Moehlman, 1982; Ralls *et al.*, 2001). Furthermore, high rates of density independent mortality have been linked in urban red foxes with drifting territoriality, absence of social suppression of reproduction, and an hypothesized disruption of the social hierarchy (Doncaster & Macdonald, 1991). In summary, frequent perturbation of dog group structure might be expected to alter the nature of social relationships, and we predict that these relationships will be qualitatively different in periods of stability where kinship bonds develop, as distinct from periods of high mortality when unrelated recruits may predominate.

In this context, it is noteworthy that between 1981 and 1983 we found only two unrelated immigrants in the HIWG. In contrast, Boitani *et al.* (Chapter 17) studied the same group between 1984 and 1987, during which time, although the total group size remained unchanged, there was a continual flux of immigrants such that only one survivor of the 1981–3 period was present in 1987.

We conclude that 1981–3 was, by chance, a less perturbed period for the HIWG, and was characterized by a move towards longstanding social ties and kinship ties, whereas the opposite circumstances prevailed in Boitani's 1984–7 study. If this hypothesis has any validity it could be that corollaries of the shift are: (1) synchronous reproduction in 1981–3 but not in 1984–7; and (2) stability of territorial configuration. Boitani *et al.* (Chapter 17) report that at approximately six-month intervals the home range borders shifted so that over three years the total range of the HIWG was roughly 30 km², whereas it was only about 10 km² at any given time. In red foxes perturbation is associated with shifting prevailing ranges (Doncaster & Macdonald, 1991). Range shifts in our sylvatic dog groups may arise because resources shift, wolf ranges shift, a change in composition of the pack alters the balance of strength, or because new recruits blend part of their previous range with that of the existing group.

Acknowledgements

This work was funded by a grant to DWM from the Waltham Centre for Pet Nutrition. We warmly acknowledge the friendship and collaboration of our colleague, Professor Luigi Boitani, and we thank him, along with Drs John Bradshaw and James Serpell for their forebearance. The manuscript benefited greatly due to comments from L. Boitani and S. Creel.

References

Beck, A. M. (1973). *The Ecology of Stray Dogs: A Study of Free-Ranging Urban Animals.* Baltimore, MD: York Press.

Bekoff, M. & Wells, M. C. (1980). The social ecology of coyotes. *Scientific American*, 242: 130–51.

Bekoff, M. & Wells, M. C. (1986). Social ecology and behavior of coyotes. *Advances in the Study of Behavior* 16: 251–338.

Belaev, D. K. & Trut, L. N. (1975). Some genetic and endocrine effects of selection for domestication in silver foxes. In *The Wild Canids*, ed. M. W. Fox. New York: Van Nostrand Reinhold, pp. 416–26.

Berman, M. & Dunbar, I. (1983). The social behavior of free-ranging suburban dogs. *Applied Animal Ethology*, 10: 5–17.

Bhunu, C. P. (2011). Impact of culling stray dogs and vaccination on the control of human rabies: a mathematical modeling approach. *International Journal of Biomathematics*, 4: 379–97.

Bino, G., Dolev, A., Yosha, D., Guter, A., King, R., Saltz, D. & Kark, S. (2010). Abrupt spatial and numerical responses of overabundant foxes to a reduction in anthropogenic resources. *Journal of Applied Ecology*, 47: 1262–71.

Blackwell, P. & Bacon, P. J. (1993). A critique of the territory inheritance hypothesis. *Animal Behaviour*, 46: 821–3.

Boitani, L. (1983). Wolf and dog competition in Italy. *Acta Zoologica Fennica*, 174: 259–64.

Boitani, L. & Ciucci, P. (1995). Comparative social ecology of feral dogs and wolves. *Ethology Ecology & Evolution*, 7: 49–72.

Boitani, L. & Fabbri, M. L. (1983). Censimento dei cani in Italia con particulari reguardo al fenomeno del randagismo. *Ricerche di Biologia delta Selvaggina* (INBS, Bologna), 73: 1–51.

Bonanni, R., Cafazzo, S., Valsecchi, P. & Natoli, E. (2010a). Effect of affiliative and agonistic relationships on leadership behaviour in free-ranging dogs. *Animal Behaviour*, 79: 981–91.

Bonanni, R., Valsecchi, P. & Natoli, E. (2010b). Pattern of individual participation and cheating in conflicts between groups of free-ranging dogs. *Animal Behaviour*, 79: 957–68.

Camenzind, F. (1978). Behavioral ecology of the coyote in the national Elk Refuge, Jackson, Wyoming. In *Coyotes: Biology, Behavior and Management*, ed. M. Bekoff. New York: Academic Press, pp. 267–94.

Carr, G. M. & Macdonald, D. W. (1986). The sociality of solitary foragers: a model based on resource dispersion. *Animal Behaviour*, 35: 1540–9.

Cooper, S. M. (1991). Optimal hunting group-size – the need for lions to defend their kills against loss to spotted hyaenas. *African Journal of Ecology*, 29: 130–6.

Coppinger, R. P. & Schneider, R. A. (1995). Evolution of working dogs. In *The Domestic Dog: Its Evolution,*

339 **David W. Macdonald and Geoffrey M. Carr**

Behaviour and Interactions with People, ed. J. Serpell. Cambridge: Cambridge University Press, pp. 21–47.

Creel, S., Creel, N. M., Mills, M. G. L. & Monfort, S. L. (1997). Rank and reproduction in cooperatively breeding African wild dogs: Behavioral and endocrine correlates. *Behavioral Ecology*, 8: 298–306.

Daniels, M. J., Beaumont, M. A., Johnson, P. J., Balharry, D., Macdonald, D. W. & Barratt, E. (2001). Ecology and genetics of wild-living cats in the north-east of Scotland and the implications for the conservation of the wildcat. *Journal of Applied Ecology*, 55: 263–72.

Daniels, T. J. (1983a). The social organization of free-ranging urban dogs. I: Non-estrous social behavior. *Applied Animal Ethology*, 10: 341–63.

Daniels, T. J. (1983b). The social organization of free-ranging urban dogs. II: Estrous groups and the mating system. *Applied Animal Ethology*, 10: 365–73.

Daniels, T. J. & Bekoff, M. (1989a). Spatial and temporal resource use by feral and abandoned dogs. *Ethology*, 81: 300–12.

Daniels, T. J. & Bekoff, M. (1989b). Population and social biology of free-ranging dogs, *Canis familiaris. Journal of Mammalogy*, 70: 754–62.

Dayan, T., Simberloff, D., Tchernov, E. & Yomtov, Y. (1992). Canine carnassials – character displacement in the wolves, jackals and foxes of Israel. *Biological Journal of the Linnean Society*, 45: 315–31.

Dayan, T., Tchernov, E., Yom-Tov, Y. & Simberloff, D. (1989). Ecological character displacement in Saharo-Arabian *Vulpes*: outfoxing Bergmann's rule. *Oikos*, 38: 146–61.

Doncaster, C. P. & Macdonald, D. W. (1991). Drifting territoriality in the red fox, *Vulpes vulpes. Journal of Animal Ecology*, 60: 423–39.

Driscoll, C. A., Macdonald, D. W. & O'Brien, S. J. (2009). From wild animals to domestic pets, an evolutionary view of domestication. *Proceedings of the National Academy of Sciences of the United States of America*, 106: 9971–8.

Fanshawe, J. H. & Fitzgibbon, C. D. (1993). Factors influencing the hunting success of an African wild dog pack. *Animal Behaviour*, 45: 479–90.

Ginsberg, J. & Macdonald, D. W. (1990). *Foxes, Wolves, Jackals and Dogs: Action Plan for the Conservation of Canids*. Gland, Switzerland: IUCN Publications.

Gittleman, J. L. (1989). Carnivore group living: comparative trends. In *Carnivore Behaviour, Ecology, and Evolution*, ed. J. L. Gittleman. London: Chapman & Hall, pp. 183–207.

Harrington, F. H., Paquet, P. C, Ryon, J. & Fentress, J. C. (1982). Monogamy in wolves: a review of the evidence. In *Wolves of the World, Perspectives of Behavior, Ecology and Conservation*, eds. F. H. Harrington & P. C. Paquet. Park Ridge, NJ: Noyes Publications, pp. 209–22.

Hersteinsson, P. & Macdonald, D. W. (1992). Interspecific competition and the geographic distribution of red and arctic foxes (*Vulpes vulpes* and *Alopex lagopus*). *Oikos*, 58: 505–15.

Jennions, M. D. & Macdonald, D. W. (1994). Cooperative breeding in mammals. *Trends in Ecology & Evolution*, 9: 89–93.

Johnson, D. D. P. (2003). Sentenced without trial: reviling and revamping the Resource Dispersion Hypothesis. *Oikos*, 101: 433–40.

Johnson, D. D. P., Jetz, W. & Macdonald, D. W. (2002). Environmental correlates of badger social spacing across Europe. *Journal of Biogeography*, 29: 411–25.

Kerby, G. & Macdonald, D. W. (1988). Social behaviour of farm cats. In *The Domestic Cat: The Biology of its Behaviour*, eds. D. Turner & P. Bateson. Cambridge: Cambridge University Press, pp. 67–81.

Kleiman, D. G. & Malcom, J. R. (1981). The evolution of male parental investment in mammals. In *Parental Care in Mammals*, eds. D. J. Gubernik & P. H. Klopfer. New York: Plenum, pp. 347–87.

Kruuk, H. (1972). *The Spotted Hyaena: a Study of Predation and Social Behavior*. Chicago, IL: University of Chicago Press.

Kruuk, H. (1975). Functional aspects of social hunting by carnivores. In *Function and Evolution in Behaviour*, eds. G. Baerends, C. Beer & A. Manning. Oxford: Clarendon Press, pp. 119–41.

Kruuk, H. & Macdonald, D. W. (1985). Group territories of carnivores: empires and enclaves. In *Behavioural Ecology: Ecological Consequences of Adaptive Behaviour*, eds. R. Sibley & R. Smith. Oxford: Blackwell Scientific Publications, pp. 521–36.

Kruuk, H. & Snell, H. (1981). Prey selection by feral dogs from a population of marine iguanas (*Amblyrhynchus cristatus*). *Journal of Applied Ecology*, 18: 197–204.

Lamprecht, J. (1978). The relationship between food competition and foraging group size in some larger carnivores. *Zeitschrift für Tierpsychologie*, 46: 337–43.

Lehman, N., Clarkson, P., Mech, L. D., Meier, T. H. & Wayne, R. (1992). A study of genetic relationships within and among wolf packs using DNA fingerprinting and mitochondrial DNA. *Behavioural Ecology & Sociobiology*, 30: 83–94.

Liberg, O., Sandell, M., Pontier, D. & Natoli, E. (2000). Density, spatial organisation and reproductive tactics in the domestic cat and other felids. In *The Domestic Cat: The Biology of its Behaviour*, eds. D. C. Turner & P. P. G. B. Bateson. Cambridge: Cambridge University Press, pp. 119–47.

Lindstrom, E. (1986). Territory inheritance and the evolution of group living in carnivores. *Animal Behaviour*, 34: 1825–35.

Loveridge, A. J., Valeix, M., Davidson, Z., Murindagomo, F., Fritz, H. & Macdonald, D. W. (2009). Changes in home range size of African lions in relation to pride size and prey biomass in a semi-arid savanna. *Ecography*, 32: 953–62.

Macdonald, D. W. (1979). Flexibility of the social organization of the golden jackal, *Canis aureus*. *Behavioral Ecology and Sociobiology*, 5: 17–38.

Macdonald, D. W. (1981). Resource dispersion and the social organisation of the red fox (*Vulpes vulpes*). In *Worldwide Furbearer Conference Proceedings*, Vol. 2, eds. J. Chapman & D. Pursley. Frostburg, MD: R.R. Donnelley, pp. 918–49.

Macdonald, D. W. (1983). The ecology of carnivore social behaviour. *Nature*, 301: 379–84.

Macdonald, D. W. (1987). *Running with the Fox*. London: Unwin Hyman.

Macdonald, D. W. (1992). *The Velvet Claw: A Natural History of the Carnivores*. London: BBC Books.

Macdonald, D. W. & Amlaner, C. J. (1980). A practical guide to radio tracking. In *A Handbook on Biotelemetry and Radio Tracking*, eds. C. J. Amlaner Jr & D. W. Macdonald. Oxford: Pergamon Press, pp. 143–59.

Macdonald, D. W., Apps, P. J., Carr, G. & Kerby, G. (1987). Social behaviour, nursing coalitions and infanticide in a colony of farm cats. *Advances in Ethology*, 28: 1–66.

Macdonald, D. W., Ball, F. & Hough, N. G. (1980a). The evaluation of home range size and configuration using radio-tracking data. In *A Handbook on Biotelemetry and Radio Tracking*, eds. C. J. Amlaner Jr & D. W. Macdonald. Oxford: Pergamon Press, pp. 405–24.

Macdonald, D. W., Barasso, P. & Boitani, L. (1980b). Foxes, wolves and conservation in the Abruzzo Mts., Italy. In *The Red Fox, Behaviour and Ecology*, ed. E. Ziman. The Hague: W. Junk, pp. 223–35.

Macdonald, D. W. & Carr, G. M. (1989). Food security and the rewards of tolerance. In *Comparative Socioecology: the Behavioural Ecology of Humans and other Mammals*, eds. V. Standen & R. A. Foley. Oxford: Blackwell Scientific Publications, pp. 75–99.

Macdonald, D. W., Courtenay, O., Forbes, S. & Mathews, F. (1999). The red fox (*Vulpes vulpes*) in Saudi Arabia: loose-knit groupings in the absence of territoriality. *Journal of Zoology*, 249: 383–391.

Macdonald, D. W., Loveridge, A. J. & Nowell, K. (2010). Dramatis personae: an introduction to the wild felids. In *Biology and Conservation of Wild Felids*, eds. D. W. Macdonald & A.J. Loveridge. Oxford: Oxford University Press, pp. 3–58.

Macdonald, D. W. & Moehlman, P. D. (1982). Cooperation, altruism and restraint in the reproduction of carnivores. In *Perspectives in Ethology*, Vol. 5, eds. P. P. G. Bateson & P. Klopfer. New York: Plenum Press, pp. 443–67.

Macdonald, D. W. & Sillero-Zubiri, C. (2004). Dramatis personae. In *Biology and Conservation of Wild Canids*, eds. D. W. Macdonald & C. Sillero-Zubiri. Oxford: Oxford University Press, pp. 3–36.

Mangalam, M. & Singh, M. (2013). Differential foraging strategies: motivation, perception and implementation in urban free-ranging dogs, *Canis familiaris*. *Animal Behaviour*, 85: 763–70.

Mela, J. S. & Weber, J. M. (1996). Social organization of red foxes (*Vulpes vulpes*) in the Swiss Jura mountains. *Zeitschrift Fur Saugetierkunde-International Journal of Mammalian Biology*, 61: 257–68.

Mills, M. G. L. (1990). *Kalahari Hyaenas: The Comparative Behavioural Ecology of Two Species*. London: Unwin Hyman.

Moehlman, P. D. (1989). Intraspecific variation in canid social systems. In *Carnivore Behavior, Ecology, and Evolution*, ed. J. L. Gittleman. Ithaca, NY: Cornell University Press, pp. 164–82.

Nesbitt, W. H. (1975). Ecology of a feral dog pack on a wildlife refuge. In *The Wild Canids*, ed. M. W. Fox. New York: Van Nostrand Reinhold, pp. 391–5.

Newman, C., Zhou, Y. B., Buesching, C. D., Kaneko, Y. & Macdonald, D. W. (2011). Contrasting sociality in two widespread, generalist, mustelid genera, *Meles* and *Martes*. *Mammal Study*, 36: 169–88.

Pal, S. K. (2001). Population ecology of free-ranging urban dogs in West Bengal, India. *Acta Theriologica*, 46: 69–78.

Pal, S. K. (2003). Reproductive behaviour of free-ranging rural dogs in West Bengal, India. *Acta Theriologica*, 48: 271–81.

Pal, S. K., Ghosh, B. & Roy, S. (1998). Dispersal behaviour of free-ranging dogs (*Canis familiaris*) in relation to age, sex, season and dispersal distance. *Applied Animal Behaviour Science*, 61: 123–32.

Paquet, P. C. (1992). Prey use strategies of sympatric wolves and coyotes in Riding-Mountain-National-Park, Manitoba. *Journal of Mammalogy*, 73: 337–43.

Poulle, M. L., Artois, M. & Roeder, J. J. (1994). Dynamics of spatial relationships among members of a fox group (*Vulpes vulpes*, Mammalia, Carnivora). *Journal of Zoology*, 233: 93–106.

Ralls, K., Pilgrim, K. L., White, P. J., Paxinos, E. E., Schwartz, M. K. & Fleischer, R. C. (2001). Kinship social relationships, and den sharing in kit foxes. *Journal of Mammalogy*, 82: 858–66.

Rood, J. (1987). Dispersal and intergroup transfer in the dwarf mongoose. In *Mammalian Dispersal Patterns: the Effects of Social Structure on Population Genetics*, eds. B. D. Chepko-Sade & Z. T. Halpin. Chicago, IL: University of Chicago Press, pp. 85–103.

Sargeant, A. B. & Allen, S. H. (1989). Observed interactions between coyotes and red foxes. *Journal of Mammalogy*, 70: 631–3.

Scott, J. P. & Fuller, J. L. (1965). *Genetics and the Social Behavior of the Dog*. Chicago, IL: University of Chicago Press.

Scott, M. D. & Causey, K. (1973). Ecology of feral dogs in Alabama. *Journal of Wildlife Management*, 37: 253–65.

Starling, M. J., Branson, N., Thomson, P. C. & Mcgreevy, P. D. (2013). "Boldness" in the domestic dog differs among breeds and breed groups. *Behavioural Processes*, 97: 53–62.

Tallents, L. A., Randall, D. A., Williams, S. D. & Macdonald, D. W. (2012). Territory quality determines social group composition in Ethiopian wolves, *Canis simensis*. *Journal of Animal Ecology*, 81: 24–35.

Tannerfeldt, M., Elmhagen, B. & Angerbjorn, A. (2002). Exclusion by interference competition? The relationship between red and arctic foxes. *Oecologia*, 132: 213–20.

van Ballenberghe, V. (1983). Two litters raised in one year by a wolf pack. *Journal of Mammalogy*, 64: 171–3.

Voigt, D. R. & Earle, B. D. (1983). Avoidance of coyotes by red fox families. *Journal of Wildlife Management*, 47: 852–7.

Wiren, A., Gunnarsson, U., Andersson, L. & Jensen, P. (2009). Domestication-related genetic effects on social behavior in chickens – Effects of genotype at a major growth quantitative trait locus. *Poultry Science*, 88: 1162–1166.

Woodroffe, R. & Macdonald, D. W. (1993). Badger sociality – models of spatial grouping. *Proceedings of the Symposia of the Zoological Society of London*, 65: 145–69.

World Health Organization (WHO) (1988). *Report of WHO Consultation on Dog Ecology Studies Related to Rabies Control*. WHO/Rabies Research 88.25.

Young, J. K., Olson, K. A., Reading, R. P., Amgalanbaatar, S. & Berger, J. (2011). Is wildlife going to the dogs? Impacts of feral and free-roaming dogs on wildlife populations. *Bioscience*, 61: 125–132.

Zabel, C. J. (1986). Reproductive behavior of the red fox (*Vulpes vulpes*): a longitudinal study of an island population. Unpublished Ph.D. dissertation. University of California, CA, USA.

Zimen, E. (1972). *Wolfe und Königspudel – Vergleichende Verhaltensbeobachtungen*. Munich: R. Piper Verlag.

17

The ecology and behavior of feral dogs: A case study from central Italy

LUIGI BOITANI, FRANCESCO FRANCISCI, PAOLO CIUCCI AND GIORGIO ANDREOLI

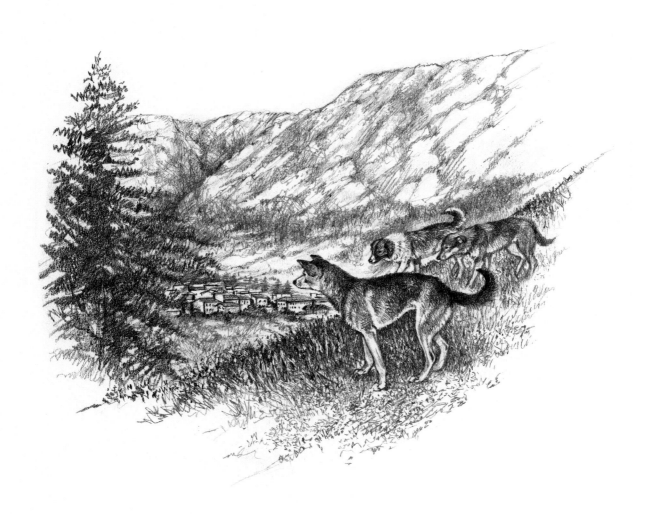

17.1   Feral dogs: A definition

What exactly is a feral dog? Dogs are not a homogeneous category and their immense diversity of phenotypes and functional specializations hinders any unambiguous classification (Boitani *et al.*, 2006). Dog categories have been proposed on the basis of a variety of natural history traits and relationships with humans: behavioral and ecological traits (Causey & Cude, 1980; Scott & Causey, 1973); origins (Daniels & Bekoff, 1989a, 1989b); rural vs. urban habitat (Berman & Dunbar, 1983); access to public property (Beck, 1973), and level of dependency on humans (WHO, 1988). This diversity of definitions contributes to the difficulty of comparing results from different studies, while the great variety of ecological contexts of urban, rural and "natural" habitats means that such comparisons may only yield a confirmation of the high ecological and behavioral flexibility of dogs.

Boitani & Fabbri (1983a), Perry (1993) and Vanak & Gompper (2009) proposed similar classifications based on dogs' associations with humans. While Perry's categories were functional to his work in managing a rabies control program, Boitani and Fabbri were more interested in the ecology of dog populations in their natural environment. Boitani & Fabbri (1983a) proposed four categories (owned restricted, owned unrestricted, stray and feral dogs) based on the type of social bond with humans, and the ecology of dogs with varying degrees of human dependency. The first two categories are similar to Perry's (1993), i.e. restricted and family dogs. A restricted dog is fully dependent on (all its needs provided intentionally), and also restricted by, humans. Family dogs have an owner on whom they depend, but may be only semi-restricted or left free to roam (Hsu *et al.*, 2003). The third category, stray dogs, is a heterogeneous group that includes dogs that still have a social bond with humans (possibly abandoned or born into human settings), and dogs with different degrees of fear/tolerance towards humans. Stray dogs live near human settings where they find food and shelter regardless of whether these resources are intentionally provided by humans or are causally associated with them (e.g. handouts, refuse tips or garbage dumps for food, structures for shelter, etc.). These dogs are a common sight across most continents and have been consistently reported by many authors; those roaming many of the large cities of the Mediterranean basin (Istanbul, Alexandria) were even described in the eighteenth century as separate subspecies (cf. Brehm, 1893). They are often called "village dogs" (Macdonald & Carr, Chapter 16; Ortolani *et al.*, 2009). Finally, the fourth category, feral dogs, includes all dogs living in a free state with no direct food or shelter intentionally supplied by humans (Causey & Cude, 1980) and showing no evidence of socialization to humans (Daniels & Bekoff, 1989a). Rather, they display strong continuous avoidance of direct human contact (Boitani & Ciucci, 1995) and a lifestyle restricted mainly to natural environments.

These four categories, however, are not exclusive. Not only is the distinction between feral, stray/neighborhood/village, and other free-roaming dogs often a matter of degree, but dogs may also change their status during their lifetimes (Boitani & Ciucci, 1995; Daniels, 1988; Daniels & Bekoff, 1989a; Hirata *et al.*, 1987; Nesbitt, 1975; Scott & Causey, 1973). Stray and feral appear to describe robust categories, at least with respect to the social dimension of the human–dog relationship. Stray dogs maintain social bonds with humans, even when they do not have an obvious owner. Feral dogs live successfully without any contact with humans and their social bonds, if any, are with other dogs.

17.2   The feralization process

As dogs can move across the four categories, it is of utmost importance to understand the causes and processes prompting changes of status, especially when the change results in moving between the stray and feral categories (Boitani *et al.*, 2006). From an evolutionary perspective, the process of feralization can be analyzed at two separate levels. At the individual level, feralization is a behavioral ontogenetic process (Daniels & Bekoff, 1989c), as shown by observations of dogs becoming feral within their lifetimes (see e.g. Boitani & Ciucci, 1995). At the population level, feralization is the domestication process in reverse (Hale, 1962; Price, 1984). Because the two perspectives focus on different levels (population and individual), they imply different temporal scales as well as different theoretical and research approaches (Daniels & Bekoff, 1989c).

Ontogenetically, changes in status may be the result of several natural and artificial factors (see Figure 17.1) and may never be definitive; that is, the process can move in either direction. An owned dog, for example, may become stray by escaping human control, by being abandoned, or simply by being born to an owned but otherwise free-roaming mother (Beck, 1975; Hsu *et al.*, 2003; Perry, 1993).

The return journey is also possible, as demonstrated by the many stray dogs adopted by humans. A stray dog can become feral when forced out of a human environment or when recruited by a feral group existing nearby (Daniels, 1988; Daniels & Bekoff, 1989a, 1989c), as was the case with eight out of 11 dogs in our study group (see below). The way back for feral dogs, though less common than the stray-owned change, has also been observed in our study, when a feral dog was experimentally rehabilitated to domestic status by one of us (P. Ciucci, unpublished data). Despite this potential fluidity, there are obvious intrinsic limitations to status changes: for example, dogs deprived of contacts with humans in the early stages of life will tend to remain shy and fearful of humans for the rest of their lives (Hare *et al.*, 2002; Serpell *et al.*, Chapter 6).

As the four dog categories are neither stable nor closed, it may also happen that dogs end up living all their lives in an indeterminate position between two categories. For example, Pal *et al.* (1998a, 1998b, 1999) and Ortolani *et al.* (2009) showed that stray/village dogs in India and Ethiopia never

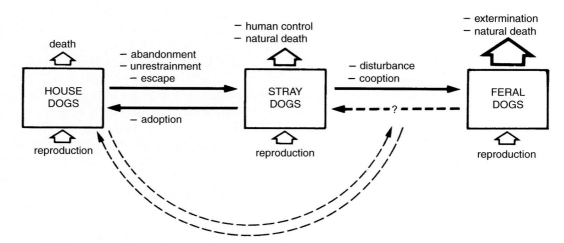

Figure 17.1 The feralization model.

managed to complete the passage from stray to truly feral animals, probably due to local ecological (dependence on human-related food and shelter) and human social conditions (human avoidance of close contact with dogs).

In summary, feralization is an intricate process that results from the complex interactions of several ecological and behavioral variables in highly diversified natural and human contexts. Therefore, any attempt to model these interactions is likely to have poor predictive power. Such a model, however, may improve our understanding of the critical factors facilitating status change in dogs, as well as helping to disentangle the various components of feralization for research purposes.

17.3   Feral dogs' occurrence in natural environments

As a result of the many opportunities dogs have to move in and out of human settlements, it is likely that feralization has been occurring since the beginning of dog domestication. The dingo in Australia and its likely ancestor, the pariah dogs of southern Eurasia, provide evidence that the feralization process was already going on several millennia ago (Clutton-Brook, Chapter 2; Zeuner, 1963). McKnight (1964) has also suggested that on the North American continent, feral dogs existed long before European contact. In the Mediterranean basin, the presence of large cities such as Istanbul and Alexandria, combined with a warm climate and ample food resources, tended to favor the subsistence of relatively fluid dog populations that shifted readily between owned, stray and feral conditions. Mediterranean lifestyles and environmental conditions appear to be particularly favorable to the support of stray and feral dog populations (e.g. relatively warm climate, availability of small game and free-ranging livestock, garbage dumps, loose interests and controls on the commons, etc.) (Boitani & Fabbri, 1983b). Currently, feral dog populations are widely reported from several regions of almost all continents except Antarctica (Boitani *et al.*, 2006) and their impact on wildlife and natural environments has been flagged as a critical issue for biodiversity conservation (e.g. Butler *et al.*, 2004; Hughes *et al.*, Chapter 18; Vanak & Gompper 2009; Young *et al.*, 2011). However, in spite of the obvious relevance of the problems caused by feral dogs to human health, wildlife conservation and livestock depredation, free-roaming dogs have been poorly investigated until recently and relatively few studies of their ecology have been reported (Barnett & Rudd, 1983; Beck, 1973; Bonanni *et al.*, 2010a, 2010b; Causey & Cude, 1980; Daniels, 1983a, 1983b; Daniels & Bekoff, 1989a, 1989b; Gipson, 1983; Macdonald & Carr, Chapter 16; Nesbitt, 1975; Pal, 2001; Pal *et al.*, 1998a, 1998b, 1999; Scott & Causey, 1973). Below we report on a study carried out on a group of feral dogs between 1984 and 1988 using radio-tracking in a mountainous area of the central Apennines (Abruzzo, Italy). In particular, we analyze parameters such as demography and sociality, reproduction and life history, space-use patterns, activity patterns and feeding habits.

17.4   Case study: The ecology of a feral dog group in central Italy

In Italy, free-roaming dogs are a familiar sight to anyone visiting the countryside. A nationwide census conducted in 1981 revealed that almost every region reported free-roaming dog populations. The national estimate was about 800 000 free-roaming dogs, mostly distributed in the central and southern regions (Boitani & Fabbri, 1983a). More recently, these estimates were confirmed by

Genovesi & Duprè (2000). Feral dogs were estimated to represent about 10% of the total (they are only a component of the more numerous population of free-roaming dogs, as these also include stray dogs and all those allowed by their owners to move freely in and out of villages and into surrounding countryside).

We studied one group of dogs in the Apennine Mountains about 100 km east of Rome. The group was selected as representative of a truly "feral" condition. We were interested in dogs living in a completely wild and free state with no direct food or shelter intentionally supplied by humans (Causey & Cude, 1980). The dogs also showed no evidence of socialization to humans (Daniels & Bekoff, 1989a), and tended to display a strong and continuous avoidance of direct human contact. Here we present data on group composition, life histories, recruitment, home range, movements and activity patterns.

17.4.1 Methods

Study area

The 250 km^2 study area was located in the Velino–Sirente mountain group, one of the Apennine ridges that crosses the Abruzzo region, comprising a flat carst highland at 1300 m elevation, surrounded by mountains up to 2490 m. This highland is crossed by the main paved road that connects the villages of Ovindoli, Rovere, Rocca di Mezzo, Rocca di Cambio, and Secinaro to the east. Several dirt roads reach side valleys and higher altitude pastures, and are mostly used in the summertime by shepherds and tourists.

The mean annual temperature is 7.6 °C with a minimum in January (−1.4 °C) and maximum in August (17.2 °C). Extreme low temperatures of the order of −20 °C are not unusual. Annual precipitation averages 90 cm for a total of 100 rain days, a third of them in the autumn. Snow depth is at its maximum in February–March, averaging 100 cm during the years 1982–4 at 1800 m altitude.

Thirty-two percent of the area is covered by beech (*Fagus sylvatica*) forests, mostly in pure stands, with other species (*Pinus nigra, Fraxinus excelsior* and *Quercus cerris*) occurring at lower altitudes. The bottom of the valley is covered by abandoned fields, or pastures and fields cultivated annually with potatoes and cereals. At 1800 m the beech forests give way to alpine meadows that have been severely degraded by centuries of livestock grazing. Large mammals were almost totally exterminated before the end of the last century. In the 1980s roe deer (*Capreolus capreolus*) were very rare, and wild boar (*Sus scrofa*) were increasing following a recent introduction. Hares (*Lepus europaeus*), squirrels (*Sciurus vulgaris*) and foxes (*Vulpes vulpes*) were common, while 6–10 wolves (*Canis lupus*) were estimated to be permanently in the area (Boitani & Fabbri, 1983b, Ciucci *et al.*, 1997). In summer, the area was also used by about 7000 sheep, mostly in the alpine pastures. At night, these were kept in stables or enclosures, often heavily guarded by shepherd dogs. Roughly 1400 cows and 200 horses were also kept in the most productive pastures of the valley.

Feral dogs were studied from February 1984 through May 1987. However, the same group of dogs had been observed repeatedly, though not intensively, since 1981, in parallel with a study reported by Macdonald & Carr (Chapter 16).

Capture and handling

Dogs were captured alive using a variety of traps depending on different trapping conditions – e.g. snow, ground texture, presence of human activities (see e.g. Boitani & Fabbri, 1983b). Baiting stations and lures were used, but most traps were set along known trails. A blow-pipe (Telinject) was used to inject the dogs intramuscularly with a mixture of xylazine hydrochloride (Rompun,

Bayer) (3 mg/kg body weight) and ketamine hydrochloride (Ketalar, Parke Davis) (4 mg/kg of body weight). This mixture made it possible to reduce the amount of liquid injected to 1.6 ml per 30 kg dog. After 15–20 minutes the dogs were sufficiently sedated to be approached and handled safely, and the anesthetic's effect lasted for about 20–30 minutes. All immobilized dogs recovered physical control quickly and apparently completely.

Classification of dog types and morphology

Visual and radio-tracking observations were used to distinguish feral dogs from other free-roaming dogs. The amount of aggression shown by trapped dogs – as used by Scott & Causey (1973) and Daniels & Bekoff (1989a, 1989b) – was not found to be consistent with the known status of dogs and was therefore discarded as a means of classification. Some feral dogs were never trapped and they were classified as feral because they consistently associated with other marked feral dogs.

Sex of unmarked feral dogs was easily determined by observing the animals and their behavior, especially their urination postures (see Bekoff, 1979). Visual observation was also used to classify the dogs into broad age classes: pups (up to 3 months), juveniles (3 months–1 year), adults (1–5 or 6 years), and old (more than 5 or 6 years). Trapped animals were aged according to the eruption and wear patterns of their dentition (Kirk, 1977), up to the limit of these techniques.

All trapped dogs were weighed and their body measurements, coat color and pattern, and breed type recorded. These external morphological characters were used to help identify possible breed combinations, as all the dogs were crossbred. At the time of the study, genetic tools were not easily available, so we did not assess the dogs genetically at the individual or breed level.

Radiotelemetry

Dogs were marked with plastic, numbered ear-tags (Rototag, Dalton, England) and the nine captured adults were fitted with radio-transmitters.[1] Radio-collared dogs were normally monitored five times a day, rotating the time when each dog was located. In addition, at least once a week, a single dog was monitored every 10 minutes for 24 hours. Radio fixes were classified as either "resting," "active" or "travelling" according to signal reception patterns. "Travelling" involved a change in location of the subject animal during the observation period. These activity classes were established by testing radio-collars on domestic dogs. Several periods of continuous, direct observation were also dedicated to particular situations. For example, during spring 1985 and spring 1986, two den sites were continuously monitored and observed from the time they were attended by the bitch. Telemetry was also used to locate and home-in on dogs so that visual observations could be made on group size, composition and behavior. Snow-tracking, sightings, wolf-howling, scat collection, as well as telemetry were used to monitor the home ranges of two wolf packs living in the area.

Life histories and group composition

The study area was continuously searched for signs of dogs, and all free-living animals were identified and located by radio-telemetry or visual observation. Frequent radio locations and snow-tracking made it possible to monitor the dogs' activities very closely, while group composition

[1]Radio-collars were assembled with an AVM SB-2 transmitter cast in dental acrylic and packed in a PVC pipe with a lithium battery and transmitting antenna; the total weight of these collars was about 300 g. Transmission was in the 150–151 MHz frequency range. Signals were received by vehicle roof-mounted and hand-held directional antennas (4 and 5 elements yagi). Location of dogs was accomplished by triangulation (Mech, 1983). Locations were plotted on topographic maps (1:25 000) and referred to a grid system where the unit was a 250×250 m^2 to account for the maximum tested error obtained in using the radio-location technique in that mountain area and on the dogs.

was monitored by direct observation. Mating times, breeding, litter sizes and mortality causes were all checked by direct observations. Litter sizes were based on the first sighting of pups, and this was usually possible within a couple of weeks after birth. Pup survival was estimated from the difference between numbers at first sightings and numbers observed over the following months.

Stray dogs from the villages were also monitored so that they could be identified when found outside their normal urban environment.

Home range and spatial patterns

The size, configuration and seasonal dynamics of the dogs' home ranges were estimated by an extension of the Harmonic Mean method (Dixon & Chapman, 1980), utilizing the HOME RANGE program (made available from E. O. Garton, Moscow, Idaho). The Harmonic Mean method allows home range to be represented as a series of contours (isopleths) as illustrated in Figure 17.2. Although isopleths have a strict mathematical meaning, their interpretation is made easier when extended to area contours including different percentages of all observations. Disproportionate use of the home range was tested for statistical significance using a one-tailed Kolmogorov–Smirnov test (Samuel et al., 1985). Counts and proportion data were analyzed with chi-square tests. Habitat use was analyzed by integrating home range contours with a land-use layer in a GIS environment.[2]

17.4.2   Results

A total of nine adult feral dogs (four males and five females) were captured and radio-collared. Four individuals were subsequently recaptured a second time. Forty pups were born during the study period, two of which (coded 14 and 25 in Table 17.1) reached adulthood.

From July 1984 to March 1987, a total of 7956 locations were recorded, of which 1387 (17%) were visual observations of radio-collared individuals, and 883 (11%) involved observations of uncollared individuals belonging to the study group. Fifty-six percent of the total records were made during the daytime, while the rest were recorded during the evening or after dark. From the original data set, a random subsample of 1618 radio-locations was utilized for the analysis of group ranging behavior, representing an average of 1.6 locations/day. Two animals were observed for longer periods (712 and 649 days, respectively), while the shortest observation period per dog was 55 days (see Table 17.1).

All dogs were crossbred. The predominant breed appeared to be the "Abruzzo" shepherd dog, together with some German shepherd and hound type animals. All were medium to large in size (weight ranging from 17 to 31 kg, mean = 22.8 kg). Small-sized dogs were never observed among feral or other free-roaming dogs. Colors varied from almost solid brownish yellow to the more common combination of white with black or brown patches.

---

[2]A subsample of the original data set was randomly selected to eliminate the bias due to sampling procedures (i.e. autocorrelation of locations and sampling efforts not equally distributed through time) and inclusion of extreme locations (i.e. outliers). We chose 95% Harmonic Mean isopleths to represent home-range boundaries, and 50% isopleths to delineate core areas (Spencer & Barret, 1984). To assess the internal anatomy of the home range, we used a GIS (ARC-INFO)/HOME RANGE integration (Boitani et al., 1989). Habitat topology included vegetative cover (woodland, open forest/shrubland complex, grassland complex, open field and farmed area), elevation, roads, villages and other areas of human activity. On a smaller scale, habitat features characterizing the feral dogs' refuge areas were identified by analyzing the portion of home range included within 25% isopleths.

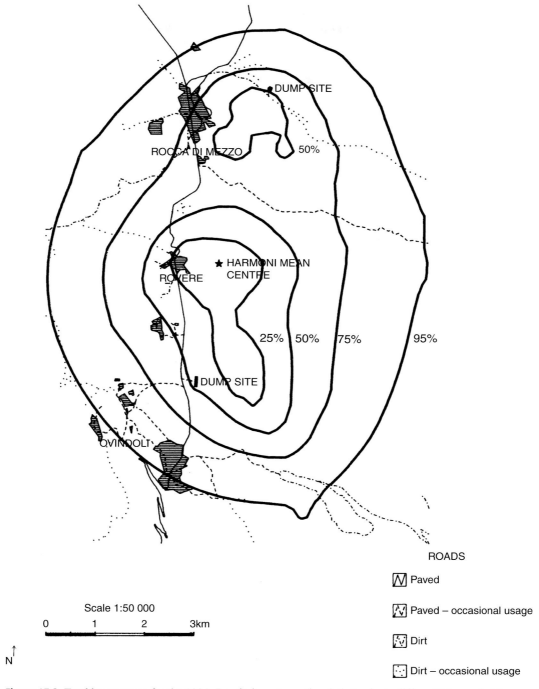

Figure 17.2 Total home range for the 1984–7 period: contours (isopleths) refer to different Harmonic Mean Centers.

Table 17.1 Feral dogs (pups excluded) of the studied group.

Animal code	Sex	Age	Origin	Cause of death	Date of death	Radio-days no.
01	f	A	R/F	Poisoned	Dec. 85	128
02	f	A	R/F	Poisoned	Dec. 84	137
03	m	A	R/F	?	June 86	117
04	m	A	F	Poisoned	Apr. 88	712
05	f	A	R	Poisoned	Apr. 88	649
06	f	J	R	Shot	Dec. 85	112
14	x	J	F	Wolves	Apr. 86	–
17	m	A	R	Poisoned	Oct. 86	55
18	f	A	R	Poisoned	Apr. 88	177
25	f	J-A	F	Poisoned	Apr. 88	–
30	m	A	R	Captured	Nov. 87	117

f, female; m, male; x, unsexed; A, adult; J, juvenile; F, feral; R, recruited

Group composition and life histories

A group of feral dogs was living in the same area since at least 1980, and in the summer of 1982 numbered at least nine adults. This group, however, was almost exterminated by poison baits set out by local people in the autumn of 1983, and the only surviving animal (male 04) became part of the present study group until the end of the study. Intensive search for tracks in areas within and outside the known range of the group indicated that the population of feral dogs we studied was relatively isolated, since no tracks were found apart from those of dogs living within the villages.

Figure 17.3 summarizes the group's history from February 1984 to the end of 1987, showing arrivals of new animals, and deaths and births that changed the pack composition during the study period. The group ranged in size from a minimum of three animals, in the fall of 1984 and spring of 1986, to a maximum of 15 dogs in the summer of 1984, when two litters (seven and four pups, respectively) joined the four adults. Overall, the group consisted of a core of two breeding pairs. The initial pairs (dogs 01 & 04 and 02 & 03) maintained their relationships until the death of one or other partner. When one partner died or disappeared, it was usually replaced by a free-roaming dog actively recruited from the villages. New pairs were then formed with newcomers (in three cases) or with a young animal from a previous litter (one case), and these new relationships were then in turn maintained until the death or disappearance of one partner. During the study period three cases of new recruits were observed (dogs 05, 18, 30) and their arrival was always associated with females being in estrus. Adult female 18 arrived accompanied by an adult male 17, who remained with the group for two months before his death. Adult female 05 arrived accompanied by her daughter (female 06) who was accepted and integrated into the group. Later, an adult male, phenotypically identical to female 06 and showing great confidence with her (probably her brother), tried repeatedly to approach and enter the group. However, he was rejected aggressively by the rest of the group, with the exception of females 05 and 06 (his probable mother and sister).

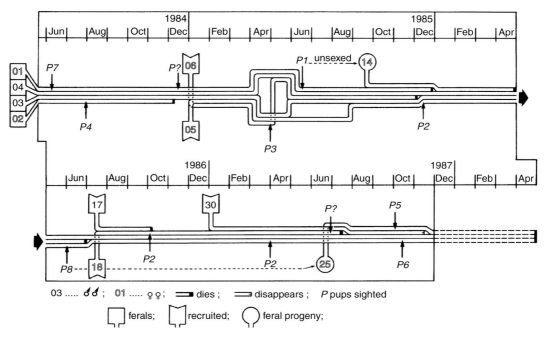

Figure 17.3 Feral dogs' group composition (all headings timed at either effective date of discovery or at start of effective individual role).

Group members always maintained very close contact, even when the den sites of the females were located far from the usual resting sites and required long journeys to visit. The two pairs split apart for a short time in 1985 when female 05 gave birth in an area about 15 km away from the usual range. Male 03 (her partner) stayed with her for about two months, although with frequent visits to the rest of the group, while the young female 06 (her daughter) stayed only 10 days before leaving and rejoining the group. Female 05 then rejoined the group almost three months later, without encountering any apparent difficulty reintegrating. Dog 30 was a persistent loner until he joined the group during the estrus period of female 05 in December 1986 (05 had lost her previous partner in June 1986). Soon after this, he became more closely associated with female 18.

In general, the group was relatively stable, basically rotating around two pairs and their offspring. Male 04 tended to act as leader of the group, in the sense that he took the lead in aggressive behavior toward intruders, and was usually last to retreat after such encounters. The group did not show competition or aggression toward unknown dogs found around villages or at the dumps or around sheep yards, but they usually showed strong aggression toward intruders trespassing in their core areas. In one extreme case, a shepherd dog from a nearby sheep yard crossed the feral group's core area and was physically attacked by the group in broad daylight. Most clashes with intruders, however, ended with furious barking and holding the ground until the intruder slowly retreated.

Temporal associations with transient dogs were observed during estrus periods, when aggressive tendencies seemed less pronounced. In the winter of 1986, for example, a male with a female in heat, both stray animals from the village of Rocca di Mezzo, joined the group (which consisted of five individuals at that time, but only one adult female) for a month. Similarly, in the winter of 1987 a group of nine stray dogs from Ovindoli met the feral dog group at the dump for several nights, sometimes spending the whole night within the group's home range, although without any apparent interaction with them.

We found no evidence that exclusive mating occurred within the group's breeding pairs, nor that the males in each pair were the fathers of the females' offspring. Estrus occurred at relatively regular 6–7 month intervals, but there was no sign of any synchronization of estrus cycles among females. Out of 12 estrus periods, six (50%) were in the spring (February to May) while the rest were scattered through most of the other months. The earliest recorded estrus and successful parturition occurred in a wild born female at 13 months of age. This female was the daughter of female 05 and she was the only wild born pup observed to reach sexual maturity and to reproduce.

Dens were not the center of activities for the rest of the group, although they were often close to the more familiar resting sites (within 100–200 m, with the exception of female 05 in spring 1985). Other members of the group only occasionally visited den sites or females with pups, and never made any significant contribution to the feeding and/or care of the mother and her young. Dens were all in natural cavities, among boulders or under large rocks.

Eleven litters were observed, involving a total of 40 pups. In addition, postmortem examination of female 02 revealed six fetuses. Out of a total of 42 pups or fetuses that were sexed, 32 (76%) were males, including extreme cases of male:female sex ratios of 5:0 and 5:1 per litter. The mean litter size at first sighting was 3.63 ($n = 11$, range 1–8 pups). Pups were difficult to observe and their carcasses were seldom found, limiting our ability to estimate mortality rates and causes. Foxes, crows and other small predators were fairly common in the area, and they may have been responsible for the rapid disappearance of any carcasses. Out of 40 pups born alive, 28 (70%) died within 70 days of birth, nine (22.5%) within 120 days, and one (2.5%) within 1 year. Only two pups (5%) survived beyond the age of 1 year. Most deaths appeared to occur when pups started moving from the den site at 2–3 months of age. However, direct evidence of death is available for only a few pups; three 70-day old pups were killed at the den by a fox. When a pup survived to juvenile age, it was always the only surviving member of its litter.

Seven adults were killed by poison baits, a 1-year-old juvenile was killed by wolves, an 18-month-old female was shot, one was captured by local people, and we do not know the fate of one adult (see Table 17.1). Male 04 was the longest living individual (6 full years in the wild), followed by female 05 (3.4 years). Recruitment of new and viable members of the group appeared to depend on free-roaming village dogs joining the group at intervals. At least four adults joined the group successfully at different stages of the group's history, and not a single pup born to the group survived to produce enough offspring to replace the losses due to mortality (see Figure 17.5).

Home range and spatial patterns

From July 1984 to May 1987 the overall home range size was 57.9 km², as shown within the 95% harmonic mean contour (see Figure 17.2). Its mean elevation was 1500 m above a sea level range of 1260–1950 m. The home range was not used uniformly, and some areas (i.e. core areas) were consistently more frequented than others.

Most of the home range lay to the east of the paved road connecting three villages located at the lower altitude of the highland. Of these, Ovindoli and Rocca di Mezzo are medium-sized villages with a permanent high level of human activity, especially during the summer and winter tourist seasons: these villages are mostly contained within the outer circle of the home range. In contrast, Rovere is a smaller village, partly abandoned at the time of the study, where human presence is at a very low level for several months a year. This village was included in the core area of the range and it was located <1 km from the center (harmonic mean) of the 1984–7 dogs' group home range.

Two garbage dumps were located in open fields near the two main villages, and these sites were neither fenced nor protected in any other way from animal utilization. Both dumps lay at the edges of the 50% contour zones (i.e. the core areas). Water was scarce but fairly homogeneously distributed throughout the area, and easily accessible. About 76% of the range was utilized from spring to fall by free-ranging livestock, mostly sheep and, to a lesser extent, horses and cattle.

To evaluate the extent to which roads influence the dogs' ranges, a buffer zone of 100 m was calculated along each paved road with more intensive traffic, and a buffer of 50 m along each less intensively used road. The total buffer area within each contour zone was then compared to each contour area. Road area as a proportion of total area declined from the 95–25% contour zones, indicating the tendency of the dogs to avoid roads. Although the proportions of the different habitat types within the 95% contour range did not differ significantly from those typical of the overall study area, there were significant differences between the inner and outer contour zones. Forest cover tended to increase, and open fields tended to decrease, toward the core areas.

Home-range size changed over the years, but without any seasonal fluctuations. Average size was 11.3 km^2 (±6.2 km^2, $n = 10$), with a minimum size of 2.2 km^2 in the summer of 1986 and a maximum of 21.2 km^2 in the summer of 1985. All seasonal ranges were in the same general area, and any variations in sizes and/or utilization patterns of the area were generally due to various occasional and unpredictable factors: e.g. disturbance by humans (hunters, shepherds, tourists), interference by other dogs or wolves, presence of large sources of carrion (cattle or horse carcasses), previous territorial knowledge of newly recruited dogs (e.g. female 05 in 1985), or disturbance at the dumps.

Individual dogs' home ranges varied considerably. An extreme case is that of female 05 during her denning period of about four months in the spring/summer of 1986. When compared to her annual home range for the same year (37.5 km^2), the denning period range represented only 4.3% (1.6 km^2), and the 25% contour area was reduced to an even greater extent (from 0.98 km^2 for the whole year to only 10 m^2 for the denning period). The den was located on a rocky and inaccessible slope at the edge of Rovere, fully protected from human disturbance, and yet with easy access to garbage disposed of by the village households. The female had to move only a few hundred meters to find all she needed to feed herself and her pups.

Three major extraterritorial excursions outside the home range occurred in the winter and spring of 1985 and they eventually led to the denning by female 05 in an area 15 km away from the usual range. These excursions, excluded from the overall home range calculations, were not apparently due to any particular factor, although in one case a visit to a nearby village dump may have provided the incentive.

The seasonal 25% core areas show a significant variability in size (see Table 17.2), confirming different range utilization patterns during different periods, although without seasonal recurrence, and mostly due to occasional, unpredictable events or circumstances. Average core area size is 5.71% of the total home range, suggesting a high level of attachment to particular sites where dogs tend to stay most of their time and where they return after excursions to other parts of the range. Twenty-five percent core areas include dens, resting sites and retreat sites, and a highly significant proportion of the non-active radio fixes were found within their limits (see Table 17.3). Shifts in core areas appeared to be largely random, although the key environmental features within them remained remarkably consistent. Three preferred core areas couldn't be identified by plotting the seasonal centers of activity:

Table 17.2 Seasonal core areas (25% isopleth).

	Fall 1984	Wint. 1984–5	Spr. 1985	Summ. 1985	Fall 1985	Wint. 1985–6	Spr. 1986	Summ. 1986	Fall 1986	Wint. 1986–7	mean ± SE
Area (km^2)	0.35	0.69	1.21	1.04	1.66	0.65	0.25	0.002	0.77	0.37	0.69 ± 0.49
% of H.R.	3.0	4.0	10.6	5.0	7.9	10.5	4.2	0.1	6.9	4.9	5.7 ±3.3

Table 17.3   Activity distribution within the home range.

	95% Iso	75% Iso	50% Iso	25% Iso
Activity				
Obs.	751	700	559	379[a]
(%)	(100)	(93.2)	(74.4)	(50.5)
No activity				
Obs.	837	803	691	489[b]
(%)	(100)	(95.9)	(85.5)	(58.4)

[a-b]$P < 0.001$.

two by the two major dumps, and one by the village of Rovere, itself a safe food and shelter source with little human interference. All seasonal centers of activity were located away from roads, other villages and areas of human activity. Core areas also have distinct territorial significance. Aggressive behavior, as indicated by barking, chasing or approaching intruders aggressively, was more frequent and more intense when encounters were closer to the core areas. Aggression toward shepherd dogs or other free-roaming dogs, as well as to our own research working dogs, was often observed within the core areas, but rarely occurred in other parts of the range. Although there is no numerical evidence for this, levels of aggression were apparently lower during estrus periods. As a consequence, these periods provided the only opportunities for the successful recruitment of new group members.

Utilization of garbage dumps reflected different levels of disturbance. The Ovindoli dump (the largest and richest of all) was located near a major road and in the middle of a large, open field often frequented by people during daylight hours. It was mostly visited by the dogs at night (70.6% of observations). In contrast, the Secinaro dump was located in a secluded and quiet, small valley where nobody ever went except the little truck carrying the garbage there every morning. The dogs quickly learned this pattern and visited the dump immediately after the truck had left (90.5% of all fixes). The Rocca di Mezzo dump had intermediate characteristics: it was large and often disturbed by human presence, but it was located in a protected side valley surrounded by forest with plenty of potential retreats. It was visited significantly more often during the daytime (68.4%). The dumps offered an unlimited source of food to the dogs: all kinds of refuse were thrown there in large quantities, including slaughterhouse leftovers. Large bones could be found all along the trails from the dumps to the dogs' resting sites. Dogs were observed feeding at the dumps for periods of up to an hour or more, usually arriving in groups or pairs rather than singly. They were also tolerant of each other as they skillfully ripped open the plastic sacs delivered freshly every morning.

During the years before our field study, local people had made several claims for damages to livestock caused by feral dogs. During the study period we saw no evidence of any killing of, or damage to, either domestic or wild animals by the feral dogs. A few chases of hares or squirrels were observed but they seemed to arise from playfulness rather than predatory behavior. Occasional dead livestock had an important impact on the dogs' activities and movements, and the group sometimes moved its center of activities to take complete and continuous advantage of such sudden and abundant food sources.

During the study period, two main packs of wolves used the area with home ranges partially overlapping those of the feral dogs. The first pack comprised five to seven individuals and had its range NE of the dogs' range, for a total of about 300 km². It partially overlapped with the northern portion (about 30%) of the dogs' home range, since the wolves also utilized the Rocca di Mezzo dump as a food source. The second pack averaged about five individuals. Its entire home range was never fully defined, since it extended well south of the study area, but it overlapped with the southern part of the dogs' range (about 35%). This pack utilized the Ovindoli dump as a food source. While no evidence of direct contact between wolves and dogs was obtained, it is possible to infer some interactions from movement patterns and behavioral observations. For instance, excursions and exploratory journeys by the dogs into the northern pack's territory coincided with the estrus periods of the wolves. In April 1986, a juvenile feral dog was killed by wolves close to the Rocca di Mezzo dump. In addition, our own imitations of wolf howling when the dogs were at the Rocca di Mezzo dump elicited immediate and strong aggressive reactions from the dogs. The two wolf packs' territories never came in contact with each other, and the central part of the dogs' home range (Rovere area) was located in the zone between the wolves' territories.

Activity and temporal patterns

A total of 7073 fixes of radio-collared animals was utilized for the analysis of activity patterns. Feral dogs "rested" for 48% of the time, and they were "active" (40%) or "travelling" (12%) for the rest of the time. Activity patterns by season and by sex show significant differences for both sexes among seasons and also, for some seasons, between sexes. Females in general travelled less and rested for longer, and this sex difference was more marked in the spring and, to a lesser extent, the fall when denning and pup-rearing kept them at the den sites. Males were more active and travelled for longer in the spring and summer. Winter activity showed a generally similar pattern for both sexes.

Female 02 during her autumn 1984 pregnancy period provided a good example of activity pattern changes: she spent only 3% of her time travelling, and this was limited to a single daily trip from the resting site to the dump and back. Most of the rest of the time she was resting (66%). Female 05 also rested most of the time (69%) during her denning period in the spring of 1985, and only 8% of her time was dedicated to her twice daily trips to the dump. During the same period, male 04 showed the highest recorded percentage of travelling (23%) as he was often checking the den and patrolling the rest of his range. His higher travelling percentage reduces the resting percentage, since the "active" category remains largely unchanged.

As expected, seasonal analysis of overall activity indicates two activity peaks coinciding with dawn and dusk, respectively. This pattern is best shown when diurnal activity is divided into six daily periods defined in relation to dawn and sunrise (see Figure 17.4). Travelling maintains its two peaks, but is evenly distributed through the other periods, including the daytime. "Active" is significantly higher during the hours of darkness. The dogs show a basic pattern of becoming active at their resting sites around sunset, travelling to the dumps, staying active around the dump areas and at lower altitudes, and then travelling back at dawn to their resting sites.

In spring, breeding activities modify the basic activity pattern and a third significant peak of activity is evident during the central part of the day. Mating, pregnancy, denning, and visits to the den sites by males influence both sexes' activities at this time. Intensive radio-tracking during breeding times showed that female activities were strongly affected. Female 02, during her pregnancy in October–November 1984, did not show any significant activity peaks throughout the 24 hours. Female 05 was closely monitored during three separate breeding periods in very different denning conditions. In the spring of 1985 when she denned by the Secinaro dump – a quiet place she could visit at any time of the day – her activity showed no significant peaks. In the fall of 1985 she denned in an abandoned stable at the edge of Rovere, and the village's garbage cans were her main source of food. Here her activity was mainly nocturnal (although, statistically speaking, not highly

Table 17.4 Diurnal and nocturnal activity distribution within habitat types.

	Wood	Meadow/scrubland	Open field
Day			
% Activity[a]	26.7	41.3	32.0
% No activity[b]	32.2	45.5	22.2
Night			
% Activity[c]	15.0	41.9	43.1
% No activity[d]	21.7	46.4	31.9

$^{a-b}P < 0.001$; $^{c-d}P < 0.001$; $^{a-c}P < 0.001$; $^{b-d}P < 0.001$

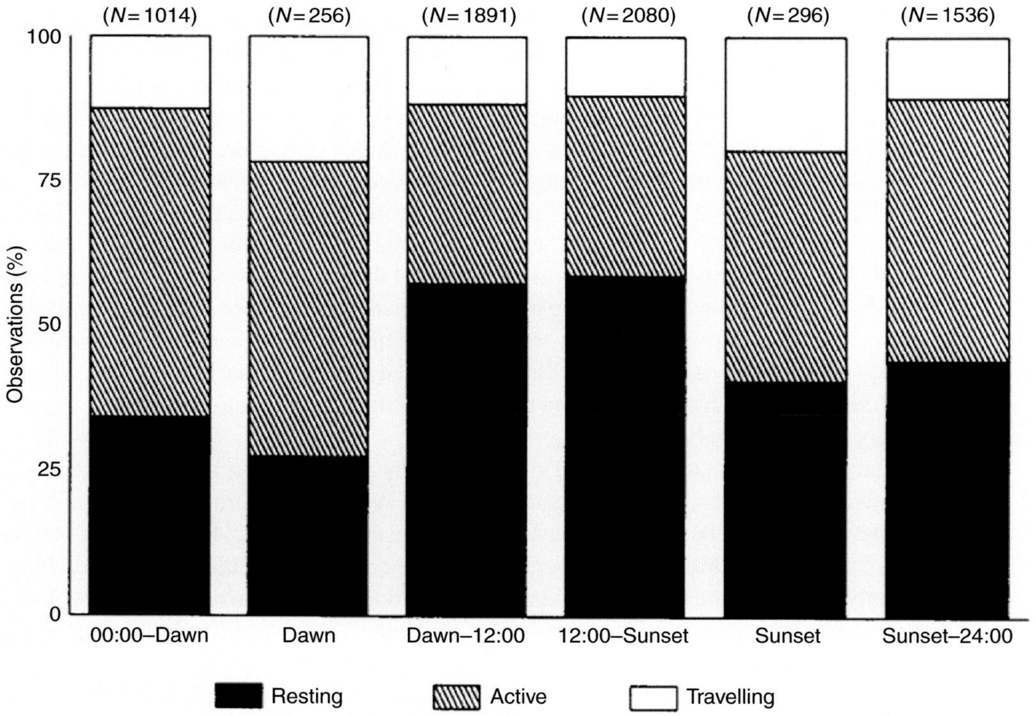

Figure 17.4 Activity distribution in different periods of the day.

significantly so). In the summer of 1986 she denned in a cave outside Rovere, where her activity was strictly (and statistically highly significantly) nocturnal.

Correlation between activity and vegetation cover (see Table 17.4) was highly significant: daytime resting was mostly confined to wooded or mixed habitat, as was "active" behavior, though to a lesser extent. During the hours of darkness, activity was more likely to occur in areas with no vegetation cover, since the dogs were travelling to the more exposed areas around dumps and villages.

17.4.3 Discussion: A broader view of feral dog ecology and behavior

Group composition

Among canids, packs are defined as social units that hunt, rear young and protect a communal territory as a stable group (Mech & Boitani, 2003). Pack members are usually related (Bekoff *et al.*, 1984). The feral dogs in our study area showed these characters only to a limited extent and they were not fully related, as is the case with most stray and feral dogs studied elsewhere (see Berman & Dunbar, 1983; Bonanni *et al.*, 2010a; Causey & Cude, 1980; Daniels & Bekoff, 1989a, 1989b; Nesbitt, 1975; Scott & Causey, 1973). The kinds of associations and social bonds formed among feral dogs do not follow the precise rules of pack living, as described for other canids (see Bekoff *et al.*, 1984; Gittleman, 1989; Kleiman & Eisenberg, 1973), and therefore the term "group" seems more appropriate than pack.

Overall dog density for the Abruzzo region, where the study area was located, is 2.59/km²: owned but uncontrolled dogs account for the bulk of animals (1.38 dogs/km²), followed by strays (0.89 dogs/km²) and feral dogs (0.32 dogs/km²) (Boitani & Fabbri, 1983a). Feral dogs are not evenly distributed over the entire region; they show a disjunct pattern of small, partially isolated populations, mainly at lower altitudes in more densely populated areas where food resources are richer, and opportunities for exchanges with village-based, stray dog populations are higher (Boitani & Fabbri, 1983a; Boitani, 1983).

Extrapolating from our group's total home-range size gives a mean density of 0.2–0.05 dogs/km² for the area as a whole, depending upon group composition. These densities are considerably lower than the densities reported for free-roaming dogs studied in conditions of strong dependence on human-related resources. For example, Cafazzo *et al.* (2010) reported a density of 30 dogs/km² in an urban environment near Rome.

Feral dog group sizes tend to be similar across a wide range of situations. Two studies in Alabama reported group sizes of 2–5 and 2–6 individuals, respectively (Causey & Cude, 1980; Scott & Causey, 1973). Daniels & Bekoff (1989b) reported 2–4 animals per group in a feral population in Arizona, and Nesbitt (1975) found a mean group size of 5–6 animals, in his 5-year study of feral dogs in Illinois. Although Boitani & Racana (1984) observed feral dogs in Basilicata (southern Italy) mostly in pairs, the group size of 3–6 adults found in the present study (Figure 17.5) tends to agree with those reported previously. Studies of urban free-roaming dogs report mainly solitary animals or pairs (Beck, 1975; Berman & Dunbar, 1983; Daniels, 1983a, 1983b; Daniels & Bekoff,

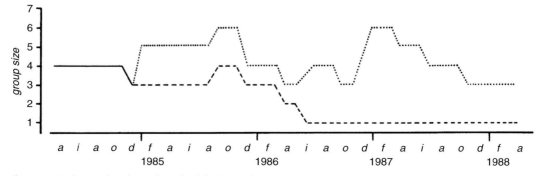

Figure 17.5 Group size dynamics of original members and their progeny (solid and dashed line), and total number including recruited stray dogs (dotted line).

1989b; Hirata *et al.*, 1986; Macdonald & Carr, Chapter 16), and there has been some debate about whether smaller group sizes in urban areas are a response to scarce (Beck, 1973; Daniels & Bekoff, 1989b) or plentiful (Berman & Dunbar, 1983) food resources. Unfortunately, neither hypothesis is supported by accurate estimates of food resource distribution. Daniels & Bekoff (1989b) recognize that patterns of social organization at urban and rural sites are based largely on dog-ownership practices. They stress the level of care and food provided by the owner as a primary reason for the lack of sociality in urban dogs. In other words, existing social bonds with owners and other humans tend to lower the dogs' motivation to form other social contacts. The higher levels of sociability among feral dogs, and the relatively strong bonds we observed among the members of our group, seem to be maintained despite the presence of abundant and easily accessible food resources. The presence of predatory wolves in areas partly overlapping the dogs' range may have provided an important pressure for group-living (see also Macdonald & Carr, Chapter 16).

Group composition (excluding pups) was relatively stable during the study period (see Figure 17.5). Although the study lasted more than three years, all of the events that resulted in a reduction or increase in group numbers appeared to occur unpredictably. All deaths were accidental or caused by human interference, while newborns from feral parents contributed almost nothing to the group's long-term stability. Recruitment of new group members from the village stray population appeared to be the most powerful force maintaining group size. At the end of the study, all but one dog in the group originated from village dogs (see Figure 17.5). The presence of breeding pairs appears essential to trigger the process of recruitment: new adults were accepted into the group only when a resident adult was left alone during the breeding period. Breeding periods in canids are accompanied by extensive social interactions that, in turn, may contribute to stronger pair bonds (Kleiman & Eisenberg, 1973). Increased social interactions may facilitate the acceptance of outsiders (most of the temporal association with dogs from the villages were observed during these periods), while the formation of strong pair bonds may be the major factor preventing further recruitment.

Although these speculations provide a promising hypothesis, they do not fully explain how a stable group size is maintained, and further data are needed on the behavioral responses of individual dogs to attempts by outsiders to approach and join the group. Macdonald & Carr (Chapter 16) propose that recruitment tends to occur in association with social disturbance. Our data support this view, if mating times are treated as periods of increased social stress.

Quantity and distribution of food resources are often cited as primary causes of social groups and determinants of group size (see Macdonald, 1983; von Schantz, 1984; Macdonald & Carr, 1989 and Chapter 16). The Resource Dispersion Hypothesis suggests that, "groups may develop in an environment where resources are dispersed such that, under certain circumstances, the smallest economically defensible territory for a pair can also sustain additional animals" (Macdonald & Carr, 1989). The theory also predicts that group size will be determined by richness of food resource patches during periods of minimum food availability. The garbage dumps in our study area provided a superabundant food supply during all seasons, and food did not appear to be a limiting resource. In such cases, group size is likely to be related more to social factors than to ecological ones. It is interesting to note that the marked philopatry of our dogs meets the general premises of the Territory Inheritance Hypothesis (Lindstrom, 1986). This hypothesis on the evolution of group living in carnivores gives greater importance to the attachment of individuals to their parents' territories, and predicts an optimal group size which agrees with that observed in our study. However, further research on feral dog ecology is needed in order to test the strength of these various alternatives.

Group-splitting was observed only in conjunction with denning and pup-rearing by female 05, and it lasted more than five months. During this period her male partner maintained close contact with the rest of the group, travelling back and forth between the den and the group's usual home range. Daniels & Bekoff (1989b) have suggested that group-splitting may serve an adaptive function for pack-living canids as a means of reducing both the burden of alloparental care on the pack, and the threat of infanticide by the dominant female. Conversely, group participation in pup-rearing is adaptive for precisely the opposite reasons, i.e. it relieves the female of the burden of caring alone for her pups, and it provides more protection for the young from predators (Kleiman & Eisenberg, 1973). In our study group, splitting appeared to be more an accidental event, linked to the finding of a new, abundant and relatively undisturbed food source (the dump at Secinaro). In all other observed cases of denning, females always reared their pups without any assistance or threats from other group members. In the absence of any adaptive advantage to group-splitting, the result is a positive pressure against it.

Reproduction and life histories

Denning and rearing pups apart from the group has been reported by Daniels (1988) and Daniels & Bekoff (1989b), although actual distances are not given. With the exception of female 05 in the spring of 1985, all other dens were within short distances from the usual resting sites. Denning females spent most of their time at the dens where they were often visited by other group members, and there was no evidence that females were actually separated from the group. Again, the presence of potential predators (including humans) may have played a role in keeping dens within the group core areas.

Rearing pups without male assistance may be an artifact of the domestication process and has been observed in urban free-roaming dogs (Pal, 2005). Domestic dogs stand alone among living canids in their almost total lack of paternal care (Kleiman & Malcolm, 1981). Domestic dogs usually breed twice a year, although artificial selection for faster reproductive rates seems to have disrupted any seasonal patterns. Feral dogs maintain the pattern with an average of 7.3 months (range 6.5–10 months) between successive estrus periods (female 01 may have bred late in 1984, but we failed to gather direct evidence for this). Since 50% of the breeding events occurred during February–May (33% in April–May), they indicate a seasonal increase in reproduction in the spring. Although this spring concentration is statistically significant, it has not been possible to demonstrate any real synchrony of breeding among females. Macdonald & Carr (Chapter 16) report a much higher level of synchrony of breeding in their dogs and relate this to a period of group stability. This hypothesis would also fit our data, and would merit further study. Increases in breeding frequency in the spring and fall were reported by Gipson (1972) and suggested as likely by Daniels & Bekoff (1989b). In terms of probability of pup survival, the time of the year when breeding occurs is critical. Wild canids in Italy give birth in April (*Vulpes vulpes*) or May (*Canis lupus*) (Boitani, 1981), and the pattern shown by feral dogs may indicate a converging strategy.

In wolves, breeding is generally restricted to a single "dominant" female (Mech, 1970), although there are reported cases of two litters being raised successfully within the same pack (Van Ballenberghe, 1983). In feral dogs we saw no indication of any attempts to control reproduction of any (subordinate) adult. All adult females reproduced, giving the pack its full potential for demographic increase.

Domestic dogs are known to have litter sizes of up to 17 pups, although 10 is the more usual upper limit (Kleiman, 1968; Kleiman & Eisenberg, 1973). A litter of five and a total of eight for two other litters have been reported for feral dogs by Nesbitt (1975), while Daniels & Bekoff (1989b) report 10 pups from two litters. Most estimates of litter size rely on numbers obtained at the first sighting of pups, which rarely occurs before they are mobile (at 3–4 weeks). Earlier mortality may therefore contribute to the smaller litter sizes of feral animals. Our mean litter size of 3.6 is lower than previously reported, and also smaller than the 5.5 pups/litter obtained by Macdonald & Carr (Chapter 16) from village dogs in the same area. Variability in age-related fecundity in different breeds may help to explain these differences.

Pup survival rates were also low compared with figures quoted elsewhere. For example, Nesbitt (1975) reports three pups surviving out of eight (37% survival); Scott & Causey (1973) describe 33% survival to 4 months and 22% survival to 1 year; Daniels & Bekoff (1989b) give a figure of 34% survival to 4 months of age for five litters; Pal (2008) reports 27% survival to 3 months of age of six litters in urban environments; and Macdonald & Carr (Chapter 16) report 16% survival up to 5 months. In the present study we obtained lower survival rates and high early mortality (70% mortality within 70 days). Two factors may contribute to increased mortality at the time when the pups becomes independent: (a) the tendency of juveniles to explore the range without adult supervision; and (b) the fact that the mother is entering a new estrus and is likely to lower her interest in previous offspring. Bekoff (1977) has proposed that a female dog entering a new estrus would benefit energetically from weaning pups from the previous litter early. The very low survival rate at 4 months of age would suggest that the majority of mortality occurs during this period of enforced early independence. Low reproductive efficiency in feral dogs can be attributed to two main causes: (a) estrus onsets are irregular and many litters are born at bad times of the year; and (b) mothers suffer the entire burden of parental care. In such conditions, it is perhaps not surprising that reproductive failures and high mortality rates are common.

With pup survival rates of only 5% after one year, it becomes easier to understand why free-roaming dogs have such difficulty maintaining their population levels. The same problem has already been noted but not explained for urban dogs (Beck, 1973; Daniels, 1983b; Pal, 2008) and for feral dogs in Arizona (Daniels & Bekoff, 1989b), and our study suggests that, without continuous recruitment of new group members from outside sources, feral groups cannot maintain their population levels.

A critical factor contributing to negative demographic balance in our feral group is their skewed sex ratio. Most urban and rural/suburban free-roaming dog populations show sex ratios skewed toward males. Beck (1973), for example, reported a ratio of 1.8:1 in favor of males in Baltimore, Maryland; Daniels (1983b) obtained a ratio of 3:1 in three study areas in Newark, New Jersey; Boitani & Racana (1984) found a ratio of 5:1 in Bella, a village of southern Italy, and a ratio of 4:1 in the surrounding rural areas; Daniels & Bekoff (1989b) found ratios of 1.6:1 and 2:1 in urban areas, and ratios of 4:1 and 3:1 in rural areas; three independent studies in Tunisia, Sri Lanka and Ecuador found male-biased sex ratios (60–65%) (WHO, 1988) and, finally, Macdonald & Carr (Chapter 16) found ratios of 4:1 and 2.6:1 in the villages of our study area. Possible reasons for such findings have already been discussed (see Beck, 1973; Daniels & Bekoff, 1989b): the unbalanced sex ratios of urban dogs result from direct selection of males as pets, and from the selective removal of females from the population, either temporarily to avoid unwanted pregnancies, or permanently by killing them as newborn puppies. Differential mortality rates for the two sexes are unlikely to occur in the absence of human interference. In one case, Daniels & Bekoff (1989b) noted a sex ratio of 1:3.5 in favor of females in a feral dog population in Arizona, in an area adjacent to an urban area. They attributed this result to the differential abandonment of female dogs by urban owners, since they could find no evidence of skewed sex ratios among puppies or of differential survival rates between the sexes.

When considering only the adult members in our group, a sex ratio of from 1:2 to 1:1.5 (group composition at various stages) in favor of females was obtained. From an initial 1:1 ratio, three females and two males were recruited from outside at various stages. Such small numbers, however, would not support the higher female abandonment hypothesis and they would not justify, in our opinion, any generalizations concerning the origins of skewed sex ratios. Two other animals that joined the group (a female and an unsexed individual) were the progeny of the feral group and their addition skewed the ratio more significantly in favor of females. This result is even more anomalous given that overall litter composition was highly skewed (3.2:1) in favor of males. Higher female survival rates would appear to be the only explanation for the observed adult sex ratio. Male-biased litter sex ratios have been reported in other canids, e.g. wolves (Mech, 1975), and wolves and hunting dogs (*Lycaon pictus*) (*International Zoo Yearbook*, vols. 5–11), but this sort of reproductive strategy would appear to have little adaptive value given the biological context of feral dogs. Further research is needed on different philopatric tendencies between the sexes, and on whether philopatry increases survival. A further interesting and open question is whether pups of the two sexes receive differential parental care.

Home range

Several environmental factors determine home range size, and human activities are among the most powerful. This is especially true for canids (Kleiman & Brady, 1978), and for dogs in particular. At the time of the study, the Harmonic Mean (HM) method proved to be the most appropriate in view of the dogs' highly flexible and diverse spatial patterns as it allowed a more accurate analysis of the home range's internal anatomy. The more internal contours reveal active selection by the dogs for lower road density and higher woodland density, and they show the strategic locations of core areas with respect to garbage dumps and villages. We know of no other study that has provided such detailed definition of the environmental and activity patterns within feral dogs' home ranges.

Within the overall home range, the group used smaller portions at any one time, shifting its core area in response to various factors, such as availability of temporary food resources (i.e. a large livestock carcass), disturbance by humans, denning activities, previous spatial use patterns of newly recruited dogs (i.e. when females 05 and 06 joined the group), unpredictable fluctuations in food availability at dumps, and possible interference from wolves. These factors had no seasonal predictability, and they appeared to occur as random events in the group's history. Daniels & Bekoff (1989a) found seasonal variations in home range related to the presence of dependent pups in one group they studied, while another group showed no such changes. Differential energetic requirements were suggested as a possible reason for the two groups' behavior (Daniels & Bekoff, 1989a), one group being slightly larger and having less food available. Scott & Causey (1973) also found a shifting of core areas depending on the presence or absence of pups. In our case, we suggest that drifting of seasonal ranges reflects not only direct environmental changes, but also the influence of previous knowledge of the area by new members of the group.

Seasonal home ranges reflected the same key environmental features of the annual range; seasonal core areas were similarly located with respect to roads, dumps, forests, villages, etc. They are more interesting, however, in relation to territorial behavior. The seasonal home range sizes we obtained (average 11.3 km^2 ± 6.2, range 2.2–21.2 km^2) are comparable with those found in previous feral dog studies. Nesbitt (1975), for example, recorded a home range of 28.5 km^2 in his 5-year study. Scott & Causey (1973) found home range sizes of 4.4–10.5 km^2 for three groups of dogs in Alabama. One solitary individual had a smaller home range of 2.8 km^2, but it also used to travel up to 1.6 km away from its usual range. Causey & Cude (1980) found a minimum home range of 18.7 km^2 for another group of dogs in Alabama. Daniels & Bekoff (1989a) reported a mean home range size of 1.6 km^2 for five feral dogs after the pups reached independence (but only 0.14 km^2 when the pups were still dependent). Their estimate, however, is based on the average of four animals located by sightings, and only one followed by radio-tracking. It is not surprising that the average for the four animals' home range was only 0.59 km^2, since the fifth had by far the largest home range of the entire study

(5.1km^2). Gipson (1983) reported the largest estimate for feral dogs' home range (70 km^2) in Alaska, but he obtained this estimate using a different method (Minimum Convex Polygon) that tends to overestimate space use and is quite sensitive to sample size. For example, the overall home range size of our feral dog group was much larger (91.7 km^2) if computed by that method.

Territorial aggression has been reported for free-roaming dogs in an urban environment (Bonanni *et al.*, 2010a, 2010b), but our feral dogs were more consistently territorial than reported previously for dogs living in a natural environment (Bekoff, 1979; Berman & Dunbar, 1983; Boitani & Racana, 1984; Daniels & Bekoff, 1989a; Scott & Fuller, 1965). In fact, we obtained evidence of territorial behavior not only in the proximity of den sites, but also within the entire core areas and at any time of the year. Similar observations have also been made by Macdonald & Carr (Chapter 16) in the same area. This high frequency of territorial behavior may be related to a somewhat higher level of social integration within the group, the higher degree of isolation from other dogs, and/or the high value of suitable core areas strategically located in proximity to quite predictable and concentrated food resources found in the dumps.

The partial overlap with two wolf pack ranges may also have increased the dogs' overall wariness and defensiveness. Although we have little evidence of direct competition between feral dogs and wolves (apart from dog 14 being killed by wolves), the partial overlap of territories and the almost identical niche they share in central Italy (Boitani, 1983) make competition for food and for space highly likely. The presence of wolves may, therefore, be an important factor shaping the dogs' home range and determining its location (Ciucci *et al.*, 1997).

Patterns of dump utilization (daytime/night) and of visits to the villages illustrate the flexibility of the group's behavior. At the individual level, the same animal was able to adopt different strategies to suit local conditions and minimize its risks. This overall adaptability should make us wary of drawing functional generalizations on the dogs' behavior and ecology based on few data or short-term studies.

Activity patterns

The tendency of dogs to show nocturnal and crepuscular activity patterns was first reported by Beck (1973) for urban dogs. During the summer, activity was mainly restricted to two periods, 7–10 p.m. and 5–8 a.m., and similar bimodal activity peaks were found by Berman & Dunbar (1983) among the dogs of Berkeley, California. Hirata *et al.* (1986) reported that the dogs of several Japanese towns were most active from midnight to 6 a.m., with a peak just before and around 6 a.m. A prominent dawn peak of activity has also been observed in free-roaming rural dogs in Virginia (Perry & Giles, 1971), while bimodal, dawn and dusk activity have been reported in several studies of feral dogs (Boitani & Racana, 1984; Causey & Cude, 1980; Daniels & Bekoff, 1989a; Scott & Causey, 1973). Nesbitt (1975) found similar temporal patterns, although he suggested that feral dogs could be active and travel all day, and that they tended to restrict themselves to the nocturnal and crepuscular hours in an attempt to avoid human contact. The movements of female 05 in three different but comparable denning situations seem to confirm Nesbitt's suggestion; when human presence was low, she moved mostly during the daytime, while she later resumed nocturnal habits when visiting the villages and the more disturbed dumps. Avoiding humans may provide an explanation for nocturnal activity, but it does not explain the bimodal pattern found for all dogs during all seasons. However, 9 out of 17 canid species are strictly nocturnal (see Bekoff *et al.*, 1981), and bimodal activity regimes have been suggested to be an innate behavioral trait, independent from any environmental pressure (Aschoff, 1966).

Wolves show seasonal activity changes, being more nocturnal in summer and both nocturnal and diurnal in winter (Mech, 1970). The activity patterns of feral dogs may reflect this ancestral flexibility. Seasonal variation has been reported previously by Scott & Causey (1973) and Beck (1973) who suggested that on hot summer days dogs preferred lying around and resting in shaded areas, resulting in the concentration of foraging activities during the night. We know of no previous study that has quantified activity variations during breeding periods.

Food sources and predation

Possible predation on wildlife and livestock has been the main impetus for feral dog studies. In North America, feral dogs have long been accused of predation on deer by the popular press, though on the basis of little evidence. In central Italy, the remains of wild boar (*Sus scrofa*), the only large ungulate in the area at the time of the study, were rarely found in dogs' scats and we never saw any evidence of predation on a live wild boar. Most previous studies of free-ranging dogs' feeding ecology have produced similar results. Perry & Giles (1971) studied owned radio-collared dogs; Causey & Cude (1980), Scott & Causey (1973) and Gipson & Sealander (1977) studied feral dogs, and all of them concluded that the dogs in their study areas were merely a nuisance, and had little overall impact on wildlife populations. Sweeney *et al.* (1971) recorded 65 experimental chases of radio-marked deer by hounds, without a single deer suffering any injury. Progulske & Baskett (1958), Corbett *et al.* (1971) and Olson (1974) experimented with trained dogs chasing deer and were unable to document a single successful hunt. A small percentage (7%) of successful chases were reported by Hawkins *et al.* (1970) in Illinois, and, in Idaho, Lowry & MacArthur (1978) reported 12 deer killed out of 39 chases. Several other authors have reported dog predation on wildlife (i.e. deer, gazelle, wild boar, hare, coyote, etc.) although most studies failed to document any serious impact on wildlife populations (Butler & du Toit, 2002; Butler *et al.*, 2004; Campos *et al.*, 2007; Denney 1974; Gavitt *et al.*, 1974; Federoff *et al.*, 1994; Herranz *et al.*, 2000; Kamler *et al.*, 2003; Manor & Saltz, 2004; Rouys & Theuerkauf, 2003; Vanak & Gompper, 2009).

On the other hand, free-roaming dogs have also been reported hunting and killing endangered and rare species, causing serious conservation concerns (see review in Young *et al.*, 2011; see also Hughes *et al.*, Chapter 18). Dog predation on vulnerable wildlife populations can have a significant negative impact at a local level and fully justifies the call for stronger controls on free-roaming dog populations (Hughes *et al.*, Chapter 18; Johnson, 2002; Lenth *et al.*, 2008; Young *et al.*, 2011).

The apparently contradictory results on the impact of feral dogs on wildlife are probably best explained by local conditions, and whether dogs had adequate alternative sources of food. It is also likely that some individual dogs or groups of dogs acquire the ability to chase and kill a particular species and maintain the habit through cultural transmission to new group members.

In Italy, the press and the conservation movement pointed to stray and feral dogs as primary predators of livestock and competitors of wild wolves, again with little supporting evidence (see Boitani, 1983). During our study we did not find any evidence of predation of livestock. Absence of livestock predation was reported by Scott & Causey (1973), and Nesbitt (1975) was unable to document a single case of livestock depredation in his five-year study. Similarly, in our study area, where cattle were free ranging over most of the area, no interference with livestock was ever observed. In contrast, Nesbitt (1975) reported that free-roaming pet dogs killed three calves in his study area, and one of us (Boitani, unpublished data) was able to document severe damage by free-roaming owned dogs on livestock in other areas of Italy. Thus, it appears that free-roaming owned and stray dogs may be the primary agents of livestock predation, although the blame tends to fall on feral dogs and wolves. This attitude is deeply rooted in the traditional perception humans have of the role of dogs as friends, and of wolves as enemies, and is difficult to counteract on the basis of often "tentative" biological evidence.

17.5   Management and conservation implications: Lessons from our work

The idea of a population of potential predators, with plenty of food resources to rely on, and with the reproductive potential given by all females producing litters twice a year, has all the makings of an ecologist's nightmare. Although not all studies of feral dogs, including our own, confirm the need for serious concerns about their impact on livestock or wildlife populations, feral dogs do have an impact on the human and natural environment. They can be effective carriers of potentially harmful diseases to both humans and wildlife (rabies, echinococcus, toxocara, parvovirus, etc.), may enhance parasite transmission (Biocca *et al.*, 1984; Corrain *et al.*, 2007; Salb *et al.*, 2008), and they can have a significant negative impact on the survival of endangered species (Hughes *et al.*, Chapter 18; Young *et al.*, 2011).

The ecological problem has a number of different dimensions, including the role of the dog as a predator, as a disease carrier, and as a competitor with biologically similar wild species (Hughes *et al.*, Chapter 18). In Italy, the ecological impact of feral dogs has been assessed in relation to wolf conservation, and potential conflicts between wolves and dogs have been identified at various levels (Boitani, 1983). The first area of conflict involves the space available for territorial ranges. Wolves in Italy mainly live in small packs (Boitani & Fabbri, 1983b), and dispersing animals play a critical role in securing the species' survival. Wolf packs tend to become highly unstable as human disturbance displaces them, and competition with stable and strong feral dog groups may prevent the wolves from establishing new pairs and new territories.

The second area of concern is for wolves and dogs' potential interbreeding. Although they belong to the same biological species, the two gene pools have been separated for many thousands of years by domestication. Evidence of "hybridization" has been reported since the early 1970s (Boitani & Fabbri, 1983a) and it has been spreading across Italy since then (Randi, 2008, Ciucci, 2012). Wolf/dog interbreeding has probably been going on for centuries, at least in Italy where shepherd dogs and wolves have been closely associated in the same habitat. Yet, paradoxically, hybridization may represent an even greater danger to the wolf today, with wolf populations naturally recolonizing their former ranges and increasing opportunities for wolf–dog encounters in human dominated contexts with abundant free-roaming dogs (e.g. Ciucci *et al.*, 2003).

The third area of conflict concerns the attitudes of humans towards wolves and dogs. In the mountain regions of central Italy, dogs are traditionally regarded as companions, and people tend to underestimate their potential impact as predators. Wolves, on the contrary, are perceived as vermin and any damage supposedly perpetrated by them is considered unacceptable. Shepherds and farmers consistently blame wolves for livestock predation, in order to get financial compensation, and as a result wolves suffer much heavier condemnation than they deserve. At present, free-roaming dogs are among the major threats to wolf conservation in Italy, and this fact adds additional weight to arguments in favor of their removal from the natural environment.

Thus, in the absence of any conceivable positive role for feral dogs, it appears obvious that it is preferable to eradicate them from natural areas. Any eradication plan aimed directly at the dogs living in the wild would be very costly and difficult to implement, since their (lethal or non-lethal) effective control would be a formidable task. In addition, it would probably not provide a permanent solution to the problem, as long as stray dogs continue to proliferate in the villages. Direct control measures are rendered even more difficult by the need to be highly selective to avoid harming other wildlife, especially competing carnivores (Boitani, 1983).

One particularly important and encouraging result from our study was the discovery that feral dogs seem to be unable to maintain their population levels without the continuous recruitment of new individuals from the stray reservoir. This evidence would indicate that the easiest and most effective way of controlling feral dogs would be by emphasizing the control of the stray population, combined with direct control of feral dogs to accelerate the process of eradication. Nesbitt's (1975) study on feral dogs following a massive removal effort of more than 100 dogs carried out a few years earlier by Hawkins *et al.* (1970) demonstrated that healthy groups of feral dogs still remained in the area despite these measures and were able to maintain the potential for a new demographic expansion.

Stray dog control is an old problem that many countries around the world are tackling with varying degrees of success (see Hiby & Hiby, Chapter 19). Direct control of stray animals is technically feasible and, in fact, is being implemented by public authorities in many towns and districts. However, unless the source of stray dogs is eliminated, an ultimate solution will never be reached. In the end, the most effective way of solving the stray dog problem is by influencing people's overall attitudes toward dog keeping.

It is likely that the management of most feral dog populations could be accomplished with little direct impact on the dogs themselves (though some direct removal must remain an inevitable management option) by approaching the problem with an intensive and effective campaign of public education. This should include a general information and education campaign, but also be focused more specifically on those human groups that are most responsible for the problem: hunters, shepherds, farmers and tourists who release, abandon or simply take inadequate care of their dogs. A complementary, indirect way to effectively regulate stray and feral dog populations is to halt their access to garbage dumps and other human-related food resources. In our study, reliable and predictable anthropogenic food sources in the form of dumps seem to represent the single, most important resource feral dogs relied upon for their continued existence. When the garbage dumps were finally eliminated in the mid 1990s, we found little evidence of feral dog groups persisting in successive years, notwithstanding the continuous availability of stray and other free-roaming dogs in the villages (Boitani *et al.*, 2006).

Acknowledgements

We thank M. L. Fabbri, J. Geppert, E. Schoenfeld, D. Talarico, and all the others who volunteered with field work assistance. F. Corsi helped with GIS and computer analysis. The project was funded by the Istituto Nazionale di Biologia della Selvaggina (INBS, now ISPRA), Bologna, and by an Earthwatch programme; their support is gratefully acknowledged. D. W. Macdonald is a long-time friend and there is no way to acknowledge properly his collaboration. An anonymous referee helped with improvements to the manuscript, and J. Serpell edited it and made it readable.

References

Aschoff, J. (1966). Circadian activity patterns with two peaks. *Ecology*, 47: 657–702.

Barnett, B. D. & Rudd, R. L. (1983). Feral dogs of the Galapagos Islands: impact and control. *International Journal for the Study of Animal Problems*, 4: 44–58.

Beck, A.M. (1973). *The Ecology of Stray Dogs: A Study of Free-ranging Urban Animals*. Baltimore, MD: York Press.

Beck, A. M. (1975). The ecology of "feral" and free-roving dogs in Baltimore. In *The Wild Canids*, ed. M. W. Fox. New York: Van Nostrand Reinhold, pp. 380–90.

Bekoff, M. (1977). Mammalian dispersal and the ontogeny of individual behavioral phenotypes. *American Naturalist*, 111: 715–32.

Bekoff, M. (1979). Scent-marking by free-ranging domestic dogs. *Biology of Behavior*, 4: 123–39.

Bekoff, M., Daniels, T. J. & Gittleman, J. L. (1984). Life history patterns and the comparative social ecology of carnivores. *Annual Review of Ecological Systematics*, 15: 191–232.

Bekoff, M., Diamond, J. & Mitton, J. B. (1981). Life history patterns and sociality in canids: body size, reproduction, and behavior. *Oecologia*, 50: 388–90.

Berman, M. & Dunbar, I. (1983). The social behavior of free-ranging suburban dogs. *Applied Animal Ethology*, 10: 5–17.

Biocca, M., Giovannini, A. Gradoni, L., Gramiccia, M., Mantovani, A., Pozio, E., Procicchiani, L. & Mantovani, A. (1984). Problemi di sanità pubblica legati ai cani randagi e inselvatichiti. *Annali Dell' Istituto di Sanita*, 20: 275–86.

Boitani, L. (1981). Lupo, *Canis lupus*. In *Distribuzione e Biologia di 22 Specie di Mammiferi in Italia*, ed. M. Pavan. Roma: CNR, pp. 61–7.

Boitani, L. (1983). Wolf and dog competition in Italy. *Acta Zoologica Fennica*, 174: 259–64.

Boitani, L. & Ciucci, P. (1995) Comparative social ecology of feral dogs and wolves. *Ethology Ecology and Evolution* 7: 49–72.

Boitani, L., Ciucci, P., Corsi, F. & Fabbri, M. L. (1989). A geographic information system (GIS) application to analyze the internal anatomy of the home range: feral dogs in the Apennines (Italy). In *Abstracts of the Fifth International Theriological Congress*, University of Rome, Rome, pp. 890–1.

Boitani, L., Ciucci, P. & Ortolani, A. (2006). Behavior and social ecology of free-ranging dogs. In *The Behavioral Biology of Dogs*, ed. P. Jensen. Wallingford, UK: CAB International, pp. 147–65.

Boitani, L. & Fabbri, M. L. (1983a). Censimento dei cani in Italia con particolare riguardo al fenomeno del randagismo. *Ricerche di Biologia della Selvaggina* (INBS, Bologna), 73: 1–51.

Boitani, L. & Fabbri, M. L. (1983b). Strategia nazionale di conservazione per il lupo (*Canis lupus*). *Ricerche di Biologia della Selvaggina* (INBS, Bologna), 72: 1–31.

Boitani, L. & Racana, A. (1984). Indagine eco-etologica sulla popolazione di cani domestici e randagi di due comuni della Basilicata. *Silva Lucana* (Bari), 3/84: 186.

Bonanni, R., Cafazzo, S., Valsecchi, P. & Natoli, E. (2010b) Effect of affiliative and agonistic relationships on leadership behavior in free-ranging dogs. *Animal Behavior*, 79: 981–91.

Bonanni, R., Valsecchi, P. & Natoli, E. (2010a) Pattern of individual participation and cheating in conflicts between groups of free-ranging dogs. *Animal Behavior*, 79: 957–68.

Brehm, A. (1893). *Tierleben*, 4 vols. Liepzig-Wien. Brisbin, I. L. (1974). The ecology of animal domestication: its relevance to man's environmental crises – past, present and future. *Association of Southeastern Biologists Bulletin*, 21: 3–8.

Butler, J. R. A. & du Toit, J. T. (2002). Diet of free-ranging domestic dogs (*Canis familiaris*) in rural Zimbabwe: Implications for wild scavengers on the periphery of wildlife reserves. *Animal Conservation*, 5: 29–37.

Butler, J. R. A., du Toit, J. T. & Bingham, J. (2004) Free-ranging domestic dogs (*Canis familiaris*) as predators and prey in rural Zimbabwe: threats of competition and disease to large wild carnivores. *Biological Conservation*, 115: 369–78.

Cafazzo, S., Valsecchi, P., Bonanni, R. & Natoli, E. (2010) Dominance in relation to age, sex and competitive contexts in a group of free-ranging domestic dogs. *Behavioral Ecology*, 21: 443–455.

Campos, C. B., Esteves, C. F., Ferraz, K., Crawshaw, P. G. & Verdade, L. M. (2007) Diet of free-ranging cats and dogs in a suburban and rural environment, south-eastern Brazil. *Journal of Zoology*, 273: 14–20.

Causey, M. K. & Cude, C. A. (1980). Feral dog and white-tailed deer interactions in Alabama. *Journal of Wildlife Management*, 44: 481–484.

Ciucci, P. (2012). Ibridazione con il cane come minaccia per la conservazione del lupo: stato delle conoscenze e criteri per l'identificazione degli ibridi. [Wolf/dog hybridization as a threat for wolf conservation: a review and criteria for the identification of hybrids]. Technical Report Life Project 10NAT/IT/00265/Ibriwolf, Roma. [In Italian].

Ciucci, P., Boitani, L., Francisci, F. & Andreoli G. (1997). Home-range, activity and movements of a wolf pack in central Italy. *Journal of Zoology (London)*, 243: 803–19.

Ciucci, P., Lucchini, V., Boitani, L. & Randi E. (2003). Dew-claws in wolves as evidence of admixed ancestry with dogs. *Canadian Journal of Zoology*, 81: 2077–81.

Corbett, R. L., Marchinton, R. L. & Hill, C. L. (1971). Preliminary study of the effects of dogs on radio-equipped deer in mountainous habitat. *Proceedings of the Annual Conference of the Southeastern Association State Game and Fish Commissioners*, 25: 69–77.

Corrain, R., Francesco, A., di Bolognini, M., Ciucci, P., Baldelli, R. & Guberti, V. (2007). Serosurvey for CPV-2, distemper virus, ehrlichiosis and leishmaniosis in free-ranging dogs in Italy. *Veterinary Record*, 160: 91–2.

Daniels, T. J. (1983a). The social organization of free-ranging urban dogs: II. Estrous groups and the mating system. *Applied Animal Ethology*, 10: 365–73.

Daniels, T. J. (1983b). The social organization of free-ranging urban dogs: I. Nonestrous social behavior. *Applied Animal Ethology*, 10: 341–63.

Daniels, T. J. (1988). Down in the dumps. *Natural History*, 97: 8–12.

Daniels, T. J. & Bekoff, M. (1989a). Spatial and temporal resource use by feral and abandoned dogs. *Ethology*, 81: 300–12.

Daniels, T. J. & Bekoff, M. (1989b). Population and social biology of free-ranging dogs, *Canis familiaris. Journal of Mammalogy*, 70: 754–62.

Daniels, T. J. & Bekoff, M. (1989c). Feralization: the making of wild domestic animals. *Behavioural Processes*, 19: 79–94.

Denney, R. N. (1974). Impact of uncontrolled dogs on wildlife and livestock. *Transactions of the North American Wildlife and Natural Resources Conference*, 39: 257–91.

Dixon, K. R. & Chapman, J. A. (1980). Harmonic mean measure of animal activity areas. *Ecology*. 61: 1040–4.

Federoff, N. E., Jakob, W. J. & Bauer, W. C. (1994) Female feral dog and two pups kill deer fawn at the Patuxent

Wildlife Research Center, Laurel, Maryland. *Maryland Naturalist*, 38: 1–2.

Gavitt, J. D., Downing, R. L. & McGinnes, B. S. (1974). Effects of dogs on deer reproduction in Virginia. *Proceedings of the Annual Conference of the Southeastern Association State Game and Fish Commissioners*, 28: 532–9.

Genovesi, P. & Dupré, E. (2000) Strategia nazionale di conservazione del Lupo (*Canis lupus*): indagine sulla presenza e la gestione dei cani vaganti in Italia. [National strategy for the conservation of the wolf (*Canis lupus*): survey on the presence and management of free-ranging dogs in Italy.] *Biologia e Conservazione della Fauna*, 104: 1–33.

Gipson, P. S. (1972). The Taxonomy, Reproductive Biology, Food Habits, and Range of Wild *Canis* (Canidae) in Arkansas. Unpublished Ph.D. dissertation, University of Arkansas, Fayetteville.

Gipson, P. S. (1983). Evaluation of behavior of feral dogs in interior Alaska, with control implications. In *Vertebrate Pest Control and Management Materials: 4th Symposium*, ed. D. E. Kaukeinen. Philadelphia, PA: ASTM Special Technical Publication, pp. 285–94.

Gipson, P. S. & Sealander, J. A. (1977). Ecological relationship of white-tailed deer and dogs in Arkansas. In *Proceedings of the 1975 Predator Symposium, Montana Forest Conservation Experimental Station*, eds. R. L. Philips & C. Jonkel. Missoula: University of Montana, pp. 3–17.

Gittleman, J. L. (ed.) (1989). *Carnivore Behavior, Ecology and Evolution*. London: Chapman & Hall.

Hale, E. B. (1962). Domestication and the evolution of behaviour. In *The Behaviour of Domestic Animals*, 2nd edition, ed. E. S. E. Hafez. London: Bailliere, Tindall & Cassell, pp. 22–42.

Hare, B., Brown, M., Williamson, C. & Tomasello, M. (2002). The domestication of social cognition in dogs. *Science*, 298: 1634–6.

Hawkins, R. E., Klimstra, W. D. & Antry, D. C. (1970). Significant mortality factors of deer in Crab Orchard National Wildlife Refuge. *Transactions of the Illinois State Academy of Sciences*, 63: 202–6.

Herranz, J., Yanes, M. & Suarez, F. (2000) Relationships among the abundance of small game species, their predators, and habitat structure on Castilla-La Mancha (Spain). *Ecologia*, 14: 219–33.

Hirata, H., Okuzaki, M. & Obara, H. (1986). Characteristics of urban dogs and cats. In *Integrated Studies in Urban Ecosystems as the Basis of Urban Planning I.*, ed. H. Obara. Special Research Project on Environmental Science (B276-R15-3). Tokyo: Ministry of Education, pp. 163–75.

Hirata, H., Okuzaki, M. & Obara, H. (1987). Relationships between men and dogs in urban ecosystem. In *Integrated Studies in Urban Ecosystems as the Basis of Urban Planning II.*, ed. H. Obara. Special Research Project on Environmental Science (B334R15-3). Tokyo: Ministry of Education, pp. 113–20.

Hsu, Y., Severinghaus, L. L. & Serpell, J. A. (2003) Dog keeping in Taiwan: its contribution to the problem of free-roaming dogs. *Journal of Applied Animal Welfare Science*, 6: 1–23.

Johnson, M. R. (2002). A new capture pen for Caribbean feral dog packs. *Intermountain Journal of Sciences*, 8: 255.

Kamler, J. F., Keeler, K., Wiens, G., Richardson, C. & Gipson, P. S. (2003) Feral dogs, *Canis familiaris*, kill coyote, *Canis latrans*. *Canadian Field-Naturalist*, 117: 123–4.

Kirk, R. W. (ed.) (1977). *Current Veterinary Therapy. Vol. VI: Small Animal Practice*. Philadelphia, PA: W. B. Saunders.

Kleiman, D. G. (1968). Reproduction in the Canidae. *International Zoo Yearbook*, 8: 1–7.

Kleiman, D. G. & Brady, C. A. (1978). Coyote behavior in the context of recent canid research: problems and perspectives. In *Coyotes*, ed. M. Bekoff. New York: Academic Press, pp. 163–88.

Kleiman, D. G. & Eisenberg, J. F. (1973). Comparisons of canid and felid social systems from an evolutionary perspective. *Animal Behavior*, 21: 637–59.

Kleiman, D. G. & Malcolm, J. R. (1981). The evolution of male parental investment in mammals. In *Parental Care in Mammals*, eds. D. J. Gubernik & P. H. Klopfer. New York: Plenum, pp. 347–87.

Lenth, B., Knight, R. & Brennan M. E. (2008). The effects of dogs on wildlife communities. *Natural Areas Journal*, 28: 218–27.

Lindstrom, E. (1986). Territory inheritance and the evolution of group living in carnivores. *Animal Behavior*, 34: 1825–35.

Lowry, D. A. & MacArthur, K. L. (1978). Domestic dogs as predators on deer. *Wildlife Society Bulletin*, 6: 38–9.

Macdonald, D. W. (1983). The ecology of carnivore social behavior. *Nature*, 301: 379–84.

Macdonald, D. W. & Carr, G. M. (1989). Food security and the rewards of tolerance. In *Comparative Socioecology: the Behavioral Ecology of Humans and Other Mammals*, eds. V. Standen & R. A. Foley. Oxford: Blackwell Scientific Publications, pp. 75–99.

Manor, R. & Saltz D. (2004). The impact of free-roaming dogs on gazelle kid/female ratio in a fragmented area. *Biological Conservation*, 119: 231–6.

McKnight, T. (1964). *Feral Livestock in Anglo–America*. Berkeley, CA: University of California Press.

Mech, L. D. (1970). *The Wolf: The Ecology and Behavior of an Endangered Species*. New York: Natural History Press.

Mech, L. D. (1975). Disproportionate sex ratios of wolf pups. *Journal of Wildlife Management*, 39: 737–740.

Mech, L. D. (1983). *Handbook of Animal Radiotracking*. Minneapolis, MN: University of Minnesota Press.

Mech, L. D. & Boitani, L. (2003) Social ecology of the wolf. In *Wolves: Behavior, Ecology and Conservation*, eds. L. D. Mech & L. Boitani. Chicago, IL: University of Chicago Press, pp. 1–34.

Nesbitt, W. H. (1975). Ecology of a feral dog pack on a wildlife refuge. In *The Wild Canids*, ed. M. W. Fox. New York: Van Nostrand Reinhold, pp. 391–5.

Olson, J. C. (1974). Movements of deer as influenced by dogs. Indiana Department of Natural Resources Job Progress Report Project W-26-R-5, Job III-b-4, pp. 1–36.

Ortolani, A., Vernooij, H. & Coppinger, R. (2009). Ethiopian village dogs: Behavioural responses to stranger's approach. *Applied Animal Behaviour Science*, 119: 210–18.

Pal, S. K. (2001). Population ecology of free-ranging urban dogs in West Bengal, India. *Acta Theriologica*, 46: 69–78.

Pal, S. K. (2005). Parental care in free-ranging dogs, *Canis familiaris*. *Applied Animal Behaviour Science*, 90: 31–47.

Pal S. K. (2008). Maturation and development of social behavior during early ontogeny in free-ranging dog puppies in West Bengal, India. *Applied Animal Behaviour Science*, 111: 95–107.

Pal, S. K., Gosh, B. & Roy, S. (1998a) Dispersal behavior of free-ranging dogs (*Canis familiaris*) in relation to age, sex, season and dispersal distance. *Applied Animal Behaviour Science*, 61: 123–32.

Pal, S. K., Gosh, B. & Roy, S. (1998b) Agonistic behavior of free-ranging dogs (*Canis familiaris*) in relation to season, sex and age. *Applied Animal Behaviour Science* 59: 331–48.

Pal, S. K., Gosh, B. & Roy, S. (1999) Inter- and intra-sexual behavior of free-ranging dogs (*Canis familiaris*). *Applied Animal Behaviour Science*, 62: 267–78.

Perry, B. D. (1993). Dog ecology in eastern and southern Africa: implications for rabies control. *Onderstepoort Journal of Veterinary Research*, 60: 429–36.

Perry, M. C. & Giles, R. H. (1971). Free running dogs. *Virginia Wildlife*, 32: 17–19.

Price, E. O. (1984). Behavioral aspects of animal domestication. *Quarterly Review of Biology*, 59: 1–32.

Progulske, D. R. & Baskett, T. S. (1958). Mobility of Missouri deer and their harassment by dogs. *Journal of Wildlife Management*, 22: 184–92.

Randi, E. (2008). Detecting hybridization between wild species and their domesticated relatives. *Molecular Ecology*, 17: 285–93.

Rouys, S. & Theuerkauf, J. (2003). Factors determining the distribution of introduced mammals in nature reserves of the southern province, New Caledonia. *Wildlife Research*, 30: 187–91.

Salb, A. L., Barkema, H. W, Elkin, B. T., Thompson, R. C. A., Whiteside, D. P., Black, S. R., Dubey, J. P. & Kutz, S. J. (2008). Dogs as sources and sentinels of parasites in humans and wildlife, northern Canada. *Emerging Infectious Disease*, 14: 60–3.

Samuel, M. D., Pierce, D. J. & Garton, E. O. (1985). Identifying areas of concentrated use within home ranges. *Journal of Animal Ecology*, 54: 711–19.

Scott, M. D. & Causey, K. (1973). Ecology of feral dogs in Alabama. *Journal of Wildlife Management*, 37: 253–65.

Scott, J. P. & Fuller, J. L. (1965). *Genetics and the Social Behavior of the Dog*. Chicago, IL: University of Chicago Press.

Spencer, W. D. & Barret, R. H. (1984). An evaluation of the harmonic mean measure for defining carnivore activity areas. *Acta Zoologica Fennica*, 171: 255–9.

Sweeney, J. R., Marchinton, R. L. & Sweeney, J. M. (1971). Responses of radiomonitored white-tailed deer chased by hunting dogs. *Journal of Wildlife Management*, 35: 707–17.

van Ballenberghe, V. (1983). Two litters raised in one year by a wolf pack. *Journal of Mammalogy*, 64: 171–3.

von Schantz, T. (1984). Carnivore social behavior – does it need patches? *Nature*, 307: 389.

Vanak, A. T. & Gompper, M. E. (2009). Dogs (*Canis familiaris*) as carnivores: their role and function in intraguild competition. *Mammal Review*, 39: 265–83.

Young, J. K., Olson K. A, Reading R. P., Amgalanbaatar S. & Berger, J. (2011). Is wildlife going to the dogs? Impacts of feral and free-roaming dogs on wildlife populations. *BioScience*, 61: 125–32.

World Health Organization (1988). *Report of WHO Consultation on Dog Ecology Studies Related to Rabies Control*. WHO/Rabies Research/88.25.

Zeuner, F. E. (1963). *A History of Domesticated Animals*. London: Hutchinson.

18 Roaming free in the rural idyll: Dogs and their connections with wildlife

JOELENE HUGHES, DAVID W. MACDONALD AND LUIGI BOITANI

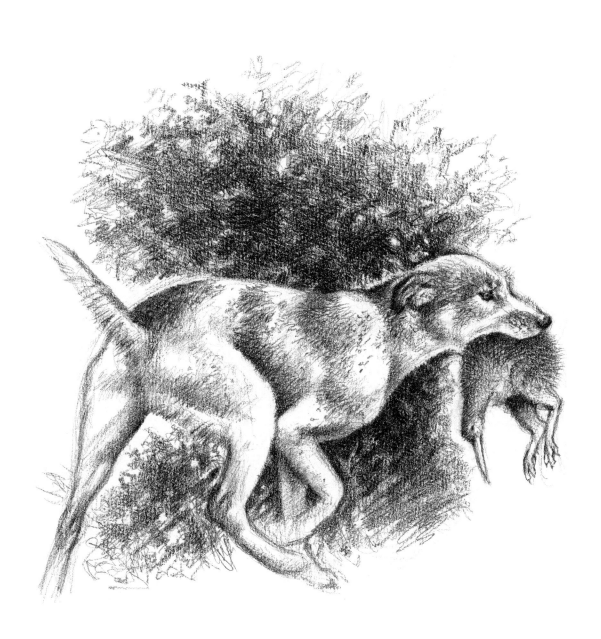

18.1   Introduction

Since the domestication of the wolf (*Canis lupus*), some 13 000–17 000 years ago, dogs (*Canis familiaris*) have become close companions to humans, and been integrated into communities, families and folklore (Driscoll & Macdonald, 2010). During that time the dog population has extended, along with humans, across every continent except mainland Antarctica, until there are now an estimated 700 million of them worldwide (Hughes & Macdonald, 2013). Today the roles of dogs in human society are complex and varied: from status symbols kept in handbags to dogs raised with the livestock they are trained to protect; from sacred icons to sources of income for breeders or racers; from waste disposers to family members, with each role resulting in different levels of integration with the human community (see Serpell, Chapter 15). The benefits of domesticated dogs to communities and human society are manifold but there are also costs to this symbiosis. It is undoubtedly true that dogs cause problems for humans – they are, for example, the most common source of rabies in the world, the cause of 99% of the 55 000 human fatalities globally (Knobel *et al.*, 2005) – and a sizeable economic cost may be incurred due to the injuries they cause (e.g. estimated $620 million a year in the US; Pimentel *et al.*, 2005). There are also costs for the dogs who may suffer from high mortality, malnutrition, disease, parasitism, starvation and abuse (Pal, 2001; Sowemimo, 2009). Indeed, where dogs are identified as a source of public health problems, governing bodies may be prompted to eradicate them in a variety of ways with attendant welfare concerns (Dalla Villa *et al.*, 2010), whilst owners may abandon or destroy puppies and adults they cannot afford (Hsu *et al.*, 2003).

Alongside these costs – and our focus in this chapter – are the problems this domestic carnivore may cause within the environments to which they are introduced, and for the wildlife species with which they interact (Hughes & Macdonald, 2013; Young *et al.*, 2011). While wildlife does exist within urban areas, it is arguable that the majority of interactions of conservation relevance between wildlife and dogs take place in rural regions, where dogs may move between human-dominated areas and the surrounding landscape (Macdonald & Carr, Chapter 16). Such movements not only cause problems for wildlife but also connect wildlife and the local human population more closely than is beneficial for either. The purpose of this review is to explore both the impacts of domestic dogs on wildlife and the solutions proposed to mitigate any problems that arise.

In rural locations the number of dogs sometimes exceeds the number of humans (Wandeler *et al.*, 1993), and generally the human:dog ratio is lower than in urban situations. The rural domestic dog population can be a mix of several sub-populations due to the varying relationships dogs may have with humans. Some dogs are restrained and completely dependent on humans, some are free-roaming but still rely on human communities to provide food and shelter, and still others require little or no human contact and may be labeled as feral (Boitani *et al.*, Chapter 17). These distinct sub-populations may exhibit different movements and behavior, fertility and survival rates, as well as being treated differently by the humans with whom they associate. Free-roaming dogs (FRDs) in particular may spend a lot of time both within the human community and in the surrounding natural habitat. These dogs may be owned and allowed to roam free during various periods in a day, or just have some semblance of attachment to a household, street or area, only infrequently, if ever, coming under human control. As such, FRDs provide a link between wildlife and humans; a linkage that results in a range of negative impacts on both (Hughes & Macdonald, 2013). Dogs effectively extend the range of harmful influences that human settlements have on natural habitats and on the wildlife that lives there, and facilitate interaction between wildlife and humans and/or their livestock.

18.2   Impact of dogs on wildlife

Domestic dogs interact with a variety of wildlife species worldwide. A recent review of published papers that mention interactions between domestic dogs and wildlife around the globe (69 papers set in 29 different countries on six continents, Table 18.1), reveals contact between dogs and a total of 64 different wildlife species (Hughes & Macdonald, 2013). Of these, only three studies concluded that the interaction with dogs was having no detrimental effects: a study that looked at prey competition between domestic dogs and Ethiopian wolves, *Canis simensis*, which found no evidence of competition (Atickem *et al.*, 2010); a study that found no consequences of hybridization between dogs and wolves (*Canis lupus*; Vilà & Wayne, 1999); and a third which found that dogs were not involved in the transmission of the parasite, *Echinococcus granulosus*, between wildlife and domestic animals in Queensland, Australia (Banks *et al.*, 2006). However, even in these contexts the dogs could not necessarily be described as a benign presence. Indeed, Atickem *et al.* (2010) gave evidence of dogs harassing wolves, in addition to unquantified predation of a number of other wildlife species, such as rock hyraxes (*Procavia capensis*), various rat-sized rodents, molerats (*Tachyoryctes spp.*), and Starck's hare (*Lepus starcki*). In all the other studies reviewed, dogs were either assumed or demonstrated to be important figures in local ecosystems.

Table 18.1   The types of interactions occurring between wildlife and free-roaming dogs (FRDs) in rural areas, as recorded from a review of current research. The FRDs appear to interact mainly with other mammals. However, this, along with the geographic distribution, is most likely due to the focus of the research rather than reflecting reality.

Interaction type	Group studied	Country/region	Reference
Competition	Mammals	General	Vanak & Gompper (2009a, 2009b)
		Italy	Ciucci and Boitani (1998)
Disease	Insects	Argentina	Acardi *et al.* (2010)
	Mammals	Africa	Bingham (2005)
		Botswana	Alexander *et al.* (1996)
		Israel	David *et al.* (2009)
		Kenya	Alexander *et al.* (1993)
			Cleaveland *et al.* (2007)
			Lembo *et al.* (2008)
			Macpherson *et al.* (1983)
		Namibia	Gowtage-Sequiera *et al.* (2009)
		Spain	Sobrino *et al.* (2009)
		Turkey	Johnson *et al.* (2006)
		Panama	Herrer *et al.* (1973)
		US	Rausch (1958)

Table 18.1 (*Cont.*)

Interaction type	Group studied	Country/region	Reference
Disturbance	Mammals	Chile	Medina-Vogel *et al.* (2007)
			Silva-Rodriguez *et al.* (2010)
		India	Vanak *et al.* (2009)
		US	Fox *et al.* (1975)
			Marks & Duncan (2009)
			Mech (1988)
			Hennessy *et al.* (1981)
		General	Engelhart & Mullerschwarze (1995)
Hybridization	Mammals	Australia	Jenkins (2006)
		Ethiopia	Sillero-Zubiri & Gotelli (1994)
		US	Freeman & Shaw (1979)
			Gipson *et al.* (1974)
Predator–prey	Amphibians	Fiji	Morley (2006)
	Birds	New Zealand	Taborsky (1988)
		Spain	Yanes and Suarez (1996)
		US	Hale (2004)
			Krogh & Schweitzer (1999)
			Marti (1994)
			McChesney & Tershy (1998)
			Miller & Leopold (1992)
			Szekely & Cuthill (2000)
			Young *et al.* (2011)
	Birds and mammals	US	Gipson & Sealander (1976)
	Invertebrates, mammals, birds, reptiles	Brazil	Campos *et al.* (2007)
	Mammals	Australia	Meek (1999)
		Brazil	Brito *et al.* (2004)
		Canada	Bergeron & Demers (1981)
		Chile	Silva-Rodriguez *et al.* (2010)
		Cote d'Ivoire	Bodendorfer *et al.* (2006)
		Cuba	Borroto-Paez (2009)
		Estonia	Maran *et al.* (2009)

Table 18.1 (*Cont.*)

Interaction type	Group studied	Country/region	Reference
		Ethiopia	Atickem *et al.* (2010)
		India	Edgaonkar & Chellam (2002)
			Jhala (1993)
		Israel	Manor & Saltz (2004)
		Mongolia	Young *et al.* (2011)
		Syria/Israel	Gingold *et al.* (2009)
		Tibet	Schaller (1998)
		US	Kamler *et al.* (2003)
			Lowry & Macarthur (1978)
			Timm & Schmidt (1989)
		Italy	Boitani *et al.* (1995)
		Venezuela	Farrell *et al.* (2000)
		Zimbabwe	Butler & Du Toit (2002)
			Butler *et al.* (2004)
	Mammals, reptiles	Brazil	Lacerda *et al.* (2009)
		US	Causey & Cude (1980)
	Mammals, reptiles, insects	India	Vanak & Gompper (2009)
	Reptiles	Costa Rica	Fowler (1979)
		Galapagos	Kruuk & Snell (1981)
		US	Madden *et al.* (2008)
		West Indies	Iverson (1978)
None	Mammals	Australia	Banks *et al.* (2006)
		Europe	Vilà & Wayne (1999)

The most common interactions were with mammals, recorded in 54 out of 69 studies (78%). Species of birds were recorded in 11 (16%) studies, reptiles in eight (12%), invertebrates in four (6%) and amphibians in one study. This is likely to be an underestimate of the true number and types of wildlife species affected in these areas due to most of the research being carried out with a focus on a particular wildlife species, or a particular habitat area, rather than focussing on the foraging behavior and ecology of the dogs themselves. Of the 64 wildlife species recorded as interacting with dogs, 63 appear on the IUCN Red List: 5% as Critically Endangered; 14% as Endangered; 14% as Vulnerable; 8% as Near Threatened; 56% were Least Concern; and 1 was unknown. Therefore, one third of the wildlife species recorded as interacting with domestic dogs are classified as globally threatened. In the majority of cases, these dog–wildlife interactions were negative. It's safe to conclude, therefore, that dogs are a potential concern for wildlife conservation.

18.2.1 Predation

There are five main routes through which FRDs are generally recorded to impact native wildlife: predation, disease transmission, disturbance, competition and hybridization (Hughes & Macdonald, 2013). Predation of wildlife by dogs is the most frequently recorded interaction and can have ruinous consequences for wildlife populations since dog populations, supported by local humans, do not necessarily decline in response to wildlife prey depletion in the way that wild predator populations do. In the early twentieth century, Lotka and Volterra independently developed simple mathematical models describing how predator and prey species interact, now known as the Lotka–Volterra model (Krebs, 2009). The Lotka–Volterra model describes how as prey populations increase, after a while, the predator population will increase, as there is more food available. However, with increasing predation due to the rising predator numbers, the prey population will decline and cause a decline in predators in response. This decline in predators consequently releases the prey from high levels of predation and the prey population can grow again. Thus, prey and predator population abundances oscillate in cycles. However, if an alternative food source is available for the predators, for example the human provision of food for dogs, or predators are continually migrating into the area, for example by dogs being continually abandoned, the abundance of predators will stay at high levels and the prey population will be constantly supressed and potentially exterminated.

Predation by dogs affects 15 of the 21 species listed as Threatened by the IUCN, including two of the three Critically Endangered species, the saiga antelope (*Saiga tatarica mongolica*; Young *et al.*, 2011) and the West Indian rock iguana (*Cyclura carinata*; Iverson, 1978). Predation may be of particular concern on islands where animals are range restricted or have not developed the necessary antipredator skills to deal with introduced carnivores. In the conservation hotspot of the Galapagos, dogs have been introduced and abandoned on several islands where they devastate populations of seabirds and reptiles (Brand Phillips *et al.*, 2012). Dogs have been identified as a potential cause of extinction of populations of the marine iguana (*Amblyrhynchus cristatus*) on Isabela, where they preferentially predated the larger individuals that remain out on rocks at night and do not flee from predators as readily as smaller ones – a behavior thought to have evolved in response to predation by the endemic Galapagos hawk (*Buteo galapagoensis*), which only preys on small iguanas (Kruuk & Snell, 1981). In Waitangi Forest in New Zealand, a single dog was thought to be responsible for the killing of over half (500 from an estimated 900) of a population of *Apteryx mantelli*, the North Island brown kiwi, in a period of six weeks (Taborsky, 1988).

Predation of wildlife species by domestic dogs may be either incidental or specific. The predation of ground-nesting larks in Spain, although opportunistic for the dogs who are hunting for rabbits, may be significant for the populations of Thekla larks (*Galerida theklae*) and short-toed larks (*Calandrella rufescens*) as 68–99% of nests are predated by foxes or dogs (Yanes and Suarez, 1996). Targeted predation of endemic mammals, such as the Conga hutia (*Capromys pilorides*) and the almiquí (*Solenodon cubanus*) occurs on 16 islands in the Cuban archipelago (Borroto-Paez, 2009). On some of the islands, dogs, originally brought in by humans in order to hunt hutias, have been abandoned (Borroto-Paez, 2009). When left to their own devices, the dogs may wait for nightfall when the more arboreal hutias come to ground to forage, and they have also been known to attack livestock (Borroto-Paez, 2009). The effect of dogs on wildlife species may only be obvious when the wildlife population is brought close to extinction. However, dogs may be affecting population dynamics even when the prey is seemingly still abundant. A compelling example is the declining population of mountain gazelles (*Gazella g. gazella*) in Israel (Manor & Saltz, 2004). In a heavily fragmented area which does not support natural predators, Manor and Saltz (2004), examined the relationship between the recruitment of gazelles, as measured by the kid:female ratio, and the presence of dogs in 12 sub-sections, taking into account evidence of human activity and vegetation available for grazing. The study was conducted from October 1998 to February 2000. During March–September 1999 Israel Nature and Parks Authority carried out a cull of dogs targeted around a dump in the study site, which reduced the dog numbers in four adjacent sub-sections. The gazelles reproduce all year round in this environment with two peaks, in April–May and September–October, and consequently the researchers were able to measure the effect of the dog cull on gazelle reproduction rates over three birthing peaks. Not only was the dog-presence index the only significant factor the authors found in determining the kid:female ratio, but during and after the cull, the kid:female ratio increased in the four sub-sections near the dump while remaining the same in the other eight sub-sections.

Predation by dogs is not necessarily a conservation concern if it does not limit the prey population. Although the effects of predation by dogs can be severe in some situations, in others dogs have been observed to be relatively ineffectual predators. For example, domestic dogs were responsible for over half of the 25% of green sea turtle nests destroyed by terrestrial predators on Tortuguero. However, this was considered a small fraction of the losses normally sustained by the marine reptile and of comparatively minor concern (Fowler, 1979). In the Gokwe Communal Land and Sengwa Wildlife Research Area in Zimbabwe, Butler *et al*. (2004) found that, compared with other large carnivores (e.g. lions, leopards and spotted hyenas), the impact of predation by dogs was limited by their inability to catch the majority of prey species due to their smaller group and body size. Moreover, rather than being competition for larger carnivores, the dogs may themselves become the prey with around 6% of the dog population being taken by leopards, lions and spotted hyaenas (Butler *et al*., 2004). Undigested food remains in scats have revealed that wolves eat dogs in Velavadar National Park, India (Jhala, 1993). Similarly, leopard scats in Comoé National Park, Côte d'Ivoire, have shown dogs to be part of this felid's diet (Bodendorfer *et al*., 2006). In both of these cases, however, they only constitute a tiny proportion of the diet (1% of wolf diet in two years, 0.3% of leopard diet in three years). Under these conditions, the presence of dogs as a food source might be considered a positive effect from a wildlife conservation perspective. In the Sanjay Gandhi National Park near Mumbai, where there is a low density of wild ungulates, dogs have become a major prey item of the leopard, constituting about 58% of the diet (Edgaonkar & Chellam, 2002). As a result of the apparent importance of dogs as prey for leopards, Edgaonkar and Chellam (2002) concluded that any action to control the dog population may deprive the leopards of an important food source (see Bhatia *et al*., 2013). This situation raises obvious welfare issues for the dogs, but such interactions between dogs and wildlife may also represent a potential threat to wild carnivores due to another factor, the potential for disease transmission (Butler *et al*., 2004).

18.2.2   Disease transmission

Disease transmission from domestic dogs to humans has long been a global health concern due to the devastating impacts of several zoonoses, in particular rabies, a disease that still remains a human health problem more than 125 years since the first successful cure by Louis Pasteur (Bourhy *et al*., 2010). Biologists have recognized the importance of diseases and population health in wildlife conservation for many decades. One of the earliest mentions of negative interactions between domestic dogs and wildlife recorded in the scientific literature was of the transmission of rabies between wild and domestic canids in Alaska (Rausch, 1958), and in Hughes & Macdonald's (2013) review of dog and wildlife interactions, disease transmission is the second most frequently recorded interaction type. However, it is only since the end of the twentieth century that this crucial issue has really begun to draw attention from the wider conservation community (Deem *et al.*, 2001; Rhodes *et al.*, 1998). Free-roaming domestic dogs are an important vector for diseases, such as rabies and canine distemper virus (CDV), which can severely impact wild species' population abundance. The effects of disease transmission between dogs and wildlife can be drastic. For example, the highly endangered Ethiopian wolf, *Canis simensis*, has suffered a number of rabies epidemics over the last 20 years that reduced the population by around 75% (Randall *et al.*, 2006). Domestic dog populations may act as a reservoir for the disease, enabling it to persist in the environment and cause repeated outbreaks in wildlife populations. This has been observed in the Serengeti where domestic dogs are now considered a critical component of the Serengeti–Mara ecosystem, acting as the reservoir for rabies and CDV in the area and causing outbreaks amongst wild carnivore populations (Cleaveland *et al.*, 2007). Research in Kenya has shown that contact with domestic dogs was a significant predictor of the exposure of African wild dogs (*Lycaon pictus*) to three of six pathogens studied – canine parvovirus, *Ehrlichia canis* and *Neospora caninum* – and a possible predictor of rabies transmission (Woodroffe *et al.*, 2012). In addition to being a potential reservoir host, the presence of dogs may alter local disease ecology. Parasites that usually cycle among wildlife species may develop a second cycle among wildlife, dogs, livestock and even humans, due to transmission between wildlife and dogs. For example, *Echinococcus spp.* are parasites that cause hydatid disease, resulting in the growth of cysts on major internal organs such as the liver, lungs and heart, and are a global human health concern. In Kenya, *Echinococcus granulosus* is thought to be transmitted between wildlife, domestic dogs, livestock and humans through the scavenging of dogs and wildlife on livestock, and through humans eating infected wildlife (Macpherson *et al.*, 1983). Zoonotic transmission of diseases between wildlife and humans or livestock, can lead to human–wildlife conflict, as well as increased parasite load for wildlife.

18.2.3   Disturbance and competition

Even if not directly affecting wildlife species through predation or disease transmission, dogs may impact wild populations indirectly through disturbance and competition. Marine otters (*Lontra felina*) in Chile sometimes take advantage of the fishing waste found around villages along the coast. This, however, brings them into the vicinity of village dogs that may chase them away (Medina-Vogel *et al.*, 2007). Being chased by dogs may exact an energetic cost from the otters, even if the dogs don't manage to catch and kill them. Furthermore, the native Chilean chilla fox (*Lycalopex griseus*), has been shown to alter its movements and foraging behavior due to the presence of domestic dogs (Silva-Rodriguez *et al.*, 2010). Domestic dogs were observed to actively harass, and even kill, the foxes, which is possible evidence of interference competition and intraguild predation observed between other canid species (Silva-Rodriguez *et al.*, 2010). Chilla foxes are generalist omnivores with a preference for open habitats and, at the landscape scale, the home ranges of chillas and dogs overlap. However, on a finer scale, the foxes show a propensity to rest in native woodland, the only habitat dogs do not visit. Foxes also avoid visiting scent stations when dogs are around, and, while housing may also represent other threats to foxes, their distribution was negatively related to the proximity to houses, where the chances of encountering dogs increased, despite there being no apparent effect on prey distribution (Silva-Rodriguez *et al.*, 2010).

In addition to direct harassment, domestic dogs may compete with other carnivores for food, either as predators or scavengers. The domestic dogs observed hunting ineffectively in the Gokwe Communal Land and Sengwa Wildlife Research Area of Zimbabwe scavenged both domestic and wild carrion in the area (Butler & Du Toit, 2002). Although not considered competitors for the larger wild predators (Butler *et al.*, 2004), as scavengers they out-competed vultures and were the most prominent members of the scavenger guild in the community lands, potentially reducing food availability for other species (Butler & Du Toit, 2002).

18.2.4 Hybridization

Dogs are known to interbreed with several species of wild canids, and hybrids are often fertile, offering the opportunity for dog genes to spread through wild populations to the point of extensive dilution of the original wild gene frequencies (Allendorf & Luikart, 2006). When hybridization is not limited to a few cases within a population but proceeds to high levels of genetic introgression (the occurrence of genes from one species in the genotype of another due to hybrids crossing with members of the parent species), it results in a so-called "hybrid swarm" (Rhymer & Simberloff, 1996), an irreversible condition of genomic extinction and loss of the original wild population. However, even a few sporadic hybrids can have deleterious effects, especially on the demography of small populations, competing with pure specimens for breeding opportunities (Allendorf & Luikart, 2006).

Wolves and dogs have probably hybridized since the early days of dog domestication (Anderson *et al.*, 2009; Clutton-Brock, 1999; Lehman *et al.*, 1991; Vilà and Wayne, 1999; vonHoldt & Driscoll, Chapter 3) and it has been suggested that hybridization between wolves and both coyotes (*Canis latrans*) and dogs have occurred repeatedly throughout the wolf's range (Roy *et al.*, 1994; Wayne *et al.*, 1995). While wolf populations were abundant and widespread, hybridization may not have been a serious conservation issue. However, the current status of many small, fragmented and low-density wolf populations along with the high (and often increasing) number of free-roaming dogs, such as found in many countries of Europe and Asia, may lead to a far more deleterious impact of hybridization. Small wolf populations and large dog numbers provide dispersing wolves with numerous opportunities for interspecific mating, particularly at the edges of their distribution (Andersone *et al.*, 2002; Randi and Lucchini, 2002). Indeed, cases of wolf–dog hybridization have been reported for several countries in Europe: Italy (Boitani *et al.*, Chapter 17; Ciucci *et al.*, 2003; Lucchini *et al.*, 2004; Randi and Lucchini, 2002; Verardi *et al.*, 2006), Sweden and Norway (Vilà *et al.*, 2003), Spain (Godinho *et al.*, 2011), Russia, Ukraine and Latvia (Andersone *et al.*, 2002), Croatia and Israel (Lucchini *et al.*, 2004), Serbia (Milenković *et al.*, 2006). Furthermore, the commercial exchange of wolf–dog hybrids, particularly prolific in North America, provides additional opportunities for wolf–dog interbreeding as these animals are frequently lost or abandoned (Hope, 1994).

Hybridization is a major concern when it affects small, endangered populations. For example, wolf–dog–coyote hybrids are the main conservation concern for the unique, reintroduced population of critically endangered red wolves (*Canis rufus*) in North Carolina, USA, and a factor in their initial decline (Kelly *et al.*, 2008). Dog–coyote hybrids are known to be frequent across large parts of the coyote range (Adams *et al.*, 2003) and taxonomic analysis of 284 skulls from animals collected in Arkansas, USA, during the period from 1968 to 1971, found 38 examples of coyote × dog hybrids, 27 coyote × red wolf hybrids and a red wolf × dog hybrid (Gipson *et al.*, 1974). As the domestic dog population of local communities continues to spread, hybridization is also a potential concern for the endangered Ethiopian wolf (*Canis simensis*), one of the rarest canids found only in seven isolated mountain ranges of the Ethiopian highlands (Sillero-Zubiri & Gottelli, 1994).

Although there is no evidence as yet of widespread wolf–dog hybrid swarms, several studies have shown that hybrids are effectively back-crossing with wolves and dogs, indicating that the potential for extensive introgression exists (Adams *et al.*, 2003; Andersone *et al.*, 2002; Lehman *et al.*, 1991; Randi *et al.*, 2000; Roy *et al.*, 1994). Especially worrisome is the case of Spain, where Godinho *et al.*

(2011) have shown, using a new extended set of genetic markers (42 microsatellites), that they could describe a significantly higher level of hybridization compared to earlier studies (Vilà *et al.*, 1997): the disturbing conclusion is that hybridization has been severely underestimated and that improved techniques may in the future reveal even more concerning results.

18.3   Management solutions

While the problems caused to wildlife by domestic dogs are increasingly recognized, there has not yet been a corresponding increase in ingenious solutions, particularly for non-disease related issues. In the review by Hughes & Macdonald (2013), the solution suggested for disease-related problems, such as transmission of rabies or CDV, was to vaccinate appropriate sections of the domestic dog or wildlife population (e.g. Lembo *et al.*, 2008; Bacon & Macdonald, 1980). Vaccination programs of this type have been demonstrated to be effective in the Serengeti (Cleaveland *et al.*, 2007) and Ethiopia (Randall *et al.*, 2006). For non-disease related conservation concerns, most of the proposed solutions involve the removal of dogs from the area while taking into account local cultural and social factors that contribute to people's perceptions and treatment of dogs. Although several studies have highlighted concerns about free-roaming domestic dogs, only a few reported any successfully implemented solutions to the problem: in New Zealand a single dog was found to be decimating a kiwi population, and was shot (Taborsky, 1988); in Fiji a Fijian frog *Platymantis vitianus* population was protected by removing all 12 free-roaming dogs from the island (Morley, 2006), and the reduction of waste reduced the abundance of dogs in a study of a Spanish agro-ecosystem (Sobrino *et al.*, 2009). Managing dog–wild canid hybrids poses uniquely difficult challenges for conservation for at least two reasons. First, the evolution and refinement of techniques used to identify hybrids from genetic evidence alters the results of genetic screening, as it becomes possible to discriminate ever finer levels of introgression (Vilà *et al.*, 2003). Second, there is no obvious or agreed threshold for morphological characters, genetic differences, or levels of introgression that should trigger a conservation response (Ciucci *et al.*, 2003; Daniels and Corbett, 2003; Godinho *et al.*, 2011; Woodall *et al.*, 1996). Consequently, translating these changing results into norms for conservation action remains a challenge.

For many conservation problems, dog removal may be the most obvious option, and in some cases feasible, as on Viwa Island, Fiji, where the total population of 12 free-roaming dogs were considered to be important predators of the Fijian frog. In collaboration with local community members, 10 dogs were socialized by humans, captured alive, and then moved to mainland Fiji. The two dogs which could not be tamed were killed (Morley, 2006). It is rare, however, that programs to remove dogs are so effective. Dog removal programs that have been carried out, generally by culling and with the objective of reducing the incidence of rabies, are considered inefficient as they rarely reach the target cull levels. For example, even removing 24% of the local dog population in a single year had no long-term effect on the population of Guayaquil, Ecuador (World Health Organisation (WHO), 1988). Furthermore, culling domestic animals is often unpopular. This unpopularity may stem from the use of inhumane methods, such as indiscriminate mass culling by means of poison rather than humane euthanasia. A general cull may also be particularly unpopular with local people in the case of FRDs that may be perceived as community or family members. Such relationships and taboos may not be obvious to people from other cultures (see Serpell, Chapter 15), and can cause resentment towards those carrying out such actions. This may, in turn, lead to loss of support for other rabies control actions, such as vaccination. Consequently lethal control programs are strongly discouraged (WHO, 1988; WHO & World Society for the Protection of Animals (WSPA), 1990). Similarly, by culling domestic animals without complete community involvement or acceptance, conservationists may also lose support for other conservation actions, both locally and with wider international stakeholders (Hiby & Hiby, Chapter 19). It is clear, therefore, that the negative impacts of domestic dogs on wildlife confront conservationists with a sensitive dilemma. Domestic dogs are intimately tied to the economic, social and cultural values of local people, and their management therefore requires interdisciplinary cooperation for successful outcomes (Lindenmayer & Hunter, 2010).

Many organizations already work with domestic dog populations in a number of countries throughout the world. Animal welfare and human health organizations have produced collaborative guidelines on dog population management (Hiby & Hiby, Chapter 19; International Companion Animal Management (ICAM) Coalition, 2008; World Organization for Animal Health (OIE), 2011; WHO and WSPA, 1990), with the aim of successfully controlling the dog population, reducing the incidence of disease, and raising the welfare of the dogs. These guidelines examine factors influencing dog population size and density; why a control program may be desirable; the ideal components of a control program; the control measures that can be used; monitoring program effects; and considerations for the future of areas where programs are implemented. Options for control include environmental control, regulation and legislation on ownership, regulation of national and international movement of dogs, and capture–neuter–release/rehome as well as euthanasia. However, many of these require significant long-term investment and have problems of their own. Programs that operate animal shelters, for example, may experience a constant influx of dogs from other areas as people from outside dump their dogs in an area where they know the animals will be cared for. As euthanizing or culling dogs has been shown to have little effect on rabies transmission, many animal welfare organizations tend toward trap–neuter–release/rehome (TNR) programs combined with vaccination. Releasing vaccinated and neutered animals back into the FRD population is thought to maintain social stability, while producing a healthier, sterilized dog population with immunity to rabies. When done well, TNR programs can achieve many desirable outcomes for public health and animal welfare. For instance, a long-term study in Jaipur, India, has shown that persistent TNR can reduce population size (Hiby & Hiby, Chapter 19; Totton *et al.*, 2010), although such programs may be more effective when combined with rehoming initiatives. However, the timescale over which TNR and rehoming programs affect population size may not be quick enough to achieve species conservation outcomes, especially if there are immediate concerns for the survival of local wildlife populations due to predation by returned animals. In circumstances where fast action is required and euthanasia is not acceptable, novel solutions will be required.

Both the WHO/WSPA (1990) and OIE (2011) guidelines recognize that dog population control may be desirable due to conflicts with wildlife. The ICAM (2008) guidelines focus on human–dog interactions but provide detailed information about implementing dog management programs. All the guidelines recognize the need for proper population assessment and accurate monitoring of management outcomes, with the WHO stating that further research is needed on domestic dog ecology, and that wildlife biologists often have the experience and ecological tools necessary to gather such information (WHO, 1988). By collaborating with people who have already developed knowledge and experience of working in conjunction with local communities in order to manage domestic dog populations, wildlife biologists have the potential to improve understanding of domestic dog ecology as well as the success of dog management and wildlife conservation programs. For example, although it is important to assess and monitor basic demographic parameters of dog populations, such as the abundance, density, sex ratios, age-class structure, and fertility and mortality rates, remarkably few studies report such information (Hughes & Macdonald, 2013), perhaps due to a lack of ecological expertise. Pooling research experience, methodologies and tools, will lead to economies of scale and better-informed management actions. Such programs will stand a greater chance of attaining the targets of wildlife conservation, animal welfare, and public health organizations.

The importance of collaboration between public health, animal welfare, conservationist, and local community groups is undeniable. The entrenched, adversarial positions sometimes adopted with regard to other domestic species, such as domestic cats (Lepczyk *et al.*, 2011), highlight the advantages to be gained when wildlife scientists, conservationists, animal protection groups, and public health advocates collaborate in formulating policy on free-roaming domestic dogs. With this in mind, we deliberately draw attention to the scale of the conservation, welfare and health issues, and urge discussion between stakeholders in pursuit of acceptable and effective solutions. As is so often the case, prevention is better than cure, so attention should be directed not only at interventions, but also at staunching the sources of problematic FRDs. From a conservation perspective, research is needed to establish whether and where concerns exist, to investigate potential conflicts, and to determine whether dogs are a neutral, deleterious or benign factor (Macdonald *et al.*, 2006). The nature of any action must be considered carefully with an appreciation of the attitudes and outcomes desired by a multitude of interested parties.

18.4 Conclusions

Free-roaming domestic dogs can cause a range of problems for the wildlife they encounter, by acting as predators, prey or competitors, through hybridization with other canids, or by transmitting diseases. These problems occur throughout the globe and depend on a variety of factors including the particular wildlife species involved, the habitat, the level of care and confinement imposed by dog owners, and the nature of the relationship between dogs and local communities. Due to the special relationship between dogs and people, culling and euthanasia are often unpopular, yet few other solutions have been developed for reducing the interaction between wildlife and dogs. Therefore, solutions to wildlife conservation problems caused by dogs require collaborative management with local people, animal welfare organizations, public health agencies, and other stakeholders with expertise in dog population management. Clear and transparent communication of desirable outcomes is necessary for all groups involved in developing a dog management program. Both short- and long-term motivations for dog population management and control will often differ between groups. The future of wildlife species in places where they are threatened by free-roaming domestic dogs is dependent on the development of novel solutions, and the engagement of all stakeholders for successful actions and outcomes.

References

Acardi, S. A., Liotta, D. J., Santini, M. S., Romagosa, C. M. & Salomon, O. D. (2010). Detection of *Leishmania infantum* in naturally infected *Lutzomyia* longipalpis (Diptera: Psychodidae: Phlebotominae) and *Canis familiaris* in Misiones, Argentina: the first report of a PCR-RFLP and sequencing-based confirmation assay. *Memorias Do Instituto Oswaldo Cruz*, 105: 796–9.

Adams, J. R., Leonard, J. A. & Waits, L. P. (2003). Widespread occurrence of a domestic dog mitochondrial DNA haplotype in southeastern US coyotes. *Molecular Ecology*, 12, 541–6.

Alexander, K. A., Kat, P. W., Munson, L. A., Kalake, A. & Appel, M. J. G. (1996). Canine distemper-related mortality among wild dogs (*Lycaon pictus*) in Chobe

National Park, Botswana. *Journal of Zoo and Wildlife Medicine*, 27: 426–7.

Alexander, K. A., Smith, J. S., Macharia, M. J. & King, A. A. (1993). Rabies in the Masai Mara, Kenya: preliminary report. *Onderstepoort Journal of Veterinary Research*, 60: 411–14.

Allendorf, F. W. & Luikart, G. (2006). *Conservation and the Genetics of Populations*. Oxford: Blackwell Publishing.

Anderson, T. M., Vonholdt, B. M., Candille, S. I. *et al.* (2009). Molecular and evolutionary history of melanism in North American gray wolves. *Science*, 323: 1339–43.

Andersone, Z., Lucchini, V., Randi, E. & Ozolins, J. (2002). Hybridization between wolves and dogs in Latvia as documented using mitochondrial and microsatellite DNA markers. *Mammalian Biology*, 67: 79–90.

Atickem, A., Bekele, A. & Williams, S. D. (2010). Competition between domestic dogs and Ethiopian wolf (*Canis simensis*) in the Bale Mountains National Park, Ethiopia. *African Journal of Ecology*, 48: 401–7.

Bacon, P. J. & Macdonald, D. W. (1980). To control rabies – vaccinate foxes. *New Scientist*, 87: 640–5.

Banks, D. J. D., Copeman, D. B. & Skerratt, L. F. (2006). *Echinococcus granulosus* in northern Queensland. 2. Ecological determinants of infection in beef cattle. *Australian Veterinary Journal*, 84: 308–11.

Bergeron, J. M. & Demers, P. (1981). The diet of the coyote (*Canis latrans*) and the wild dog (*Canis familiaris*) in south Quebec. *Canadian Field-Naturalist*, 95: 172–7.

Bhatia, S., Athreya, V., Grenyer, R. & Macdonald, D. W. (2013). Understanding the role of representations of human–leopard conflict in Mumbai through media-content analysis. *Conservation Biology*, 27: 588–94.

Bingham, J. (2005). Canine rabies ecology in southern Africa. *Emerging Infectious Diseases*, 11: 1337–42.

Bodendorfer, T., Hoppe-Dominik, B., Fischer, F. & Linsenmair, K. E. (2006). Prey of the leopard (*Panthera pardus*) and the lion (*Panthera leo*) in the Comoe and Marahoue National Parks, Cote d'Ivoire, West Africa. *Mammalia*, 70: 231–46.

Boitani, L., Francisci, F., Ciucci, P. & Andreoli, G. (1995). Population biology and ecology of feral dogs in central Italy. In *The Domestic Dog: Its Evolution, Behaviour and Interactions with People*, ed. J. Serpell. Cambridge: Cambridge University Press, pp. 216–44.

Borroto-Paez, R. (2009). Invasive mammals in Cuba: an overview. *Biological Invasions*, 11: 2279–90.

Bourhy, H., Dautry-Varsat, A., Hotez, P. J. & Salomon, J. (2010). Rabies, still neglected after 125 years of vaccination. *Plos Neglected Tropical Diseases*, 4: 3.

Brand Phillips, R., Wiedenfeld, D. A. & Snell, H. L. (2012). Current status of alien vertebrates in the Galapagos Islands: invasion history, distribution, and potential impacts. *Biological Invasions*, 14: 461–480.

Brito, D., Oliveira, L. C. & Mello, M. A. R. (2004). An overview of mammalian conservation at Poco das Antas Biological Reserve, southeastern Brazil. *Journal for Nature Conservation (Jena)*, 1: 219–28.

Butler, J. R. A. & Du Toit, J. T. (2002). Diet of free-ranging domestic dogs (*Canis familiaris*) in rural Zimbabwe: implications for wild scavengers on the periphery of wildlife reserves. *Animal Conservation*, 5: 29–37.

Butler, J. R. A., Du Toit, J. T. & Bingham, J. (2004). Free-ranging domestic dogs (*Canis familiaris*) as predators and prey in rural Zimbabwe: threats of competition and disease to large wild carnivores. *Biological Conservation*, 115: 369–78.

Campos, C. B., Esteves, C. F., Ferraz, K., Crawshaw, P. G. & Verdade, L. M. (2007). Diet of free-ranging cats and dogs in a suburban and rural environment, south-eastern Brazil. *Journal of Zoology*, 273: 14–20.

Causey, M. K. & Cude, C. A. (1980). Feral dog and White-tailed deer interactions in Alabama. *Journal of Wildlife Management*, 44: 481–4.

Ciucci, P. & Boitani, L. (1998). Wolf and dog depredation on livestock in central Italy. *Wildlife Society Bulletin*, 26: 504–14.

Ciucci, P., Lucchini, V., Boitani, L. & Randi, E. (2003). Dew-claws in wolves as evidence of admixed ancestry with dogs. *Canadian Journal of Zoology–Revue Canadienne de Zoologie*, 81: 2077–81.

Cleaveland, S., Mlengeya, T., Kaare, M. *et al.* (2007). The conservation relevance of epidemiological research into carnivore viral diseases in the Serengeti. *Conservation Biology*, 21: 612–22.

Clutton-Brock, J. (1999). *A Natural History of Domesticated Mammals*. Cambridge: Cambridge University Press.

Dalla Villa, P., Kahn, S., Stuardo, L. *et al.* (2010). Free-roaming dog control among OIE-member countries. *Preventive Veterinary Medecine*, 97: 58–63.

Daniels, M. J. & Corbett, L. (2003). Redefining introgressed protected mammals: when is a wildcat a wild cat and a dingo a wild dog? *Wildlife Research*, 30: 213–18.

David, D., Dveres, N., Yakobson, B. A. & Davidson, I. (2009). Emergence of dog rabies in the northern region of Israel. *Epidemiology and Infection*, 137: 544–8.

Deem, S. L., Karesh, W. B. & Weisman, W. (2001). Putting theory into practice: wildlife health in conservation. *Conservation Biology*, 15: 1224–33.

Driscoll, C. A. & Macdonald, D. W. (2010). Top dogs: wolf domestication and wealth. *Journal of Biology (London)*, 9: 10.

Edgaonkar, A. & Chellam, R. (2002). Food habit of the leopard, *Panthera pardus*, in the Sanjay Gandhi National Park, Maharashtra, India. *Mammalia*, 66: 353–360.

Engelhart, A. & Mullerschwarze, D. (1995). Responses of beaver (*Castor canadensis* Kuhl) to predator chemicals. *Journal of Chemical Ecology*, 21: 1349–64.

Farrell, L. E., Roman, J. & Sunquist, M. E. (2000). Dietary separation of sympatric carnivores identified by molecular analysis of scats. *Molecular Ecology*, 9: 1583–90.

Fowler, L. E. (1979). Hatching success and nest predation in the Green sea turtle, *Chelonia mydas*, at Tortuguero, Costa Rica. *Ecology*, 60: 946–55.

Fox, M. W., Beck, A. M. & Blackman, E. (1975). Behavior and ecology of a small group of urban dogs (*Canis familiaris*). *Applied Animal Ethology*, 1: 119–37.

Freeman, C. R. & Shaw, J. H. (1979). Hybridization in Canis (Canidae) in Oklahoma. *The Southwestern Naturalist*, 24: 485–99.

Gingold, G., Yom-Tov, Y., Kronfeld-Schor, N. & Geffen, E. (2009). Effect of guard dogs on the behavior and reproduction of gazelles in cattle enclosures on the Golan Heights. *Animal Conservation*, 12: 155–62.

Gipson, P. S. & Sealander, J. A. (1976). Changing food habits of wild *Canis* in Arkansas with emphasis on coyote hybrids and feral dogs. *American Midland Naturalist*, 95: 249–53.

Gipson, P. S., Sealander, J. A. & Dunn, J. E. (1974). The taxonomic status of wild *Canis* in Arkansas. *Systematic Zoology*, 23: 1–11.

Godinho, S. J., Laneza, L., Blanco, J. C. *et al.* (2011). Genetic evidence for multiple events of hybridization between wolves and domestic dogs in the Iberian Peninsula. *Molecular Ecology*, 20: 5154–66.

Gowtage-Sequiera, S., Banyard, A. C., Barrett, T., Buczkowski, H., Funk, S. M. & Cleaveland, S. (2009). Epidemiology, pathology and genetic analysis of a canine distemper epidemic in Namibia. *Journal of Wildlife Diseases*, 45: 1008–20.

Hale, A. M. (2004). Predation risk associated with group singing in a neotropical wood-quail. *The Wilson Bulletin*, 116: 167–71.

Hennessy, D. F., Owings, D. H., Rowe, M. P., Coss, R. G. & Leger, D. W. (1981). The information afforded by a variable signal: constraints on snake-elicited tail flagging by California ground squirrels. *Behaviour*, 78: 188–226.

Herrer, A., Christensen, H. A. & Beumer, R. J. (1973). Detection of leishmanial activity in nature by means of sentinel animals. *Transactions of the Royal Society of Tropical Medicine and Hygiene*, 67: 870–9.

Hope, J. (1994). Wolves and wolf hybrids as pets are big business – but a bad idea. *Smithsonian*, 25: 34–44.

Hsu, Y., Severinghaus, L. L. & Serpell, J. A. (2003). Dog keeping in Taiwan: its contribution to the problem of free-roaming dogs. *Journal of Applied Animal Welfare Science*, 6: 1–23.

Hughes, J. & Macdonald, D. W. (2013). A review of the interactions between free-roaming domestic dogs and wildlife. *Biological Conservation*, 157: 341–351.

ICAM (2008). *Humane Dog Population Management Guidance*. International Companion Animal Management Coalition.

Iverson, J. B. (1978). Impact of feral cats and dogs on populations of West Indian rock iguana, *Cyclura carinata*. *Biological Conservation*, 14: 63–73.

Jenkins, D. J. (2006). *Echinococcus granulosus* in Australia, widespread and doing well! *Parasitology International*, 55: S203–6.

Jhala, Y. V. (1993). Predation on blackbuck by wolves in Velavadar National Park, Gujarat, India. *Conservation Biology*, 7: 874–81.

Johnson, N., Un, H., Vos, A., Aylan, O. & Fooks, A. R. (2006). Wildlife rabies in western Turkey: the spread of rabies through the western provinces of Turkey. *Epidemiology and Infection*, 134: 369–75.

Kamler, J. F., Keeler, K., Wiens, G., Richardson, C. & Gipson, P. S. (2003). Feral dogs, *Canis familiaris*, kill coyote, *Canis latrans*. *Canadian Field-Naturalist*, 117: 123–4.

Kelly, B. T., Beyer, A. & Phillips, M. K. (2008). *Canis rufus* [Online]. http://dx.doi.org/10.2305/IUCN.UK. 2008.RLTS .T3747A10057394.en [accessed July 11, 2011].

Knobel, D. L., Cleaveland, S., Coleman, P. G. *et al.* (2005). Re-evaluating the burden of rabies in Africa and Asia. *Bulletin of the World Health Organization*, 83: 360–8.

Krebs, C. J. (2009). *Ecology: The Experimental Analysis of Distribution and Abundance*. New York: Pearson Benjamin Cummings.

Krogh, M. G. & Schweitzer, S. H. (1999). Least terns nesting on natural and artificial habitats in Georgia, USA. *Waterbirds: The International Journal of Waterbird Biology*, 22: 290–6.

Kruuk, H. & Snell, H. (1981). Prey selection by feral dogs from a population of marine iguanas (*Amblyrhynchus cristatus*). *Journal of Applied Ecology*, 18: 197–204.

Lacerda, A. C. R., Tomas, W. M. and Marinho, J. (2009). Domestic dogs as an edge effect in the Brasilia National Park, Brazil: interactions with native mammals. *Animal Conservation*, 12: 477–87.

Lehman, N., Eisenhawer, A., Hansen, K. *et al.* (1991). Introgression of coyote mitochondrial DNA into sympatric North American gray wolf populations. *Evolution*, 45: 104–19.

Lembo, T., Hampson, K., Haydon, D. T. *et al.* (2008). Exploring reservoir dynamics: a case study of rabies in the Serengeti ecosystem. *Journal of Applied Ecology*, 45: 1246.

Lepczyk, C. A., Van Heezik, Y. & Cooper, R. J. (2011). An issue with all-too-human dimensions. *The Wildlife Professional*, 5.

Lindenmayer, D. & Hunter, M. (2010). Some guiding concepts for conservation biology. *Conservation Biology*, 24: 1459–68.

Lowry, D. A. & Mcarthur, K. L. (1978). Domestic dogs as predators on deer. *Wildlife Society Bulletin*, 6: 38–9.

Lucchini, V., Galov, A. & Randi, E. (2004). Evidence of genetic distinction and long-term population decline in wolves (*Canis lupus*) in the Italian Apennines. *Molecular Ecology*, 13: 523–36.

Macdonald, D. W., King, C. M. & Strachan, R. (2006). Introduced species and the line between biodiversity conservation and naturalistic eugenics. In *Key Topics in Conservation Biology*, eds. D. W. Macdonald & K. Service. Oxford: Blackwell, pp. 186–205.

Macpherson, C. N. L., Karstad, L., Stevenson, P. & Arundel, J. H. (1983). Hydatid disease in the Turkana District of Kenya. 3. The significance of wild animals in the transmission of *Echinococcus granulosus*, with particular reference to Turkana and Masailand in Kenya. *Annals of Tropical Medicine and Parasitology*, 77: 61–73.

Madden, D., Ballestero, J., Calvo, C., Carlson, R., Christians, E. & Madden, E. (2008). Sea turtle nesting as a process influencing a sandy beach ecosystem. *Biotropica*, 40: 758–65.

Manor, R. & Saltz, D. (2004). The impact of free-roaming dogs on gazelle kid/female ratio in a fragmented area. *Biological Conservation*, 119: 231–6.

Maran, T., Põdra, M., Põlma, M. & Macdonald, D. W. (2009). The survival of captive-born animals in restoration programmes: case study of the endangered European mink, *Mustela lutreola. Biological Conservation,* 142: 1685–92.

Marks, B. K. & Duncan, R. S. (2009). Use of forest edges by free-ranging cats and dogs in an urban forest fragment. *Southeastern Naturalist,* 8: 427–36.

Marti, C. D. (1994). Barn owl reproduction: patterns and variation near the limit of the species' distribution. *The Condor,* 96: 468–84.

McChesney, G. J. & Tershy, B. R. (1998). History and status of introduced mammals and impacts to breeding seabirds on the California channel and northwestern Baja California islands. *Colonial Waterbirds,* 21: 335–47.

Mech, L. (1988). *The Arctic Wolf: Living With The Pack.* Stillwater, MN: Voyageur Press.

Medina-Vogel, G., Boher, F., Flores, G., Santibañez, A. & Soto-Azat, C. (2007). Spacing behavior of marine otters (*Lontra felina*) in relation to land refuges and fishery waste in Central Chile. *Journal of Mammalogy,* 88: 487–94.

Meek, P. D. (1999). The movement, roaming behaviour and home range of free-roaming domestic dogs, *Canis lupus familiaris,* in coastal New South Wales. *Wildlife Research,* 26: 847–55.

Milenković, M., Habijan-Mikes, V. & Matic, R. (2006). Cases of spontaneous interbreeding of wolf and domestic dog in the region of southeast Banat (Serbia). *Archives of Biological Sciences, Belgrade* 58: 225–31.

Miller, J. & Leopold, B. (1992). Population influences: predators. In *The Wild Turkey: Biology and Management,* ed. J. Dickinson. Harrisburg, PA: Stackpole, pp. 119–28.

Morley, C. (2006). Removal of feral dogs *Canis familiaris* by befriending them, Viwa Island, Fiji. *Conservation Evidence,* 3: 3.

OIE (2011). Stray dog population control. In *Terrestrial Animal Health Code,* 20th edition, ed. OIE. Paris: OIE, World Organisation for Animal Health.

Pal, S. K. (2001). Population ecology of free-ranging urban dogs in West Bengal, India. *Acta Theriologica,* 46: 69–78.

Pimentel, D., Zuniga, R. & Morrison, D. (2005). Update on the environmental and economic costs associated with alien-invasive species in the United States. *Ecological Economics,* 52: 273–88.

Randall, D. A., Marino, J., Haydon, D. T. *et al.* (2006). An integrated disease management strategy for the control of rabies in Ethiopian wolves. *Biological Conservation,* 131: 151–162.

Randi, E. & Lucchini, V. (2002). Detecting rare introgression of domestic dog genes into wild wolf (*Canis lupus*) population by Bayesian admixture analyses of microsatellite variation. *Conservation Genetics,* 3: 31–45.

Randi, E., Lucchini, V., Christensen, M. F. *et al.* (2000). Mitochondrial DNA variability in Italian and East European wolves: detecting the consequences of small population size and hybridization. *Conservation Biology,* 14: 464–73.

Rausch, R. (1958). Some observations on rabies in Alaska, with special reference to wild Canidae. *The Journal of Wildlife Management,* 22: 246–260.

Rhodes, C. J., Atkinson, R. P. D., Anderson, R. M. & Macdonald, D. W. (1998). Rabies in Zimbabwe: reservoir dogs and the implications for disease control. *Philosophical Transactions of the Royal Society of London Series B – Biological Sciences,* 353: 999–1010.

Rhymer, J. M. & Simberloff, D. (1996). Extinction by hybridization and introgression. *Annual Review of Ecology and Systematics,* 27: 83–109.

Roy, M. S., Geffen, E., Smith, D., Ostrander, E. A. & Wayne, R. K. (1994). Patterns of differentiation and hybridization in North American wolf-like canids, revealed by analysis of microsatellite loci. *Molecular Biology and Evolution,* 11: 553–70.

Schaller, G. B. (1998). *Wildlife of the Tibetan Steppe.* Chicago, IL and London: University of Chicago Press.

Sillero-Zubiri, C. & Gottelli, D. (1994). *Canis simensis. Mammalian Species,* 485: 1–6.

Silva-Rodriguez, E. A., Ortega-Solis, G. R. & Jimenez, J. E. (2010). Conservation and ecological implications of the use of space by chilla foxes and free-ranging dogs in a human-dominated landscape in southern Chile. *Austral Ecology,* 35: 765–77.

Sobrino, R., Acevedo, P., Escudero, M. A., Marco, J. & Gortazar, C. (2009). Carnivore population trends in Spanish agrosystems after the reduction in food availability due to rabbit decline by rabbit haemorrhagic disease and improved waste management. *European Journal of Wildlife Research,* 55: 161–5.

Sowemimo, O. A. (2009). The prevalence and intensity of gastrointestinal parasites of dogs in Ile-Ife, Nigeria. *Journal of Helminthology,* 83: 27–31.

Szekely, T. & Cuthill, I. C. (2000). Trade-off between mating opportunities and parental care: brood desertion by female Kentish plovers. *Proceedings: Biological Sciences,* 267: 2087–92.

Taborsky, M. (1988). Kiwis and dog predation: observations at Waitangi State Forest. *Notornis,* 35: 197–202.

Timm, R. & Schmidt, R. (1989). Management problems encountered with livestock guarding animals at the University of California, Hopland Field Station. *Great Plains Wildlife Damage Control Workshop,* 9: 54–8.

Totton, S. C., Wandeler, A. I., Zinsstag, J. *et al.* (2010). Stray dog population demographics in Jodhpur, India following a population control/rabies vaccination program. *Preventive Veterinary Medicine,* 97: 51–7.

Vanak, A. T. & Gompper, M. E. (2009a). Dietary niche separation between sympatric free-ranging domestic dogs and Indian foxes in Central India. *Journal of Mammalogy,* 90: 1058–65.

Vanak, A. T. & Gompper, M. E. (2009b). Dogs *Canis familiaris* as carnivores: their role and function in intraguild competition. *Mammal Review,* 39: 265–83.

Vanak, A. T., Thaker, M. & Gompper, M. E. (2009). Experimental examination of behavioural interactions between free-ranging wild and domestic canids. *Behavioral Ecology and Sociobiology,* 64: 279–87.

Verardi, A., Lucchini, V. & Randi, E. (2006). Detecting introgressive hybridisation between free-ranging domestic dogs and wild wolves (*Canis lupus*) by admixture linkage disequilibrium analysis. *Molecular Ecology*, 15: 2845–55.

Vilà, C., Savolainen, P., Maldonado, J. E. *et al*. (1997). Multiple and ancient origins of the domestic dog. *Science*, 276: 1687–9.

Vilà, C., Walker, C., Sundqvist, A. K. *et al*. (2003). Combined use of maternal, paternal and bi-parental genetic markers for the identification of wolf-dog hybrids. *Heredity*, 90: 17–24.

Vilà, C. & Wayne, R. K. (1999). Hybridization between wolves and dogs. *Conservation Biology*, 13: 195–8.

Wandeler, A. I., Matter, H. C., Kappeler, A. & Budde, A. (1993). The ecology of dogs and canine rabies: a selective review. *Revue Scientifique et Technique-Office International des Epizooties*, 12: 51–71.

Wayne, R. K., Lehman, N. & Fuller, T. K. (1995). Conservation genetics of the Gray Wolf. In *Ecology and Conservation of Wolves in a Changing World*, eds. L. N. Carbyn, S. H. Fritts & D. R. Seip. Edmonton, Canada: Canadian Circumpolar Institute.

WHO (1988). *Report of Dog Ecology Studies Related to Rabies. WHO/Rab.Res/88.25*. Geneva, Switzerland: World Health Organization.

WHO & WSPA (1990). *Guidelines for Dog Population Management*. Geneva, Switzerland: World Health Organisation and World Society for the Protection of Animals, London.

Woodall, P. F., Pavlov, P. & Twyford, K. L. (1996). Dingoes in Queensland, Australia: skull dimensions and the identity of wild canids. *Wildlife Research*, 23: 581–7.

Woodroffe, R., Prager, K. C., Munson, L. *et al*. (2012). Contact with domestic dogs increases pathogen exposure in endangered African wild dogs (*Lycaon pictus*). *Plos One*, 7, 9.

Yanes, M. & Suarez, F. (1996). Incidental nest predation and lark conservation in an Iberian semiarid shrubsteppe. *Conservation Biology*, 10: 881–7.

Young, J. K., Olson, K. A., Reading, R. P., Amgalanbaatar, S. & Berger, J. (2011). Is wildlife going to the dogs? Impacts of feral and free-roaming dogs on wildlife populations. *Bioscience*, 61: 125–32.

19 Dog population management

ELLY F. HIBY AND LEX R. HIBY

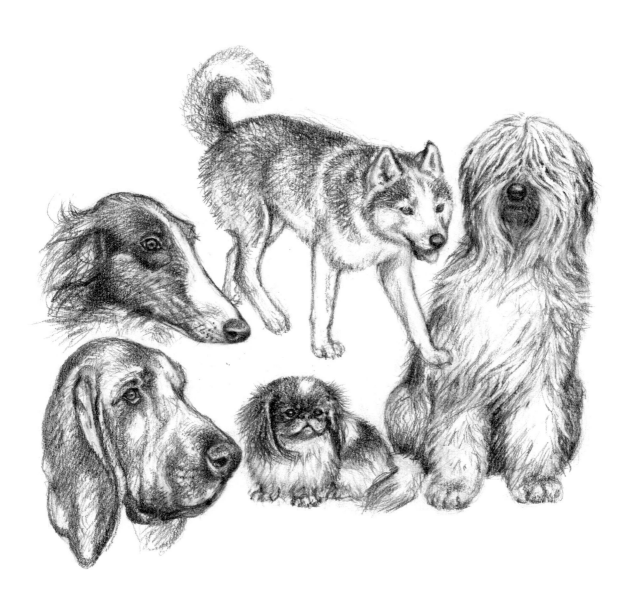

19.1   Introduction

Dogs enjoy a unique niche within a human dominated ecology. Fulfilling a range of roles, they are a part of human society around the world. There is an estimated worldwide dog population of 500–700 million distributed unevenly throughout the human population (Hughes & Macdonald, 2013; Matter & Daniels, 2000). Ratios of dogs to humans can vary from a reported 1:1.1 in the Philippines (Beran, 1982) to 1:45 in Zambia (de Balogh et al., 1993). However, for most populations the ratio is between 1:3 and 1:10 (Davlin & VonVille, 2012).

As the first species to be domesticated, dogs have developed the most intimate and complex relationship with humans (Serpell, 1996). The closeness of this relationship means that dogs are uniquely dependent on humans, with a severely limited ability to survive and reproduce in their absence (Macdonald & Carr, Chapter 16; Boitani et al., Chapter 17). It also means that they are vulnerable to any changes in this relationship that may accompany changes in human society, a notable example being urbanization. Bradshaw (2011) describes today's pet dogs as being on the verge of a crisis, struggling to meet the demands of being well-behaved urban pets when they have, until very recently, been bred for a rural working lifestyle. One consequence of urbanization, highly visible outside of Western Europe and North America, is the presence of dogs roaming on city streets, also known sometimes as *stray, street* or *free-roaming* dogs. The presence of roaming dogs can bring a range of problems, including disease risks, nuisance behaviors and welfare problems, not least through road traffic accidents. The methods used to control the population, even where efforts are made to reduce animal suffering, may also present an unacceptable situation to society. These issues, plus others, provide the motivation for humane dog population management.

The structure of the dog population is also complex. Figure 19.1, copied from ICAM Coalition (2007), illustrates the division of the population into a number of subpopulations and the routes of transition between those subpopulations. The diagram shows how a roaming dog may be a survivor of a litter born to a roaming female "on the street," an owned dog not currently confined, or a dog that was once owned but has been abandoned. In essence a roaming dog is simply a dog that is not currently under direct control or is not currently restricted by a physical barrier (ICAM, 2007). A common misconception is that roaming dogs are "unowned," when often this is not the case. Importantly, this definition reflects the inevitable relevance of dog owners when addressing the problem of roaming dogs. Similarly, once the fluidity of the dog population is understood it becomes clear that, in order to have an impact on any one of the sub-populations, it will be necessary to address the dog population holistically.

19.2   Impact of human behavior on dog ecology and dynamics around the world

The composition of the dog population in terms of its sub-populations varies depending on location. In a review of studies on dog population demographics from 18 different countries predominately in the global south, Davlin & VonVille (2012) reported that the ratio of ownerless dogs to owned dogs was generally very low but with higher proportions of ownerless dogs reported in South Asia (Matter et al., 2000; Sudarshan et al., 2001). Underlying this variation is the factor of human attitudes and behavior towards dogs.

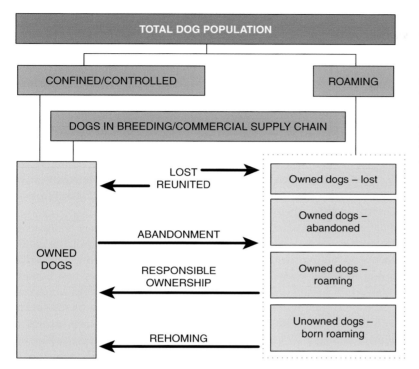

Figure 19.1 Diagrammatic representation of the sub-populations into which the total dog population can be partitioned. Note that these categories are fluid and dogs move between categories, as indicated by the arrows. (Reproduced with permission from ICAM Coalition, 2007, *Humane Dog Population Management Guidance.*)

The term *carrying capacity* refers to the number of animals a particular habitat can support through the provision of locally available resources, such as food, water and whelping sites. When using this term in relation to dogs, it is the behavior of people that will have the greatest impact on the availability of important resources and hence the number of dogs (Wandeler *et al*., 1988). For example, in a study in Tunisia, the percentage of dogs that were found to be truly ownerless was normally between 7.0% and 8.3% (Wandeler *et al*., 1993); anything above 10% was unusual and only ever found in close proximity to aggregated and accessible resources such as garbage sites. Questionnaire surveys revealed that dog owners would kill unwanted puppies (WHO, 1988), and that feeding of dogs that were not your own was presumably rare. The survival and reproductive success (ability to reproduce and raise offspring to recruitment) of ownerless dogs in this situation was low and the population of ownerless dogs was maintained largely by additions from the owned population.

In India, people commonly feed dogs on the streets and hence the proportion of roaming dogs that have no single owner is unusually high. However, in these cases it can be argued that, although these dogs do not have a single referral household that claims ownership, they are often not considered as completely unowned and may not be unwanted. A commonly used term for these dogs is "community dogs." This tolerance and care of dogs supports their survival and reproductive success, and hence these populations may be able to maintain their numbers without constant additions from the owned dog population.

Another human behavior that differs between countries is the level of confinement imposed on owned dogs. In many countries, most of the observed roaming dog population is not ownerless but simply comprises owned dogs that are currently roaming freely outside the owner's property. For example, in Sri Lanka, only one third of owned dogs were found to be confined on private property

(Wandeler *et al.*, 1993); in Mexico 32% of dogs were reported by their owners to be allowed to roam freely leaving 68% confined (Flores-Ibarra & Estrella-Valenzuela, 2004), and in Boliva only 15% were always restricted (Suzuki *et al.*, 2008). This can be contrasted with Western Europe or North America where confinement and leashing when outside private property is the norm and often required by law. Allowing your dog to roam may seem unusual to a developed world dog owner. However, there may be a range of motivations for this – for example, wanting to allow the dog opportunities to express natural behaviors such as socialization and exploration; avoiding problem (natural) behaviors such as barking or digging when confined and bored; for functional reasons such as acting as watch dogs for the wider community, or protecting crops in the immediate vicinity from pests (commonly rodents, but also monkeys and deer); or simply because fencing property is not a cultural norm. Exploring the motivations for allowing dogs to roam and, hence, finding suitable options to increase confinement that respect both the needs of owners and animal welfare, is an area that has received little research interest to date but could contribute significantly to dog population management.

The extent of dog population management efforts will also have a significant impact on the visibility of roaming dogs. In the developed world, a system of dog wardens, temporary holding facilities and rehoming centers function to remove roaming dogs from the streets and provide a place for owners to bring a dog when it is no longer wanted. Ideally, these dogs will be found new homes, although in many cases the number of dogs exceeds the adoption rate and healthy dogs are euthanized. Where this system is sufficiently well resourced and functional, dogs roaming on the streets become a rare sight. This can be contrasted to the developing world where such systems are not in place, or are limited in the number of dogs they can cope with, and hence dogs are left roaming on the streets and owners will abandon their unwanted dogs at other convenient public locations.

In summary, dog populations and their dynamics differ greatly across the world and there is no "typical" situation that dictates a single approach to dog population management. Differences in the environment and, most significantly, differences in human attitudes, behavior, and cultural traditions require each situation to be considered on its own merits.

19.3   Limiting factors for dog population size

The complexity of the relationship between dogs and humans, the complexity of dog population structure, and variations between geographical locations would seem to make population management a daunting task. However, in simple terms, such programs are aiming to manage the size of the dog population to ensure it fits comfortably within the available environment. Where dogs have access to adequate resources and without any restriction on reproduction, their population will grow until it reaches carrying capacity, at which point it becomes limited by a reduction in survival. This reduction in survival may be due to malnutrition and disease, or culling by the authorities or local people, when dogs exceed what is wanted or tolerated. Thus, irrespective of the structure of the dog population and its relationship to the human population, failure to control reproduction will lead ultimately to low average survival within the dog population. Controlling reproduction does not necessarily mean sterilization because owners who confine their dogs can prevent access to females in "heat." In Northern Europe, for example, the proportion of sterilized dogs is low but unplanned litters are relatively rare because dogs are carefully controlled. Where dogs have the opportunity to roam freely, however, some form of contraception or sterilization of females will form part of any control program.

The approach of controlling population size through decreased reproduction rather than increased mortality is preferable in almost all situations. However, it is also important to consider other problems presented by dog populations beyond only their size and breeding related behaviors.

19.4   The dog "problem"

Although dogs provide many benefits to people, not least as companions, where humans fail to care for or manage them effectively, unwanted dogs and those owned dogs allowed to roam can present problems. Recognizing these problems and understanding why they occur, including the human attitudes and behavior underlying any lack of care or management, helps population managers focus their efforts where they are most needed. One of the most commonly recognized problems is that of zoonoses: diseases that can be passed between non-human animals and humans. Dogs are known to be involved in the transmission of several zoonoses (Macpherson *et al.*, 2012). However, probably the most feared is rabies, which kills over 55 000 people per year worldwide (Knobel *et al.*, 2005), and over 95% of these deaths are due to a bite from a rabid dog (WHO, 2005). Even when disease transmission is not implicated, dog bites are a serious concern. In the UK, dog bites are estimated to lead to hospitalizations costing £3.9 million per year (RSPCA, 2010).

Predation or harassment of wildlife (see Hughes *et al.*, Chapter 18) and livestock by dogs may also be an issue. However, in areas where carnivorous wildlife exist, domestic dogs tend to represent a minority of the overall predation of livestock. For example, domestic dogs are responsible for less than 10% of reported predation on cattle in the USA (NASS, 2011). Furthermore, livestock guarding dogs have been successfully used to prevent wildlife predation in some countries; 73% of Namibian farmers reported significant decreases in wildlife predation following introduction of livestock guarding dogs (Marker *et al.*, 2005). Even where these encounters between dogs and other species do not lead to direct injury, there may be issues of disease transmission. This can be a particular concern in the case of vulnerable species of wild canids, such as the Ethiopian wolf (*Canis simensis*) (Hughes *et al.*, Chapter 18; Randall *et al.*, 2006). However, it is the non-life threatening issue of nuisance (including barking at night, defecating in public areas, and knocking over garbage cans) that seems to be cited most commonly by local authorities as a cause for public complaints against dogs (Bancroft, 1974).

Welfare problems of the dogs themselves are also often mentioned as a motivation for population management. The sight of dogs sick with mange or distemper, or injured in road traffic accidents, is clearly distressing. In many countries the methods currently used to control the population are themselves a welfare problem. Inhumane methods of killing, such as strychnine poisoning, electrocution, and drowning; inhumane methods of catching such as wire nooses; and poorly equipped and managed holding facilities can all present very severe welfare problems (Dalla Villa *et al.*, 2010; World Organization for Animal Health (OIE), 2013). Even where humane methods have been employed to avoid causing suffering, euthanasia itself is often considered an unacceptable waste of animal life. In the USA, the number of dogs and cats euthanized in government and non-governmental shelters is estimated by the Humane Society of the United States at between 3 and 4 million per year (HSUS, 2012). This is widely considered as socially unacceptable and, as a result, significant investment is made in dog population management to reduce this unwanted or "surplus" dog population. The current Humane Society estimate is a significant improvement from the estimate of 13.5 million dogs and cats euthanized in 1973 (Scarlett, 2004).

19.4.1   Assessing the dog "problem" and its causes to inform focused management

The perceived problems caused or encountered by dogs will clearly differ between countries, especially between those of the developing and developed world, with endemic rabies in one country and a high level of euthanasia of shelter dogs in another. In order to ensure dog population management is as effective and efficient as possible, it is important to identify and focus on these specific problems and ask where these dogs that present – or suffer – these problems come from. What are the sources of the dogs that are roaming, sick, euthanized in shelters, or carrying disease? What are the human attitudes and behavior that tend to give rise to these sources? By focusing on the dog "problem" and conducting a root cause analysis to understand the source of the problem and, importantly, assessing how people influence this source, the management program will stand the best chance of making a positive change. Understanding the source will indicate what actions are needed, and inform how best to run these activities, such as how best to access dogs for reproduction control in a way that encourages responsible human behavior.

Differences will also exist within countries; for example, between urban and rural areas, between different states or regions, or between different ethnic and religious groups. In the US, key differences are found in the demographics of dogs and cats entering different shelters and hence programs to reduce shelter intake and euthanasia rates need to be context specific (Marsh, 2010). Following detailed surveys of shelters in the USA, Wenstrup & Dowidchuk (1999, p. 308) stated that, "incoming animal demographics vary dramatically by shelter, implying high variance in localized problems, root causes, and efficacy of shelter activity to date." As a result, the authors warn that, if blanket policies or recommendations are applied across these shelters, the impact on the number of animals coming in or being rehomed is likely to be limited. To avoid potential waste of resources, the relinquished animal population and the root causes for its relinquishment must be assessed for each shelter, and policies developed specifically with that shelter in mind.

Unfortunately, assessments that ask fundamental questions about root causes are rare. Instead, assumptions tend to predominate, including the belief that there are simply too many dogs and that by killing enough of them there will be fewer dogs and the problems will be solved. Or that a simple solution that worked in one location can be imported and replicated to the same effect somewhere else. In reality, there is no "one-size-fits-all" in dog population management.

In order to understand local dog population dynamics, a period of observation and assessment is required, taking advantage of street surveys, questionnaires and focus groups. Following this process will help to test current assumptions. Close involvement with local communities will help with data collection and meaningful interpretation, and should also lead to designing dog population management programs that have full community support and engagement.

19.5   Dog population management programs

Assessments of dog-related problems and their root causes are best conducted by teams that endeavor to engage relevant stakeholders in the process to ensure that the analysis is not biased by any one viewpoint, and is as accurate as possible. Stakeholders will include responsible authorities such as municipalities, non-governmental organizations (NGOs) already engaged in this work, professions such as veterinarians and physicians who may treat the dogs and people affected by dogs, as well as a sample of dog owners. Further guidance on this process can be found in the ICAM Coalition (2007) *Humane Dog Population Management Guidelines*.

Using this process of initial assessment to analyze which objectives are required locally will clearly lead to different management programs in different parts of the world. For example, in the developing world, management programs may be more focused on reducing the risks of zoonotic diseases such as rabies through vaccination of dogs. Conversely, in the developed world, microchipping with registration and neutering of owned dogs may be focused on reducing intake to shelters and hence reducing euthanasia rates. In essence there is no one management program that works for all.

The majority of successful dog population management programs have adopted a comprehensive approach, combining a range of activities to best effect. For example, in the USA during the 1970s and 1980s, a program that combined education on responsible pet ownership, improved legislation, and increased access to low-cost spay and neuter led to a halving of the percentage of healthy dogs euthanized in US shelters (Rowan & Williams, 1987). In comparison, some population management programs promote a single approach, such as spay/neuter campaigns only. Although an apparently simple "pill" may be easier for governments and the general public to swallow, it runs the risk of being less impactful as it does not address the many causes and sources of unwanted dogs (Frank & Carlisle-Frank, 2007). A neutered dog, for example, can still carry zoonotic diseases, can still engage in problematic behavior, and may still not meet the expectations of an unprepared or inexperienced dog owner. This concept of using a comprehensive approach is not new. Carding (1969) noted the need for simultaneous actions in an early publication on the management of stray dog populations.

Adopting a humane approach to dog population management is essential. Dogs are sentient beings with a capacity to suffer and their welfare is therefore a matter of concern. It is also advantageous to adopt a humane approach in order to ensure maximum dog owner cooperation and public support for the program. Once the impact of human behavior on the dynamics of dog populations is accepted, it becomes clear that encouraging the support and action of local people will be as important to the program as direct intervention on dogs such as neutering, vaccination and rehoming.

The following sections describe actions that may be required as part of a comprehensive program to manage a dog population. Although many of these actions involve direct intervention on the animals themselves, delivery of these actions will involve people, most commonly dog owners and carers. Hence community engagement for the purposes of changing human behavior for the better will be an enduring requirement.

A range of professionals will typically be responsible for conducting dog population management activities, although veterinarians and animal control officers are especially important. These may be employed privately, by NGOs, or by government and will be involved in several of the actions described below. These professionals will find themselves on the "front line," interacting directly with the dogs and their owners, and responsible for imparting advice on population management. Such pivotal roles deserve particular support in terms of education and infrastructure. In addition, these professionals, and the government policy makers they respond or report to, can contribute significantly to developing and evaluating population management actions.

19.5.1   Reproduction control

When seeking to limit the growth of an animal population, reproduction control is a valuable alternative to reducing survival. In addition, when carefully targeted, reproduction control aims to prevent the birth of those dogs that were likely to have been unwanted. It also has benefits in reducing undesirable reproductive behaviors, such as fighting around females in "heat," and associated health risks such as transmissible venereal tumours (Bronden et al., 2010).

Bringing reproduction under control is commonly achieved through surgical sterilization. However, some non-surgical options are currently available and many more are under development (Briggs & Rhodes, 2010; www.acc-d.org). The development of an affordable non-surgical option, even one that provides a limited period of contraception and could be combined with regular vaccination, would be highly beneficial, especially in the developing world where resources and veterinary capacity limit current use of surgical sterilization. However, it should be noted that sterilization alone is not a requirement for effective dog population management. In some northern and central European countries the percentage of sterilized dogs is very low but dogs are carefully controlled, especially when in oestrus, and hence there are few unwanted litters. This level of responsible ownership has ensured that the dog population is well managed.

When sterilization is used, it is necessary to target this intervention carefully to where it is most needed. Female dogs are the limiting factor in population growth, and a further focus on those females that have been revealed to be the source of unwanted dogs will be most effective. When selecting and targeting dogs for sterilization, two commonly held assumptions can become problematic: one is that ownerless dogs are reproductively successful, and the other is that all roaming dogs are unowned. Evidence suggests that ownerless dogs usually have very low reproductive success and their populations are generally maintained through constant immigration from the owned dog population (see e.g. Boitani et al., Chapter 17). Also, due to lack of confinement, many or most free-roaming dogs are actually owned. The importance of these findings relates to their impact on how reproduction control should be delivered, i.e. by accessing dogs via their owners or by catching them. Such choices may seem at first to be an unimportant detail. However, consider the potential impact of catching an owned dog on the street for sterilization and release, without first consulting the owner. Owners may become justifiably angry that their dogs have been altered without their consent, but perhaps more concerning in the long-term is the lost opportunity to engage people with their dog through the intervention; potentially improving attachment through increased engagement may be implicated in later decisions to not abandon the dog or to intervene when the dog is unwell or lost. The decision to sterilize a dog includes motivations to protect the animal's individual welfare, but also to address its role in reducing the potential problems that dog populations present. There are also issues relating to post-operative care. To exclude an owner from these important discussions and animal care needs is to miss a unique opportunity to increase responsible ownership and improve public understanding and behavior. Further, accessing dogs for reproduction control allows for the option of owners contributing to the financial costs of these services. This may help increase the perceived value of veterinary services and support their long-term sustainability.

All of these factors are known to vary between countries and locations and, hence, it is important that assumptions about reproductive success and ownership of roaming dogs are tested locally using appropriate methods such as questionnaires, dog observation surveys, and focus groups. However, elucidating the true status of different sub-populations of dogs may prove difficult and time-consuming. Hence, a precautionary principle should be used starting with the premise that all roaming dogs are owned. Dogs can then be accessed for sterilization through their owners (and carers, see Box 19.1); some owners may wish to retain specific dogs for breeding, which should be respected since eliminating the dog population is not the goal. The wider population of dogs should also be monitored to assess the reach of sterilization activities as well as helping with decisions regarding which additional dogs need to be captured and sterilized. At worst, the sterilization of truly ownerless dogs may be delayed by this approach. But in most cases a sufficient number of dogs will be reached through their owners and carers, and involvement in the process will have encouraged a greater sense of responsibility and understanding in the owners and better post-operative care for the dogs.

Currently, little attention is paid to the impact that different options for accessing dogs has on owner behavior and attitudes. This is, however, a growing concern for governments and charities that invest in these services, and further research in this area would be highly beneficial. The example provided (Box 19.1 and Figure 19.2) from Colombo, Sri Lanka, describes how an initial assessment was used to elucidate the ownership status of roaming dogs, leading to the selection of a range of methods of reaching dogs for sterilization that encouraged responsible behavior by people.

Box 19.1 Community carers and Dog Managed Zones in Colombo, Sri Lanka

An assessment of the dog population in Colombo using questionnaires and street dog observation surveys, conducted in 2007, revealed that approximately half the roaming dogs had a single referral household and owner. Further, the local community were seen interacting positively with apparently unowned dogs, and these dogs seemed relaxed and happy in their environment. The project team (comprising the Veterinary Department of the Colombo Municipal Council, local NGO the Blue Paw Trust, and international NGO the World Society for the Protection of Animals) took the decision to access dogs for free surgical sterilization in three ways:

– Via dog owners using a mobile clinic and several routes of public awareness, including street theater, to ensure owners understood the benefit of sterilization and where and when to access these services.
– By engaging a community liaison officer experienced in communicating with local people to recruit community carers; these were people in the local community sympathetic to the local dogs that would agree to help access these dogs for sterilization and provide postoperative care.
– By developing the concept of Dog Managed Zones for business and government buildings where roaming dogs were, at least partially, living off refuse and handouts from people who worked in these buildings. These organizations agreed to develop feeding and watering stations for the dogs in low-risk areas of their grounds and improve their fencing in order to prevent further immigration of dogs. In return the project sterilized, vaccinated and treated these dogs.

By these three approaches to accessing dogs the project aimed to improve responsible dog ownership through their delivery of sterilization. Street surveys in 2010 revealed that, in 22 of the 32 wards surveyed, the percentage of roaming dogs sterilized was 70% or above. Further, there was a visible improvement in dog welfare as indicated by a reduction in the proportion of dogs in poor body condition from 30% in 2007 to less than 10% in 2010; both time and neuter status were found to have a significant positive effect on body condition ($R_2 = 0.44$, df = 65, $p < 0.001$). Similarly, there was a decrease in dogs with visible skin conditions from 46% in 2007 to 15% in 2010; again both time and neuter status were found to have a significant effect on the percentage of the population that had no skin condition ($R_2 = 0.44$, df = 64, $p < 0.001$) (WSPA mid-term 2010 report, unpublished).

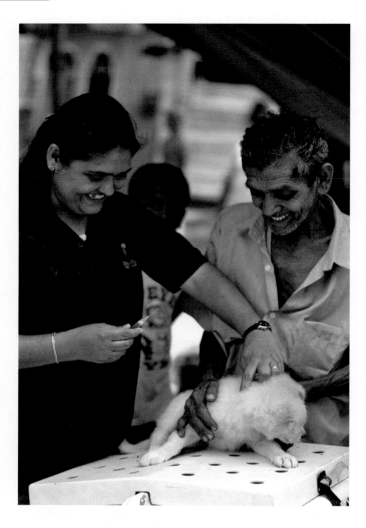

Figure 19.2 Blue Paw Trust Community liaison officer conducting rabies vaccination of an owned puppy at a mobile clinic site.

In general, engaging the local community as much as possible in delivering reproduction control should be beneficial for long-term sustainability, where the goal is for all dogs to have some form of responsible owner or carer who is willing to access health care for the dog including reproduction control. Even where a dog seems initially to have no referral household, engaging the local community in catching and handling the dog for reproduction control, and providing post-intervention care, could start them on the journey towards considering themselves responsible for that dog's welfare.

The number of sterilizations required to limit the growth of a population is normally given in terms of the proportion of the female population that needs to be sterile, but it is more informative to consider the rate at which the sterilizations need to be performed. The very simplest case is for a population of annually breeding females that reach sexual maturity at one year of age (which approximates to the situation in northern India) and where the percentage of the remaining unsterilized females that need to be sterilized each year to maintain the population at a desired level is given by $100\left(1 - \dfrac{1}{FLS_j + S}\right)$ leading to $100\left(1 - \dfrac{1 - S}{FLS_j}\right)$ as the percentage of sterile females in the population. Here L is the average number of female pups per litter, S is adult survival, S_j is survival from birth to recruitment (age at first breeding) and F is the fraction of recruited females that have a litter during a breeding season.

As a simple example, if $F = 1$, $L = 3$, $S = 0.7$ and a third of the female pups survive to recruitment then 41% of unsterilized females need to be sterilized per year, leading to 70% of the total population of females being sterile. It is straightforward to adapt such equations to real-world situations by incorporating the effects of, for example, using contraception that is less than 100% effective or only temporarily effective.[1]

Even from these simple equations we see that the rate at which sterilizations are to be done depends on juvenile and adult survival in the population at the level at which it is to be maintained, which may be quite different to survival in the original population close to its carrying capacity. The consequence of this is that, apart from a rapid initial decrease in numbers of pups and lactating females, the rate of decrease in total roaming dogs tends to slow as survival increases.

Although fewer sterilizations are required to control small populations compared to large ones, as a percentage of the number of remaining unsterilized females the rate is independent of population size. In programs that rely exclusively on catching without the cooperation of the owner or carer community, the effort required to find unsterilized females does not decrease in line with the reduction in population size. Indeed, effort may increase as only females with the ability to escape capture remain. The way that females are to be accessed should be organized with these likely outcomes in mind. Rapid reduction in total roaming dog numbers is unlikely, and, when a desirable reduction has been achieved, a significant effort to maintain that reduction will be required.

19.5.2 Education

Education of dog owners about the needs of their dogs and appropriate care is a key part of all successful programs, since improvement in responsible dog ownership will have a positive impact on nearly all dog population "problems." The aims of education are to improve dog welfare, reduce potential disease risks through preventative measures such as vaccination and parasite control, and improve approaches to dog acquisition, retention, reproduction and rehoming. Children are particularly important targets for such educational initiatives as they are commonly closely involved with dog care, and also commonly over-represented in dog bite statistics (e.g. Ozanne-Smith *et al.*, 2001).

Education of professionals, such as veterinarians and animal control officers, may also be valuable, and this is commonly referred to as "capacity building." These professionals are often dealing directly with the problems presented and suffered by dogs. They also play a potentially influential role in guiding the public in appropriate and responsible dog care. In many parts of the developing world these professionals are poorly prepared and equipped to deal with humane dog population management and, hence, training and ongoing support is likely to be required (see Box 19.2).

19.5.3 Legislation

The combination of government policies, legislation at central government level, and local government regulations can together provide a legislative framework that ensures key principles, such as respect for animal welfare, while also providing flexibility for local adaptation. From a government

[1] Calculation software for, and derivation of, these equations is available from: www.conservationresearch.org.uk

Box 19.2 Animal Control Officer (ACO) training, Brazil

In many countries, ACOs are an undeveloped profession and the staff employed to fulfil this role have had minimal prior training or support. As a consequence, ACOs' handling techniques and attitudes commonly lack respect for animal welfare or for their potentially influential position in the local community. It is not uncommon for the behavior of these staff towards animals and the public to be a source of public complaints and animosity. In recognition of this challenge in Brazil, the Institute of Education and Population Management (ITEC) developed a course for ACOs that work within the many government Zoonosis Control Centers where stray dogs are impounded. The ACOs from several municipalities are brought together for one week for a series of lectures, activities and technical training sessions. The strength of this course is that it not only provides training in technical skills and knowledge of subjects such as zoonosis control, but also addresses attitudes towards animals and empowers the ACOs to recognise the contributions they can make to animal welfare and public health. The aim is to change the behavior of ACOs towards animals and the public, and to encourage them to adopt the role of champions for animal welfare and humane zoonosis control. Observed impacts at the Zoonosis Control Centers have included the adoption of more humane methods of culling, initiation of sterilization services at the centers, improved welfare of impounded animals, an increase in the adoption of dogs from centers, and an increase in the use of owner education to reduce numbers of roaming dogs as opposed to catching roaming dogs without engaging with owners.

perspective, legislation and local regulations should outline how dog population management should be conducted and who is responsible for its implementation, including who is responsible for enforcement and penalties for infractions. Key areas for legislation include protection of dogs from cruelty, dog control (professionals, infrastructure and protocols), dog supply (breeders, markets and pet stores), dog registration, identification and disease control.

Legislation should clearly support responsible behavior that provides a benefit to the wider community and penalizes behavior that is damaging. Detailed regulations on dog ownership may not be suitable for legislation. Instead, this can be outlined in supporting guidance such as Codes of Practice, where minimum standards to comply with legislation are provided along with "best practices" that may not be required by law but are to be encouraged. An example of one such Code of Practice is New Zealand's *Code of Welfare for Dogs in New Zealand*, issued in support of the Animal Welfare Act (1999), which provides guidance on how to comply with the legislative requirements of the Act. The code gives general information, minimum standards, and recommendations for best practice under each type of important dog-related behavior, from purchasing or adoption through to specific actions such as exercise, preventing infectious disease, and performing euthanasia. Failure to meet a minimum standard in this code may be used as evidence to support a prosecution for an offence under the Animal Welfare Act. However, the code was also designed as an educational tool following the concept of education first and compliance will follow. Hence the recommendations for best practice in this code have no legal effect and are included to encourage higher standards of animal welfare.[2] Education is used here as the principal tool to encourage responsible behavior

[2] www.biosecurity.govt.nz/animal-welfare/codes/dogs

required for compliance with legislation, either through campaigns targeting specific behavior, or via broader programs in which the public is made aware of the Codes of Practice.

19.5.4 Disease and parasite control

Control of diseases and parasites in dogs helps to ensure good animal welfare, as well as protecting public health, in the case of zoonoses such as rabies, echinococcus and leishmaniasis (see Macpherson *et al.*, 2012 for a review of canine zoonoses). A preventative approach to disease and parasite control, as opposed to only surveillance and treatment, will be better for animal welfare, in particular with invariably fatal diseases such as rabies, and is also likely to be more cost-effective. The World Organization for Animal Health (OIE), for example, states that just 10% of the current costs of rabies post-exposure treatment for humans would be enough to eliminate rabies in the domestic animal reservoir through mass vaccination (Vallat, 2011). As preventative approaches usually require repeated interventions, such as vaccination or deworming, it is again important to engage owners fully to ensure that they appreciate the importance of these measures for both animal and human health and welfare. This may be especially true for parasite control such as deworming for echinococcus with praziquantel which must be done every few weeks.

In some situations, control of zoonotic diseases will be a priority above all other perceived problems of dogs. Hence disease control activities may be required to take precedence in early phases while other actions are introduced later to create a more holistic approach to dog population management (see Box 19.3 and Figure 19.3).

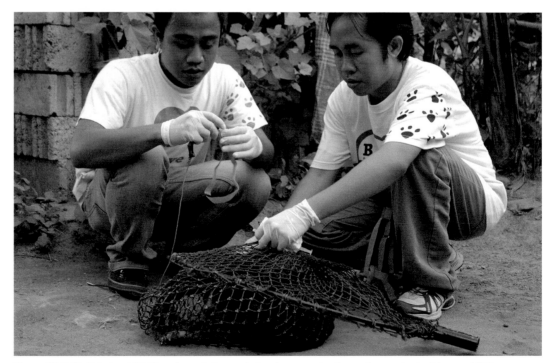

Figure 19.3 Bali Animal Welfare Association veterinarians vaccinating a dog against rabies, and fitting a collar to the dog to indicate it has been vaccinated, through the fenestrations of a dog catching net. (Reproduced with permission of World Animal Protection.)

Box 19.3 Bali

The island province of Bali was historically rabies free until late 2008, when several people living on the southern peninsula died with symptoms clinically consistent with rabies. An incursion is thought to have occurred approximately 8 months earlier, when a fisherman from nearby Sulawesi landed on the peninsula with a dog that was incubating rabies. In the two administrative regencies initially affected (Denpasar and Badung), the Balinese government began culling roaming dogs with strychnine and vaccinating dogs at fixed posts using locally manufactured vaccine, requiring a booster after three months. However, because Balinese dogs are infrequently handled by their owners and dog vaccination is rarely conducted, this fixed post-vaccination approach reached a minority of dogs and very few received the required booster (approximately 40% and 25% respectively, Agung *et al.*, 2013). An additional problem was that vaccinated dogs were not marked and, because owned dogs on Bali are rarely confined (over 90% of the roaming dog population is actually owned), many of these vaccinated roaming dogs were also culled. Dog movement was also potentially an issue; the first case of canine rabies in the previously uninfected region of Gianyar was due to an owner moving his dog from the infected Tabanan region where roaming dogs were being culled. Over 100 000 dogs were reported to have been culled from an estimated starting population of over 400 000 following the outbreak, but this emergency response failed to contain rabies and by September 2010 the virus had been confirmed in 221 villages (30.5%) throughout Bali. Dog culling was halted on agreement that an island-wide mass vaccination campaign was adopted as the primary rabies control measure with financial support from international donors. The majority of dogs were accessed by expert dog handlers using nets, and with the vaccination delivered via injection through the fenestrations of the net. However, those dogs that could be handled were held by their owners. During the first phase of mass culling, the average number of confirmed rabid dogs per month was 45, this fell to 11 per month and then 6 per month during the first and second island-wide vaccination campaigns (Agung *et al.*, 2013). Similarly, when comparing the last 6 months of mass culling (April–September 2010) and the first 6 months of mass vaccination (October 2010–March 2011) human rabies deaths fell by 35% and dog rabies cases fell by 76%.

19.5.5 Rehoming centers

In some locations, roaming dog populations are relatively well accepted and the goal of management can be to produce a healthy and safe population through reproduction control and basic health services. Elsewhere, roaming dogs will be unacceptable and will need to be collected and removed from public areas. Dogs that have been removed from the street need to be held for a period of time to allow them to be reunited with their owners before potentially being offered for rehoming. In many countries, most dogs will be relinquished to rehoming centers by their owners when they can no longer keep them. Rehoming centers hence provide an important social function, but they should

> ### Box 19.4 Rehoming centers in the USA
>
> Dogs roaming freely on public property are not acceptable in the USA and hence a network of rehoming centers, also known as shelters, exists across the country run by private organizations, governments and non-governmental organizations. The dogs in these shelters are either relinquished by owners or found as strays. The reach and public awareness of this service has meant that roaming dogs are rarely seen on US streets. In the 1970s over 20% of US dog and cat populations were euthanized in shelters in the USA (Rowan & Williams, 1987); recently this figure was estimated at 2.6% (APPA, 2008). The sheltering community has worked hard to decrease intake to shelters and hence the number of dogs that are euthanized. Key actions that have led to these improvements include: increased sterilization with emphasis on acting before first litter and before rehoming in the case of shelter dogs, this has been supported by low-cost programs run through shelter clinics, local vets and mobile veterinary units; identification of dogs to support reuniting them with their owners if they become lost; PR campaigns to encourage adoption; and education on dog behavior to ensure dog owners have realistic expectations of their dogs and invest in appropriate socialization and training (Marsh, 2010).

not be considered an easy option. Poorly run facilities can cause significant animal welfare problems and can quickly become overcrowded and unable to perform their function of taking in unwanted dogs. They are also expensive to run and very difficult to close once opened (see Box 19.4). Before a commitment is made to create such a facility, it is therefore advisable to hold sufficient funds for building and running costs for at least one year as capital, and have a clear and realistic plan for sustainability. Alternatives to rehoming centers include fostering schemes in which dogs are temporarily kept within a household by volunteers while permanent homes are found. Such programs may be more cost effective and better for animal welfare than kenneling in rehoming centers.

When running holding facilities, rehoming centers or fostering networks, euthanasia will be required for animals that are suffering from incurable illness, injury or severe behavioral problems that prevent them being rehomed. Dogs that are not coping well enough with the facilities to maintain a reasonable quality of life are also possible candidates for euthanasia. Ultimately, a successful dog population management program should aim to create a situation in which all healthy animals can be found a good home. In reality, however, most countries will not be able to achieve this ideal situation immediately and will need to work towards it, accepting that some healthy animals will be euthanized as not enough homes exist that can provide a good level of welfare. Whenever euthanasia is used, it must employ humane methods that ensure the animal moves into unconsciousness and death without suffering (ICAM Coalition, 2007, 2011).

19.6   The power of monitoring and evaluation

Worldwide, a significant investment is made every year in managing dog populations and yet very little data is collated or reported on the outcomes of these efforts. The importance of such data is not only to justify this level of public and private spending but also to learn what has been most effective and what has failed in order to improve future management. A notable exception has been the recent efforts in the USA to collate data from shelters across the nation in order to identify what has worked and what future actions are needed to further reduce shelter euthanasia rates (Marsh, 2010).

Effective data collection starts with clear identification of objectives and this links directly back to the initial requirement to assess each situation locally in order to understand the dog "problem" and what needs to be changed. Objectives could be to reduce the number of roaming dogs, improve roaming dog health, or reduce the incidence of a specific disease such as rabies. Appropriate data will need to be collected to measure the progress of objectives alongside data reflecting relevant actions. For example, if the objective is to reduce the number of roaming dogs, data can be collected through regular street dog observation counts to assess progress, while concurrent monitoring of the number of dogs sterilized will provide a measure of action that is predicted to contribute to this objective. Data relating to human attitudes and practices relating to dogs will also be needed, in recognition of the core role that human individuals play in dog population dynamics. Regular evaluation of the data should provide an indication of whether the effort expended has achieved the desired outcomes and which actions have proved most fruitful.

It is important that data collection is not a burdensome task but is devised to be as easy as possible to ensure that data collection is sustained over a long enough period to allow patterns to emerge. Time also needs to be allocated for analysis and interpretation of findings in collaboration with those involved in data collection to ensure they can see how meaningful their work has been (see Box 19.5; ICAM Coalition, 2015).

Box 19.5 Monitoring and evaluation in Jaipur, India

A catch, neuter, vaccination and return (CNVR) intervention has been conducted by the NGO, *Help in Suffering*, in the Rajasthan city of Jaipur, India since 1996. An average of 2500 female dogs have been spayed and vaccinated per year, while male dogs have been vaccinated and young males also castrated.

Estimates of the total number of roaming dogs in a city of this size require large-scale surveys and will be affected by growth and development of the city over the duration of the intervention. To directly monitor the effectiveness of the intervention, biannual index of abundance counts have therefore been conducted in the "Pink City," which is the historical center of Jaipur and therefore a region unlikely to undergo significant further development. Counts are made while walking a standard route between 06.30 and 09.00 a.m. at the same two times of year. The dogs seen are recorded as females, males and pups and further subdivided into those with ear notches (i.e. sterilized and vaccinated or vaccinated only) and those without. The counts show a rapid initial decline in the number of pups followed by a slow decline in the total number of dogs. Over the period 1997–2002 the total dog population observed on these routes declined by 28% (Reece & Chawla, 2006) and unpublished data shows a continuing decline, leading to a stable population over the last five years at about half its initial size.

Human rabies cases seen by the hospital servicing people within the intervention area also declined from a maximum of 10 cases per year within the period starting in 1992 to zero cases from October 2000 until the study completed in December 2002. During the same period there was a continued incidence of rabies outside the intervention area (Reece & Chawla 2006). The reduction in human rabies deaths follows a reduction in rabies in dogs, the principal reservoir for rabies in this part of the world.

Reece *et al.* (2013) show a decline in the incidence of human dog bite cases of 4.91 bites per month over the period January 2003 to June 2011, despite an annual increase in the human population of 4.95% over the same period, providing further evidence of a decrease in the number of roaming dogs in the city as a whole. The increase in the percentage of sterilized females may also have contributed to the reduction of bite incidence frequency because bite frequency is seasonally correlated with breeding, and many bites are the result of children interacting with pups on the street.

Detailed clinical records have also been maintained from the outset, including the age class and reproductive state of each dog spayed, date and region of capture (and hence release), any existing medical conditions and treatments, and reasons for euthanasia if not released. The data revealed the existence and timing of the reproductive season (Chawla & Reece 2002), which has subsequently been shown to match that of other cities in northern India (Hiby *et al.*, 2011).

The dogs released following the operation are permanently marked using a small notch in the margin of the ear-flap. In addition, an individually unique mark is tattooed on the inner surface of the ear. Accidental recapture over the years of dogs marked in this way allowed the average annual survival of spayed females to be estimated (Reece *et al.*, 2008), which in turn allowed the size of the ear-notched female component of the roaming dog population to be estimated from the release records for each region of the city. Street counts recording the percentage of females that are ear-notched could then provide estimates of the current number of female roaming dogs. The staff employed to catch roaming dogs for sterilization are particularly efficient at such counts because they are skilled at judging the sex and ear-notched state of roaming dogs at a distance. With the counter travelling on the pillion seat of a motorcycle, long tracks can be covered to average out regional variation in the percentage of ear-notched dogs. Such street counts can also be used to highlight particular areas of the city where the percentage of dogs notched is unusually low and hence guide future catching efforts.

19.7   Conclusions

Through the process of domestication, dogs have evolved to become a species that depends heavily on humans for their survival. Hence we have a particular responsibility to manage their populations humanely both to protect dog welfare and to ensure that the benefit of dogs to human society outweighs the potential risks. A common principle of dog population management is the idea of regulating dog numbers through reproduction control so as to avoid the suffering and high mortality that results when a population reaches carrying capacity. However, reproduction control alone is insufficient, and a comprehensive approach including education, legislation, disease and parasite control, and rehoming is usually required to maintain good dog welfare and reduce risks and nuisance to people.

As human attitudes and behavior towards dogs varies geographically and over time, dog demographics and the problems that their populations can present to human society also vary. This diversity means that, although reproduction control will be a common requirement, a one-size-fits-all system of dog population management is unlikely to be successful. Initial assessments employing a combination of methodologies can be used to develop effective management programs tailored to local contexts. Of particular importance is the requirement for population management programs to be designed to maximise the involvement of dog owners and other members of the community to ensure a sustainable change in dog-related attitudes and practices. These will include controlling the reproduction of dogs as well as providing consistent and appropriate care for dogs to maintain good health and welfare status.

Several areas of technology may help advance population management actions in the future, including the development of non-surgical methods of sterilization or contraception – particularly for females – that are safe and affordable. Improved methods of marking dogs as sterilized or contracepted would also be advantageous. These must be safe and painless for the dog, and ideally be visible from a distance and provide individual identification. Mapping and data collection innovations could also support effective monitoring and evaluation.

The landscape in which dog population management functions is changing. Both the physical environment and the relationship between people and dogs is resulting in new challenges. High-density urban living and fast-moving traffic leaves little private or public space for dogs to roam and express their normal behavior. Changes in the perception of public spaces, and what constitutes a clean and healthy environment, may decrease tolerance for roaming dogs that were once considered a normal part of the community. Increase in companionship as the principal function of dog ownership and associated changes in what owners desire in terms of behavior and physical characteristics of dogs may lead to different pressures on breeding, as has been illustrated by the recent pedigree dog breeding crisis in the UK (Bradshaw, 2011; Hubrecht *et al.*, Chapter 14). In response, dog population management will need to evolve. Program implementers will need to evaluate the impact of their programs, and trends in the environment, regularly in order to review root causes of continuing or emerging problems and adjust their actions accordingly.

References

Agung, G. P., Hampson, K., Girardi, J. *et al.* (2013). Response to a rabies epidemic in Bali, Indonesia. *Emerging Infectious Diseases Dispatch*, 19: 648–51.

American Pet Products Association (APPA) (2008). National Pet Owners Survey 2007–2008. [Online]. Available: www.americanpetproducts.org

Bancroft, R. L. (1974). America's Mayors and Councilmen: their problems and frustrations. *Nation's Cities*, 12: 14–22.

Beran, G. W. (1982). Ecology of dogs in the Central Philippines in relation to rabies control efforts. *Comparative Immunology, Microbiology and Infectious Diseases*, 5: 265–70.

Bradshaw, J. S. (2011). *In Defense of Dogs*. London: Penguin Books.

Briggs, J. & Rhodes, L. (2010). Non-surgical sterilization: priorities and challenges (abstract). *Proceedings of the 4th International Symposium on Non-Surgical Contraceptive Methods of Pet Population Control*, Dallas, Texas, April 8–10.

Bronden, L. B., Nielsen, S. S., Toft, N. & Kristensen, A. T. (2010). Data from the Danish veterinary cancer registry on the occurrence and distribution of neoplasms in dogs in Denmark. *Veterinary Record*, 166: 586–90.

Carding, A. H. (1969). The significance and dynamics of stray dog populations with special reference to the UK and Japan. *Journal of Small Animal Practice*, 10: 419–46.

Chawla, S. K. & Reece, J. F. (2002). Timing of oestrus and reproductive behaviour in Indian street dogs. *Veterinary Record*, 150: 450–1.

Dalla Villa, P., Kahn, S., Stuardo, L. *et al.* (2010). Free-roaming dog control among OIE-member countries. *Preventive Veterinary Medecine*, 97: 58–63.

Davlin, S. L. & VonVille, H. M. (2012). Canine rabies vaccination and domestic dog population characteristics in the developing world: a systematic review. *Vaccine*, 30: 3492–502.

De Balogh, K. K., Wandeler, A. I., Meslin, F. X. (1993). A dog ecology study in an urban and a semi-rural area of Zambia. *Onderstepoort Journal of Veterinary Research*, 60(4): 437–43.

Flores-Ibarra, M. & Estrella-Valenzuela, G. (2004). Canine ecology and socioeconomic factors associated with dogs unvaccinated against rabies in a Mexican city across the US-Mexico border. *Preventive Veterinary Medicine*, 62: 79–87.

Frank, J. M. & Carlisle-Frank P. L. (2007). Analysis of programs to reduce overpopulation of companion animals: do adoption and low-cost spay/neuter programs merely cause substitution of sources? *Ecological Economics*, 62: 740–6.

Hiby, L. R., Reece, J. F., Wright, R. *et al.* (2011). A mark-resight survey method to estimate the roaming dog population in three cities in Rajasthan, India. *BMC Veterinary Research*, 7: 46.

Hughes, J. & Macdonald, D. W. (2013). A review of the interactions between free-roaming domestic dogs and wildlife. *Biological Conservation*, 157: 341–51.

Humane Society of the United States (HSUS) (2012). U.S. shelter and adoption estimates for 2011–2012. [Online]. Available: www.humanesociety.org/issues/pet_overpopulation/facts/overpopulation_estimates.html [accessed May 2012].

International Companion Animal Management (ICAM) Coalition (2007). Humane dog population management guidance. [Online]. Available: www.icam-coalition.org [accessed May 2012].

International Companion Animal Management (ICAM) Coalition (2011). The welfare basis for euthanasia of dogs and cats and policy development. [Online]. Available: www.icam-coalition.org [accessed May 2012].

International Companion Animal Management (ICAM) Coalition (2015). Are we making a difference? A guide to monitoring and evaluating dog population and management interventions. [Online]. Available: www.icam-coalition.org [accessed September 11, 2016].

Knobel, D. L., Cleaveland, S., Coleman, P. G. *et al.* (2005). Re-evaluating the burden of rabies in Africa and Asia. *Bulletin of the World Health Organization*, 83: 360–368.

Macpherson, C. N. L., Meslin, F. X. & Wandeler, A. I. (2012). *Dogs, Zoonoses and Public Health*, 2nd edition. Oxford and New York: CABI Publishing.

Marker, L. L., Dickman, A. J. & Macdonald, D. W. (2005). Perceived effectiveness of livestock-guarding dogs placed on Namibian farms. *Rangeland Ecology & Management*, 58: 329–36.

Marsh, P. (2010). *Replacing Myth with Math: Using Evidence-based Programs to Eradicate Shelter Overpopulation*. Concord, NH: Town and Country Reprographics. [Online]. Available: www.shelteroverpopulation.org [accessed May 2012].

Matter, H. C. & Daniels, T. J. (2000). Dog ecology and population biology. In *Dogs, Zoonoses and Public Health*, eds. C. N. L. Macpherson, F. X. Meslin & A. I. Wandeler. Wallingford, UK: CABI International, pp. 17–62.

Matter, H. C., Wandeler, A. I., Neuenschwander, B. E., Harischandra, L. P. & Meslin, F. X. (2000). Study of the dog population and the rabies control activities in the Mirigama area of Sri Lanka. *Acta Tropica*, 75: 95–108.

National Agricultural Statistics Service (NASS) of the United States Department of Agriculture (USDA) (2011). *Cattle Death Loss Report*, released May 12, 2011. [Online]. Available: www.nass.usda.gov/Publications/Reports_By_Title/index.asp [accessed May 2014].

National Animal Welfare Advisory Committee (2010). *Animal Welfare (Dogs) Code of Welfare 2010*. Wellington: Animal Welfare Directorate, MAF Biosecurity New Zealand.

OIE (2013). Stray dog population control. Terrestrial Animal Health Code, chapter 7.7. [Online]. Available: www.oie.int/index.php?id=169&L=0&htmfile=chapitre_1.7.7.htm [accessed May 2014].

Ozanne-Smith J., Ashby, K. & Stathakis, V. Z. (2001). Dog bite and injury prevention – analysis, critical review, and research agenda. *Injury Prevention*, 7: 321–6.

Randall, D. A., Marino, J., Haydon, D. T. *et al.* (2006). An integrated disease management strategy for the control of rabies in Ethiopian wolves. *Biological Conservation*, 131: 151–62.

Reece, J. F. & Chawla, S. K. (2006). Control of rabies in Jaipur, India, by the sterilization and vaccination of neighbourhood dogs. *The Veterinary Record*, 159: 379–83.

Reece, J. F., Chawla, S. K., Hiby, E. F. & Hiby, L.R. (2008). Fecundity and longevity of roaming dogs in Jaipur, India. *BMC Veterinary Research*, 4: 6.

Reece, J. F., Chawla, S. K. & Hiby, A. R. (2013). Decline in human dog-bite cases during a street dog sterilization program in Jaipur, India. *The Veterinary Record*, 172(18): 473–6. http://doi:10.1136/vr.101079

Rowan, A. & Williams, J. (1987). The success of companion animal management programs: a review. *Anthrozoos*, 1: 110–22.

RSPCA (2010). Improving dog ownership: the economic case for dog licensing. [Online]. Available: www.rspca.org.uk/ImageLocator/LocateAsset?asset=document&assetId=1232721594783&mode=prd [accessed May 2012].

Scarlett, J. M. (2004). Pet population dynamics and animal shelter issues. In *Shelter Medicine for Veterinarians and Staff*, eds. L. Miller & S. Zawistowski. Ames, IA: Blackwell, pp. 11–24.

Serpell, J. (1996). *In the Company of Animals: A Study of Human–Animal Relationships*, 2nd edition. Cambridge: Cambridge University Press.

Sudarshan, M. K., Mahendra, B. J. & Narayan, D. H. (2001). A community survey of dog bites: anti-rabies treatment, rabies and dog population management in Bangalore City. *Journal of Communicable Diseases*, 33: 245–51.

Suzuki, K., Pereira, J. A., Frias, L. A. *et al.* (2008). Rabies vaccination coverage and profiles of the owned-dog population in Santa Cruz de la Sierra, Bolivia. *Zoonoses and Public Health* 55: 77–83.

Vallat, B. (2011). The OIE's commitment to fight rabies worldwide. Rabies: a priority for humans and animals. *OIE Bulletin*, 3: 1–2.

Wandeler, A. I., Budde, A., Capt, S., Kappeler, A. & Matter, H. C. (1988). Dog ecology and dog rabies control. *Reviews of Infectious Diseases*, 10: S684–8.

Wandeler, A. I., Matter, H. C., Kappeler, A. & Budde, A. (1993). The ecology of dogs and canine rabies: a selective review. *Revue Scientifique et Technique (International Office of Epizootics)*, 12: 51–71.

Wenstrup, J. & Dowidchuk, A. (1999). Pet overpopulation: data and measurement issues in shelters. *Journal of Applied Animal Welfare Science*, 2: 303–19.

World Health Organization (WHO) (1988). *Report of the WHO Consultation on Dog Ecology Studies Related to Rabies Control*. WHO/Rab.Res/88.25

World Health Organization (WHO) (2005). *Expert Consultation on Rabies: First Report. Technical Report Series, 931*. Geneva: WHO.

20

Epilogue: The tail of the dog

JAMES SERPELL

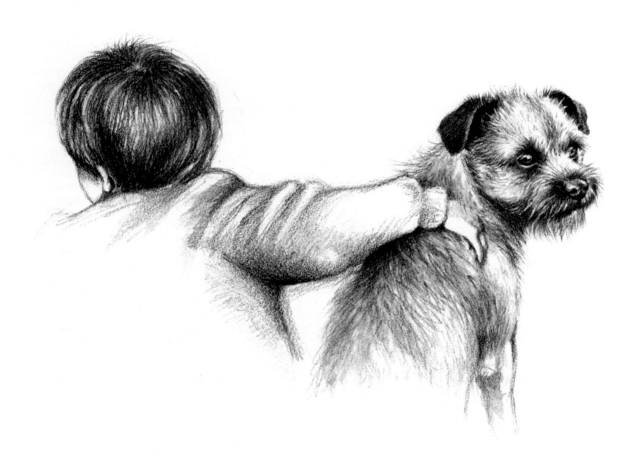

20.1   Origins and evolution

One of the disconcerting ironies of science is that often the more we discover about a particular topic the less we seem to know about it. In the concluding chapter of the first edition of this book, I reported confidently that the dog was domesticated from the grey wolf (*Canis lupus*) at least 12 000 years ago, and that future discoveries would probably reveal precisely when, where and how this happened (Serpell, 1995). Despite the passage of 20 years, however, and the many remarkable new advances in archaeology and molecular genetics reviewed in this new edition (see Clutton-Brock, Chapter 2; vonHoldt & Driscoll, Chapter 3), the scientific debate concerning the origin(s) of the dog continues to rage without any clear consensus emerging as to the most likely time and place of domestication, whether it occurred only once or multiple times, or even the reasons why our ancestors decided to share their lives with this large and potentially dangerous carnivore in the first place (Drake *et al.*, 2015; Larson *et al.*, 2012; Skoglund *et al.*, 2015; Thalman *et al.*, 2013). Whether the discovery of new archaeological remains, or further advances in morphometrics and/or genetic sequencing will eventually settle these questions still remains to be seen.

Widely accepted ideas regarding the selective processes that led to the emergence of the domestic dog from its ancestor(s) may also need revision. Twenty years ago, Coppinger & Schneider (1995) made a compelling case that much of the variation in the working behavior and head shape of dogs was a coordinated product of different levels of selection for juvenile or puppy-like aspects of behavior (neoteny/pedomorphosis), an argument that seemed to resonate with the canine science community at the time. Now, these authors, together with Kathryn Lord, propose a decidedly different view; namely, that breed-specific dog behavior patterns, the shapes of their faces and jaws, and even the quality and color of their coats are all regulated by a population of embryonic cells known as "neural crest cells," and that these cells act, "as a conduit through which breed-specific adaptations are implemented" (Lord *et al.*, Chapter 4).

This idea is reinforced by a recent article by Wilkins *et al.* (2014), who argue that all of the disparate features associated with what they call "the domestication syndrome" – e.g. short muzzles, smaller teeth, floppy ears, curled tails, piebald coat color, more frequent estrus cycles, reduced secretion of adrenal hormones, and behavioral docility – are derived developmentally from these same neural crest cells, and that the single factor that links them all is the intense selection for "tameness" (or, more correctly, *tameability*) that is assumed to have accompanied domestication. When the domestic environment selects for a tamer phenotype, or so this story goes, it actually selects for gene variants that produce mild deficits in the action of the neural crest cells that govern the development of the adrenal glands which are, in turn, responsible for the secretion of the stress hormones associated with so-called *flight or fight* reactions. Because these are embryonic cells, however, any deficits tend to affect all of the organs and tissues derived from them, and not just the adrenals. Thus, many of the dog-like features that we tend to think of as "adaptations" to domestic life may not be adaptations at all, but rather inadvert by-products of functional deficits in neural crest cells caused by selection for tameability.

Lord *et al.* take this fascinating idea a stage further by arguing that it isn't just selection for tameability that produces these complex pleiotropic effects but pretty much any selected change in behavioral phenotype, such as the markedly different expressions of foraging/hunting behavior seen among sled dogs, herding dogs and livestock guarding dogs, respectively. If this theory holds, however, it could be argued that Coppinger & Schneider's (1995) original pedomorphosis idea is not entirely misguided. For example, if the behavioral differences between dogs and wolves, and between different breeds of dog, are due primarily to different degrees of retardation in the development of adult behavior patterns, and if behavior and functional morphology are linked embryologically via the cells of the neural crest, then selection for an immature behavioral phenotype – such as a disinclination to hunt or a prolonged sensitive period for socialization – might also be expected to produce correlated immaturity in neural crest-derived anatomy and physiology. Either way, these ideas generate a host of intriguing questions regarding the mechanisms of evolutionary change, and dogs would appear to provide an ideal model for investigating them.

20.2   Behavior, cognition and training

These novel evolutionary insights may go some way toward explaining the surprising lack of progress geneticists have made when it comes to identifying the genes underpinning the extraordinary behavioral diversity of domestic dogs (van den Berg, Chapter 5). If selection for a relatively simple temperament trait such as tameness acts through genes that regulate the expression of embryonic stem-like cells, thereby resulting in multiple phenotypic effects across the developing organism, then the search for particular genes that regulate particular behavior patterns is likely to be somewhat akin to the pursuit of wild geese. The notion that selection for minor delays in the development of the HPA axis could also lead to rapid and profound evolutionary changes in behavior and morphology within a species (e.g. Belyaev et al., 1985; Trut et al., 2004) also emphasizes the need for more research on behavioral development in dogs, and on breed-specific differences in the timing of the developmental program in particular (see Serpell et al., Chapter 6). The domestic dog may also prove to be a valuable model for studying the role of epigenetics in altering the expression of the genes that regulate the development of neural crest-derived organs and tissues (see Hu et al., 2014). Additionally, there are abundant practical reasons for studying the impact of early environments on the development of behavior in dogs (Serpell et al., Chapter 6). Canine behavioral problems are thought to be the number one cause of premature relinquishment and/or euthanasia in companion dogs, and the single largest reason why young working dogs are released from breeding and training programs. Dogs that bite are a significant public health concern, while dogs that are chronically anxious or fearful have a dramatically reduced quality of life. Heritability estimates for such behaviors in dogs are typically low to moderate, suggesting that much if not most of the variance in such traits is environmentally induced (van den Berg, Chapter 5). Yet far greater efforts and resources are directed toward the search for "genes for behavior" than are devoted to understanding the more accessible developmental causes of such problems.

The success of future genetic and developmental studies will continue to depend on the use of reliable and accurate measures of canine behavioral phenotypes. The gold standard of behavioral measurement is the so-called "focal animal" observation – that is, the careful observation and recording of essentially everything an animal does within a given, representative time-frame (Martin & Bateson, 2001). Unfortunately, because most dogs live inside people's homes where they are difficult, and sometimes impossible, to observe for extended periods, it is necessary to develop different kinds of measurement techniques in order to study their behavior. Most such techniques involve measuring behavior by proxy using information provided by a person – usually the dog's owner or handler, or an expert such as a veterinarian or show judge – who has extensive knowledge of either the individual dog or the breed as a whole (Hsu & Serpell, 2003; Serpell & Duffy, 2014). Hart & Hart (Chapter 7) explore the latter approach with their analysis of differences in the behavior of 80 different breeds of dog based on the expert assessments of 168 small animal veterinarians.

This approach not only identified significant breed differences in behavior for every trait measured, but was also able to group breeds into related clusters that tended to overlap those based on genetic affinities (e.g. Parker *et al.*, 2004). Looking forward, efforts to cross-validate these different proxy measures of dog behavior with each other and with independent behavioral observations will be tremendously helpful.

Wolves evolved within the context of interactions with other wolves, and their social behavior and cognitive abilities reflect this history. Domestic dogs, in contrast, have evolved in the context of a mixed-species social organization in which interactions with humans were probably at least as important to survival and reproductive success as interactions with other dogs. We would therefore expect domestic dogs to differ from wolves in terms of how they solve problems and engage and communicate with others. This simple observation raises doubts concerning the extent to which the behavior or mental capacities of dogs can be properly understood or explained using a theoretical framework derived from studies of their non-domesticated relatives. With respect to social behavior and communication, for example, dogs are far more variable than wolves (Bradshaw & Rooney, Chapter 8), as might be expected given the widely different roles they have played in human society and the enormous variation in functional morphology and behavior that has resulted from this. Yet many self-styled dog experts continue to advocate a one-size-fits-all approach to dog-related problems and issues based on this animal's supposedly wolf-like propensities. As a result, the field of canine behavior has become a partisan battleground, particularly with respect to human-directed aggression and the extent to which genetic predispositions or environmental circumstances contribute to instances of dog bite (Lockwood, Chapter 9). Controversies over reputedly "dangerous" dog breeds, and the recent rise and fall of so-called *breed-specific legislation*, are manifestations of this societal conflict over the causes of, and solutions to, canine problems. Hopefully, future research will help to quantify the true extent of breed differences in behavior, as well as the impact (if any) of legislative breed bans on the prevalence of serious dog bites.

Behavioral comparisons with wild canids have also dogged the field of training and behavior modification. Several chapters in this new edition emphasize the proven effectiveness and humaneness of positive reinforcement as a training method for dogs – i.e. rewarding dogs when they do things right *versus* punishing them for doing things wrong (Bradshaw & Rooney, Chapter 8; Reisner, Chapter 11; Zawistowski & Reid, Chapter 12). Some of these authors also draw obvious parallels between the use of punishments and more old-fashioned philosophies of training that emphasize the need to assert control, using force if necessary, to establish a hierarchy of "dominance" in which the person is the authority figure or "alpha" and the dog is the respectful subordinate who knows his place in the social order. Unfortunately, due to the extraordinary level of media attention that dogs now command, the public debate about training methods has also become increasingly polarized and politicized, with some at the liberal and progressive end of the spectrum arguing that social dominance in dogs is a "myth" and that the use of any kind of aversive stimulus in training is abusive, and those at the more conservative, authoritarian extreme exhorting dog owners to become "pack leaders" while advocating a range of coercive or even violent tactics to enforce control and obedience.

In reality, the truth probably lies somewhere in between. The notion that social dominance in wolves is largely an artifact of keeping unrelated individuals in captivity where they cannot disperse (e.g. Mech, 2008) may have some validity, but it needs to be emphasized that this is also the social context in which the majority of domestic dogs are obliged to live their lives. Moreover, when left to their own devices, free-living dogs and wolves do form and maintain social hierarchies, even though rank order within such groups seems to be maintained primarily by younger individuals deferring to their elders rather than by top-down physical enforcement by "alpha" animals (Bekoff, 2012; Cafazzo *et al.*, 2010). On the other hand, thousands of years of selection by humans has likely resulted in the gradual suppression of dominance-related aggression directed towards people, at least among the medium-size to larger breeds (Duffy *et al.*, 2008; McGreevy *et al.*, 2013). Clearly, more work is needed to clarify the role (if any) of dominance in interactions between humans and their dogs.

Using wolves as the template for domestic dog social behavior may be misleading, but comparisons between wild and domestic canids have nevertheless become a key ingredient of the emerging field of canine cognitive science (Range & Viranyi, Chapter 10). Interest in dogs' social-cognitive skills stems from the notion that, because dogs are adapted to living and cooperating with humans, they may provide clues to the evolution of human cognitive capacities. However, designing experiments to test for human-like cognition while ruling out simpler processes has proven to be challenging, and it remains unclear the extent to which the observed abilities of dogs represent evolved adaptations to domestic life or the effects of early environment during development. Cognitive comparisons of "identically reared" dogs and wolves are also fraught with difficulties because these two species may be predisposed to engage with the world in different ways, and their human handlers may be predisposed to respond to them differently. In future research, it may be more productive to focus on individual and breed differences in the cognitive capacities of dogs alone, given the large range in individual abilities within breeds, and the widely different cognitive skills selected for across them. Early comparative work on breed differences in behavior (e.g. Scott & Fuller, 1965) played a seminal role in the development of the field of canine science, and it may be time to revisit these types of studies in light of modern advances in molecular genetics, behavioral phenotyping, and multivariate statistical techniques.

20.3   Dog–human interactions

Notwithstanding doubts about dogs' capacities to understand and empathize with people, it is clear that humans – or at least many humans – are enormously attached to their dogs, and not just for the practical services they provide. In the USA alone, people share their homes and their lives with some 70–80 million of these animals, most of which serve no obvious instrumental or practical purpose. This raises intriguing questions about the possible social, emotional and medical benefits that people may gain from these interspecies partnerships (see Hart & Yamamoto, Chapter 13). Despite all the positive media hype, however, the scientific evidence for the benefits of human–dog interactions is still equivocal, and it remains unclear whether the occasional negative findings reflect a lack of efficacy, poor study design, or something more nuanced to do with the varied characteristics of the individuals (both human and animal) who participate in these relationships (Herzog, 2011; Serpell, 2009). The same is true of most dog-assisted therapeutic interventions, including the use of so-called "emotional support dogs." To be convincing, future studies in this area will need to be prospective in design, take into account the overall heterogeneity of the people and animals involved, and include appropriate control groups. A better understanding of the underlying mechanisms would also be helpful. Recent work suggests that the "bonding" hormone oxytocin may provide a key to explaining some of the psychosocial benefits of canine companionship (Handlin *et al.*, 2012; Nagasawa *et al.*, 2015). However, more work is needed to clarify why some dogs appear to be better at producing such effects than others, and why different humans are more or less susceptible to their charms.

In spite of all the talk of *mutually beneficial* dog–human interactions, the health and welfare of dogs is sometimes severely compromised by their relations with people, and, compared with farm and laboratory animals, there is a dearth of research dedicated to understanding and measuring the welfare of domestic dogs (see Hubrecht *et al.*, Chapter 14). For example, when hobby breeders in the nineteenth century began isolating dog breeds genetically, and breeding for form rather than function, they began a process that has now resulted in a host of health and welfare problems for many purebred dogs. A better understanding of the true prevalence of such problems in the pet dog population, as well as the seemingly arbitrary aesthetic preferences that maintain them, would be valuable. Even basic questions concerning what is "natural" for dogs, in terms of their physical and social needs, have barely been addressed, perhaps partly because different breeds of dog may have different welfare requirements. Working dog breeds, for example, are often highly motivated to perform the particular behaviors for which they have been selected over thousands of years (Bradshaw, 2011; Lord *et al.*, Chapter 4). Yet we know almost nothing about how their welfare is affected when these internally motivated actions are thwarted by societal constraints or their owners' incompatible life-styles. Experimental studies are therefore needed to determine how much dogs of different breeds and backgrounds are prepared to "pay" to gain access to particular resources and activities. Similarly, studies that focus on understanding the affective states of dogs living under different conditions – e.g. house pets, kenneled dogs, working dogs, etc. – could also provide valuable welfare insights. It is widely believed that behavior problems are the number one reason why dogs are disowned or surrendered to shelters, but how much of this is due to dogs being poorly adapted to modern life or simply the result of inadequate early socialization is still largely unknown.

The welfare of dogs is a global problem that is ultimately determined by the local and regional attitudes and behavior of human beings. Improvements in canine welfare are therefore, to some extent, conditional on understanding the practical, social and symbolic roles that dogs play in different cultures and societies around the world. As symbols, dogs appear to combine and embody a curious mix of admirable and despicable traits that greatly influence people's attitudes toward them (Serpell, Chapter 15). The capacity of dogs to form strong familial attachments for humans during an extended period of early development – even in the face of rejection and punishment – endows them with an unusual degree of "personhood" compared with most other domestic species. In some cultural contexts, this has encouraged a highly positive image of dogs as loyal family members. In others, this same human affinity has become a liability, promoting an image of the dog as an outcast or "pariah' – a victim of its own depravity and a violator of human social norms and taboos. Because of their influence on the treatment of dogs, these interactions between dog behavior and cultural perceptions merit greater attention, particularly in relation to the management of free-roaming dog populations (Hiby & Hiby, Chapter 19).

20.4   Life on the margins

As a domestic species, dogs live habitually in association with humans. But the strength of this association varies greatly from place to place. In many regions of the world, particularly in developing countries, free-roaming dogs live on the fringes of human society where they are obliged to fend at least partly for themselves. The two chapters by Macdonald & Carr (Chapter 16) and Boitani *et al.* (Chapter 17) provide fascinating insights into the natural history, ecology and behavior of such dogs living in the mountains of central Italy. Several important lessons can be gleaned from this work. First, that even among those groups of dogs that are spatially independent and avoidant of humans, survival and reproduction is still contingent on more-or-less continuous access to human garbage dumps. Little if any active predation of either livestock or wildlife is ever observed. Second, it is clear that, due to high rates of adult and pup mortality, these feral or semi-feral dog communities are unsustainable without periodic recruitment from the owned dog population. Such observations tend to challenge the popular belief that dogs evolved originally as commensal scavengers (e.g. Coppinger & Coppinger, 2001), and suggest that this ecological niche is at best a marginal one in which dogs typically struggle to survive and reproduce successfully. These studies also raise questions about how much of the observed variation in behavior displayed by domestic dogs is truly adaptive and how much is a product of history/phylogeny. For example, the lack of predation shown by these Italian dogs may represent an adaptive response to the presence of superabundant garbage, or it may reflect the fact that most of them are descended from mountain shepherd dogs in which predatory behavior has been strongly selected against by humans (see Lord *et al.*, Chapter 4).

While the feral and free-roaming dogs of central Italy show little inclination to hunt, dogs do pose a significant predation threat to wildlife – including endangered wildlife – in other parts of the world (see Hughes *et al.*, Chapter 18). Furthermore, unlike wild predators whose population size and reproductive capacity is ultimately constrained by prey abundance, dogs who are provisioned by humans can theoretically hunt prey species to extinction without necessarily limiting their own success. Free-roaming dogs may also compete for prey with native predators, and, even in the absence of active predation, may have a disruptive influence on wildlife, either by interrupting important activities or by blocking their access to valuable resources. Canine interactions with wild animals also increase opportunities for the transmission of diseases, such as rabies, distemper and *echinococcus*, between dogs and wildlife, and between wildlife and the humans and livestock with which dogs commonly associate. Finally, in some areas of the world, roaming dogs may hybridize with wild canids resulting in loss of genetic integrity in the wild population. A better understanding of the particular situations and circumstances in which free-roaming dogs pose serious threats to wildlife would be helpful for guiding effective management strategies.

In addition to the risks they pose to wildlife, free-roaming dogs also cause abundant problems for humans and their livestock animals, including infectious disease and parasite transmission, bites and attacks, traffic accidents, and general nuisance due to barking, fecal pollution and so on (Hiby & Hiby, Chapter 19). Yet, despite all these problems, people throughout much of the developing world tolerate the continued existence of these animals, and often at surprisingly high densities. The reality is that most humans seem to like dogs, even when they may have very different views about what constitutes proper dog–human relations. This leads to an extraordinary degree of local and regional variation in dog numbers and distribution; in patterns of dog ownership, restraint, and levels of care; in the willingness of people to touch or handle dogs; and in their levels of exposure to zoonotic disease and other dog-associated risks. These dog-related attitudes and behavior are key determinants of both the acceptability and the ultimate success of any proposed dog population management strategy, and their origins should be investigated.

20.5   Conclusions

The domestic dog is a remarkably adaptable and resilient animal that has undoubtedly prospered biologically through its long partnership with humans. Many would argue that humans have also prospered through their relations with dogs – that we have, so to speak, co-evolved to create a *mutualistic* association in which each species benefits from coexistence and cooperation with the other. While this may be true up to a point, it is apparent that most of the evolutionary adaptation to this new niche has been accomplished by dogs rather than humans. Considering the brief time-span during which it occurred, the transition from the wolf to, say, the French bulldog is extraordinary by any standards, and it provides a stunning illustration of just how rapidly and dramatically an organism's morphology and behavior can change when faced with novel ecological opportunities and selection pressures. The process is also ongoing. Confronted by the capricious and ever-changing demands of humans, dogs are continuing to adapt and evolve, albeit with varying degrees of success. In this sense, the domestic dog truly belongs alongside Darwin's famous finches as another remarkable biological model for understanding the dynamics of evolutionary change.

Although a source of fascination to evolutionary biologists, the often noted physical and behavioral diversity of dogs ought to discourage generalizations about the nature of these animals. Yet much of the scientific and lay literature continues to talk about the domestic dog as a relatively homogeneous taxon, as if a finding or observation derived from, say, Siberian huskies is necessarily relevant or applicable to Anatolian shepherds or Maltese terriers. Notwithstanding the understandable urge to simplify a complex world, the staggering heterogeneity of dogs should be celebrated rather than ignored because of its significant implications for virtually every branch of canine science, including evolution, genetics, behavior, training, cognition, ecology, welfare, and interactions with humans. Future research in all of these disparate fields will be greatly enriched by acknowledging and exploring this diversity.

References

Bekoff, M. (2012). Social dominance is not a myth: wolves, dogs, and other animals. *Psychology Today*, February 15. [Online]. Available: www.psychologytoday.com/blog/animal-emotions/201202/social-dominance-is-not-myth-wolves-dogs-and-other-animals

Belyaev, D. K., Plyusnina, I. Z. & Trut, L. N. (1985). Domestication in the silver fox (*Vulpes vulpes*): Changes in physiological boundaries of the sensitive period of primary socialization. *Applied Animal Behaviour Science*, 32: 253–68.

Bradshaw, J. S. (2011). *In Defense of Dogs*. London, UK: Penguin Books.

Cafazzo, S., Valsecchi, P., Bonanni, R. & Natoli, E. (2010). Dominance in relation to age, sex, and competitive contexts in a group of free-ranging domestic dogs. *Behavioral Ecology*. http://doi:10.1093/beheco/arq001

Coppinger, R. & Coppinger. L. (2001). *Dogs: A Startling New Understanding of Canine Origin, Behavior & Evolution*. New York: Scribner.

Coppinger, R. P. & Schneider, R. (1995). Evolution of working dogs. In *The Domestic Dog: Its Evolution, Behaviour and Interactions with People*, ed. J. Serpell. Cambridge: Cambridge University Press, pp. 21–47.

Drake, A. G., Coquerelle, M. & Colombeau, G. (2015). 3D morphometric analysis of fossil canid skulls contradicts the suggested domestication of dogs during the late Paleolithic. *Science Reports*, 5: 8299. http://doi:10.1038/srep08299.

Duffy, D. L., Hsu, Y. & Serpell, J. A. (2008). Breed differences in canine aggression. *Applied Animal Behaviour Science*, 114: 441–60.

Handlin, L., Nilsson, A., Ejdebäck, M., Hydbring-Sandberg, E. & Uvnäs-Moberg, K. (2012). Associations between psychological characteristics of the human-dog relationship and oxytocin and cortisol levels. *Anthrozoös*, 25: 215–28.

Herzog, H. (2011). The impact of pet ownership on human health and psychological well-being: fact, fiction or hypothesis? *Current Directions in Psychological Science*, 20: 236–9.

Hu, N., Strobl-Mazzula, P. H. & Bronner, M. E. (2014). Epigenetic regulation in neural crest development. *Developmental Biology*, 396: 159–68.

Hsu, Y. & Serpell, J. A. (2003). Development and validation of a questionnaire for measuring behavior and temperament traits in pet dogs. *Journal of the American Veterinary Medical Association*, 223: 1293–300.

Larson, G., Karlsson, E. K., Perri, A. et al. (2012). Rethinking dog domestication by integrating genetics, archeology, and biogeography. *Proceedings of the National Academy of Sciences USA*, 109: 8878–83.

Martin, P. R. & Bateson, P. P. G. (2001). *Measuring Behaviour: An Introductory Guide*, 2nd edition. Cambridge: Cambridge University Press.

McGreevy, P. D., Georgevsky, D., Carrasco, J., Valenzuela, M., Duffy, D. L. & Serpell, J. A. (2013). Dog behavior co-varies with height, bodyweight and skull shape. *PLoS ONE* 8: e80529. http://doi:10.1371/journal.pone.0080529

Mech, L. D. (2008). Whatever happened to the term "alpha wolf"? *International Wolf*, Winter: 4–8: www.wolf.org/

Nagasawa, M., Mitsui, S., En, S. et al. (2015). Oxytocin-gaze positive loop and the coevolution of human-dog bonds. *Science*, 348: 333–6.

Parker, H. G., Kim, L. V., Sutter, N. B. *et al.* (2004). Genetic structure of the purebred domestic dog. *Science*, 304: 1161–4.

Scott, J. P. & Fuller, J. L. (1965). *Genetics and the Social Behavior of the Dog*. Chicago, IL: University of Chicago Press.

Serpell, J. A. (1995). *The Domestic Dog: Its Evolution, Behaviour and Interactions with People*. Cambridge: Cambridge University Press.

Serpell, J. A. (2009). Having our dogs and eating them too: why animals are a social issue. *Journal of Social Issues*, 65: 633–44.

Serpell, J. A. & Duffy, D. L. (2014). Breeds and their behavior. In *Domestic Dog Cognition and Behavior*, ed. A. Horowitz. Berlin: Springer-Verlag, pp. 31–57.

Skoglund, P., Ersmark, E., Palkopoulou, E. & Dalén, L. (2015). Ancient wolf genome reveals an early divergence of domestic dog ancestors and admixture into high-latitude breeds. *Current Biology*, 25: 1–5.

Thalmann, O., Shapiro, B., Cui, P. *et al.* (2013) Complete mitochondrial genomes of ancient canids suggest a European origin of domestic dogs. *Nature*, 342: 871–4.

Trut, L. N., Plyusnina, I. Z. & Oskina, I. N. (2004). An experiment on fox domestication and debatable issues of evolution of the dog. *Russian Journal of Genetics*, 40: 794–807.

Wilkins, A. S., Wrangham, R. W. & Tecumseh-Fitch, W. (2014). The "Domestication Syndrome" in mammals: a unified explanation based on neural crest cell behavior and genetics. *Genetics*, 197: 795–808.

INDEX

Printed in the United States
By Bookmasters